Human Respiratory Viral Infections

Human Respiratory Viral Infections

Editor: Albie Graham

AMERICAN
MEDICAL PUBLISHERS
www.americanmedicalpublishers.com

AMERICAN
MEDICAL PUBLISHERS
www.americanmedicalpublishers.com

Cataloging-in-Publication Data

Human respiratory viral infections / edited by Albie Graham.
p. cm.
Includes bibliographical references and index.
ISBN 979-8-88740-565-0
1. Respiratory infections. 2. Respiratory infections--Research.
3. Respiratory organs--Diseases. I. Graham, Albie.
RC740 .N49 2023
616.2--dc23

American Medical Publishers,
41 Flatbush Avenue,
1st Floor, New York,
NY 11217, USA

ISBN 979-8-88740-565-0 (Hardback)

Contents

Preface

The world is advancing at a fast pace like never before. Therefore, the need is to keep up with the latest developments. This book was an idea that came to fruition when the specialists in the area realized the need to coordinate together and document essential themes in the subject. That's when I was requested to be the editor. Editing this book has been an honour as it brings together diverse authors researching on different streams of the field. The book collates essential materials contributed by veterans in the area which can be utilized by students and researchers alike.

Human respiratory viral infections are diseases caused by a range of viruses having similar characteristics, which negatively affect the respiratory system and respiratory tract. The viruses that cause respiratory viral infections encompass parainfluenza viruses, respiratory adenoviruses, influenza viruses and respiratory syncytial virus (RSV). These spread directly through coughing or sneezing, which results in the transmission of viruses when they are then inhaled. They can also spread indirectly by coming in contact with contaminated surfaces, hands, handkerchiefs, toys, etc. Some common symptoms of respiratory viral infections are fever, headache, chills, loss of appetite, body ache and weakness. There are various complications associated with respiratory viral infections, including pneumonia, tonsillitis, bronchitis and laryngitis. Their treatment involves administration of antiviral agents, such as amantadine and ribavirin. This book provides detailed a understanding of human respiratory viral infections. A number of latest researches have been included to keep the readers up-to-date with the global concepts in this area of study. The book will prove to be immensely beneficial to students and researchers engaged in the study of these infections.

Each chapter is a sole-standing publication that reflects each author´s interpretation. Thus, the book displays a multi-facetted picture of our current understanding of application, resources and aspects of the field. I would like to thank the contributors of this book and my family for their endless support.

Editor

1

MicroRNAs: Mediators and Therapeutic Targets to Airway Hyper Reactivity after Respiratory Syncytial Virus Infection

Shuwen Feng, Dongxin Zeng, Junwen Zheng and Dongchi Zhao*

Department of Pediatrics, Children's Digital Health and Data Center, Zhongnan Hospital of Wuhan University, Wuhan, China

***Correspondence:**
Dongchi Zhao
zhao_wh2004@hotmail.com

Respiratory syncytial virus (RSV) is the most important pathogen correlated to the first-time infant wheezing and later recurrence after its primary infection. RSV infection promotes the bronchial smooth muscle sensitivity to leukotrienes (LTs) in acute stage, causes the extensive inflammatory reaction and the aggregation of Th2-like cells during respiratory tract obstruction. Infants and young children infected with RSV exhibit an increased susceptibility to the exposure of exogenous allergens, easy to suffer from the recurrent wheezing, which prompts that the body is still in a state of inflammation or immunological bias. However, the pathological mechanism is unclear. The recent researches demonstrate that abnormal expression of non-coding microRNAs (miRNAs) can be detected from the peripheral blood and airway tract epithelial of RSV infected infants, which participate the regulation of immune cells polarization and LTs synthesis. Improving the immune tolerance can significantly relieve the airway inflammation and broncho-spasm caused by RSV. In this review, we discuss recent advances in understanding the mechanism of RSV-induced inflammatory reaction and immune dysfunction leading to airway hyper-reactivity. Further, we summarize the potential molecular basis that, in this process, miRNAs, which are produced by airway epithelial cells or peripheral blood mononuclear cells, directly or in the form of exosome to regulate the inflammation programs as well as the function, differentiation and proliferation of immune cells. miRNAs may become a potential bio-marker of detecting severe RSV infection and a novel target of early intervention and therapeutic strategy in recurrent wheezing or asthma related to RSV infection.

Keywords: microRNAs, airway hyper reactivity, immune dysfunction, respiratory syncytial virus, immune tolerance

INTRODUCTION

Respiratory syncytial virus (RSV), a single-stranded, negative-sense RNA virus belonging to the genus *Orthopneumovirus* of the new family *Pneumoviridae*, is the most common etiological agent for acute lower respiratory infection (ALRI) in infants aged less than 24 months. The clinical course contains both the wheezing (bronchiolitis) during acute infection period and the secondary airway hyperactivity (AHR) in the late life (Bisgaard, 2003; Zheng et al., 2015a; Frias et al., 2018;

Petrarca et al., 2018). The infection of RSV is restricted in airways, viral replication results in the recruitment of inflammatory cells, releasing inflammatory factors which contribute to the airway edema, sputum accumulation, smooth muscle spasm, leading to the airway obstruction manifested as wheezing (Johnson et al., 2007; Shirey et al., 2014). Furthermore, in infants infected with RSV, the T helper 17 cell (Th17)/regulatory T-cell (Treg) imbalance, and the over-expression of Th2-like cytokines make the airway inflammatory reaction getting worse, particularly in preterm newborns, RSV infections are more likely to become severe cases (Mangodt et al., 2015).

Usually, AHR lasts for months or even years after the acute infection stage is one of the significant clinical features in infants primary challenged by RSV, who exhibit an increased susceptibility to the exogenous allergens and reinfection to evoke asthma, especially in those severe enough to cause hospitalization, which is highly associated with the development of asthma and allergic sensitization up to age 7 (Sigurs et al., 2000; Nenna et al., 2015). However, the pathological mechanism could not be appropriately explained so far. In recent years, the use of leukotriene receptor antagonist (LTRA) to prevent asthmatic attack has got certain effect (Bisgaard, 2003), which suggests that an alteration of leukotriene receptors (TLRs) expression pattern, possible the up-regulation of LTR in smooth muscle cells and enhanced sensitivity to leukotrienes (LTs), may be an important event that could contribute to the development of the histopathology in RSV infected individuals (Liu et al., 2015). Wheezing induced by primary RSV infections in early childhood is specifically time-ordered, it is quite often before 2 years old, then reduced, and obviously less occurs after 5, which is in agreement with the process of lymphocytes differentiation and functional maturation during childhood (Simoes et al., 2018). MicroRNAs (miRNAs) are small, non-coding, regulatory RNAs which can induce message RNA (mRNA) degradation or translational repression of their target genes. miRNA species have recently emerged as gene expression regulators that play a modulatory role in virus infection by modifying host responses in inflammatory and immune cells as well as airway epithelial cells (Globinska et al., 2014; Werz et al., 2017). It has been shown that abnormal expression of miRNAs can be detected from the peripheral blood and airway tract of RSV infected infants, involved in the regulation of 5-lipoxygenase (5-LO) activity and lymphocyte differentiation (Othumpangat et al., 2012; Simpson et al., 2014; Busch et al., 2015; Su et al., 2016; Wang et al., 2017; Werz et al., 2017).

Given this, it could be inferred that, during an interval of time after acute infection, RSV could trigger inflammatory programs, and subsequently comes the decreased host immune tolerance and hyper-function of Th2-like cells, which might be the pathological basis of the chronic airway inflammation. In view of miRNA plays an important role in RSV-related AHR, further studies are required to identify the possible molecular basis of abnormal behaviors of immune and inflammatory cells, in which miRNAs could act as inflammatory mediators and can be used as the potential bio-markers as well as the therapeutic targets.

RSV-INDUCED INFLAMMATORY REACTION AND IMMUNE DYSFUNCTION

Globally, RSV is the most common pathogen identified in infants with ALRI (Shi et al., 2015). The feature in histopathological studies of children with RSV-ALRI is mucus inflammatory exudation and small airway filled with dense plugs composed of mucus, fibrin, and debris from leukocytes and sloughed bronchial epithelial cells, which is the primary cause of airway stenosis and obstruction, smooth muscle spasm of bronchioles also plays a role (Cortjens et al., 2016). Activation and release of inflammatory mediators promoted by virus infection could induce enhanced immune reaction, which brings about immune dysfunction and further exacerbated immunopathology (Schmidt et al., 2018).

During the activation of innate immunity by airway epithelial cells (AECs) upon RSV infection, AECs can sense RSV components through pattern recognition receptors (PRRs), including Toll-like receptors (TLRs) and retinoic acid-inducible gene I (RIG-I)-like receptor (RLR) family members which are coupled to various pathways that control the activation of the corresponding transcription factors, such as IRF-3 and NF-kB (Zheng et al., 2015b; Tian et al., 2017). Subsequently, the generation of an early innate immune response, including secretion of cytokines and antiviral molecular, is induced (Rossi and Colin, 2015; Lay et al., 2016). A serious of studies have shown that RSV infection stimulates RIG-I and TLR3 in AECs to produce thymic stromal lymphopoitein (TSLP), which enhances the immune response mediated by Th2 cells and promotes allergic inflammation and asthma (Lee et al., 2012; Feng et al., 2017). TSLP, an interleukin-7 (IL-7)-like cytokine derived from epithelial cells, is considered as a master switch in Th2 mediated immune responses, and is believed to play a key role in allergic asthma. It could promote the cytokine production in mast cells and the maturation of dendritic cells (DCs) during the sensitization/priming stage of innate and adaptive allergic responses, while it supports Th2 CD4+T-cell proliferation and also induces cytokine production during the challenge stage (Ziegler and Liu, 2006). In the TSLP/DC/OX40L pathway, TSLP triggers the Th2 mediated allergic cascade by induction of OX40-ligand (OX40L) on DCs, may contribute to asthma pathogenesis and airway inflammation by modulating level of CD4+CD25+Treg cells and the profile of inflammatory cytokines (Murakami-Satsutani et al., 2014; Feng et al., 2017). In the process of phagocytic recruitment and lymphocytic aggregation, virus could induce host cells to produce non-coding RNAs which interfere with the post-transcriptional biological activity of host mRNA, and also play an important role in the form of exosome to regulate target genes via blood circulation (Anderson et al., 2016; Hasegawa et al., 2018). miRNAs exert an extensive regulatory influence on the production of inflammatory mediators, the stimulation of pattern recognition receptors expressions in epithelial cells, as well as the oriented differentiation of immune cells (Lay et al., 2016; Peng et al., 2018).

The underlying mechanisms contributed to asthma in children who underwent RSV wheezing episodes in early life are proposed. Firstly, RSV infection could induce a Th2-like effector phenotype in Treg cells, attenuating their capacity to promote tolerance to inhaled allergens by means of GATA-3 activation and Th2 cytokine production in FOXP3+ Treg cells (Chauhan et al., 2015; Hirose et al., 2017; Schmidt et al., 2018). Simultaneously, RVS may also induce the secretion of TSLP in epithelial cells, in addition to the possible role in RSV immunopathology, epithelium-derived cytokines IL-25 and IL-33 are also associated to an allergic Th2 response (Lay et al., 2016). Furthermore, the enhanced expression of thymus and activation-regulated chemokines (TARC) and OX40L of mature DCs activated by TSLP could promote Th2 polarization/proliferation in thymus and exacerbate the local inflammatory response (Hirose et al., 2017). In the meanwhile, TSLP directly or selectively impairs IL-10 production of FOXP3+ Treg cells and inhibited their suppressive activity (Chauhan et al., 2015). Therefore, initiation of inflammation program, hyper-function of Th2-like cells, as well as decreased immune tolerance, might be the crucial links to wheezing recurrence correlated to RSV infection, while miRNAs participate the regulation of both T-cells function and 5-LO synthesis procedures (**Figure 1**).

RSV INFECTION REGULATES INFLAMMATION MEDIATED BY miRNAs

Multiple non-coding RNAs take part in the regulation of post-transcriptional activity, of which, miRNAs are small, single-stranded, regulatory RNAs. With a length of 19–24 nt, it mediates the post-transcriptional silence of its target genes through incorporation into the RNA-include silencing complex (RISC) and then directing this complex to the 3′untranslated region (3′UTR) or open reading frame (ORF) of the target gene's mRNA (Ross et al., 2007). For most interactions, miRNAs act as rheostats to make optimum-scale adjustments to specific protein output (Baek et al., 2008).

miRNAs-Related Regulation of LTs Bio-Activity

Respiratory syncytial virus infection causes cysteinyl leukotrienes (CysLTs) increase in the bronchoalveolar lavage fluids and lung tissue (Musiyenko et al., 2009). Subsequently, sensitized with mite allergen, enhanced the allergic inflammation following allergen challenge, and this was accompanied by elevations in lung dendritic cells and CysLTs (Werz et al., 2017). Leukotrienes are lipid mediators produced from arachidonic acid (AA) with a broad variety of bioactivities in allergic inflammation and immune responses, which are over 1000 times more powerful than histamine (Liu et al., 2015). LTs are divided into two types, one is LTB4, considered as a potent chemoattractant for most subsets of leukocytes, whereas the another CysLTs are potent bronchoconstrictors that have effects on airway remodeling (Matsuse et al., 2007; Liu and Yokomizo, 2015). LTs exert their biological effects by binding to LTRs, to induce smooth muscle spasm, increased microvascular permeability, mucosal edema, mucous hypersecretion, migration of granulocytes to lung and their adhesion to endothelium, degranulation, release of lysosomal enzymes, etc., which are of vital importance in asthma airway inflammation. LTRs belong to G protein-coupled receptors (GPCRs), produced predominantly by immune and inflammatory cells, their expressions have also been detected in airway smooth muscle cells, endothelial cells as well as peripheral tissues and organs (Wang et al., 2014). In response to various biological stimuli, arachidonic acid is released from membrane phospholipids and transformed into LTs via multistep enzymatic reactions (Liu and Yokomizo, 2015). Arachidonic acid is first oxidized at the C-5 position by the dual enzymatic activity of 5-LO to yield 5-hydroxyperoxyeicosatetraenoic acid (5- HpETE) followed by an unstable intermediate, leukotriene A4 (LTA4). LTA4 is either converted to LTB4 by or conjugated to reduced glutathione to produce CysLT (LTC4). LTC4 is then exported from the cell and converted to LTD4 and LTE4, the most stable CysLTs, by extracellular peptidases. Among the multiple process of enzymatic reactions, 5-LO is the key enzyme which has been most widely studied, expressed mainly in granulocytes, macrophages and mast cells, catalyzing the conversion from arachidonic acid to LTs (Busch et al., 2015).

Regulation of LTs bio-activity mainly includes two kinds of pathway: LTRAs and 5-LO inhibitors (Werz et al., 2017). The former blocks the organ response to LTs via selective binding with receptors in bronchial smooth muscles and competitively inhibiting effects of CysLTs, such as montelukast, showed the effect on controlling wheeze induced by RSV infection (Peng et al., 2014). The latter inhibits LTs synthesis via interfering 5-LO pathway (Liu et al., 2015). miRNAs modulate LTs synthesis by regulating 5-LO activity, and the effect of miRNAs derived from different cell lines seem to be cell type- and stimulus-specific, which might contribute to maintain physical function of LTs in normal circumstances. Busch et al. (2015) had revealed that the miRNA-19a-3p and miR-125-5p are involved in the regulation of leukocyte functions and immune responses by regulation 5-LO transcriptional efficiency (**Figure 2**). Antagonizing miR-19a-3p in PHA-stimulated T cells leads to an increase in 5-LO mRNA expression, and treatment of differentiated monocytic MM6 cells with antagomirs for miR-19a-3p and miR-125b-5p also increases 5-LO protein expression. And upregulation of LTRs was found in both human allergic nasal mucosa and asthmatic bronchial mucosa (Zhu et al., 2005; Shirasaki et al., 2013). LTB4, via leukotriene receptor 1 signaling, increases macrophage expression of miR-155, miR-146b, and miR-125b, in which, LTB4-mediated miR-155 generation was attributable to the protein-1 activation. Antagomirs against miR-155 and miR-146b prevented both the LTB4-mediated decrease in SOCS-1 and increase in MyD88, in which controls macrophage activation (Wang et al., 2014).

These researches above imply that RSV infection could interfere miRNAs expression to regulate LTs synthesis, which mediates airway hyperresponsiveness (Zago et al., 2014). In primary RSV infection, RSV could induce the expression of specific miRNAs which lead to upregulation of LTs bio-activity,

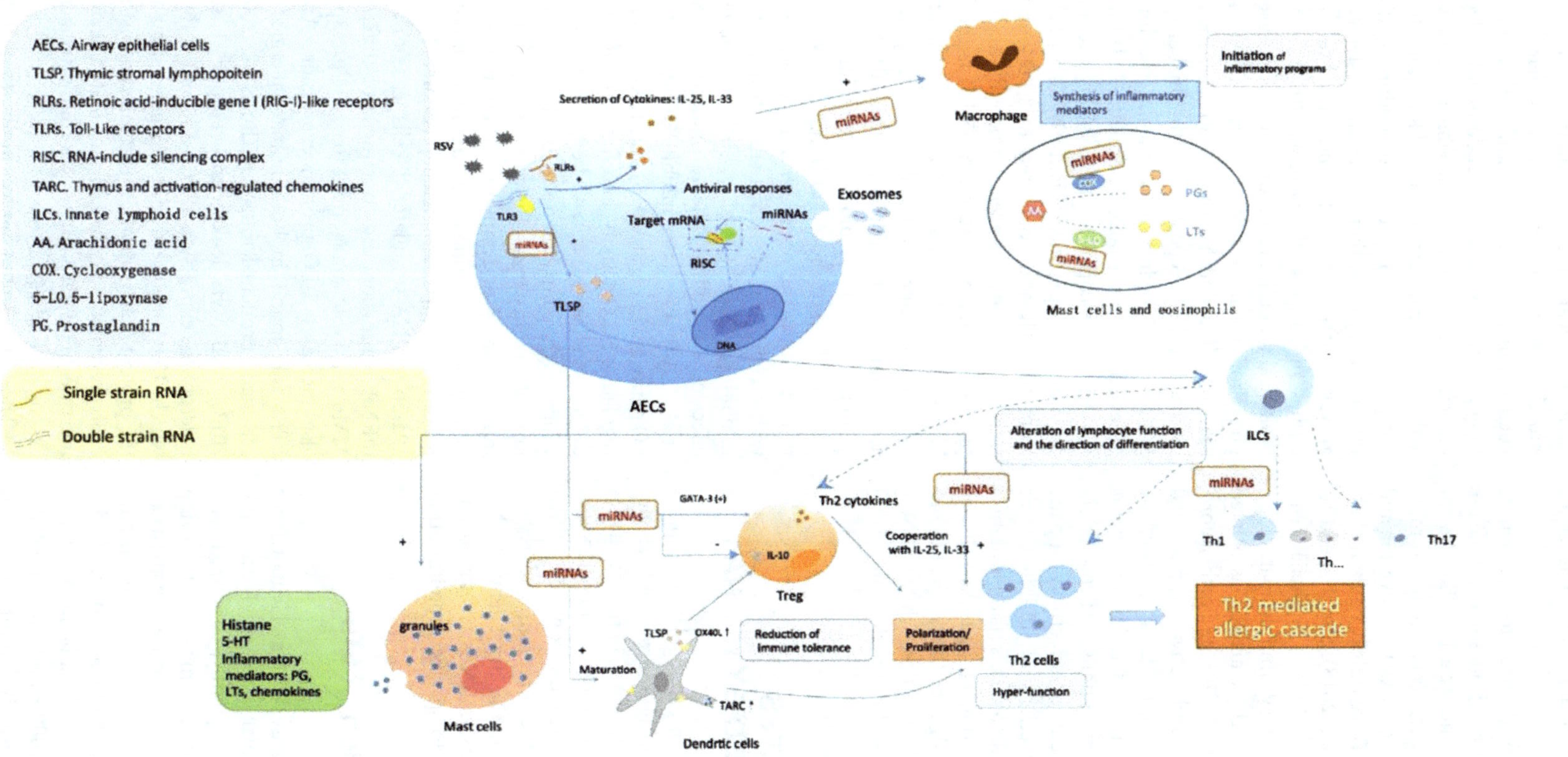

FIGURE 1 | Respiratory syncytial virus (RSV) infection causes AHR formation mediated by miRNAs. The viral single-stranded RNAs and double-stranded RNAs components during RSV replication were recognized by pattern recognition receptors in AECs, subsequently induce the secretion of cytokines and antiviral responses. In the meanwhile, the upregulation/downregulation of miRNAs began to take part in regulating the expression of target genes, such as TSLP, one of the most important factors in allergic inflammation, which might have an impact on multiple inflammation and immunologic process: degranulation of mast cells, activation and maturation of DCs, alteration of lymphocyte function and differentiation, weakness of Treg cells, polarization/proliferation of Th2 cells, etc. Furthermore, miRNAs also played a role in the activation of monocyte-macrophage via interfering PGs and 5-LO synthesis to produce inflammatory mediators. All these led to the initiation of aberrant inflammatory programs and immune dysfunction correlated to AHR post-RSV infection.

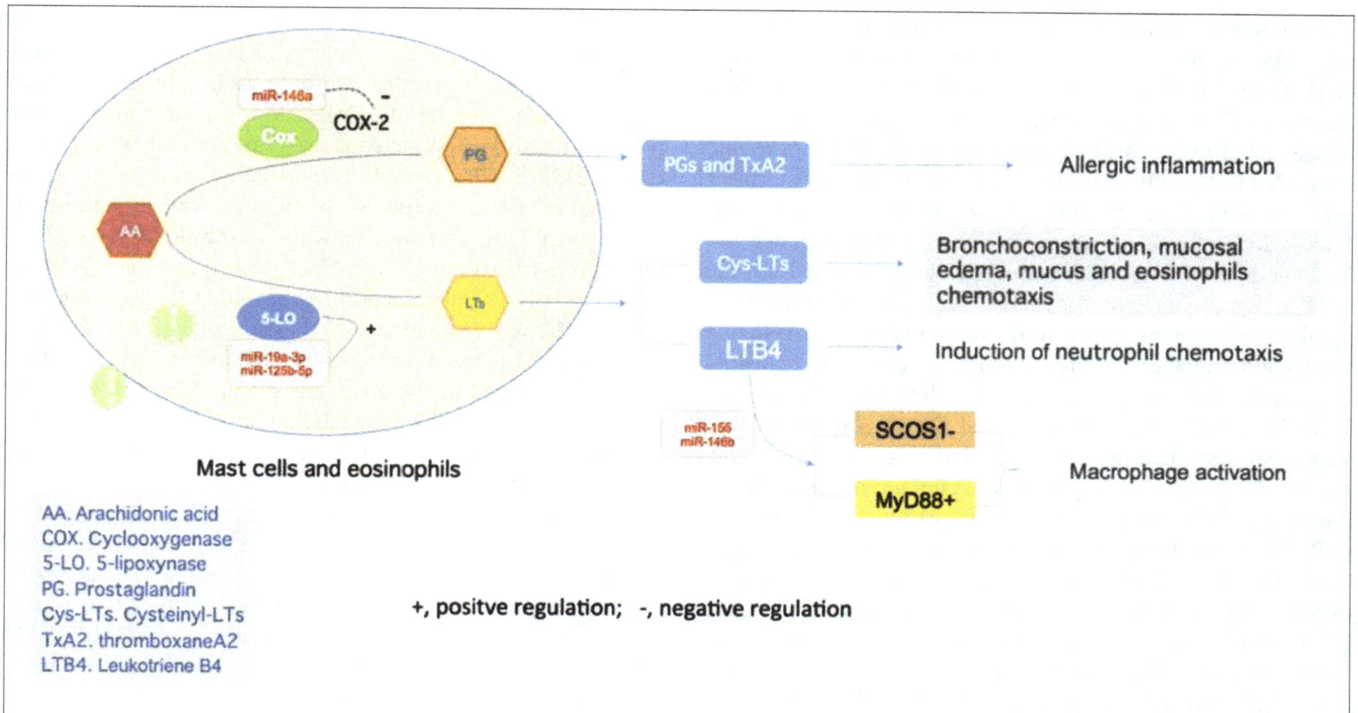

FIGURE 2 | Regulations of inflammation reaction mediated by miRNAs. miR-146a negatively regulates the Cox-2 activity to influence the alteration from AA to PG, and later become TxA2, which is related to allergic inflammation. On the other hand, activity of 5-LO is under the regulation of miR-19a-3p and miR-125b-5p, which promote the production of LTs. These two types of LTs, CysLTs, and LTB4, act as bronchoconstrictors or chemoattractant to take an essential part in inflammation. The latter one could also promote the expression of miR-155 in macrophage, which target on both SCOS1 and MyD88 to control macrophage activation and airway remodeling.

contributing to inflammatory reactions and wheezing during acute infectious period. Continuous impacts may exist after primary infection, probably the upregulation of LTRs or influence on differentiation and function of immunocytes, which brings about chronic airway inflammation. Further studies are required to explore mechanisms of RSV-induced miRNAs expression and AHR.

miRNAs Participate in Regulation of Innate Immune

miRNAs could take part in the regulation of early innate immune and initiation of inflammatory responses. Of which, macrophages are the major cellular component of the innate immune system, and play an important role in the recognition of microbes, particulates, immunogens and the regulation of inflammatory responses (Pappas et al., 2013). The central conserved region of RSV G protein modulates virus replication and the pattern of host gene expression by downregulating miRNAs let-7i to active IFN-λ secretion, which could induce innate antiviral responses in epithelial cells (Bakre et al., 2017). It has been demonstrated that miRNAs regulate M1 and M2 macrophage polarization through targeting adaptor proteins and transcription factors in various pathways to participate in inflammatory program modulation (Banerjee et al., 2013; Wang et al., 2014; Essandoh et al., 2016; Bras et al., 2017; Self-Fordham et al., 2017). Besides, miR-27a could negatively regulate the IL-10-dependent signal transducer and activator of transcription 3 (STAT3) phosphorylation, thereby relieve TLR2 and TLR4 driven inflammatory responses (Xie et al., 2014). STAT3 drives the development of Th17 cells and the cytokine production by Th2 and Th17 cells, and the activation of STAT3 pathway is closely related to the development of airway inflammation, which contribute a lot to asthma (Gavino et al., 2016). miR-19b can reduce airway remodeling, airway inflammation, and degree of oxidative stress by inhibiting STAT3 signaling through TSLP downregulation in a mouse asthma model (Ye et al., 2017). In addition, studied show that miRNAs modulate DCs development as well as their maturation process, antigen presentation capacity and cytokine release to take part in immune regulation, which link the innate and adaptive immune systems (Smyth et al., 2015).

ALTERATION OF IMMUNOCYTE FUNCTION MEDIATED BY miRNAs

Respiratory syncytial virus replication could influence the expression of multiple genes related to immunity via miRNAs regulation, leading to alteration of lymphocytic function (Anderson et al., 2016). miRNAs are crucial regulators of type 2 innate lymphoid cells (ILC2s) biological function that mediate similar but non-identical programs of post-transcriptional gene regulation in innate and adaptive lymphocytes. It was identified in mice that the miR-17∼92 cluster is required to maintain

ILC2 homeostasis and function *in vivo* (**Figure 3**). The over-expression of miR-17∼92 could promote the ILC2s production of IL-13 and IL-5 in response to IL-33 driven inflammation, and these cells could be detected in sputum and bronchoalveolar lavage (BAL) in human asthma (Singh et al., 2017). Activation of ILC2s in responds to IL-33, IL-25, and TSLP act as a role in the initiation and maintenance of chronic airway inflammation. Mice lacking of miR-17∼92 expression exhibit growth defect in ILC2s and decreased cytokine expression in respond to IL-33 and TSLP, which could relieve the allergic lung inflammation induced by allergens. Among them, miR-19a augments Th2 cytokines production and allergic inflammation via coordinate regulation of cytokine and antigen receptor signaling pathways [NF-κB, JAK-STAT, and PI(3)K] (Simpson et al., 2014). Another research suggested that tight and fine regulation of miR-23∼27∼24 clusters in T cells is required to maintain optimal effector function and to prevent aberrant immune responses. miR-24 and miR-27 collaboratively limit Th2 responses through targeting IL-4 and GATA3 in both direct and indirect manners. Although over-expression of the entire miR-23 cluster negatively impacts other Th lineages, enforced expression of miR-24, in contrast to miR-23 and miR-27, actually promotes the differentiation of Th1, Th17, and induced regulatory T cells (Cho et al., 2016). miR-31 increases the sensitivity of T cells to type I interferon, which interferes with effector T cell function and increases the expression of several proteins related to T cell dysfunction (Moffett et al., 2017). The nasal epithelial cell-derived miR-146a could induce the expression of IL-10 in monocytes, which suppresses the activities of CD4+ effector T cells and the Th2 polarization, and relieves allergic reactions induced by virus (Luo et al., 2015). Besides, upregulation of let-7d can be detected in epithelial cells of nasal mucosa in children with RSV infection (Inchley et al., 2015). In the meanwhile, let-7 miRNAs, possibly in the manner of exosome, play a significant role in the regulation of allergic airway inflammation by regulating the expression of IL-13 in Th2 cells (Kumar et al., 2011; Panganiban et al., 2012).

Our former research demonstrated that differential expression of miRNAs existed in the peripheral blood of infants with RSV infection, including the upregulation miRNAs (miR-106b-5p, miR-181a-5p, miR-20b-5p, miR-342-3p, and miR-652-3p) and the downregulation miRNAs (miR-122-5p, miR-320e, miR-320d, miR-877-5p, miR-92b-5p, and let-7c-5p) (Wang et al., 2017). Among them, miR-92b-5p and let-7c-5p have been reported in relation to G1/S and G2/M in cell circle, and they might regulate cell proliferation by targeting cyclins such as E2F1, CcnE, Cdc6, CcnB1, and Cdc25C (Markopoulos et al., 2017). RSV replication induces let-7i upregulation in epithelial cells while let-7b upregulation in DCs. And it appears to manipulate host pathways and nuclear transcription related to proliferation and differentiation through regulation of expression of these miRNAs

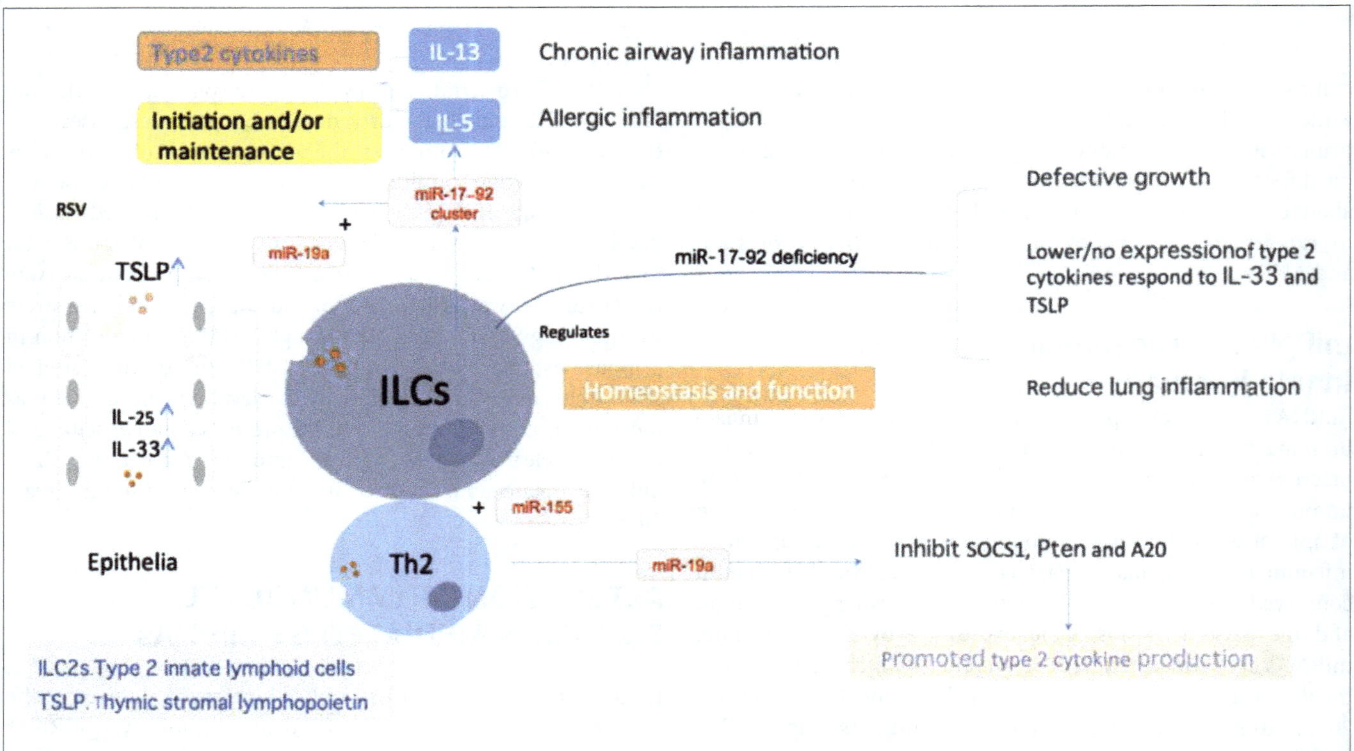

FIGURE 3 | miRNAs regulate ILC2 homeostasis and function. miRNA expression was essential in maintaining ILCs homeostasis and function, particularly the miR-17∼92 cluster. Epithelium-derived cytokines IL-33, IL-25, and TSLP could activate ILCs to promote type2 cytokines production, which plays a role in the initiation and maintenance of chronic airway inflammation. During the process, miR-17∼92 promoted IL-13 and IL-5 production in response to IL-33 and ILC2-driven type 2 inflammation. miR-17∼92 deficiency will result in the defective growth in ILCs, decrease the respond to IL-33 and TSLP, and reduced lung inflammation. Besides, miR-155 is indispensible for the development of ILCs-homologous Th2 cells. miR-19a could promote type2 cytokine production of Th2 cells through targeting of the signal inhibitors Pten, SCOS1 and A20.

in relation to the interferon response (Thornburg et al., 2012). Abnormal expression of miR-let-7 family in epithelial cells and lymphocytes might be closely related to airway inflammation and lymphocyte dysfunction during RSV infection. From the above, the physical expression of miRNAs is of vital importance in maintaining immunocyte function in lung and regulating Th2 cell homing. Aberrant expression of miRNAs evoked by viral infection, involving gene expression related to regulating immunocyte differentiation and immune tolerance, is in great association with asthma induction. miRNAs associated to airway hyperresponsiveness propelled by RSV infection are shown in **Table 1**.

miRNAs ARE INVOLVED IN LYMPHOCYTE PROLIFERATION AND DIFFERENTIATION

Viral infection also influences host lymphocytes polarization mediated by miRNAs (Ren et al., 2016; Haralambieva et al., 2018). Studies on involvement of miRNAs in lymphocyte differentiation, maturation, proliferation and apoptosis have made some progress, but the mechanism is still not very clear (Kroesen et al., 2015). Elevating evidences suggest that an expanding list of individual miRNAs and co-expressed miRNA clusters have been shown to have significant effects on T cell fate decisions and immune functions: miR-21, miR-155, and miR-17∼92 participate in T cell differentiation, activation and lifespan, and miR-23, ∼24, ∼27 family is involved in effector T cell differentiation and function maturation (Baumjohann and Ansel, 2013; Jeker and Bluestone, 2013; Cho et al., 2016). miR-142-3p regulates CD4+CD25+T cell proliferation by targeting the expression of glycoprotein A repetitions predominant, then inhibits Treg cell proliferation and reduces immune tolerance (Zhou et al., 2013). The adaptive immune response mediated by central immune organ is also under the regulation of miRNA. For instance, miR-155 is engaged in antigen presentation and B and T cell development. Differential expression of miRNAs exists in different stage of differentiation of the same cell. miR-150 has been only found in mature resting T and B lymphocytes, it is less or not expressed in their precursors. Memory T lymphocytes showed high expression of miR-146a, while less expressed in prime T cells, which suggests miRNAs participating in maintaining specific cellular immune. Moreover, experimental evidence suggests that miR-146a targets the Fas-associated death domain and affects activation-induced cell death (Globinska et al., 2014). Recent researches show that T lymphocytes could produce miRNAs transferred to DCs in the form of exosome miRNA, regulating gene expression of recipient cells in the process of antigen presentation. miRNA-containing exosome, passing on messages by circulating vesicles, is the third approach of intercellular communication with the exception of cell contact-depending and soluble molecules-mediated signaling, and it also takes part in antigen presentation, cell migration and differentiation to regulate immune responses (Okoye et al., 2014; Robbins and Morelli, 2014). Among which, miR-21, miR-150, miR-320, and Let-7 family are the more common exosomes.

About 2500 miRNAs have been detected in human peripheral blood, and a great deal of which have a cell-specific expression pattern. In physical conditions, there is a significant difference of miRNAs distribution in the blood, serum, plasma and exosome, even in different cell subsets. Among them, expression of miRNA precursors in neutrophils, monocytes and NK cells is quite rich, whereas CD4+ and CD8+ cells express the least (Juzenas et al., 2017). Phagocytes have a rich membrane system and could produce multiple miRNAs-containing exosomes. But there is still scarce knowledge about the way of these exosomes to participate in oriented differentiation of lymphocytes in the process of antigen presentation. Human miR-let-7 family plays an important role in the regulation of cell differentiation by directly or indirectly targeting genes related to cell cycle (Ambros, 2004; Roush and Slack, 2008). Let-7 family contains 13 isoforms, whose gene sequence and function are highly conserved in various animal species (Lee et al., 2016). Self-renewal could be inhibited in DGCR8 deletion embryotic stem cell when let-7 was inserted (Adlakha and Seth, 2017). In addition, let-7 inhibition could promote the transformation from un-differential somatic cells to induced pluripotent stem cells (iPSCs). Also, miRNA let-7b regulates neural stem cell proliferation and differentiation via interaction with stem cell regulator TLX and cell circle regulator CyclinD1 (Zhao et al., 2010). Since then, let-7 family is of great importance in self-differentiation and self-renewal of stem cells acting as regulators. Furthermore, miR-let-7d produced by Treg cells was released in the form of exosome and then transmitted to Th1 cells to suppress its proliferation and function (Okoye et al., 2014). Therefore, RSV infection induces a lot of differential expression miRNAs, which not only participate the acute stage inflammatory reaction, but act as triggers to the dysfunction of immunological bias, which might correlate to the recurrent wheezing post virus infection in later life.

miRNAs ARE POTENTIAL COMPONENTS ASSOCIATED WITH THE DEVELOPMENT OF RECURRENT WHEEZING EVOKED BY RSV INFECTION

Combined with the above mentioned, it could be inferred that there are two vital pathological basis of wheezing recurrence after RSV infection: firstly, RSV acute infection promotes the initiation of inflammatory programs mediated by macrophages and DCs, increased activity of LT synthetase as well as upregulation of LTRs. Secondly, aberrant differentiation and dysfunction of lymphocytes resulting in the immune bias could contribute the recurrent wheezing. During the pathological process, differential expression of miRNAs and/or exosomes induced by RSV replication could be the initial inducers and bridge factors.

In the circumstance that viruses were cleared by host immune system after RSV infection, respiratory tissues and lymphocytes still maintain the state of hyper-reactivity and chronic inflammation (**Figure 4**) (Obando-Pacheco et al., 2018; Simoes et al., 2018). And the over-expression of inflammatory mediators and their receptors promote the response intensity

TABLE 1 | miRNAs distribution and function related to ARH caused by RSV infection.

miRNA classification	Cell type	Target	Function	Reference
miR-let-7f and miR-24	Epithelial cells, Calu-3 cell	IFNλ+	Virus replication and host gene expression pattern	Simpson et al., 2014
miR-221	Bronchial epithelial cells	NGF and TrKA	Modulates RSV replication	Othumpangat et al., 2012
miR-124, miR-24, and miR-744	A549	P38,MAPK-	Inhibits of Respiratory Virus Infection	McCaskill et al., 2017
miR-19a-3p and miR-125b-5p	Hematopoietic cell	5-LO	5-LO expression	Busch et al., 2015
miR-674-5p	Hepatocyte	5-LO	Harbors a potential binding region for 5-LO	Su et al., 2016
miR-155, miR-146b, and miR-125b	Macrophage	SOCS1−, MyD88+	Macrophage activation	Wang et al., 2014
miR-195	Macrophage	–	Inhibits TLR2 pathway	Bras et al., 2017
miR-125a-5p	Macrophage	KLF13	M2 polarization	Banerjee et al., 2013
miR-27a	Macrophage	IL-10, STAT3	Inhibits STAT3 phosphorylation	Xie et al., 2014
miR-19b	–	TSLP, STAT3	Inhibits STAT3 through TSLP	Ye et al., 2017
miR-146a	Monocyte	IL-10	Induces IL-10	Luo et al., 2015
	Fibroblasts	NF-kappaB	Suppress COX-2 protein expression	Zago et al., 2014
miR17∼92	ILCs	–	Proliferation, differentiation of T and B cells	Simpson et al., 2014; Singh et al., 2017
miR-19a, miR-19b	ILCs, Th2	A20, SOCS1, Pten	Promotes IL-13 and IL-5 production	Singh et al., 2017
miR-23∼27∼24	T lineages		Regulates Th 2 immunity	Cho et al., 2016
miR-24, miR-27	Th2	IL-4, STAT3	Limits Th2 response	Xie et al., 2014
miR-23 and miR-27	T lineages	TGF-β	Limits the differentiation of Th17 and iTreg	Cho et al., 2016
miR-24	T lineages	Smad7, TGF-β	Promotes the differentiation of Th17 and iTreg	
miR-31	CD8+ T cells	NFAT	Increases the sensitivity of T cells to type I IFN	Moffett et al., 2017
miR-142-3p	CD25+ CD4 T Cells	Glycoprotein A	Reduces immune tolerance	Zhou et al., 2013
miR-let-7 family	Epithelial cells, DCs, etc.	–	Regulates allergic inflammation	Roush and Slack, 2008; Kumar et al., 2011; Lee et al., 2016;

to exogenous stimulus. Infant wheezing correlated to RSV infection is obviously age-specific. Children under age of 5 have an immaturity of lymphocyte distribution and function, the predominance of inflammation related to Th2 response, and the function decline of Treg cells, which could be corrected with age (Christiaansen et al., 2016). On account that RSV induces differential expression of miRNAs, and activity of LT syntheses is under regulation of specific miRNAs (Busch et al., 2015), it could be inferred that miRNAs induced by primary RSV infection contribute to the high-sensitivity to allergen. So far, there are still many obstacles to be clarified. For example, whether the continuous aberrant expression of miRNAs after RSV infection has an influence in unphysiologic alteration of inflammation factors expression in bronchial smooth cells, which leads to the state of inflammatory sensitization, or miRNAs are only the transient action on it, and when and how the immunologic bias is redressed with age. As for lymphocytes, particular for immature lymphocytes during early childhood, the aberrant expression of miRNAs might have an effect on lymphocyte differentiation and function. Acting as inducers, RSV infection could promote synthesis of inflammatory mediators and upregulation of LTRs in airway smooth muscle cells via regulation of miRNAs, and then increase the host reactivity to exogenous stimulus, which is related to wheezing severity. Modulation of lymphocyte differentiation by miRNAs or exosomes could reduce the host immune tolerance with enhanced sensitization of exogenous stimulus, which is related to wheezing frequency.

Differentiation of Treg cells could be suppressed by RSV infection, whereas the amount of CD4+CD25+Foxp3+ Treg cells reduces over age in premature infants. That the declining tendency could be improved by high-dose of intravenous immunoglobin (IVIG) (Liu et al., 2018), which is in accordance with the mechanism of immune regulation in clinical therapy that IVIG is used for the severe RSV infected pneumonia (Groothuis et al., 2011). RSV infection in early life has been considered as an independent high-risk factor of recurrent wheezing or asthma.

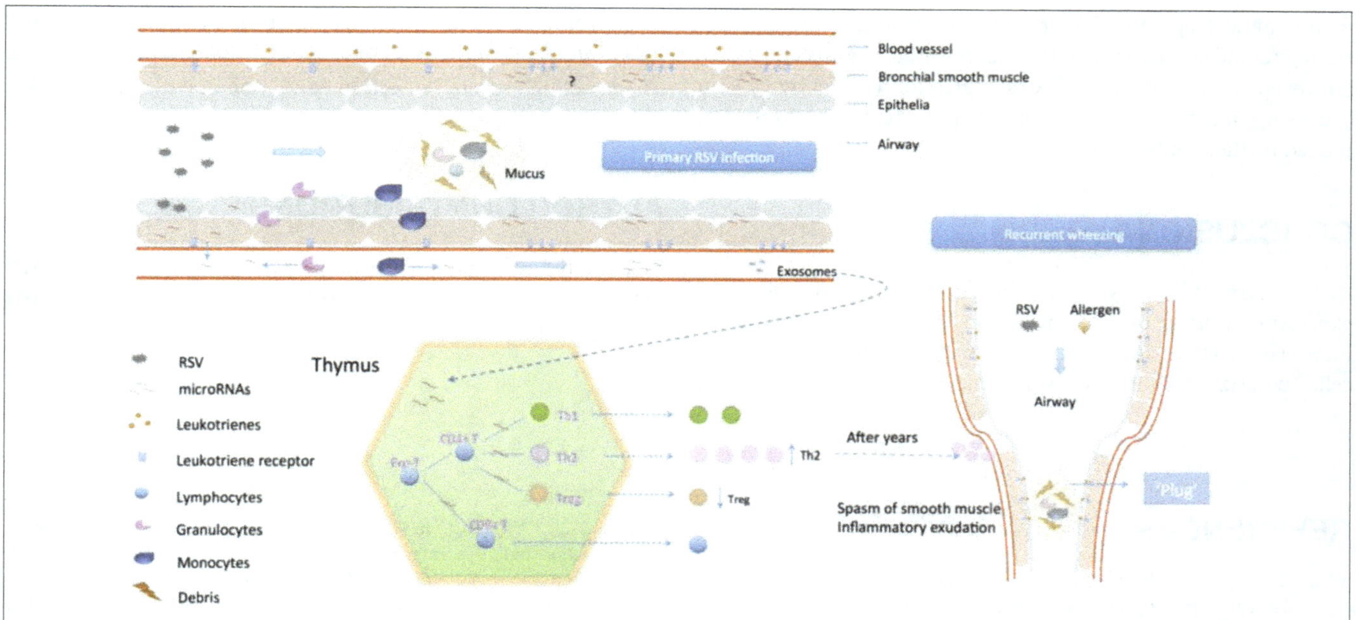

FIGURE 4 | The potential mechanism of primary RSV infection associates to recurrent wheezing. RSV infection could enhance the intensity of reaction to inflammatory mediators in airway smooth muscle via differential miRNAs expression, which regulate the activity of LTs/PGs synthetase and upregulate their receptors distribution. Also, modulation of lymphocyte differentiation by miRNAs or exosomes could promote Th2 cells differentiation and proliferation and impair Treg cells to inhibit host immune tolerance, leading to enhanced sensitization of exogenous stimulus.

However, for lack of knowledge of factors taking parts in the development of AHR, there has been less effective therapeutic strategies to prevent or retard the occurrence of later life wheezing (Fonseca et al., 2018).

miRNAs ARE POTENTIAL TARGETS OF DESIGNING miRNAs-BASED THERAPEUTIC STRATEGY FOR VIRAL INDUCED AHR

To date, miRNAs are potential therapeutic targets via either inhibiting viral genome or promoting host antiviral genes signaling (Peng et al., 2018), not only for RSV, but also for the other respiratory virus infections. New evidence has emerged on the potential role of miRNAs in influenza A virus (IAV)-induced host antivirus responses and in the modulation of the production of cytokines (Nguyen et al., 2018). For instance, miR-323-5p, miR-491-5p, and hsa-miR-654-5p directly bind to IAV H3N2 PB1 RNA, exerting an inhibitory effect on IAV replication in MDCK cells. Hsa-let-7c reduces viral replication by targeting and degrading M1 cRNA. hsa-miR-485-5p targets both RIG-I and viral PB1 to prevent spurious activation of antiviral signaling and suppress influenza virus infection. Treatment with the agomir delivery suppressed viral replication and effectively improved protection against lethal challenge with PR8 (H1N1) in mice. Besides, IAV infection decreases the expression of histone deacetylase 1 (HDAC1) that plays an important role in the activation of type-I IFN response against IAV infection. The use of miRNAs to target host factors that are utilized by viruses to promote infection and virus replication is a developing antiviral strategy, as it is hypothesized to overcome the selective pressure and subsequent drug resistance seen with direct virus-targeting antivirals (McCaskill et al., 2017). Host-targeting antiviral miRNAs could provide a complementary strategy for controlling infection, and they further illuminate host factors that are important in respiratory virus infections. Understanding the role of these small molecules in the antiviral immune response and identification of potential miRNAs-targeted genes may help to clarify the mechanisms of virus–host interaction and lead to the development of new antivirus treatments (Globinska et al., 2014). Targets of lead candidates, miR-124, miR-24, and miR-744, were identified within the p38 mitogen-activated protein kinase (MAPK) signaling pathway, and this work identified MAPK-activated protein kinase 2 as a broad-spectrum antiviral target required for both influenza and RSV infection. For three of these miRNAs, a portion of their antiviral activity was attributed to their suppression of the p38 MAPK pathway and MK2 in particular (Kim et al., 2017).

miRNAs play an essential role in the development of airway hyper reactivity, taking part in the regulation of inflammatory programs and induction of immune tolerance reduction. Nevertheless, identification of pathological basis needs further studies. In ALRI cases with RSV infection, detection of certain miRNAs expression may become a novel method to evaluate the severity of illness, which probably have the guiding significance to severity rating, especially in preterm newborn cases. Also, targeting specific miRNAs may be the potential prevention method or therapeutics strategy for infant wheezing related to RSV infection. Therefore, miRNAs target on the regulation of LTs synthesis and lymphocytes polarization will be promising treatment strategy for RSV-related AHR in future, and the strategy could also be applied to other respiratory virus infections. However, whether those miRNAs expression caused by RSV in acute stage infection act as transient or persistent impact on ARH is need further study in future.

CONCLUSION

In summary, in this review, we discuss the miRNAs differential expression caused by RSV infection, which are involving in interfering LTs synthesis enzyme activity, deciding the immune cells polarization and causing immunological homeostasis bias, contribute to ARH in later life related to post-RSV infection. miRNAs could be the potential bio-marker of detecting severe infection and therapeutic targets for RSV.

AUTHOR CONTRIBUTIONS

SF collected references, drawn the figures, and wrote this paper. DZe and JZ participated in the writing and discussion. DZh wrote and organized this paper.

REFERENCES

Adlakha, Y. K., and Seth, P. (2017). The expanding horizon of MicroRNAs in cellular reprogramming. *Prog. Neurobiol.* 148, 21–39. doi: 10.1016/j.pneurobio.2016.11.003

Ambros, V. (2004). The functions of animal microRNAs. *Nature* 431, 350–355. doi: 10.1038/nature02871

Anderson, L., Jorquera, P. A., and Tripp, R. A. (2016). MicroRNA profiling from RSV-infected biofluids, whole blood, and tissue samples. *Methods Mol. Biol.* 1442, 195–208. doi: 10.1007/978-1-4939-3687-8-14

Baek, D., Villen, J., Shin, C., Camargo, F. D., Gygi, S. P., and Bartel, D. P. (2008). The impact of microRNAs on protein output. *Nature* 455, 64–71. doi: 10.1038/nature07242

Bakre, A. A., Harcourt, J. L., Haynes, L. M., Anderson, L. J., and Tripp, R. A. (2017). The Central Conserved Region (CCR) of Respiratory Syncytial Virus (RSV) G protein modulates host miRNA expression and alters the cellular response to infection. *Vaccines* 5:E16. doi: 10.3390/vaccines5030016

Banerjee, S., Cui, H., Xie, N., Tan, Z., Yang, S., Icyuz, M., et al. (2013). miR-125a-5p regulates differential activation of macrophages and inflammation. *J. Biol. Chem.* 288, 35428–35436. doi: 10.1074/jbc.M112.426866

Baumjohann, D., and Ansel, K. M. (2013). MicroRNA-mediated regulation of T helper cell differentiation and plasticity. *Nat. Rev. Immunol.* 13, 666–678. doi: 10.1038/nri3494

Bisgaard, H. (2003). A randomized trial of montelukast in respiratory syncytial virus postbronchiolitis. *Am. J. Respir. Crit. Care Med.* 167, 379–383. doi: 10.1164/rccm.200207-747OC

Bras, J. P., Silva, A. M., Calin, G. A., Barbosa, M. A., Santos, S. G., and Almeida, M. I. (2017). miR-195 inhibits macrophages pro-inflammatory profile and impacts the crosstalk with smooth muscle cells. *PLoS One* 12:e0188530. doi: 10.1371/journal.pone.0188530

Busch, S., Auth, E., Scholl, F., Huenecke, S., Koehl, U., Suess, B., et al. (2015). 5-lipoxygenase is a direct target of miR-19a-3p and miR-125b-5p. *J. Immunol.* 194, 1646–1653. doi: 10.4049/jimmunol.1402163

Chauhan, A., Singh, M., Agarwal, A., and Paul, N. (2015). Correlation of TSLP, IL-33, and CD4 + CD25 + FOXP3 + T regulatory (Treg) in pediatric asthma. *J. Asthma* 52, 868–872. doi: 10.3109/02770903.2015.1026441

Cho, S., Wu, C. J., Yasuda, T., Cruz, L. O., Khan, A. A., Lin, L. L., et al. (2016). miR-23∼27∼24 clusters control effector T cell differentiation and function. *J. Exp. Med.* 213, 235–249. doi: 10.1084/jem.20150990

Christiaansen, A. F., Syed, M. A., Ten, E. P., Hartwig, S. M., Durairaj, L., Kamath, S. S., et al. (2016). Altered Treg and cytokine responses in RSV-infected infants. *Pediatr. Res.* 80, 702–709. doi: 10.1038/pr.2016.130

Cortjens, B., de Boer, O. J., de Jong, R., Antonis, A. F., Sabogal Piñeros, Y. S., Lutter, R., et al. (2016). Neutrophil extracellular traps cause airway obstruction during respiratory syncytial virus disease. *J. Pathol.* 238, 401–411. doi: 10.1002/path.4660

Essandoh, K., Li, Y., Huo, J., and Fan, G. C. (2016). MiRNA-mediated macrophage polarization and its potential role in the regulation of inflammatory response. *Shock* 46, 122–131. doi: 10.1097/SHK.0000000000000604

Feng, S., Zhang, L., Bian, X. H., Luo, Y., Qin, G. H., and Shi, R. M. (2017). Role of the TSLP/DC/OX40L pathway in asthma pathogenesis and airway inflammation in mice. *Biochem. Cell Biol.* 96, 306–316. doi: 10.1139/bcb-2017-0126

Fonseca, W., Lukacs, N. W., and Ptaschinski, C. (2018). Factors affecting the immunity to respiratory syncytial virus: from epigenetics to microbiome. *Front. Immunol.* 9:226. doi: 10.3389/fimmu.2018.00226

Frias, A. J., Buechel, H. M., Neupane, A., and D'Cruz, L. M. (2018). Invariant natural killer T-cell development and function with loss of microRNA-155. *Immunology* 153, 238–245. doi: 10.1111/imm.12836

Gavino, A. C., Nahmod, K., Bharadwaj, U., Makedonas, G., and Tweardy, D. J. (2016). STAT3 inhibition prevents lung inflammation, remodeling, and accumulation of Th2 and Th17 cells in a murine asthma model. *Allergy* 71, 1684–1692. doi: 10.1111/all.12937

Globinska, A., Pawelczyk, M., and Kowalski, M. L. (2014). MicroRNAs and the immune response to respiratory virus infections. *Expert Rev. Clin. Immunol.* 10, 963–971. doi: 10.1586/1744666X.2014.913482

Groothuis, J. R., Hoopes, J. M., and Hemming, V. G. (2011). Prevention of serious respiratory syncytial virus-related illness. II: immunoprophylaxis. *Adv. Ther.* 28, 110–125. doi: 10.1007/s12325-010-0101-y

Haralambieva, I. H., Kennedy, R. B., Simon, W. L., Goergen, K. M., Grill, D. E., Ovsyannikova, I. G., et al. (2018). Differential miRNA expression in B cells is associated with inter-individual differences in humoral immune response to measles vaccination. *PLoS One* 13:e0191812. doi: 10.1371/journal.pone.0191812

Hasegawa, K., Perez-Losada, M., Hoptay, C. E., Epstein, S., Mansbach, J. M., Teach, S. J., et al. (2018). RSV vs. rhinovirus bronchiolitis: difference in nasal airway microRNA profiles and NFkappaB signaling. *Pediatr. Res.* 83, 606–614. doi: 10.1038/pr.2017.309

Hirose, K., Iwata, A., Tamachi, T., and Nakajima, H. (2017). Allergic airway inflammation: key players beyond the Th2 cell pathway. *Immunol. Rev.* 278, 145–161. doi: 10.1111/imr.12540

Inchley, C. S., Sonerud, T., Fjaerli, H. O., and Nakstad, B. (2015). Nasal mucosal microRNA expression in children with respiratory syncytial virus infection. *BMC Infect. Dis.* 15:150. doi: 10.1186/s12879-015-0878-z

Jeker, L. T., and Bluestone, J. A. (2013). MicroRNA regulation of T-cell differentiation and function. *Immunol. Rev.* 253, 65–81. doi: 10.1111/imr.12061

Johnson, J. E., Gonzales, R. A., Olson, S. J., Wright, P. F., and Graham, B. S. (2007). The histopathology of fatal untreated human respiratory syncytial virus infection. *Mod. Pathol.* 20, 108–119. doi: 10.1038/modpathol.3800725

Juzenas, S., Venkatesh, G., Hubenthal, M., Hoeppner, M. P., Du, Z. G., Paulsen, M., et al. (2017). A comprehensive, cell specific microRNA catalogue of human peripheral blood. *Nucleic Acids Res.* 45, 9290–9301. doi: 10.1093/nar/gkx706

Kim, R. Y., Horvat, J. C., Pinkerton, J. W., Starkey, M. R., Essilfie, A. T., Mayall, J. R., et al. (2017). MicroRNA-21 drives severe, steroid-insensitive experimental asthma by amplifying phosphoinositide 3-kinase-mediated suppression of histone deacetylase 2. *J. Allergy Clin. Immunol.* 139, 519–532. doi: 10.1016/j.jaci.2016.04.038

Kroesen, B. J., Teteloshvili, N., Smigielska-Czepiel, K., Brouwer, E., Boots, A. M., van den Berg, A., et al. (2015). Immuno-miRs: critical regulators of T-cell development, function and ageing. *Immunology* 144, 1–10. doi: 10.1111/imm.12367

Kumar, M., Ahmad, T., Sharma, A., Mabalirajan, U., Kulshreshtha, A., Agrawal, A., et al. (2011). Let-7 microRNA-mediated regulation of IL-13 and allergic airway inflammation. *J. Allergy Clin. Immunol.* 128, 1077.e10–1085.e10. doi: 10.1016/j.jaci.2011.04.034

Lay, M. K., Bueno, S. M., Galvez, N., Riedel, C. A., and Kalergis, A. M. (2016). New insights on the viral and host factors contributing to the airway pathogenesis caused by the respiratory syncytial virus. *Crit. Rev. Microbiol.* 42, 800–812. doi: 10.3109/1040841X.2015.1055711

Lee, H., Han, S., Kwon, C. S., and Lee, D. (2016). Biogenesis and regulation of the let-7 miRNAs and their functional implications. *Protein Cell* 7, 100–113. doi: 10.1007/s13238-015-0212-y

Lee, H. C., Headley, M. B., Loo, Y. M., Berlin, A., Gale, M. J., Debley, J. S., et al. (2012). Thymic stromal lymphopoietin is induced by respiratory syncytial virus-infected airway epithelial cells and promotes a type 2 response to infection. *J. Allergy Clin. Immunol* 130, 1187.e–1196.e. doi: 10.1016/j.jaci.2012.07.031

Liu, F., Ouyang, J., Sharma, A. N., Liu, S., Yang, B., Xiong, W., et al. (2015). Leukotriene inhibitors for bronchiolitis in infants and young children. *Cochrane Database Syst. Rev.* 2015:CD010636. doi: 10.1002/14651858.CD010636.pub2

Liu, M., and Yokomizo, T. (2015). The role of leukotrienes in allergic diseases. *Allergol. Int.* 64, 17–26. doi: 10.1016/j.alit.2014.09.001

Liu, P., Li, L., Fan, P., Zheng, J., and Zhao, D. (2018). High-dose of intravenous immunoglobulin modulates immune tolerance in premature infants. *BMC Pediatr.* 18:74. doi: 10.1186/s12887-018-1055-5

Luo, X., Han, M., Liu, J., Wang, Y., Luo, X., Zheng, J., et al. (2015). Epithelial cell-derived micro RNA-146a generates interleukin-10-producing monocytes to inhibit nasal allergy. *Sci. Rep.* 5:15937. doi: 10.1038/srep15937

Mangodt, T. C., Van Herck, M. A., Nullens, S., Ramet, J., De Dooy, J. J., Jorens, P. G., et al. (2015). The role of Th17 and Treg responses in the pathogenesis of RSV infection. *Pediatr. Res.* 78, 483–491. doi: 10.1038/pr.2015.143

Markopoulos, G. S., Roupakia, E., Tokamani, M., Vartholomatos, G., Tzavaras, T., Hatziapostolou, M., et al. (2017). Senescence-associated microRNAs target cell cycle regulatory genes in normal human lung fibroblasts. *Exp. Gerontol.* 96, 110–122. doi: 10.1016/j.exger.2017.06.017

Matsuse, H., Hirose, H., Tsuchida, T., Fukahori, S., Fukushima, C., Mizuta, Y., et al. (2007). Effects of respiratory syncytial virus infection on dendritic cells and cysteinyl leukotrienes in lung tissues of a murine model of asthma. *Allergol. Int.* 56, 165–169. doi: 10.2332/allergolint.O-06-476

McCaskill, J. L., Ressel, S., Alber, A., Redford, J., Power, U. F., Schwarze, J., et al. (2017). Broad-spectrum inhibition of respiratory virus infection by microRNA mimics targeting p38 MAPK signaling. *Mol. Ther. Nucleic Acids* 7, 256–266. doi: 10.1016/j.omtn.2017.03.008

Moffett, H. F., Cartwright, A., Kim, H. J., Godec, J., Pyrdol, J., Aijo, T., et al. (2017). The microRNA miR-31 inhibits CD8(+) T cell function in chronic viral infection. *Nat. Immunol.* 18, 791–799. doi: 10.1038/ni.3755

Murakami-Satsutani, N., Ito, T., Nakanishi, T., Inagaki, N., Tanaka, A., Vien, P. T. X., et al. (2014). IL-33 promotes the induction and maintenance of Th2 immune responses by enhancing the function of OX40 ligand. *Allergol. Int.* 63, 443–455. doi: 10.2332/allergolint.13-OA-0672

Musiyenko, A., Correa, L., Stock, N., Hutchinson, J. H., Lorrain, D. S., Bain, G., et al. (2009). A novel 5-lipoxygenase-activating protein inhibitor, AM679, reduces inflammation in the respiratory syncytial virus-infected mouse eye. *Clin. Vaccine Immunol.* 16, 1654–1659. doi: 10.1128/CVI.00220-09

Nenna, R., Ferrara, M., Nicolai, A., Pierangeli, A., Scagnolari, C., Papoff, P., et al. (2015). Viral load in infants hospitalized for respiratory syncytial virus bronchiolitis correlates with recurrent wheezing at thirty-six-month follow-up. *Pediatr. Infect. Dis. J.* 34, 1131–1132. doi: 10.1097/INF.0000000000000825

Nguyen, T. H., Liu, X., Su, Z. Z., Hsu, A. C., Foster, P. S., and Yang, M. (2018). Potential role of microRNAs in the regulation of antiviral responses to influenza infection. *Front. Immunol.* 9:1541. doi: 10.3389/fimmu.2018.01541

Obando-Pacheco, P., Justicia-Grande, A. J., Rivero-Calle, I., Rodriguez-Tenreiro, C., Sly, P., Ramilo, O., et al. (2018). Respiratory syncytial virus seasonality: a global overview. *J. Infect. Dis.* 217, 1356–1364. doi: 10.1093/infdis/jiy056

Okoye, I. S., Coomes, S. M., Pelly, V. S., Czieso, S., Papayannopoulos, V., Tolmachova, T., et al. (2014). MicroRNA-containing T-regulatory-cell-derived exosomes suppress pathogenic T helper 1 cells. *Immunity* 41, 89–103. doi: 10.1016/j.immuni.2014.08.008

Othumpangat, S., Walton C., and Piedimonte, G. (2012). MicroRNA-221 modulates RSV replication in human bronchial epithelium by targeting NGF expression. *PLoS One* 7:e30030. doi: 10.1371/journal.pone.0030030

Panganiban, R. P., Pinkerton, M. H., Maru, S. Y., Jefferson, S. J., Roff, A. N., and Ishmael, F. T. (2012). Differential microRNA expression in asthma and the role of miR-1248 in regulation of IL-5. *Am. J. Clin. Exp. Immunol.* 1, 154–165.

Pappas, K., Papaioannou, A. I., Kostikas, K., and Tzanakis, N. (2013). The role of macrophages in obstructive airways disease: chronic obstructive pulmonary disease and asthma. *Cytokine* 64, 613–625. doi: 10.1016/j.cyto.2013.09.010

Peng, S., Wang, J., Wei, S., Li, C., Zhou, K., Hu, J., et al. (2018). Endogenous cellular microRNAs mediate antiviral defense against influenza a virus. *Mol. Ther. Nucleic Acids* 10, 361–375. doi: 10.1016/j.omtn.2017.12.016

Peng, W. S., Chen, X., Yang, X. Y., and Liu, E. M. (2014). Systematic review of montelukast's efficacy for preventing post-bronchiolitis wheezing. *Pediatr. Allergy Immunol.* 25, 143–150. doi: 10.1111/pai.12124

Petrarca, L., Nenna, R., Frassanito, A., Pierangeli, A., Leonardi, S., Scagnolari, C., et al. (2018). Acute bronchiolitis: influence of viral co-infection in infants hospitalized over 12 consecutive epidemic seasons. *J. Med. Virol.* 90, 631–638. doi: 10.1002/jmv.24994

Ren, J. P., Ying, R. S., Cheng, Y. Q., Wang, L., El, G. M., Li, G. Y., et al. (2016). HCV-induced miR146a controls SOCS1/STAT3 and cytokine expression in monocytes to promote regulatory T-cell development. *J. Viral Hepat.* 23, 755–766. doi: 10.1111/jvh.12537

Robbins, P. D., and Morelli, A. E. (2014). Regulation of immune responses by extracellular vesicles. *Nat. Rev. Immunol.* 14, 195–208. doi: 10.1038/nri3622

Ross, J. S., Carlson, J. A., and Brock, G. (2007). miRNA: the new gene silencer. *Am. J. Clin. Pathol.* 128, 830–836. doi: 10.1309/2JK279BU2G743MWJ

Rossi, G. A., and Colin, A. A. (2015). Infantile respiratory syncytial virus and human rhinovirus infections: respective role in inception and persistence of wheezing. *Eur. Respir. J.* 45, 774–789. doi: 10.1183/09031936.00062714

Roush, S., and Slack, F. J. (2008). The let-7 family of microRNAs. *Trends Cell Biol.* 18, 505–516. doi: 10.1016/j.tcb.2008.07.007

Schmidt, M. E., Knudson, C. J., Hartwig, S. M., Pewe, L. L., Meyerholz, D. K., Langlois, R. A., et al. (2018). Memory CD8 T cells mediate severe immunopathology following respiratory syncytial virus infection. *PLoS Pathog.* 14:e1006810. doi: 10.1371/journal.ppat.1006810

Self-Fordham, J. B., Naqvi, A. R., Uttamani, J. R., Kulkarni, V., and Nares, S. (2017). MicroRNA: dynamic regulators of macrophage polarization and plasticity. *Front. Immunol.* 8:1062. doi: 10.3389/fimmu.2017.01062

Shi, T., Balsells, E., Wastnedge, E., Singleton, R., Rasmussen, Z. A., Zar, H. J., et al. (2015). Risk factors for respiratory syncytial virus associated with acute lower respiratory infection in children under five years: systematic review and meta-analysis. *J. Glob. Health* 5:020416. doi: 10.7189/jogh.05.020416

Shirasaki, H., Kanaizumi, E., Seki, N., Fujita, M., Kikuchi, M., and Himi, T. (2013). Localization and up-regulation of cysteinyl leukotriene-2 receptor in human allergic nasal mucosa. *Allergol. Int.* 62, 223–228. doi: 10.2332/allergolint.12-OA-0490

Shirey, K. A., Lai, W., Pletneva, L. M., Karp, C. L., Divanovic, S., Blanco, J. C. G., et al. (2014). Role of the lipoxygenase pathway in RSV-induced alternatively activated macrophages leading to resolution of lung pathology. *Mucosal Immunol.* 7, 549–557. doi: 10.1038/mi.2013.71

Sigurs, N., Bjarnason, R., Sigurbergsson, F., and Kjellman, B. (2000). Respiratory syncytial virus bronchiolitis in infancy is an important risk factor for asthma and allergy at age 7. *Am. J. Respir. Crit. Care Med.* 161, 1501–1507. doi: 10.1164/ajrccm.161.5.9906076

Simoes, E., Bont, L., Manzoni, P., Fauroux, B., Paes, B., Figueras-Aloy, J., et al. (2018). Past, present and future approaches to the prevention and treatment of respiratory syncytial virus infection in children. *Infect. Dis. Ther.* 7, 87–120. doi: 10.1007/s40121-018-0188-z

Simpson, L. J., Patel, S., Bhakta, N. R., Choy, D. F., Brightbill, H. D., Ren, X., et al. (2014). A microRNA upregulated in asthma airway T cells promotes

TH2 cytokine production. *Nat. Immunol.* 15, 1162–1170. doi: 10.1038/ni.3026

Singh, P. B., Pua, H. H., Happ, H. C., Schneider, C., von Moltke, J., Locksley, R. M., et al. (2017). MicroRNA regulation of type 2 innate lymphoid cell homeostasis and function in allergic inflammation. *J. Exp. Med.* 214, 3627–3643. doi: 10.1084/jem.20170545

Smyth, L. A., Boardman, D. A., Tung, S. L., Lechler, R., and Lombardi, G. (2015). MicroRNAs affect dendritic cell function and phenotype. *Immunology* 144, 197–205. doi: 10.1111/imm.12390

Su, K., Wang, Q., Qi, L., Hua, D., Tao, J., Mangan, C. J., et al. (2016). MicroRNA-674-5p/5-LO axis involved in autoimmune reaction of Concanavalin A-induced acute mouse liver injury. *Toxicol. Lett.* 258, 101–107. doi: 10.1016/j.toxlet.2016.06.010

Thornburg, N. J., Hayward, S. L., and Crowe, J. J. (2012). Respiratory syncytial virus regulates human microRNAs by using mechanisms involving beta interferon and NF-kappaB. *mBio* 3:e00220-12. doi: 10.1128/mBio.00220-12

Tian, B., Yang, J., Zhao, Y., Ivanciuc, T., Sun, H., Garofalo, R. P., et al. (2017). BRD4 couples NF-kappaB/RelA with airway inflammation and the IRF-RIG-I amplification loop in respiratory syncytial virus infection. *J. Virol.* 91:e00007-17. doi: 10.1128/JVI.00007-17

Wang, S., Liu, P., Yang, P., Zheng, J., and Zhao, D. (2017). Peripheral blood microRNAs expression is associated with infant respiratory syncytial virus infection. *Oncotarget* 8, 96627–96635. doi: 10.18632/oncotarget.19364

Wang, Z., Filgueiras, L. R., Wang, S., Serezani, A. P., Peters-Golden, M., Jancar, S., et al. (2014). Leukotriene B4 enhances the generation of proinflammatory microRNAs to promote MyD88-dependent macrophage activation. *J. Immunol.* 192, 2349–2356. doi: 10.4049/jimmunol.1302982

Werz, O., Gerstmeier, J., and Garscha, U. (2017). Novel leukotriene biosynthesis inhibitors (2012-2016) as anti-inflammatory agents. *Expert Opin. Ther. Pat.* 27, 607–620. doi: 10.1080/13543776.2017.1276568

Xie, N., Cui, H., Banerjee, S., Tan, Z., Salomao, R., Fu, M., et al. (2014). miR-27a regulates inflammatory response of macrophages by targeting IL-10. *J. Immunol.* 193, 327–334. doi: 10.4049/jimmunol.1400203

Ye, L., Mou, Y., Wang, J., and Jin, M. L. (2017). Effects of microRNA-19b on airway remodeling, airway inflammation and degree of oxidative stress by targeting TSLP through the Stat3 signaling pathway in a mouse model of asthma. *Oncotarget* 8, 47533–47546. doi: 10.18632/oncotarget.17258

Zago, M., Rico, D. S. A., Hecht, E., Rousseau, S., Hamid, Q., Eidelman, D. H., et al. (2014). The NF-kappaB family member RelB regulates microRNA miR-146a to suppress cigarette smoke-induced COX-2 protein expression in lung fibroblasts. *Toxicol. Lett.* 226, 107–116. doi: 10.1016/j.toxlet.2014.01.020

Zhao, C., Sun, G., Li, S., Lang, M. F., Yang, S., Li, W., et al. (2010). MicroRNA let-7b regulates neural stem cell proliferation and differentiation by targeting nuclear receptor TLX signaling. *Proc. Natl. Acad. Sci. U.S.A.* 107, 1876–1881. doi: 10.1073/pnas.0908750107

Zheng, J., Yang, P., Tang, Y., Pan, Z., and Zhao, D. (2015a). Respiratory syncytial virus nonstructural proteins upregulate SOCS1 and SOCS3 in the different manner from endogenous IFN signaling. *J. Immunol. Res.* 2015, 1–11. doi: 10.1155/2015/738547

Zheng, J., Yang, P., Tang, Y., and Zhao, D. (2015b). A respiratory syncytial virus persistent-infected cell line system reveals the involvement of SOCS1 in the innate antiviral response. *Virol. Sin.* 30, 190–199. doi: 10.1007/s12250-015-3597-0

Zhou, Q., Haupt, S., Prots, I., Thummler, K., Kremmer, E., Lipsky, P. E., et al. (2013). miR-142-3p is involved in CD25+ CD4 T cell proliferation by targeting the expression of glycoprotein A repetitions predominant. *J. Immunol.* 190, 6579–6588. doi: 10.4049/jimmunol.1202993

Zhu, J., Qiu, Y. S., Figueroa, D. J., Bandi, V., Galczenski, H., Hamada, K., et al. (2005). Localization and upregulation of cysteinyl leukotriene-1 receptor in asthmatic bronchial mucosa. *Am. J. Respir. Cell Mol. Biol.* 33, 531–540. doi: 10.1165/rcmb.2005-0124OC

Ziegler, S. F., and Liu, Y. J. (2006). Thymic stromal lymphopoietin in normal and pathogenic T cell development and function. *Nat. Immunol.* 7, 709–714. doi: 10.1038/ni1360

2

Association of the Human Bocavirus with Tonsil Squamous Cell Carcinomas

Merle Höpken[1,2], Isabel Förster[2], Steffen Maune[1], Michael Brockmann[2], Oliver Schildgen[2] and Verena Schildgen[2]**

[1] Klinik für Hals-, Nasen- und Ohrenheilkunde, Kliniken der Stadt Köln, Klinikum der Privaten Universität Witten/Herdecke mit Sitz in Köln, Cologne, Germany, [2] Institut für Pathologie, Kliniken der Stadt Köln, Klinikum der Privaten Universität Witten/Herdecke mit Sitz in Köln, Cologne, Germany

Background: The human bocavirus (HBoV) is known to persist latently in the infected host cells and seems to replicate its DNA via the DNA damage response system, which is frequently defect in tumors and correlates with microsatellite instability (MSI). Because HBoV is able to persist in the infected tissues, induces pro-fibrotic and pro- cancerogenic cytokines *in vivo* and *in vitro*, and is detected in colorectal and lung tumors, the virus may be involved in cancerogenesis at least as a cofactor. Recently it was shown that the adenotonsillar tissue is an important site of HBoV1 persistence and replication. Considering the background that approximately 60% of oropharyngeal cancers were thought to be attributable to a HPV infection, a co-participation of HBoV in terms of a chronic virus infection might play a role in the cancerogenesis of tonsil tumors.

Methods: Formalin-fixed, paraffin-embedded tonsil tumor samples were screened for HBoV and HPV DNA. Positive tissue sections were afterward subjected to fluorescence *in situ* hybridization (FISH) analysis to identify HBoV and HPV infected cells. By use of an *in vitro* cell culture model with primary tonsil fibroblasts, keratinocytes, and lymphocytes infected by HBoV we tried to find the target cells of virus replication. MSI testing was based on a previously published protocol using a de-multiplexed PCR followed by fluorescent detection of PCR products in a capillary sequencing device.

Results: In total 62 of 103 (60, 19%) of the tonsil squamous cell carcinomas tested positive for HBoV DNA and 66 of 103 (66%) samples were identified as HPV positive. The FISH analysis revealed both double infection of HPV and HBoV in the same cells as well as single infections of both viruses within the tumor tissue. Twenty-two of 62 HBoV positive tumors tested HPV negative, 40 of 62 tissue sections were HBoV and HPV positive. We analyzed 21 out of the 62 HBoV positive tumors for MSI. Of those four tonsils displayed MSI in at least 1 of 10 microsatellite markers.

Conclusion: Our findings support the hypothesis that human bocavirus infections as a cofactor may have an impact on tumor development in tonsils, although it still remains possible that HBoV solely displays a tumor tropism.

Keywords: human bocavirus, tonsil squamous cell carcinoma, oncogenesis, persistence, primary cell culture

INTRODUCTION

Since the identification of human bocavirus 1 in nasopharyngeal aspirates in 2005, evidence is increasing that the HBoV1, belonging to the *Bocaparvovirus* genus of the *Parvoviridae* family, is associated with respiratory tract infections and gastrointestinal infections (Allander et al., 2005; Huang et al., 2012). It is presumed that besides causing acute infections HBoV is persisting in a replicative but subclinical state, and is a pathogen rather than an innocent bystander (Proenca-Modena et al., 2014). Previous studies suggest that HBoV is associated with some lung and colorectal tumors and prove that the bocavirus persistence is increased in cancer patients (Schildgen et al., 2013). In 20% of colorectal and lung cancers formalin-fixed paraffin-embedded (FFPE) tissues human bocavirus DNA could be detected. Li et al. (2007) revealed, that HBoV DNA commonly occurs in the serum of cancer patients and that the prevalence is significantly higher in this group than in that of the healthy control group (Addie et al., 2012). It is also known that HBoV persists in adenotonsillar tissue, which is considered as the major replication site *in vivo* by some researchers (Clement et al., 2009). Proenca-Modena et al. (2014) detected human bocavirus in 31.1% of 172 hypertrophic adenoids or tonsils from children. Szalmas et al. (2013) reported that the presence of HBoV displays a statistically significant correlation to Otitis media with effusion cases associated with adenoid hypertrophy. It could be shown that HBoV1 can persist in the infected host in form of cccDNA structures, similar to the human hepatitis B virus (HBV), leading to a chronic inflammation and culminating in organ-fibrosis (Lusebrink et al., 2011; Schildgen et al., 2014).

This observations are supported by a preceding study, which demonstrated that profibrotic and pro-cancerogenic chemokines are upregulated *in vitro* and *in vivo*, suggesting that HBoV is directly or indirectly involved in tumorigenesis (Khalfaoui et al., 2016). In addition, given the fact that the incidence of human papillomavirus associated oropharyngeal cancer is increasing especially in developed countries, the search for infectious agents playing a role in human carcinogenesis in the range of the oropharyngeal tract and their identification are important issues (Marur and Forastiere, 2008). In the case of HPV infection of the oropharynx it is presumed that the process toward malignant conversion is covering a long latency period between primary infection and cancer emergence (zur Hausen, 1999). Due to the latent, chronic inflammation provoked by oncogenic viruses this mechanism could be similar in the presence of a chronic HBoV infection (Wang et al., 2008; Zeisel et al., 2015). As animal models are still lacking for the exploration of HBoV infections, cell culture experiments and the analysis of clinical cohorts are necessary to elucidate the pathophysiology of replication, interaction with cells and other viruses and possible oncogenic effects. Taken together the previous findings lead us to the hypothesis that HBoV also persists in adult tonsillar tissue and may be even associated with oropharyngeal, especially tonsillar cancers.

Abbreviations: FFPE tissue, formaldehyde-fixed paraffin-embedded tissue; FISH, fluorescence *in situ* hybridization; Geq, genome equivalents; HBoV 1, human bocavirus 1; HBV, hepatitis B virus; HEK cells, human embryonic kidney cells; HPV, human papilloma virus; MMP-9, matrix-metalloproteinase 9; MOI, multiplicity of infection; MSI, microsatellite instability.

MATERIALS AND METHODS

Aim of the present study was to address the questions whether HBoV can be detected in tonsillar squamous cell carcinomas, whether there is a correlation of HPV and HBoV infection in tonsillar tumors and whether both viruses infect the same cells. Furthermore, we cultivated primary keratinocytes, fibroblasts, and lymphocytes of tonsil tissue and infected them with virulent HBoV particles to ascertain which the target cells for virus replication are. In addition, we tested the hypothesis that the interaction between HBoV and the host genome, in concert with the fact that the viral replication is dependent on the DNA damage repair response (Deng et al., 2016, 2017), may influence the microsatellite stability in tonsillar tumors.

Ethics Statement

All procedures were performed in accordance with the declaration of Helsinki and according to a vote of the ethical committee of the Private University of Witten/Herdecke (Vote No. 151/2016). This vote was specifically approved for the current study. There is a written informed consent of all patients, whose primary cells were used. Pediatric patients were included exclusively with parental written informed consent. For the retrospective and double blinded part of the study no written consent was required. The study cohort consisted of adult patients (tumors and primary cells) and children (primary cells).

Patient Samples

Hundred and three FFPE tonsillar cancer sections and 20 chronically inflamed tonsil sections were selected from archived samples from our routine clinical laboratory. Primary tonsil cells were gained by routinely performed tonsillectomy in adult patients ($n = 11$).

PCR Based Detection of Viral Nucleic Acids

DNA from FFPE tissue samples of 103 tonsillar cancers and 20 chronic inflamed tonsils was extracted using the Maxwell 16 FFPE tissue kit (Promega, Mannheim, Germany) according to the manufacturer's protocol. All samples were analyzed with the RespiFinder Smart22 (Pathofinder, Netherlands) being able to detect 22 respiratory pathogens, including HBoV and Adenovirus. HPV detection was performed by the HPV 3.5 LCD-Array (Chipron, Berlin, Germany) according to the manufacturer recommendations. HBoV real-time PCR was performed as previously described (Khalfaoui et al., 2016).

HBoV and HPV Detection by FISH Analysis

All FFPE tonsil tumor samples that tested positive for HBoV by the Respifinder assay ($n = 62$) were subjected to FISH analyses for the detection of HBoV1 and HPV 16.

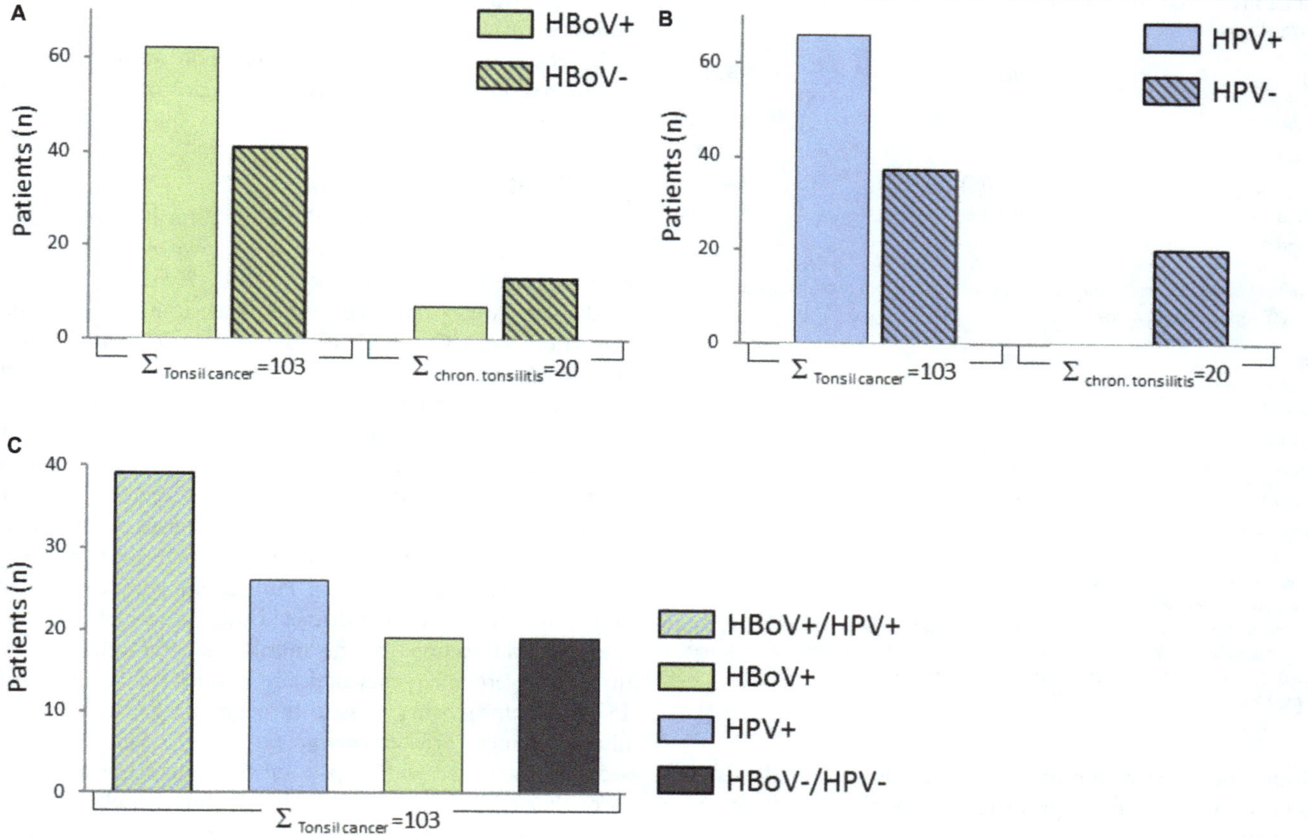

FIGURE 1 | Column diagrams showing the overview on the patient cohort. **(A)** Shows the rate of HBoV positivity in the tumor cohort compared to patients with chronic tonsilitis. **(B)** Shows the rate of HPV positivity in the tumor cohort compared to patients with chronic tonsillitis. **(C)** Shows the rate of HBoV/HPV coinfections and mono-infections in the entire tumor cohort.

Fluorescence *in situ* hybridization was performed as follows: FFPE tumor tissues were cut into slices of 3-µm and mounted on slides. Slides were treated according to the ZytoLight SPEC ALK/EML4 TriCHeck probe protocol (ZytoVision, Bremerhaven, Germany) following the manufacturers' recommendations as previously published (Schildgen et al., 2013), with the modification that HBoV and HPV specific probes were mixed in a ratio of 1:1 (2 pM each). The HBoV probe was designed to hybridize near the terminal region of the HBoV genome and labeled with rhodamine red (Eurofins MWG Operon, Ebersberg, Germany). To identify the genome of the human papilloma virus 16 a commercially available

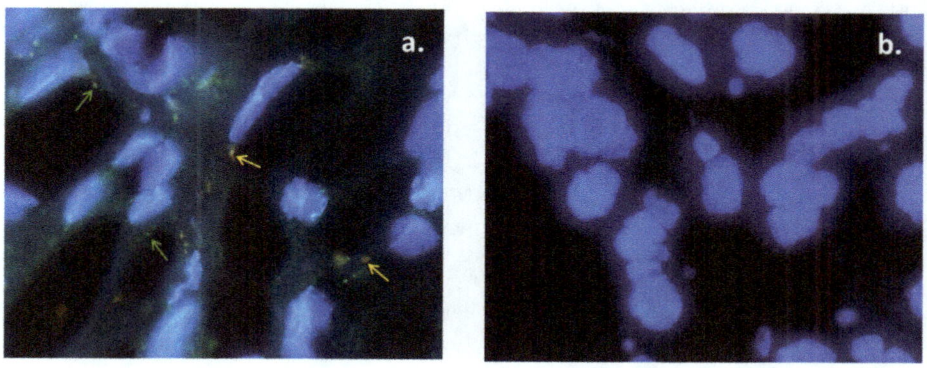

FIGURE 2 | Examples of FISH analysis of a tonsillar tumor being positive for HPV and HBoV by RespifinderSmart22 and the HPV 3.5 LCD-Array. Rhodamine red indicates the human bocavirus DNA, whereas FITC indicates human papillomavirus 16 DNA. The blue DAPI staining indicates the cell nuclei. **(a)** HBoV positive tumor. **(b)** HBoV negative tumor.

TABLE 1 | Case numbers and percentages of HBoV **(A)** and HPV **(B)** according to tumor stages.

(A)	HBoV +	HBoV –
Stage 1	5 (41.7%)	7 (58.3%)
Stage 2	2 (28.5%)	5 (71.5%)
Stage 3	17 (68.0%)	8 (32.0%)
Stage 4a	30 (54.5%)	25 (45.5%)
Stage 4b	3 (100%)	0 (0%)

Pearson correlation coefficient $r_{Pearson}$ = 0.913; coefficient of determination r^2 = 0.8335; very high correlation.

(B)	HPV +	HPV –
Stage 1	4 (33.3%)	8 (66.7%)
Stage 2	5 (83.3%)	1 (16.7%)
Stage 3	16 (66.7%)	8 (33.3%)
Stage 4a	37 (64.9%)	20 (35.1%)
Stage 4b	3 (100%)	0 (100%)

Pearson correlation coefficient $r_{Pearson}$ = 0.9213; coefficient of determination r^2 = 0.8487; very high correlation.
By using the one-tailed t-test for two dependent means there is a trend for an increase in the number of HBoV-positives in higher tumor stages (value of $p = 0.09051$ at $p \leq 0.10$ in the HBoV positive group vs. $p = 0.114027$ at $p \leq 0.10$ in the HBoV negative group).

biotin labeled HPV 16 probe (PanPath, Budel, Netherlands) was used. At this point the protocol was modified again, because the tissue was then incubated in Avidin-FITC (PanPath, Budel, Netherlands) for 30 min at 37°C before counterstaining of the cell nuclei with DAPI (DCS, Hamburg, Germany) to make HPV fluorescently visible.

Microscopic analyses and documentation was performed on a Zeiss Axioplan microscope using the AxioVixion 4.8 software (Zeiss, Jena, Germany).

Cell Culture

All cultures were performed with 1% v/v Penicillin/Streptomycin (10^4 U/ml each, BioWhittaker/Lonza, Switzerland) at 37°C. Human embryonic kidney 293 (HEK 293) cells for virus production were obtained from American Type Culture Collection (ATCC via LGC Standards, Wesel, Germany) and were cultured according to ATCC's recommendations. Primary tonsil keratinocytes, fibroblasts, and lymphocytes were obtained from 11 patients suffering from chronic tonsillitis immediately after routine tonsillectomy. Written informed consent was obtained in all cases in agreement with the ethical vote for this study. Resected tonsils were directly placed in 37°C warm keratinocyte growth medium (KGM BulletKit, Lonza, Switzerland). Further on lymphatic follicles and epithelial tissues were dissected using a scalpel. Afterward, the epithelial sections of the tonsils were minced in a Petri dish and were then enzymatically dissociated in trypsin for 15 min before being passed through an EASYstrainer cell filter (Greiner, Frickenhausen, Germany). The lymphocyte section was treated with trypsin for 5 min and was also passed through an EASYstrainer cell filter. While lymphocytes were cultured in six-well plates as suspension cultures in RPMI medium, keratinocytes and fibroblasts were cultured on

TABLE 2 | Overview on the results of MSI testing in 21 HBoV positive tumor samples eligible for the analyses.

HBoV (+ tonsillar tumor	BAT 25	BAT 26	APC	D17s250	D2s123	D13s153	BAT 40	Mycl	D18s58	D10s197
1	wt	wt	wt	wt	wt	wt	wt	wt	wt	wt
2	wt	wt	wt	wt	wt	wt	wt	wt	wt	wt
3	wt	wt	wt	wt	wt	wt	wt	wt	wt	wt
4	wt	wt	wt	wt	wt	wt	wt	wt	wt	wt
5	wt	instable	wt	wt	instable	instable	wt	wt	instable	wt
6	wt	wt	wt	wt	wt	wt	wt	wt	wt	wt
7	wt	wt	wt	wt	wt	wt	wt	wt	wt	wt
8	wt	wt	wt	wt	wt	wt	wt	wt	wt	wt
9	wt	wt	wt	wt	wt	wt	wt	wt	wt	wt
10	wt	wt	wt	wt	wt	wt	wt	wt	wt	wt
11	wt	wt	wt	wt	wt	wt	wt	wt	wt	wt
12	wt	wt	wt	wt	wt	wt	wt	wt	wt	wt
13	wt	wt	wt	instable	instable	wt	wt	wt	wt	wt
14	wt	wt	wt	wt	wt	wt	wt	instable	wt	wt
15	wt	wt	wt	wt	wt	wt	wt	wt	wt	wt
16	wt	wt	wt	wt	wt	wt	wt	wt	wt	wt
17	wt	wt	wt	wt	wt	wt	wt	wt	wt	wt
18	wt	wt	wt	wt	wt	wt	wt	wt	wt	wt
19	wt	wt	wt	wt	wt	wt	wt	wt	wt	wt
20	wt	wt	wt	wt	wt	instable	wt	wt	wt	wt
21	wt	wt	wt	wt	wt	wt	wt	wt	wt	wt

wt, wild type.

collagen-coated six-well plates (coated with 1 ml of 30 mg collagen solved in 500 ml deionized water and 100 μl glacial acetic acid) grown in keratinocyte growth medium (KGM BulletKit, Lonza, Switzerland) or epithelial growth medium (EGM BulletKit, Lonza, Switzerland), respectively. Microscopic analyses and documentation were performed on a Zeiss Primo Vert microscope using the AxioVision 4.8 software (Zeiss, Jena, Germany).

Virus Infection

Infectious human bocavirus was produced and quantified essentially as described earlier by Huang et al. (2012). The infection of the tonsillar cultures was performed in 90% confluent fibroblast and keratinocytes cell dishes, which was reached after 2–3 weeks of cultivation. The fibroblast infection was performed in triplicate, whereas the keratinocyte infection was conducted twice (in triplicate for one patient and as single infection for a second patient). The fibroblasts and keratinocytes were infected at MOI 0.5 with HBoV1 Geq in 3 ml cell medium, released from the apical surface of HEK293 cells after transfection of the full length HBoV1 plasmid pIHBoV1. The lymphocyte suspension cultures were infected at MOI 0.5 with HBoV1 inoculum immediately after preparation. Lymphocytes were previously counted by Luna-FL Fluorescence cell counter (Logos Biosystems, South Korea). The lymphocyte infection was also performed in triplicate (9 lymphocyte cultures, obtained from three different patients). Fibroblasts were harvested 12 days, keratinocytes and lymphocytes 10 days post-infection. The supernatant of the keratinocyte culture was removed and kept for quantitative HBoV1 PCR on days 1, 2, 3, 4, 5, 6, 7, and 8 following infection. The supernatant of the fibroblast culture was harvested on days 1, 3, 6, and 12 following infection, the lymphocyte culture supernatant on days 1, 3, 6, 8, and 10 following infection. HBoV DNA was extracted with the Maxwell RNA kit, which allows simultaneous DNA and RNA extractions from liquid samples (Promega, Darmstadt, Germany). Afterward the supernatant and the harvested cells were subjected to a real-time HBoV-1 PCR for a quantitative analysis of viral genomes.

Microsatellite Instability

Microsatellite instability testing was based on a previously published protocol using a multiplex PCR followed by fluorescent detection of PCR products in a capillary sequencing device. Ten microsatellites were included in the protocol, namely BAT25, BAT26, BAT40, APC, D17s250, D2s123, D13s153, D18s58, D10s197, and MycI. The protocol was de-multiplexed and established on the QiaXcel Advanced system (Qiagen, Hilden, Germany) (Forster et al., 2018).

Statistical Analyses

In order to test if a higher tumor stage correlates with the detection of HBoV, Pearson correlation coefficient $r_{Pearson}$ and the coefficient of determination r^2, and the statistical significance were calculated with the one-sided Student's *t*-test and a chi-square test.

RESULTS

In total, 62 of 103 (60.19%) of tonsil squamous cell carcinomas and 7 of 20 (35%) of chronically inflamed tonsils tested positive for HBoV DNA by the RespiFinder Smart22 PCR (**Figure 1A**). In 66 of 103 (66%) tonsil tumors, but in none (0%) of the 20 chronically inflamed tonsils HPV DNA could be identified (**Figure 1B**). In 40 of 103 (38.8%) tonsil tumors there was a coinfection of HPV and HBoV. In 26 of 103 (25.2%) we could register a single HPV infection and in 19 of 103 (18.4%) a single HBoV infection (**Figure 1C**). All samples were negative for the other 21 airway pathogens tested by the RespiFinder assay.

To ascertain whether HPV and HBoV DNA are present in the same cells of the tumor tissue an HBoV specific FISH assay was applied (**Figure 2**). The HPV type 16 FISH assay established for routine diagnostic was in agreement with the results of the HPV PCR, too. In 24 of 40 co-infected tumor sections (60%) the fluorescent signals of HPV 16 and HBoV DNA could be detected in the same cells, implying that the two viruses infected the same host cell. In contrast we found virus persistence in different cells in 13 of 40 co-infected tumor samples (32.5%) which means that FITC signals (indicating HPV DNA) and rhodamine red signals (indicating HBoV 1 DNA) were spread as distinct separated signals all over the tumor sections.

In 3 of 40 tumors (7.5%) we could observe a heterogeneous image with double infected cells and single infections in the same section. In 22 cases (35.4%) of all HBoV positive samples (single and co-infections) the presence of human bocavirus DNA could be determined. In accordance with the PCR based analyses HPV DNA was not detected in the chronic tonsillitis tissue sections. The signals were not always located in the nucleus, but appeared to be in the cytoplasm, as indicated by merging the different color channels. Moreover, multiple signals per cell were registered, indicating that multiple copies of HBoV DNA are present in the cells due to replication or, as a matter of speculation, due to persisting episomes.

Furthermore we found a correlation between the presence of human bocavirus and the tonsil tumor stage. We noticed higher bocavirus prevalence in tumor sections with progressed tumor stages. By using the one-tailed *t*-test for two dependent means a trend for the increase in the number of HBoV-positives in higher tumor stages was observed (value of $p = 0.09051$ at $p \leq 0.10$ in the HBoV positive group vs. $p = 0.114027$ at $p \leq 0.10$ in the HBoV negative group) (**Table 1A**), whereas there was no higher HPV prevalence in higher tumor stages (**Table 1B**).

In addition, we analyzed 21 out of the 62 HBoV positive tumors (single HBoV infected and HPV coinfected) for MSI (**Table 2**), because only for these tumors a tumor-free control tissue was available to compare the microsatellite status of tumor and otherwise healthy tissue. Of those, only four tonsils displayed microsatellite instabilities in at least 1 of 10 microsatellite markers, as exemplarily shown in **Figure 3**.

Because it was postulated that HBoV is likely persisting in tonsillar tissue and that this kind of tissue is assumed to be the major replication site *in vivo*, we performed a series of cell culture experiments with primary tonsil cells, directly obtained after tonsillectomy. Routinely resected, chronic infected

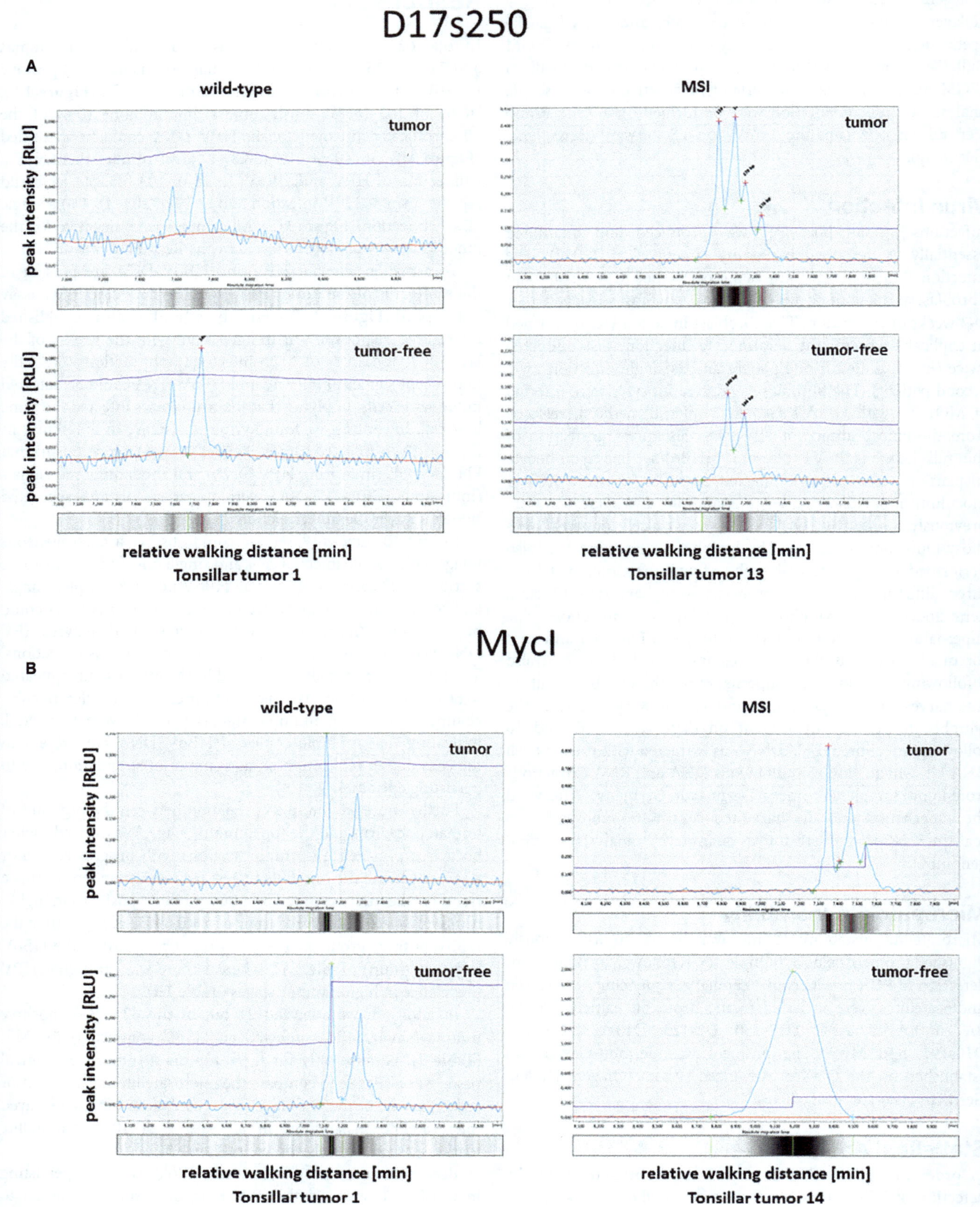

FIGURE 3 | Analyses of microsatellite instability in tonsillar tumors. The electropherograms show selected microsatellites in tumor and the corresponding healthy control tissue. **(A)** MSI for D17s250. **(B)** MSI for MycI.

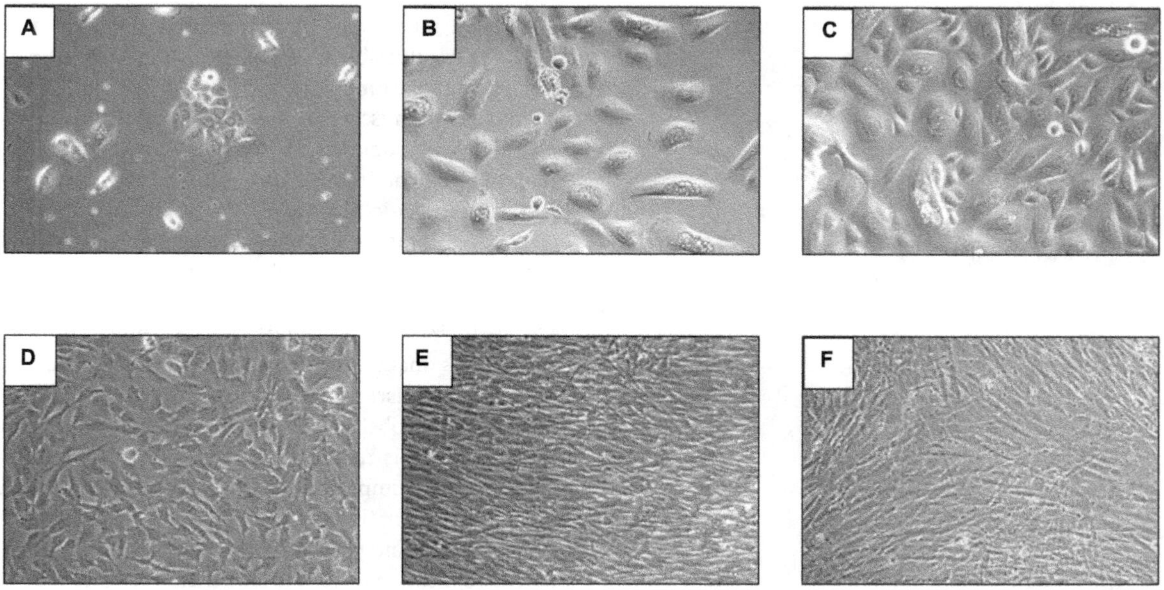

FIGURE 4 | Microscopic pictures were taken with 100x magnification with phase contrast. The upper part of the figure shows keratinocytes of the tonsil 8 days **(A)**, 3 weeks **(B)**, and 4 weeks **(C)** after cultivation in KGM medium. The lower pictures show fibroblasts of the tonsil 5 days **(D)**, 10 days **(E)**, and 14 days **(F)** after cultivation in KGM medium.

tonsils were brought to the laboratory immediately after surgery and fibroblasts, keratinocytes, and lymphocytes were prepared. To evaluate the most appropriate coating keratinocytes were cultured on laminin, fibronectin, and collagen coated plates and it turned out that collagen is the most effective coating for tonsillar keratinocytes. Nevertheless cultivating of tonsil keratinocytes was successful in solely 2 of 11 patients. These cells were infected with an HBoV inoculum with MOI 1 referred to Geq in triplicate and the amount of virus genome was determined kinetically up to day 12. Regarding the cell morphology of the isolated keratinocytes and fibroblasts, which is exemplarily shown in **Figure 4**, no difference between infected and non-infected cells could be observed (not shown). In one infected well of one patient we observed a virus replication after 3 days in accordance with the typical virus growth curve (**Figure 5**). However, in the remaining three HBoV infected cultures of the other patient there was no virus replication measurable. Virus replication in fibroblasts and lymphocytes was not detectable, indicating that this cell types are not permissive for HBoV.

DISCUSSION

It was postulated that HBoV persists in tonsillar tissues which are deemed to be the major replication site during the natural infection *in vivo* (Clement et al., 2009). Therefore, we addressed the question of HBoV also plays a role in tonsillar carcinoma.

In our study including 103 tonsil squamous cell carcinomas and 20 chronic infected tonsils, we detected human bocavirus DNA in 60.2% (n = 62) of all tonsillar tumors and in 37% (n = 7) of all chronic tonsillitis tissues. The data presented suggest that there is an association between the presence of HBoV and oropharyngeal squamous cell cancer, especially tonsillar carcinomas. The prevalence of HBoV is statistically significant higher in tonsillar tumor sections than in chronically inflamed tonsils (p = 0.037 by Chi-square test), which not only confirms the hypothesis that HBoV may be a causative pathogen in coinfection, but as well might imply that HBoV may be involved in cancerogenesis. Up to now it is not clearly verified whether HBoV persists in tumors as episomes in form of cccDNA, or whether it is integrated into the human genome but there are several studies concluding that the cccDNA structures, found in patients infected with HBoV may be viral genomes persisting in the cells (Kapoor et al., 2011; Lusebrink et al., 2011). This mechanism would be similar to the human hepatitis B virus (HBV), a virus with high oncogenic potential because of its capacity to induce chronic inflammation, leading to liver fibrosis and consequently supporting cancerogenesis (Schildgen et al., 2014). We could register multiple copies of HBoV DNA in the tumor cells due to replication or, as a matter of speculation, due to persisting episomes. This observation fits with our earlier observations when analyzing non-small lung cancers and colorectal tumors (Schildgen et al., 2013). Additionally, the role of human parvovirus as a potential contributor to carcinogenesis has been discussed for parvovirus B19 with the reasonable suspicion that the virus is a causative agent of lung and colon adenocarcinomas due to chronic inflammation (Tabata et al., 2005; Li et al., 2007). We could carefully speculate that HBoV as a single stranded DNA virus, persisting probably in form of cccDNA structures, can act in a similar way or utilizes related mechanisms like HBV. As no further respiratory pathogens were detected in the tonsillar tumors, the likelihood of a causal involvement of HBoV in the development of tonsillar tumors is increased.

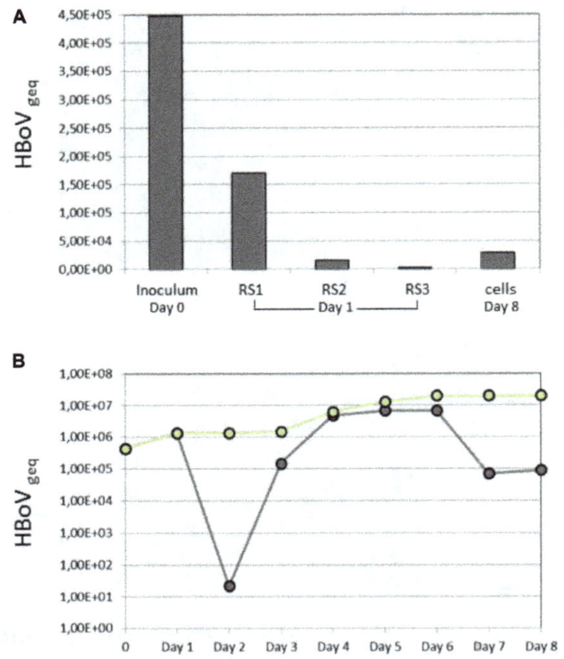

FIGURE 5 | Virus kinetics following infection of keratinocytes with HBoV. The supernatant was harvested from day 1 to day 8 post-infection. **(A)** Shows the amount of HBoV (geq) in the inoculum as well as in the three rinsing steps (RS1-3) at day 1 after infection. Finally, 2.8×10^4 HBoV geq were detected cell-bound at day 8. **(B)** Shows the accumulated viral load (geq) (green) and the daily produced viral load (geq) (gray) in the supernatant, respectively.

It is known that the incidence of human papillomavirus-associated oropharyngeal cancer is increasing especially in developed countries up to 60 to 80% (Kim, 2016; Marur and Forastiere, 2016). This is why we analyzed and compared the presence of HPV in conjunction with HBoV DNA in tonsillar tumor tissue. PCR analyses of our study revealed a coinfection rate of 37.8% in tonsillar carcinomas and our data show that in 60% of these HPV and HBoV positive tumors the viral genomes occur within the same cells. Taking into account that it is not known which infection take place initially, this may mean that synergistic effects arise, which change the mode of cancerogenesis.

Further, we hypothesized that due to the fact that HBoV infections make use and modulate the DNA damage repair systems, HBoV positive tumors could be associated with increased MSI. Thereby, we assumed that especially if the viral DNA would integrate into the host's genome MSI could be more frequently. Our data, in contrast, demonstrate that HBoV-positivity of tonsillar tumors does not go ahead with MSI, thus there appears to be no such interaction.

Regarding the target cells for infection it appears that lymphocytes and fibroblasts do not seem to be permissive for the virus, as we confirmed in triplicate in cultured fibroblasts and lymphocytes. As we could observe virus replication following HBoV infection of cultured keratinocytes in only one patient, this data must be interpreted very carefully due to the insufficient number of experiment repetitions, but they may give a first hint that keratinocytes represent a HBoV permissive cell in the tonsil. The lack of repetitions of the infection was mainly caused by the fact that culturable keratinocytes could only be isolated to a sufficient extent from 2 of 11 tonsils, of which only cells from one patient were permissive for the virus.

The observation that HBoV can persist in infected tonsil squamous cell carcinomas and chronic infected tonsils, similar to other oncogenic viruses, has to be discussed from different perspectives. One could indeed speculate that HBoV is only a harmless bystander, which just benefits of accelerated cell proliferation. The hypothesis that HBoV solely uses the cancer cells as their place of replication is supported by previous observations made with other parvoviruses. The majority of known parvoviruses is dependent on the cell cycle and are capable of replicating, probably exclusively, in actively replicating cells (in S phase). For this reason, they thrive in cancerous cells, often giving the false impression of being oncogenic (Canuti et al., 2014). In addition, there is indeed a well-established relationship between cancer and parvoviruses but this is most likely the result of viral replication reactivation in the replicating cancer calls, causing an increased viral load and therefore a higher prevalence in cancer patients, compared to healthy subjects (Cotmore et al., 2014; Kishore and Kishor, 2014; Phan et al., 2016; Qiu et al., 2017). In addition, some parvoviruses are known to be oncolytic, a fact that strongly argues against our hypothesis that HBoV is involved in tumorigenesis (Marchini et al., 2015). In contrast, as an argument for our hypothesis, it has to noted that the group of Jianming Qiu from Kansas has shown that HBoV appears to be the first known autonomous parvovirus whose replication appears to be independent of the cell cycle, which is different from the parvoviruses mentioned above (Deng et al., 2016, 2017).

However, we could not detect HBoV in breast, cervical or renal tumors (Schildgen et al., 2013), although virus spreading in many cases occurs via viremia. Due to this fact the previous assumption becomes more unlikely. On the other hand it is also possible that HBoV could have an active or passive role in development of these tumors due to chronic inflammation, but because of lacking antibodies up to now it is not known which kind of viral proteins in the respective tumors are expressed and how they interact with cellular proteins. For this reason this hypothesis remains a matter of speculation but is supported by the increased prevalence of HBoV detection in higher tumor stages, the profibrotic and pro-cancerogenic cytokine patterns of HBoV infected in CuFi-8 air-liquid interphase cell cultures, HBoV positive BALs (Khalfaoui et al., 2016), and the recent results of a whole transcriptome sequencing approach of HBoV-infected HAE-cultures, which revealed beside others evidence for bocaviral involvement in tumorigenesis of head-and-neck cancers (Schildgen et al., submitted).

CONCLUSION

With the restriction that a single study can only contribute to isolated aspects of carcinogenesis without providing the necessary comprehensive view, these observations lead to the conclusion that human bocavirus appears to be a factor with an unknown role in tonsil squamous cell cancer development. Although it remains to be investigated which cell type within the tonsil acts as a target of HBoV and its replication, it seems possible that the keratinocytes are able to propagate HBoV1. Independently, it turned out that HBoV and HPV occur in the same cells and their possible synergistic interaction with other environmental or inherited factors that eventually lead to malignant progression, will make it difficult if not impossible to classify solely a single agent as the causative factor (zur Hausen and de Villiers, 2014). Therefore, the present study is a good indicator for the direction of further studies, highly desirable to elucidate the role of HBoV in pathogenesis of oropharyngeal cancer. Finally, the fact that no increased MSI is observed in tonsillar tumors makes it unlikely that the virus interacts directly with the host genome but more likely persists in episomal form.

AUTHOR CONTRIBUTIONS

MH and VS performed culturing and infection experiments. MH and OS performed and analyzed FISH experiments. MH and SM were responsible for all clinical procedures. MB was responsible for all pathology-related diagnostics including tumor staging. OS and VS have planned the study. MH, OS, and VS wrote the manuscript. VS supervised the study. IF performed MSI testing and analyses.

ACKNOWLEDGMENTS

The authors are grateful to the volunteer patients who agreed to the usage of resected tonsils for scientific purposes.

REFERENCES

Addie, D. D., McDonald, M., Audhuy, S., Burr, P., Hollins, J., Kovacic, R., et al. (2012). Quarantine protects Falkland Islands (Malvinas) cats from feline coronavirus infection. *J. Feline Med. Surg.* 14, 171–176. doi: 10.1177/1098612X11429644

Allander, T., Tammi, M. T., Eriksson, M., Bjerkner, A., Tiveljung-Lindell, A., and Andersson, B. (2005). Cloning of a human parvovirus by molecular screening of respiratory tract samples. *Proc. Natl. Acad. Sci. U.S.A.* 102, 12891–12896. doi: 10.1073/pnas.0504666102

Canuti, M., Williams, C. V., Gadi, S. R., Jebbink, M. F., Oude Munnink, B. B., Jazaeri Farsani, S. M., et al. (2014). Persistent viremia by a novel parvovirus in a slow loris (*Nycticebus coucang*) with diffuse histiocytic sarcoma. *Front. Microbiol.* 5:655. doi: 10.3389/fmicb.2014.00655

Clement, N., Battaglioli, G., Jensen, R. L., Schnepp, B. C., Johnson, P. R., St George, K., et al. (2009). Prevalence of human bocavirus in human tonsils and adenoids. *Emerg. Infect. Dis.* 15, 1149–1150. doi: 10.3201/eid1507.090102

Cotmore, S. F., Agbandje-McKenna, M., Chiorini, J. A., Mukha, D. V., Pintel, D. J., Qiu, J., et al. (2014). The family parvoviridae. *Arch. Virol.* 159, 1239–1247. doi: 10.1007/s00705-013-1914-1

de Villiers, E. M. (2014). Cancer "causation" by infections–individual contributions and synergistic networks. *Semin. Oncol.* 41, 860–875. doi: 10.1053/j.seminoncol.2014.10.003

Deng, X., Xu, P., Zou, W., Shen, W., Peng, J., Liu, K., et al. (2017). DNA damage signaling is required for replication of human bocavirus 1 DNA in dividing HEK293 cells. *J. Virol.* 91:e01831-16.

Deng, X., Yan, Z., Cheng, F., Engelhardt, J. F., and Qiu, J. (2016). Replication of an autonomous human parvovirus in non-dividing human airway epithelium is facilitated through the DNA damage and repair pathways. *PLoS Pathog.* 12:e1005399. doi: 10.1371/journal.ppat.1005399

Forster, I., Brockmann, M., Schildgen, O., and Schildgen, V. (2018). Microsatellite instability testing in colorectal cancer using the QiaXcel advanced platform. *BMC Cancer* 18:484. doi: 10.1186/s12885-018-4400-z

Huang, Q., Deng, X., Yan, Z., Cheng, F., Luo, Y., Shen, W., et al. (2012). Establishment of a reverse genetics system for studying human bocavirus in human airway epithelia. *PLoS Pathog.* 8:e1002899. doi: 10.1371/journal.ppat.1002899

Kapoor, A., Hornig, M., Asokan, A., Williams, B., Henriquez, J. A., and Lipkin, W. I. (2011). Bocavirus episome in infected human tissue contains non-identical termini. *PLoS One* 6:e21362. doi: 10.1371/journal.pone.0021362

Khalfaoui, S., Eichhorn, V., Karagiannidis, C., Bayh, I., Brockmann, M., Pieper, M., et al. (2016). Lung infection by human bocavirus induces the release of profibrotic mediator cytokines In Vivo and In Vitro. *PLoS One* 11:e0147010. doi: 10.1371/journal.pone.0147010

Kim, S. M. (2016). Human papilloma virus in oral cancer. *J. Korean Assoc. Oral Maxillofac. Surg.* 42, 327–336. doi: 10.5125/jkaoms.2016.42.6.327

Kishore, J., and Kishor, D. (2014). Can Parvovirus B19 infection be naturally oncolytic: clinical findings raise such a possibility in leukaemic children. *Indian J. Med. Res.* 139, 952–953.

Li, Y., Wang, J., Zhu, G., Zhang, X., Zhai, H., Zhang, W., et al. (2007). Detection of parvovirus B19 nucleic acids and expression of viral VP1/VP2 antigen in human colon carcinoma. *Am. J. Gastroenterol.* 102, 1489–1498. doi: 10.1111/j.1572-0241.2007.01240.x

Lusebrink, J., Schildgen, V., Tillmann, R. L., Wittleben, F., Bohmer, A., Muller, A., et al. (2011). Detection of head-to-tail DNA sequences of human bocavirus in clinical samples. *PLoS One* 6:e19457. doi: 10.1371/journal.pone.0019457

Marchini, A., Bonifati, S., Scott, E. M., Angelova, A. L., and Rommelaere, J. (2015). Oncolytic parvoviruses: from basic virology to clinical applications. *Virol. J.* 12:6. doi: 10.1186/s12985-014-0223-y

Marur, S., and Forastiere, A. A. (2008). Head and neck cancer: changing epidemiology, diagnosis, and treatment. *Mayo Clin. Proc.* 83, 489–501. doi: 10.4065/83.4.489

Marur, S., and Forastiere, A. A. (2016). Head and neck squamous cell carcinoma: update on epidemiology. Diagnosis, and treatment. *Mayo Clin. Proc.* 91, 386–396. doi: 10.1016/j.mayocp.2015.12.017

Phan, T. G., Dreno, B., da Costa, A. C., Li, L., Orlandi, P., Deng, X., et al. (2016). A new protoparvovirus in human fecal samples and cutaneous T cell lymphomas (mycosis fungoides). *Virology* 496, 299–305. doi: 10.1016/j.virol.2016.06.013

Proenca-Modena, J. L., Paula, F. E., Buzatto, G. P., Carenzi, L. R., Saturno, T. H., Prates, M. C., et al. (2014). Hypertrophic adenoid is a major infection site of human bocavirus 1. *J. Clin. Microbiol.* 52, 3030–3037. doi: 10.1128/JCM.00870-14

Qiu, J., Soderlund-Venermo, M., and Young, N. S. (2017). Human Parvoviruses. *Clin. Microbiol. Rev.* 30, 43–113. doi: 10.1128/CMR.00040-16

Schildgen, V., Khalfaoui, S., and Schildgen, O. (2014). Human Bocavirus: from common cold to cancer? Speculations on the importance of an episomal genomic form of human bocavirus. *Rev. Med. Microbiol.* 25, 113–118.

Schildgen, V., Malecki, M., Tillmann, R. L., Brockmann, M., and Schildgen, O. (2013). The human Bocavirus is associated with some lung and colorectal cancers and persists in solid tumors. *PLoS One* 8:e68020. doi: 10.1371/journal.pone.0068020

Szalmas, A., Papp, Z., Csomor, P., Konya, J., Sziklai, I., Szekanecz, Z., et al. (2013). Microbiological profile of adenoid hypertrophy correlates to clinical diagnosis in children. *Biomed. Res. Int.* 2013:629607. doi: 10.1155/2013/629607

Tabata, T., Okada, Y., and Kondo, T. (2005). [Lung cancer with polyarthropathy due to Parvovirus B19: report of a case]. *Kyobu geka Jpn. J. Thorac. Surg.* 58, 1181–1183.

Wang, J. H., Zhang, W. P., Liu, H. X., Wang, D., Li, Y. F., Wang, W. Q., et al. (2008). Detection of human parvovirus B19 in papillary thyroid carcinoma. *Br. J. Cancer* 98, 611–618. doi: 10.1038/sj.bjc.6604196

Zeisel, M. B., Lucifora, J., Mason, W. S., Sureau, C., Beck, J., Levrero, M., et al. (2015). Towards an HBV cure: state-of-the-art and unresolved questions–report of the ANRS workshop on HBV cure. *Gut* 64, 1314–1326. doi: 10.1136/gutjnl-2014-308943

zur Hausen, H. (1999). Immortalization of human cells and their malignant conversion by high risk human papillomavirus genotypes. *Semin. Cancer Biol.* 9, 405–411. doi: 10.1006/scbi.1999.0144

3

Morbidity and Mortality Associated with Respiratory Virus Infections in Allogeneic Hematopoietic Cell Transplant: Too Little Defense or Harmful Immunity?

Anne Birgitta Versluys [1]* *and Jaap Jan Boelens* [2]

[1] *Blood and Marrow Transplantation Program, Princess Maxima Center for Pediatric Oncology, Utrecht, Netherlands,* [2] *Stem Cell Transplant and Cellular Therapies Program, Pediatrics, Memorial Sloan Kettering Cancer Center, New York, NY, United States*

Correspondence:
Anne Birgitta Versluys
a.b.versluijs@prinsesmaximacentrum.nl

The impact on morbidity and mortality of Community Acquired Respiratory Virus (CARV) infections in patients undergoing Allogeneic Hematopoietic Cell Transplant (HCT) is widely studied. Here we give an overview of the current literature on the incidence and chance of progression to severe disease in this highly immune compromised population. We discuss the issue whether it is predominantly direct viral damage that causes clinical deterioration, or that it is in fact the allogeneic immuneresponse to the virus that is most important. This is an important question as it will guide therapeutic decision making. It asks for further collaborative studies focusing on sensitive surveillance with PCR techniques and relating clinical data with parameters of immune reconstitution.

Keywords: respiratory virus infection, allogeneic transplant of hematopoietic stem cells, alloimmunity and transplantation, lung disease, outcome

INTRODUCTION

Community acquired respiratory virus infections (CARV) include a variety of viruses such as rhinovirus, coronavirus, respiratory syncytial virus (RSV), influenza virus, Para influenza virus, and metapneumo virus. CARV infections range from asymptomatic carriership to significant respiratory disease. Prevalence of CARV largely depends on season, detection mode, age of patient and immune status (Shah et al., 2012; Hirsch et al., 2013; Green, 2017). Influenza and RSV have significant seasonal variation, whereas Para influenza or rhinovirus cause disease year round (Green, 2017). Highly sensitive diagnostic techniques like polymerase chain reaction (PCR) for the detection of viral DNA and RNA reveal a high prevalence of CARV in the normal population. In healthy children attending day care prevalence is as high as 40% (Moe et al., 2016). In children admitted to hospital for respiratory disease 43–75% are tested PCR positive, almost twice as high as in adults admitted to hospital for respiratory disease (Ching et al., 2018). In the immune compromised pediatric population the prevalence of CARV is around 50–80% (Fazekas et al., 2012) with mostly mild symptoms at time of detection.

There are many reports on CARV prior to, or early after, Hematopoietic Cell Transplantation (HCT). Recently a large multicenter retrospective analysis in 1,560 pediatric HCT recipients showed an incidence of 16.6% symptomatic CARV infections within 1 year after transplant (Fisher et al., 2017). Surveillance studies in the same population on Nasopharyngeal Aspirates (NPA) routinely performed prior to transplant showed an incidence of 50% (Versluys et al., 2010).

Most studies discuss the risk of progression to viral pneumonia, for various types of CARV. Only few groups looked at long term outcome. Results are conflicting, reported risk of progression is 5–75% (Bredius et al., 2004; Hirsch et al., 2013; Chemaly et al., 2014b; Fisher et al., 2017; Green, 2017). HCT is a curative treatment for several malignant and non-malignant childhood diseases. Its success is limited by infections, allo-immunity and toxic events. Respiratory viruses contribute to post-transplantation morbidity and mortality in different ways.

Here we provide an overview of recent literature on CARV in the HCT setting, focusing on the risk of progressive viral lung disease, the role of viruses in the lung microbiome and the potential viral trigger for allo-immunity after HCT.

COMMUNITY ACQUIRED RESPIRATORY VIRUSES AND HCT

Reported incidence of **RSV** in HCT-recipients varies between 1 and 17% (Shah et al., 2012; Robinson et al., 2015; Fisher et al., 2017), depending largely on season, patients' age and detection methods. Progression to LRTI occurs in 18–55% (Shah et al., 2012; Kim et al., 2014; Fisher et al., 2017), with risk factors for progression related to age, donor source, use of steroids, immune status, and concomitant infections (Renaud et al., 2013; Chemaly et al., 2014b; Kim et al., 2014; Shah et al., 2014). Mortality rates are around 10% (Chemaly et al., 2014a; Robinson et al., 2015; Fisher et al., 2017) It is important to notice the in most pediatric studies, RSV-positive patients were treated with the antiviral drug ribavirin (Molinos-Quintana et al., 2013), with anti-RSV monoclonal antibodies (palivizumab) or with non-specific intravenous immunoglobulins (IVIG) (El-Bietar et al., 2016), or with a combination (Chávez-Bueno et al., 2007). Aerosolized ribavirin and IVIG is recommended for adult HCT recipients with RSV LRTI (Dignan et al., 2016; Waghmare et al., 2016).

Para influenza virus (PIV) in HCT recipients is systematically reviewed by Shah et al. (2016a). The incidence of PIV in HCT recipients is 5% (range 0.2–19%), 36% progressing to LRTI. Significant predictors of LRTI progression were infection within 100 days after HCT, lymphocytopenia/neutropenia at the onset of infection, use of corticosteroids, younger age, and respiratory co-infections. Reported overall mortality is 10% (0–37%), in PIV-LRTI 27%. There is currently no licensed therapy for PIV pneumonia.

Influenza is diagnosed in approximately 1–5% of HCT recipients, and in up to 33% of patients with respiratory symptoms in the flu-season. Progression to viral pneumonia occurs in 14–30% of patients, and is associated with mortality in 10–28% (Fisher et al., 2017; Green, 2017). These numbers are strongly influenced by seasonal outbreaks and the subtype of the influenza virus. Risk factors for progressive influenza disease are lymphocytpenia/neutropenia and steroid use (Kmeid et al., 2016). In contrast to many other respiratory viruses, influenza can be treated with neuraminidase inhibitors (Waghmare et al., 2016; Green, 2017).

Human rhino virus (hRV)is the most common cause of respiratory virus infections in both immunocompetent and immunocompromised individuals. Reported incidence in HCT recipients is 8–36% (Versluys et al., 2010; Shah et al., 2012; Campbell et al., 2015; Fisher et al., 2017). For a long time there was uncertainty about the ability of hRV to cause lower respiratory tract disease. Recent studies however, suggest that hRV may be a clinically significant pathogen with the potential to cause serious pulmonary disease in HCT recipients (Campbell et al., 2015; Seo et al., 2015, 2017; Versluys et al., 2017) with risk of progression to LRTI of 9–24% (Shah et al., 2012; Campbell et al., 2015; Fisher et al., 2017) and hRV related mortality of 4–33% (Shah et al., 2012; Campbell et al., 2015; Fisher et al., 2017).

There is increasing interest in the pathogenecity of **human metapneumo virus (hMPV)**. In a systematic review (Shah et al., 2016b) Shah et al. summarized all published data on hMPV in patients with hematologic malignancies or undergoing HCT. About one third of described cases were children. They report an overall incidence of 5% (range 0–40%), with a risk for progression to LRTI of 34% (range 0–100%) and a mortality rate of 6% (0–17%) in the total hMPV positive group, and 27% in the hMPV-LRTI group.

Other respiratory viruses like **bocavirus (BoV)** and **coronavirus (CoV)** in HCT setting, are scarcely studied. Prevalence of either BoV or CoV is 26% in the adult HCT population with respiratory symptoms. A significant proportion of the CoV infected patients required hospitalization, and some progressed to LRTI. In contrast, BoV detection was rare and almost always related to co-pathogens (Pinana et al., 2018). A surveillance study on BoV in children found 10% of children with RTI to be PCR positive, as well as 17% of the healthy controls; thus showing a high prevalence of the virus without necessarily causing disease. Progression to lower infection however was associated with higher BoV load and viremia, suggesting a pathogenic role in a subgroup of patients (Christensen et al., 2010).

Figure 1 shows the incidence of CARV in mainly adult HCT population, and the impact of CARV on LRTI and mortality. Profound immunosuppression in patients undergoing HCT obviously leads to a greater risk of infection, with prolonged shedding of the virus, a higher chance of transmission of disease and a greater risk of progression to severe lower respiratory tract disease. As antiviral therapy is only effective in the minority of the respiratory viruses, and vaccines are not widely available, prevention is very important.

The working group of the fourth European conference on infections in leukemia (ECIL-4) reviewed the literature on CARV in leukemic patients and patients after HCT (Hirsch et al., 2013). For prevention they recommend infection control measures like good personal hygiene, avoiding contact with individuals with a respiratory tract infection and restricting young children from visiting patients. Administration if IVIG preparations in patients with hypogammaglobulinemia (IgG < 4 g/l), and the use of intravenous monoclonal antibody specific for the RSF-F protein (palivizumab) during RSV outbreaks may be considered. They do not advocate routine screening for CARV. Deferral of chemotherapy or conditioning should be considered,

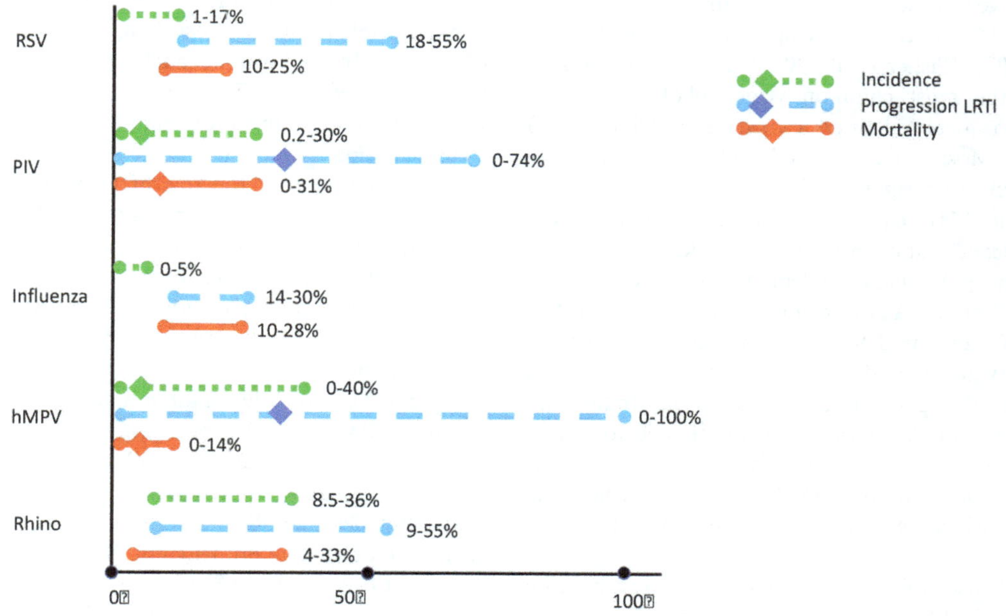

FIGURE 1 | Incidence of common respiratory viral infections (CRV) and associated progression to Lower Respiratory Tract Infections (LRTI) and mortality in HCT recipients. Updated from Shah et al. (2012), based on (Versluys et al., 2010; Shah et al., 2012; Chemaly et al., 2014b; Campbell et al., 2015; Robinson et al., 2015; Fisher et al., 2017; Green, 2017).

as well as treatment for RSV and HPIV only in the HCT setting.

In 2016 a joint working group in the UK (Dignan et al., 2016) has reviewed the available literature and made recommendations for the diagnosis and management of respiratory viral infections in patients with hematological malignancies or those undergoing hematopoietic stem cell transplantation. As far as prevention is concerned they come to the same conclusions as ECIL-4, and add the recommendation for influenza vaccinations in household contacts and medical staff, and post-exposure prophylaxis with oseltamivir in HCT patients who have been in contact with influenza.

RESPIRATORY VIRUSES AFTER HCT AND CLINICAL OUTCOME

In a recent large prospective study, including 458 adults and children undergoing allogeneic HCT, clinical outcomes associated with respiratory viruses (RV) detected prior to HCT were analyzed (Campbell et al., 2015). Multiplex PCR testing for RV was done on nasal washes or nasopharyngeal swabs. In 25% of patients a RV was detected, 22% of them being asymptomatic. In the pediatric subgroup, defined as aged < 18 years, the prevalence of RV was higher (46%), with a larger proportion being without symptoms (37%). The RV positive patients were significantly younger and had higher risk underlying disease with lower lymphocyte count. Overall mortality at day 100 was significantly higher in RV-patients than in non-RV patients (15.5 vs. 7.9%; HR 2.4; 95% CI 1.3–4.5; $p = 0.07$). In 27% of the deceased patients the cause of death was thought to be directly related to the pre-HCT RV, no data are given about the cause of death in the other patients. Patients with Rhinovirus performed worse compared to the other RV. This may be partly explained by the fact that most patients with RSV or influenza where treated with antiviral therapy or had their transplant delayed. Data on longer follow up are lacking (Campbell et al., 2015).

Hutspardol et al. retrospectively studied treatment related mortality (TRM) and long-term pulmonary complications in 32 children who had respiratory symptoms and a RV detected within 100 days after allogeneic HCT. The overall frequency of documented RV infections was 6.5%, half of the patients presented with signs of a LRTI and mortality rate at day 100 was 13%. Cause of death was pneumonitis/ARDS in all, with symptoms occurring on day 11–98 after HCT. During follow up (4.3 years, range 1.4–11.8) no chronic pulmonary complications nor allo-immune lung syndrome was observed (Hutspardol et al., 2015).

With regard to long term pulmonary function Chien et al. studied 1,130 adult HCT recipients by performing routine pulmonary function tests years after HCT. Airflow obstruction, defined as an annualized decline in FEV1 of more than 5%, occurred in 26% of patients and had impact on overall mortality. Higher age at transplant, GVHD category, pulmonary function pre-transplant and the occurrence of a respiratory virus infection within the first 100 days after HCT were significant risk factors for airflow obstruction (Chien et al., 2003). Erard et al. further studied the association of RV and airflow decline, and found that this was particularly true in patients after LRTI caused by parainfluenza virus or respiratory syncytial virus (Erard et al., 2006).

In a retrospective study among 1,560 pediatric HCT recipients in 9 US centers 16.6% acquired symptomatic RV within the first year after HCT (Fisher et al., 2017). In line with others, rhinovirus was the most common virus, followed by RSV and PIV. RV was detected after a median of 56 (11–151) days after HCT. Most children had URTI only, in patients with hMPV there was significantly more LRTI. During 3 months follow up 15% required mechanical ventilation and 14% had significant pulmonary sequelae like bronchiolitis obliterans, subacute pulmonary problems and other not specified pulmonary complications. All cause mortality among RV positive patients was 11%, compared to 5% in the non-CARV group. Recent steroid exposure and RV detection within 60 days after HCT were poor prognostic factors for morbidity and death. At least 50% of death were not attributable to CARV infection. The timing of the events is also remarkable, as 61% of deaths occurred more than 30 days after diagnosing CARV infection, which is at least 3 months after HCT for most.

The widespread use of PCR diagnostics has led to an increase in the detection of CARV in patients undergoing HCT. Many of these patients become symptomatic and a significant proportion develops LRTI. There is a clear increased risk for mortality in CARV positive patients. Hence, prevention and development of anti-viral drugs are of great importance.

However, one could debate about the reason for severe morbidity and mortality in CARV positive patients. How do you diagnose progressive viral infection? The CARV will not be cleared for months because of the immunocompromised state of the host after HCT, so finding positive PCRs is not convincing enough. Timing of (progression of) symptoms in relation to immune reconstitution might be helpful in answering the question if it is progression of viral damage or if the donor derived immunity actually is targeting the lung.

RESPIRATORY VIRUSES (RV) AND ALLOIMMUNITY

In last decade more and more evidence has emerged that "triggered" alloreactivity may play a crucial role in toxicity and mortality. This holds true for HCT, but is also recognized in solid organ transplantation. In the context of lung transplantation several studies have examined the role of RV in the development of chronic lung allograft dysfunction (CLAD), a form of chronic rejection of the lung (Kumar et al., 2005, 2010; Fisher et al., 2016). Many, but not all, reported an association between RV and CLAD. Pooled analyses of studies on RV and CLAD (Vu et al., 2011) did not confirm the association, mainly due to the heterogeneity of studies and limitations in design, diagnostic techniques and definitions. Fisher et al. tried to overcome these limitations by studying a more homogenous cohort of lung transplant recipients, using modern molecular assays to detect RV and applying consensus definitions of CLAD (Fisher et al., 2016). In 250 patients, 50 (20%) developed CLAD at a median of 95 weeks (interquartile range (IQR): 53–157 weeks). In 79 patients (31.6%) a respiratory viral episode was seen, after a median of 19 weeks post lung transplantation (IQR: 9–63 weeks). In multivariate analysis RV was associated with CLAD (HR1.9, 95% CI 1.1–3.5; $p = 0.03$). This association was stronger the more proximate the RV occurred after lung transplantation.

Our group studied the role of respiratory viruses (RV) in immune mediated lung disease after HCT, analogous to this phenomenon as described after lung transplantation (Versluys et al., 2010, 2017). The host-vs.- graft chronic allograft rejection in lung transplantation is in many ways comparable to the graft-vs.- host inflammation in hematopoietic cell transplantation.

In a cohort of 179 children undergoing allogeneic HCT routine NPA and BAL sampling for the presence of RV was done prior to transplant. RV was found in 61% (41% in BAL/NPA, 20% in NPA-only). Rhinovirus was the most frequently detected RV (42%). Allo-immune lung syndrome (Allo-LS), defined as Bronchiolitis Obliterans Syndrome (BOS) or Idiopathic Pneumonia Syndrome (IPS), occurred in 13%, after a median of 8.5 weeks (1–28 weeks). RV-positivity in BAL was a predictor for Allo-LS (HR 3.8, 95% CI 1.4–10.7; $p = 0.01$). No other predictors were found. The hypothesis is that RV causes epithelial damage and triggers an allogeneic immune response leading to severe lung disease. So the lung disease does not occur primarily from progressive viral infection during the period of low immunity, but from allo-immune mediated damage weeks after HCT.

This inflammatory aspect of disease might explain the reported benefit of steroid use on the risk of mechanical ventilation among HCT recipients with influenza (Choi et al., 2011), and the controversy on risks of steroid use in case of CARV after HCT (Waghmare et al., 2016).

VIRUSES AND THE RESPIRATORY MICROBIOME

More and more is known about the role of microbiota in human health. So far research has largely focused on the gut microbiome, also in the context of GvHD. But the microbial ecosystem at other body sites, including the respiratory tract is attracting growing attention. Host and environmental factors influencing the respiratory microbiota include genetics, microbial exposure (birth mode, feeding type, day care), vaccination, infections and antibiotics (Man et al., 2017). Viral infection interacts with the microbiome by disrupting the airway epithelial barrier facilitating bacterial adhesion, liberating host derived nutrients and decreasing muco-ciliary clearance. In addition respiratory viruses can modulate innate and adaptive immune responses promoting bacterial colonization (Man et al., 2017). Moreover, it is becoming clear that the virome should be seen as a part of the microbiome, that affects the function of the host immune system (Cadwell, 2015). The role of a disturbed respiratory microbiome/virome in lung disease is postulated for asthma and chronic obstructive pulmonary disease (COPD) (Zou et al., 2016).

DISCUSSION

Impact of CARV on outcomes after HCT is an intriguing topic where pathogenesis is not completely understood. Is the poor immune system associated with progressive infection? Does allo-immunity play a crucial role in lung toxicity?

Most studies describe data on symptomatic patients where CARV is detected at time of symptoms. Only few studies report on pre-HCT sampling, although we know a large proportion of our patients is CARV positive with only mild symptoms. Time of (worsening) of symptoms, warranting viral diagnostics and thus detecting the CARV, is often weeks after HCT. Are these nosocomial acquired viruses, or were these virus already present and giving symptoms after a certain period of time? Are the viruses acquired after discharge? But then immunity is usually restored to a certain degree.

From various infectious diseases, like RSV bronchiolitis (Fonseca et al., 2018), immune reconstitution inflammatory syndrome (IRIS) in HIV patients (with cryptococcal meningitis, CMV retinitis or BCG-itis) (Walker et al., 2015) or IRIS in non-HIV immunesuppressed patients with immune recovery (followed by worsening of treated tuberculosis, idiopatic pneumonia or hepatitis) (Sueki et al., 2018), we know the harmful effect of immune response on the patient. The debate about inappropriate immune response on infectious triggers is especially intriguing in the allogeneic setting.

The definition criteria for alloimmune mediated lung syndromes (Panoskaltsis-Mortari et al., 2011; Jagasia et al., 2015) describe the clinical, radiologic and functional aspects of lung pathology, with exclusion of other evident causes of this phenotype, like heart failure and infection, including respiratory virus infection. One can argue if this holds true for respiratory viruses detected by PCR. The detection modes have become much more sensitive over time, so the impact of positive findings on the disease criteria should be reevaluated. In the HCT population with its high prevalence of RV, these viruses will have a long persistence making them detectable for weeks after initial infection, with uncertain meaning for their role in pathology.

An interesting paper in this matter was recently published by Seo et al. (2015). In 69 patients with IPS, they went back to BAL samples at time of diagnosis, and applied more sensitive diagnostics for microbial pathogens. In 56% of patients an occult pathogen was found, 36% being a respiratory virus. All patients were treated with steroids because of IPS. Overall mortality was higher in the group of patients with an occult pathogen, than in the group without. The authors conclude that these patients had had to be excluded as IPS patients, that they had infectious pneumonia and that steroid treatment had adversely influenced their outcome.

However, as we are not informed about RV status pre-HCT, this could also be persisting RV after HCT, triggering immune-mediated lung disease (IPS). In that situation steroids are beneficial in the treatment at the moment of clinical deterioration.

In conclusion, despite the growing awareness of CARV infections in HCT patients, well-designed studies are lacking that systematically evaluate diagnostic and therapeutic strategies of CARV. Only then we will be able to better understand the direct viral impact and the indirect alloimmune pathology, both largely influencing clinical outcome of patients.

Detailed longitudinal studies, combining data from microbioma/virioma surveillance with data on immunerecovery after HCT and clinical outcome are needed to better understand pathogeneic mechanisms involved in lung disease and CARV after HCT. This insight should largely influence the therapeutic decision of delaying transplant, treating RV and most important increasing or decreasing immune suppression after transplant.

AUTHOR CONTRIBUTIONS

All authors listed have made a substantial, direct and intellectual contribution to the work, and approved it for publication.

REFERENCES

Bredius, R. G., Templeton, K. E., Scheltinga, S. A., Claas, E. C., Kroes, A. C., and Vossen, J. M. (2004). Prospective study of respiratory viral infections in pediatric hemopoietic stem cell transplantation patients. *Pediatr. Infect. Dis. J.* 23, 518–522. doi: 10.1097/01.inf.0000125161.33843.bb

Cadwell, K. (2015). The virome in host health and disease. *Immunity* 42, 805–813. doi: 10.1016/j.immuni.2015.05.003

Campbell, A. P., Guthrie, K. A., Englund, J. A., Farney, R. M., Minerich, E. L., Kuypers, J., et al. (2015). Clinical outcomes associated with respiratory virus detection before allogeneic hematopoietic stem cell transplant. *Clin. Infect. Dis.* 61, 192–202. doi: 10.1093/cid/civ272

Chávez-Bueno, S., Mejías, A., Merryman, R. A., Ahmad, N., Jafri, H. S., and Ramilo, O. (2007). Intravenous palivizumab and ribavirin combination for respiratory syncytial virus disease in high-risk pediatric patients. *Pediatr. Infect. Dis. J.* 26, 1089–1093. doi: 10.1097/INF.0b013e3181343b7e

Chemaly, R. F., Ghantoji, S. S., Shah, D. P., Shah, J. N., El Taoum, K. K., Champlin, R. E., et al. (2014a). Respiratory syncytial virus infections in children with cancer. *J. Pediatr. Hematol. Oncol.* 36, e376–e381. doi: 10.1097/MPH.0000000000000086

Chemaly, R. F., Shah, D. P., and Boeckh, M. J. (2014b). Management of respiratory viral infections in hematopoietic cell transplant recipients and patients with hematologic malignancies. *Clin. Infect. Dis.* 59(Suppl. 5), S344–S351. doi: 10.1093/cid/ciu623

Chien, J. W., Martin, P. J., Gooley, T. A., Flowers, M. E., Heckbert, S. R., Nichols, W. G., et al. (2003). Airflow obstruction after myeloablative allogeneic hematopoietic stem cell transplantation. *Am. J. Respir. Crit. Care Med.* 168, 208–214. doi: 10.1164/rccm.200212-1468OC

Ching, N. S., Kotsanas, D., Easton, M. L., Francis, M. J., Korman, T. M., and Buttery, J. P. (2018). Respiratory virus detection and co-infection in children and adults in a large Australian hospital in 2009-2015. *J. Paediatr. Child Health.* doi: 10.1111/jpc.14076. [Epub ahead of print].

Choi, S. M., Boudreault, A. A., Xie, H., Englund, J. A., Corey, L., and Boeckh, M. (2011). Differences in clinical outcomes after 2009 influenza A/H1N1 and seasonal influenza among hematopoietic cell transplant recipients. *Blood* 117, 5050–5056. doi: 10.1182/blood-2010-11-319186

Christensen, A., Nordbo, S. A., Krokstad, S., Rognlien, A. G., and Dollner, H. (2010). Human bocavirus in children: mono-detection, high viral load and viraemia are associated with respiratory tract infection. *J. Clin. Virol.* 49, 158–162. doi: 10.1016/j.jcv.2010.07.016

Dignan, F. L., Clark, A., Aitken, C., Gilleece, M., Jayakar, V., Krishnamurthy, P., et al. (2016). H. Haemato-oncology Task Force of the British Committee for Standards in, B. British Society for, T. Marrow, and U.K.C.V.N. the, BCSH/BSBMT/UK clinical virology network guideline: diagnosis and management of common respiratory viral infections in patients undergoing treatment for haematological malignancies or stem cell transplantation. *Br. J. Haematol.* 173, 380–393. doi: 10.1111/bjh.14027

El-Bietar, J., Nelson, A., Wallace, G., Dandoy, C., Jodele, S., Myers, K. C., et al. (2016). RSV infection without ribavirin treatment in pediatric hematopoietic stem cell transplantation. *Bone Marrow Transplant.* 51, 1382–1384. doi: 10.1038/bmt.2016.124

Erard, V., Chien, J. W., Kim, H. W., Nichols, W. G., Flowers, M. E., Martin, P. J., et al. (2006). Airflow decline after myeloablative allogeneic hematopoietic cell transplantation: the role of community respiratory viruses. *J. Infect. Dis.* 193, 1619–1625. doi: 10.1086/504268

Fazekas, T., Eickhoff, P., Rauch, M., Verdianz, M., Attarbaschi, A., Dworzak, M., et al. (2012). Prevalence and clinical course of viral upper respiratory tract infections in immunocompromised pediatric patients with malignancies or after hematopoietic stem cell transplantation. *J. Pediatr. Hematol. Oncol.* 34, 442–449. doi: 10.1097/MPH.0b013e3182580bc8

Fisher, B. T., Danziger-Isakov, L., Sweet, L. R., Munoz, F. M., Maron, G., Tuomanen, E., et al. (2017). A multicenter consortium to define the epidemiology and outcomes of inpatient respiratory viral infections in pediatric hematopoietic stem cell transplant recipients. *J. Pediatric Infect. Dis. Soc.* doi: 10.1093/jpids/pix051. [Epub ahead of print].

Fisher, C. E., Preiksaitis, C. M., Lease, E. D., Edelman, J., Kirby, K. A., Leisenring, W. M., et al. (2016). Symptomatic respiratory virus infection and chronic lung allograft dysfunction. *Clin. Infect. Dis.* 62, 313–319. doi: 10.1093/cid/civ871

Fonseca, W., Lukacs, N. W., and Ptaschinski, C. (2018). Factors affecting the immunity to respiratory syncytial virus: from epigenetics to microbiome. *Front. Immunol.* 9:226. doi: 10.3389/fimmu.2018.00226

Green, M. L. (2017). Viral pneumonia in patients with hematopoietic cell transplantation and hematologic malignancies. *Clin. Chest Med.* 38, 295–305. doi: 10.1016/j.ccm.2016.12.009

Hirsch, H. H., Martino, R., Ward, K. N., Boeckh, M., Einsele, H., and Ljungman, P. (2013). Fourth European Conference on Infections in Leukaemia (ECIL-4): guidelines for diagnosis and treatment of human respiratory syncytial virus, parainfluenza virus, metapneumovirus, rhinovirus, and coronavirus. *Clin. Infect. Dis.* 56, 258–266. doi: 10.1093/cid/cis844

Hutspardol, S., Essa, M., Richardson, S., Schechter, T., Ali, M., Krueger, J., et al. (2015). Significant transplantation-related mortality from respiratory virus infections within the first one hundred days in children after hematopoietic stem cell transplantation. *Biol. Blood Marrow Transplant.* 21, 1802–1807. doi: 10.1016/j.bbmt.2015.06.015

Jagasia, M. H., Greinix, H. T., Arora, M., Williams, K. M., Wolff, D., Cowen, E. W., et al. (2015). National Institutes of Health Consensus Development Project on criteria for clinical trials in chronic graft-versus-host disease: I. The 2014 diagnosis and staging working group report. *Biol. Blood Marrow Transplant.* 21, 389e1–401e1. doi: 10.1016/j.bbmt.2014.12.001

Kim, Y. J., Guthrie, K. A., Waghmare, A., Walsh, E. E., Falsey, A. R., Kuypers, J., et al. (2014). Respiratory syncytial virus in hematopoietic cell transplant recipients: factors determining progression to lower respiratory tract disease. *J. Infect. Dis.* 209, 1195–1204. doi: 10.1093/infdis/jit832

Kmeid, J., Vanichanan, J., Shah, D. P., El Chaer, F., Azzi, J., Ariza-Heredia, E. J., et al. (2016). Outcomes of influenza infections in hematopoietic cell transplant recipients: application of an immunodeficiency scoring index. *Biol. Blood Marrow Transplant.* 22, 542–548. doi: 10.1016/j.bbmt.2015.11.015

Kumar, D., Erdman, D., Keshavjee, S., Peret, T., Tellier, R., Hadjiliadis, D., et al. (2005). Clinical impact of community-acquired respiratory viruses on bronchiolitis obliterans after lung transplant. *Am. J. Transplant.* 5, 2031–2036. doi: 10.1111/j.1600-6143.2005.00971.x

Kumar, D., Husain, S., Chen, M. H., Moussa, G., Himsworth, D., Manuel, O., et al. (2010). A prospective molecular surveillance study evaluating the clinical impact of community-acquired respiratory viruses in lung transplant recipients. *Transplantation* 89, 1028–1033. doi: 10.1097/TP.0b013e3181d05a71

Man, W. H., de Steenhuijsen Piters, W. A., and Bogaert, D. (2017). The microbiota of the respiratory tract: gatekeeper to respiratory health. *Nat. Rev. Microbiol.* 15, 259–270. doi: 10.1038/nrmicro.2017.14

Moe, N., Pedersen, B., Nordbo, S. A., Skanke, L. H., Krokstad, S., Smyrnaios, A., et al. (2016). Respiratory virus detection and clinical diagnosis in children attending day care. *PLoS ONE* 11:e0159196. doi: 10.1371/journal.pone.0159196

Molinos-Quintana, A., Pérez-de Soto C., Gómez-Rosa, M., Pérez-Simón, J. A., and Pérez-Hurtado, J. M. (2013). Intravenous ribavirin for respiratory syncytial viral infections in pediatric hematopoietic SCT recipients. *Bone Marrow Transplant.* 48, 265–268. doi: 10.1038/bmt.2012.134

Panoskaltsis-Mortari, A., Griese, M., Madtes, D. K., Belperio, J. A., Haddad, I. Y., Folz, R. J., et al. (2011). An official American Thoracic Society research statement: noninfectious lung injury after hematopoietic stem cell transplantation: idiopathic pneumonia syndrome. *Am. J. Respir. Crit. Care Med.* 183, 1262–1279. doi: 10.1164/rccm.2007-413ST

Pinana, J. L., Madrid, S., Perez, A., Hernandez-Boluda, J. C., Gimenez, E., Terol, M. J., et al. (2018). Epidemiologic and clinical characteristics of coronavirus and bocavirus respiratory infections after allogeneic stem cell transplantation: a prospective single-center study. *Biol. Blood Marrow Transplant.* 24, 563–570. doi: 10.1016/j.bbmt.2017.11.001

Renaud, C., Xie, H., Seo, S., Kuypers, J., Cent, A., Corey, L., et al. (2013). Mortality rates of human metapneumovirus and respiratory syncytial virus lower respiratory tract infections in hematopoietic cell transplantation recipients. *Biol. Blood Marrow Transplant.* 19, 1220–1226. doi: 10.1016/j.bbmt.2013.05.005

Robinson, J. L., Grenier, D., MacLusky, I., and Allen, U. D. (2015). Respiratory syncytial virus infections in pediatric transplant recipients: A Canadian paediatric surveillance program study. *Pediatr. Transplant.* 19, 659–662. doi: 10.1111/petr.12553

Seo, S., Renaud, C., Kuypers, J. M., Chiu, C. Y., Huang, M. L., Samayoa, E., et al. (2015). Idiopathic pneumonia syndrome after hematopoietic cell transplantation: evidence of occult infectious etiologies. *Blood* 125, 3789–3797. doi: 10.1182/blood-2014-12-617035

Seo, S., Waghmare, A., Scott, E. M., Xie, H., Kuypers, J. M., Hackman, R. C., et al. (2017). Human rhinovirus detection in the lower respiratory tract of hematopoietic cell transplant recipients: association with mortality. *Haematologica* 102, 1120–1130. doi: 10.3324/haematol.2016.153767

Shah, D. P., Ghantoji, S. S., Ariza-Heredia, E. J., Shah, J. N., El Taoum, K. K., Shah, P. K., et al. (2014). Immunodeficiency scoring index to predict poor outcomes in hematopoietic cell transplant recipients with RSV infections. *Blood* 123, 3263–3268. doi: 10.1182/blood-2013-12-541359

Shah, D. P., Ghantoji, S. S., Mulanovich, V. E., Ariza-Heredia, E. J., and Chemaly, R. F. (2012). Management of respiratory viral infections in hematopoietic cell transplant recipients. *Am. J. Blood Res.* 2, 203–218.

Shah, D. P., Shah, P. K., Azzi, J. M., and Chemaly, R. F. (2016a). Parainfluenza virus infections in hematopoietic cell transplant recipients and hematologic malignancy patients: a systematic review. *Cancer Lett.* 370, 358–364. doi: 10.1016/j.canlet.2015.11.014

Shah, D. P., Shah, P. K., Azzi, J. M., El Chaer, F., and Chemaly, R. F. (2016b). Human metapneumovirus infections in hematopoietic cell transplant recipients and hematologic malignancy patients: a systematic review. *Cancer Lett.* 379, 100–106. doi: 10.1016/j.canlet.2016.05.035

Sueki, H., Mizukawa, Y., and Aoyama, Y. (2018). Immune reconstitution inflammatory syndrome in non-HIV immunosuppressed patients. *J. Dermatol.* 45, 3–9. doi: 10.1111/1346-8138.14074

Versluys, A. B., Rossen, J. W., van Ewijk, B., Schuurman, R., Bierings, M. B., and Boelens, J. J. (2010). Strong association between respiratory viral infection early after hematopoietic stem cell transplantation and the development of life-threatening acute and chronic alloimmune lung syndromes. *Biol. Blood Marrow Transplant.* 16, 782–791. doi: 10.1016/j.bbmt.2009.12.534

Versluys, B., Bierings, M., Murk, J. L., Wolfs, T., Lindemans, C., Vd Ent, K., et al. (2017). Infection with a respiratory virus before hematopoietic cell transplantation is associated with alloimmune-mediated lung syndromes. *J. Allergy Clin. Immunol.* 141, 697–703.e8. doi: 10.1016/j.jaci.2017.03.055

Vu, D. L., Bridevaux, P. O., Aubert, J. D., Soccal, P. M., and Kaiser, L. (2011). Respiratory viruses in lung transplant recipients: a critical review and pooled analysis of clinical studies. *Am. J. Transplant.* 11, 1071–1078. doi: 10.1111/j.1600-6143.2011.03490.x

Waghmare, A., Englund, J. A., and Boeckh, M. (2016). How I treat respiratory viral infections in the setting of intensive chemotherapy or hematopoietic cell transplantation. *Blood* 127, 2682–2692. doi: 10.1182/blood-2016-01-634873

Walker, N. F., Scriven, J., Meintjes, G., and Wilkinson, R. J. (2015). Immune reconstitution inflammatory syndrome in HIV-infected patients. *HIV AIDS* 7, 49–64. doi: 10.2147/HIV.S42328

Zou, S., Caler, L., Colombini-Hatch, S., Glynn, S., and Srinivas, P. (2016). Research on the human virome: where are we and what is next. *Microbiome* 4:32. doi: 10.1186/s40168-016-0177-y

4

Comparative Genomic Analysis of Re-emergent Human Adenovirus Type 55 Pathogens Associated with Adult Severe Community-Acquired Pneumonia Reveals Conserved Genomes and Capsid Proteins

Zetao Cheng[1†], Yuqian Yan[1†], Shuping Jing[1], Wen-Gang Li[2], Wei-Wei Chen[2], Jing Zhang[1], Min Li[1], Shan Zhao[1], Na Cao[1], Junxian Ou[1], Suhui Zhao[1], Xianbo Wu[1], Bin Cao[3*] and Qiwei Zhang[1,4*]*

[1] Guangzhou Key Laboratory of Drug Research for Emerging Virus Prevention and Treatment, Guangdong Provincial Key Laboratory of Tropical Disease Research, School of Public Health, Southern Medical University, Guangzhou, China, [2] Treatment and Research Center for Infectious Diseases, 302 Military Hospital of China, Beijing, China, [3] Department of Pulmonary and Critical Care Medicine, China-Japan Friendship Hospital, Beijing, China, [4] Dermatology Hospital, Southern Medical University, Guangzhou, China

***Correspondence:**
Xianbo Wu
xianbowu@qq.com
Bin Cao
caobin_ben@vip.163.com
Qiwei Zhang
zhang.qiwei@yahoo.com

† These authors have contributed equally to this work.

Human adenovirus type 55 (HAdV-B55) is a recently identified acute respiratory disease (ARD) pathogen in HAdV species B with a recombinant genome between renal HAdV-B11 and respiratory HAdV-B14. Since HAdV-B55 first appeared in China school in 2006, no more ARD cases associated with it had been reported until 2011, when there was an outbreak of adult severe community-acquired pneumonia (CAP) in Beijing, China. Reported here is the bioinformatics analysis of the re-emergent HAdV-B55 responsible for this outbreak. Recombination and protein sequence analysis re-confirmed that this isolate (BJ01) was a recombinant virus with the capsid hexon gene from HAdV-B11. The selection pressures for the three capsid proteins, *i.e.,* hexon, penton base, and fiber genes, were all negative, along with very low non-synonymous (dN) and synonymous (dS) substitutions/site (<0.0007). Phylogenetic analyses of the whole genome and the three major capsid genes of HAdV-B55 revealed the close phylogenetic relationship among all HAdV-B55 strains. Comparative genomic analysis of this re-emergent HAdV-B55 strain (BJ01; 2011) with the first HAdV-B55 strain (QS-DLL; 2006) showed the high genome identity (99.87%), including 10 single-nucleotide non-synonymous substitutions, 11 synonymous substitutions, 3 insertions, and one deletion in non-coding regions. The major non-synonymous substitutions (6 of 10) occurred in the protein pVI in its L3 region, which protein has different functions at various stages of an adenovirus infection, and may be associated with the population distribution of HAdV-B55 infection. No non-synonymous substitutions were found in the three major capsid proteins, which proteins are responsible for type-specific neutralizing antibodies. Comparative genomic analysis of the re-emergent HAdV-B55 strains associated with adult severe CAP revealed conserved genome and capsid proteins, providing the foundation for the development of effective vaccines against this pathogen. This study also facilitates the further investigation of HAdV-B55 epidemiology, molecular evolution, patterns of pathogen emergence and re-emergence, and the predication of genome recombination between adenoviruses.

Keywords: human adenovirus type 55, recombination, comparative genomics, severe community-acquired pneumonia, China

INTRODUCTION

Human adenoviruses (HAdV) are associated in humans with a broad spectrum of clinical diseases, such as acute respiratory disease (ARD), community-acquired pneumonia (CAP), as well as conjunctivitis, gastrointestinal, opportunistic infections in immune-deficient individuals, and possibly, obesity (Dingle and Langmuir, 1968; Chu and Pavan-Langston, 1979; Wood, 1988; Dhurandhar et al., 1992; Kojaoghlanian et al., 2003; Hakim and Tleyjeh, 2008). Since the first HAdV isolate was found in 1953 (Hilleman et al., 1953; Rowe et al., 1953), more than 80 HAdV genotypes have been identified and classified into seven species (A to G) using the whole-genome sequence as the typing standard[1] (Jones et al., 2007; Ishiko et al., 2008; Walsh et al., 2009, 2010, 2011; Liu et al., 2011, 2012; Matsushima et al., 2011, 2012, 2013; Robinson et al., 2011, 2013b; Seto et al., 2011; Dehghan et al., 2012; Singh et al., 2012, 2013; Zhou et al., 2012; Alissa Alkhalaf et al., 2014; Hage et al., 2015; Hashimoto et al., 2018). HAdV species B are further divided into subspecies B1 (HAdV-B3, -B7, -B16, -B21, and -B50) and B2 (HAdV-B11, -B14, -B34, -B35, and -B55) according to their restriction enzyme digestion patterns (Wadell et al., 1980). Subspecies B1 cause respiratory disease except for HAdV-B50. The members in subspecies B2 cause renal or urinary tract disease, except for HAdV-B14 and -B55, which are associated with ARD (Echavarria, 2008).

Human adenoviruses are usually typed according to serum neutralization and hemagglutination-inhibition tests, both of which are associated with the three major capsid proteins, *i.e.*, hexon, fiber, and penton base. Based on partial characterization of its hexon and fiber epitopes, as well as the restriction enzyme patterns (Zhang Q. et al., 2016), HAdV-B55 was first identified as HAdV-B11a (Hierholzer et al., 1974). This virus may have occurred earlier from an ARD outbreak in a military training base (Spain, 1969), and subsequently re-emerged in several outbreaks of ARD in Turkey (2004), Singapore (2005) discontinuously (Hierholzer et al., 1974; Chmielewicz et al., 2005; Zhu et al., 2009; Kajon et al., 2010; Li et al., 2014; Lu et al., 2014). Complete genome analysis suggested that this new type, HAdV-B55, is a Trojan horse, which contains a recombinant genome from both a renal pathogen, HAdV-B11, which provides the antigenic epitope, and a respiratory pathogen, HAdV-B14, which confers the cell tropism, biological and pathogenicity properties (Walsh et al., 2010). The strain QS-DLL is the first completely characterized HAdV-B55 based on the whole genomic analysis (Walsh et al., 2010). It caused an ARD outbreak in China, from March to April 2006, with 254 patients affected, of which 247 were students in a senior high school and one died during this outbreak (Zhu et al., 2009).

Since this first isolate QS-DLL of HAdV-B55 was identified in 2006 (Yang et al., 2009; Walsh et al., 2010), no more ARD cases associated with this virus had been reported in China until 2011, when 16 HAdV-B55-like strains were identified based on partial gene sequencing in a CAP outbreak in Beijing, China in February and March (Cao et al., 2014). Of these, strain BJ01 was isolated from a throat swab of a 29-year-old adult who presented with severe CAP (Gu et al., 2012). The whole genome (34,773 bp) of strain BJ01 (Human adenovirus B human/CHN/BJ01/2011/55[P14H11F14]) was sequenced using the Sanger method, following PCR amplification of targeted overlapping regions. (GenBank accession number JX491639). (Zhang et al., 2012a). In this study, comparative genomic analysis of this re-emergent HAdV-B55 strain (BJ01) with the first HAdV-B55 strain (QS-DLL), as well as the bioinformatic analysis of HAdV-B55 strains circulating recently were performed. The findings will contribute to the studies of the evolution and epidemiology of HAdV-B55, as well as provide both the foundation for the development of effective vaccines and public health strategies against this pathogen.

MATERIALS AND METHODS

Cells, Virus Stock, and Genomic DNA Extraction

This specimen was originally isolated from a throat swab of an adult diagnosed with severe CAP at Beijing Chao-Yang Hospital of China (March 2011) (Gu et al., 2012; Zhang et al., 2012a). Written informed consent was obtained from the patient. The protocol was approved by the Ethics Committee of Beijing Chao-Yang Hospital, Capital Medical University in accordance with the Declaration of Helsinki. The throat swab was inoculated and cultured in A549 cells (ATCC), and grown in Dulbecco's minimum essential medium supplemented with 100 IU/ml penicillin, 100 μg/ml streptomycin, and 2% (v/v) fetal calf serum, at an atmosphere of 5% (v/v) carbon dioxide. Viral genomic DNA was extracted from infected A549 cells, as described earlier (Le et al., 2001). PCR amplification and molecular typing was performed according to the previous study (Han et al., 2013).

Genome Sequencing and Annotation

The genome of strain BJ01 was sequenced using a Sanger primer-walking method, following PCR amplification of targeted overlapping regions (Zhang et al., 2012a,b). Both 5′- and 3′-ends (including both inverted terminal repeats)

[1] http://hadvwg.gmu.edu

were sequenced directly by 5′ primer Ad14-LTRS1 (5′-ACAGAAGACTTTCACACGGT-3′) and 3′ primer Ad14-LTRS2 (5′-GGTCCCTCTAAATACACATACA-3′), respectively, using extracted genomic DNA as sequencing template. The sequence data provided average three- to fivefold coverage of the genome. Ambiguous sequences and gaps were re-amplified and re-sequenced. All the sequencing ladders were assembled using the SEQMAN (DNAStar; Madison, WI). The genome was further annotated according to the previous report (Walsh et al., 2010).

Genome Recombination Analysis

Genome sequence recombination analysis was done using Simplot 3.5.1[2] , including the options of Simplot and Bootscan analysis (Lole et al., 1999). The software MAFFT was used to align the HAdV-B sequences[3]. The parameters of gap opening penalty (1.53), Offset value (0), and the Scoring matrix for nucleotide sequences (200 PAM/k = 2) were set by default. The LAGAN (Limited Area Global Alignment of Nucleotides) program of mVISTA was used for the pair-wise comparisons of genomes[4] (Brudno et al., 2003).

Phylogenetic Analysis

Phylogenetic analysis was performed by Molecular Evolutionary Genetics Analysis (MEGA) 5.0.5[5] (Tamura et al., 2007). Phylogenetic trees with 1,000 bootstrap replications were constructed using a maximum-composite-likelihood method. All the other parameters were set by default.

Substitution Rate Analysis of HAdV-B55 Hexon, Penton Base, and Fiber Genes

The numbers of non-synonymous (dN) and synonymous (dS) substitutions per site between sequences and dN/dS ratios were calculated. The analysis was performed with MEGA 5.05 (Tamura et al., 2011) using the Nei–Gojobori model (Nei and Gojobori, 1986). The nucleotide sequences from 23 hexon, 43 fiber, and 17 penton base genes available in GenBank were included.

All the genome sequences included for substitution rate analysis were summarized in **Table 1**. For HAdV-B55, additional genome typing details were also presented. The sequences of the hexon, penton base, and fiber genes were either extracted from the genome files or deposited as single gene entries.

Sequences Used in the Study

The HAdV sequences of the hexon, penton base, fiber genes, and the genomes used for phylogenic analyses were retrieved from GenBank and summarized in **Table 1**, with additional sequence origin details if available (strain names, countries, years and GenBank accession numbers). The prototype strains were also used.

[2]https://sray.med.som.jhmi.edu/scroftware/simplot/

[3]http://mafft.cbrc.jp/alignment/server/

[4]http://genome.lbl.gov/vista/lagan/submit.shtml

[5]http://www.megasoftware.net/index.html

RESULTS

Nucleotide Sequence Analysis of HAdV-B55 Strain BJ01

The genome data of strain BJ01 was deposited into GenBank (accession number JX491639), and named formally as "Human adenovirus 55 isolate HAdV-B/CHN/BJ01/2011/55[P14H11F14]", further referred to as "BJ01".

Figure 1 presented the genomic organization and transcription map of strain BJ01. The genome contained four early, two intermediate, and five late transcription units, and 34,773 bp in length, with a base composition of 26.16% A, 25.08% T, 24.38% G, 24.39% C, and a GC content of 48.76%, which was similar with the other members of subspecies B2 (mean of 49%) (Seto et al., 2010a). A total of 39 coding sequences were identified (**Table 2**). The 137-bp ITR of strain BJ01 was identical to that of the first HAdV-B55 strain (QS-DLL; 2006) (Walsh et al., 2010).

Protein Sequence Analysis of HAdV-B55 Strain BJ01

The amino acid sequence percent identities of the proteins of HAdV-B55 strain BJ01 were presented in **Table 3**. Selected proteins of the representative prototypes in each HAdV species, including all species B adenoviruses, were used for comparison. The amino acid sequence analysis revealed that the proteins of strain BJ01 had the highest amino acid percent identities with that of HAdV-B14 (strain de Wit) except for the hexon protein, which is responsible for virus characterization by serum neutralization. The hexon protein of strain BJ01 had the highest amino acid identity with HAdV-B11 (98.4%), rather than HAdV-B14 (92.2%). The amino acid sequence identities indicated that strain BJ01 is a recombinant between HAdV-B14 and HAdV-B11, with the HAdV-B11 hexon gene inserted chimeric into the HAdV-B14 genome backbone (**Table 3**). Interestingly, E3 11.7 kDa protein of HAdV-B55 strain BJ01 had the same amino acid sequence identity with both HAdV-B14 and HAdV-B35, indicating that these three types share the conserved and similar E3 11.7 kDa protein. Among all the proteins analyzed, the highest sequence diversity was found in the fiber gene of all the seven species.

Nucleotide Substitution Rates and Selection Pressures for HAdV-B55 Major Capsid Protein Genes

The synonymous and non-synonymous substitutions as well as the selection pressures for the three major capsid protein genes of HAdV-B55 were examined and compared. All the dN/dS ratios of the three genes were less than 1 (**Table 4**). This is to be expected because the evolution is dominated by negative selection, which removes mutations harmful to fitness (Zhao et al., 2014). Specifically, the hexon gene had least non-synonymous substitutions per site and the lowest ratio of dN/dS (0.06254). The non-synonymous substitutions and dN/dS ratio of the fiber gene was also low. However,

TABLE 1 | The genome, hexon, penton base anc fiber sequences of adenovirus species A-G used in this study.

Type	Strain	Year isolated	Country	Sequence	GenBank accession no.
HAdV-A12	Huie	1954	USA	Genome	AC_000005
HAdV-B3	GB	1953	USA	Genome	AY599834
HAdV-B7	Gomen	1952	USA	Genome	AY594255
HAdV-B11	Slobitski	1956	USA	Genome	NC_011202
HAdV-B11a*	ak37	2001	EGY	Genome	JX423385
	1222	2005	SGN	Genome	FJ597732
	AK36	2005	ARG	Genome	JX423384
HAdV-B14	de Wit	1955	Netherlands	Genome	AY803294
HAdV-B55	BJ01[#]	2011	CHN	Genome	JX491639
	CQ-814	2010	CHN	Genome	JX123027
	BD6728	2013	CHN	Genome	KJ883520
	TJ-2013-90	2013	CHN	Genome	KF908851
	CQ-2903	2012	CHN	Genome	JX123029
	QS-DLL	2006	CHN	Genome	FJ643676
	BD6729	2013	CHN	Genome	KJ883521
	QZ01	2011	CHN	Genome	KJ883522
	CQ-1657	2011	CHN	Genome	JX123028
	XZ2012-492	2012	CHN	Genome	KC857701
	Hebei/BD01	2012	CHN	Genome	KP896478
	Liaoning/LS01	2013	CHN	Genome	KP896483
	Tianjin/TJ01	2013	CHN	Genome	KP896484
	JS201501	2015	CHN	Genome	KX289874
	60-GD-2016	2016	CHN	Genome	KY070248
	AFMC 16-0011	2016	S. Korea	Genome	KX494979
	AH-CHN/CZ-TC8	2012	CHN	Hexon	KC551973
	HAdV11-QS	2010	CHN	Hexon	DQ874353
	SHX-P01	2011	CHN	Hexon	KC999882
	Shanxi-Y16	2011	CHN	Hexon	KF911353
	BJ10	2013	CHN	Hexon	KM458628
	87	2016	CHN	Fiber	KY070249
	60	2016	CHN	Fiber	KY070250
	59	2016	CHN	Fiber	KY070251
	81	2016	CHN	Fiber	KY070252
	111	2016	CHN	Fiber	KY070253
	161	2016	CHN	Fiber	KY070254
	169	2016	CHN	Fiber	KY070255
	73	2016	CHN	Fiber	KY070256
	123	2016	CHN	Fiber	KY070257
	80	2016	CHN	Fiber	KY070258
	BJ10	2013	CHN	Fiber	KP270921
	YT2011_12-44	2011	CHN	Fiber	KC510748
	YT2011_12-115	2011	CHN	Fiber	KC510749
	BJ2011_6-80	2011	CHN	Fiber	KC510750
	YT2011_12-31	2011	CHN	Fiber	KC510751
	BJ2011_10-54	2011	CHN	Fiber	KC510752
	BJ2011_7-35	2011	CHN	Fiber	KC510753
	BJ2011_10-25	2011	CHN	Fiber	KC510754
	BJ2011_1-32	2011	CHN	Fiber	KC510755
	BJ2011_4-28	2011	CHN	Fiber	KC510756
	BJ2011_10-39	2011	CHN	Fiber	KC510757
	BJ2011_1-31	2011	CHN	Fiber	KC510758

(Continued)

TABLE 1 | Continued

Type	Strain	Year isolated	Country	Sequence	GenBank accession no.
	BJ2011_1-29	2011	CHN	Fiber	KC510759
	BJ2011_1-100	2011	CHN	Fiber	KC510760
	BJ2011_1-98	2011	CHN	Fiber	KC510761
	YT2011_12-42	2011	CHN	Fiber	KC510762
HAdV-B16	ch.79	1955	USA	Genome	AY601636
HAdV-B21	AV-1645	1956	Saudi Arabia	Genome	AY601633
SAdV-21	Bertha	1954	USA	Genome	AC_000010
HAdV-B34	Compton	1972	USA	Genome	AY737797
HAdV-B35	Holden	1973	USA	Genome	AY128640
HAdV-B50	Wan	1988	USA	Genome	AY737798
HAdV-B66	87-922	1987	ARG	Genome	JN860676
HAdV-B68	Arg 827/04	2004	ARG	Genome	JN860678
HAdV-C1	Adenoid 71	1953	USA	Genome	AF534906
HAdV-D9	Hicks	1954	USA	Genome	AJ854486
HAdV-E4	RI-67	1952	USA	Genome	AY594253
HAdV-F40	Dugan	1979	Netherlands	Genome	NC_001454
HAdV-G52	T03-2244	2003	USA	Genome	DQ923122

*They are either deposited as single gene entries in GenBank or extracted from the genome files. #The HAdV-B55 genome analyzed in the present study. *They are likely typed as HAdV-B55 according to the genome sequences.*

it was relatively higher than that of the penton base and hexon genes. Overall, the major capsid proteins of HAdV-B55, hexon, penton base, and fiber, are highly conserved when compared with other types, such as HAdV-B7 (Zhao et al., 2014).

Genome Recombination Analysis of HAdV-B55 Strain BJ01

The software mVISTA-LAGAN was used to compare the genome sequence identity between HAdV-B55 strain BJ01, HAdV-B11, and -B14. The visualization alignment showed that HAdV-B55 BJ01 had higher genome sequence identity with HAdV-B14 (98.879%) globally than with HAdV-B11 (97.605%), except for the L3 region (the hexon gene), where strain BJ01 had higher sequence identity with HAdV-B11 than HAdV-B14 (**Figure 2A**). This indicates that HAdV-B55 BJ01 was a recombinant composed of the HAdV-B14 genome backbone and the chimeric HAdV-B11 hexon.

Recombination analysis of both the genome and the hexon gene of HAdV-B55 strain BJ01 along with other HAdV-B viruses were shown in **Figures 2B–D**. Simplot analysis strongly indicates that there was a recombination event between HAdV-B14 and HAdV-B11 (**Figure 2B**). Apparently, except for the hexon region, BJ01 had the highest similarity with HAdV-B14 instead of HAdV-B11 (**Figure 2B**). Bootscan analysis of the genome further confirmed the recombination (**Figure 2C**). The fine-resolution Bootscan analysis of the divergent hexon genes showed that the recombination event was within the hexon gene. Loop 1 (HVR1–6; nt 407 to 1,034) and Loop 2 (HVR7; nt 1,363 to 1,484) were derived from HAdV-B11 (the green regions). The other portions

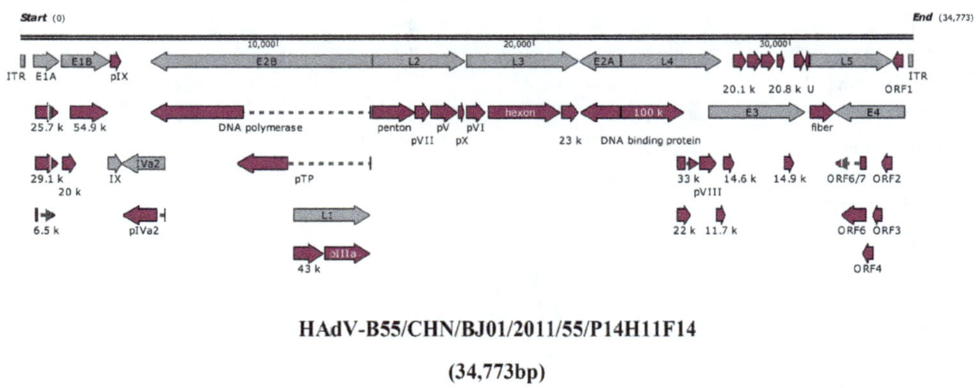

FIGURE 1 | Transcriptional map and genome organization of HAdV-B55 strain BJ01. The genome is indicated by two black horizontal lines marked at 10,000 bp intervals. Early, intermediate, and late transcription units are designated by gray arrows, while the red designates coding regions. Arrows reflect the transcriptional orientation of the coding transcripts.

were derived from HAdV-B14, so was the rest of the genome (**Figure 2D**).

Phylogenetic Analysis of the Whole Genome, the Hexon, Penton Base, and Fiber Genes of the HAdV-B55

The phylogenetic analysis of the whole genomic sequences confirmed that the genomes of HAdV-B members were closely related to each other, forming a clade (**Figure 3A**). HAdV-B55 was closer to HAdV-B14 than HAdV-B11 genome (**Figure 3A**), which was consistent with the global pairwise alignment result in **Figure 2A** and the genome percent identities between the two types (98.879% vs 97.605%). The phylogenetic analysis of the fiber base and penton base genes drew the same conclusion as the whole genomes: they were closer to HAdV-B14 than HAdV-B11 (**Figures 3C,D**). However, the phylogenetic tree of the hexon genes showed a different distribution: HAdV-B55 was closer to HAdV-B11 than HAdV-B14 (**Figure 3B**), which was consistent with the Bootscan analysis in **Figures 2C,D** as well as with the amino acid percent identities of the hexon protein (the highest identity with HAdV-B11: 98.4%) (**Table 3**).

TABLE 2 | The genome sequence annotation of HAdV-B55 strain BJ01.

Region	Product	Location
E1A	29.1 kDa protein	58–1166,1251–1459
E1A	25.7 kDa protein	587–1073,1251–1459
E1A	6.5 kDa protein	587–658,1251–1355
E1B	20 kDa protein	1629–2171
E1B	54.9 kDa protein	1934–3418
pIX	pIX protein	3501–3920
IVa2	IVa2 protein	3989–5322,5601–5613
E2B	DNA polymerase	5092–8664,13645–13653
E2B	pTP	8463–10424,13645–13653
L1	43 kDa protein	10671–11831
L1	pIIIa	11857–13620
L2	penton base protein	13701–15374
L2	protein VII	15379–15957
L2	protein V precursor	16000–17055
L2	protein X	17084–17314
L3	protein VI	17395–18135
L3	hexon protein	18251–21091
L3	23 kDa protein	21131–21760
E2A	DNA binding protein	21838–23394
L4	100 kDa hexon-assembly associated protein	23425–25863
L4	33 kDa protein	25595–25913,26083–26444
L4	22 kDa protein	25595–26170
L4	protein VIII	26494–27177
E3	11.7 kDa protein	27177–27494
E3	14.6 kDa protein	27448–27843
E3	18.4 kDa protein	27828–28328
E3	20.1 kDa protein	28348–28893
E3	20.8 kDa protein	28911–29462
E3	10.1 kDa protein	29506–29781
E3	14.9 kDa protein	29786–30190
E3	15 kDa protein	30183–30590
U	U protein	30614..30778
L5	fiber protein	30793–31770
E4	Orf6/7 protein	31806–32057,32780–32953
E4	Orf6 protein	32054–32953
E4	Orf4 protein	32856–33224
E4	Orf3 protein	33233–33586
E4	Orf2 protein	33583–33972
E4	Orf1 protein	34017–34394

Comparative Genomic Analysis of the First Two HAdV-B55 Strains Emerged in China: QS-DLL and BJ01

Comparative genomics analysis showed that strain BJ01 had a high genome identity with strain QS-DLL (99.87%). However, when compared between the two genomes in high resolution detail, 22 single-nucleotide substitutions, 3 insertions and one deletion were identified between the two genomes. (**Table 5**).

Twenty-one of twenty-two single-nucleotide substitutions were located in coding sequences from eight regions (E1B, E2B, L1, L2, L3, E2A, L4, E3). Ten single-nucleotide substitutions were non-synonymous substitutions, while 11 were synonymous substitutions (**Table 5**). Of the 10 non-synonymous substitutions, six were located in the pVI protein in the L3 region (**Figure 4**), which is one of the four cement proteins of HAdVs (IIIa, VI, VIII, and IX). Three of the six single-nucleotide non-synonymous substitutions (A66G, R68K, and V81F) occurred close to the N-terminal domain of protein VI, of which, two (A66G and R68K) were located within one of the two hexon binding domains. The other four non-synonymous substitutions were located in the 20kDa Protein, 55kDa Protein, Terminal Protein Precursor, and 14.9kDa Protein, respectively (**Table 5**). The 11 synonymous nucleotide substitutions were present in the 20kDa Protein, 55kDa Protein, DNA polymerase, 43kDa Protein, pV, pVI, Hexon, DNA Binding Protein, 100kDa Hexon-assembly Associated Protein, 11.7kDa Protein, and 20.1kDa Protein, respectively (**Table 5**). The capsid protein genes were highly conserved between the two strains isolated 5 years apart. There was only one single-nucleotide mutation (T to C) in the hexon gene, which resulted in a synonymous substitution (L to L). Both the penton base and fiber genes of the two strains were identical with each other.

Compared with the genome of strain QS-DLL, strain BJ01 had nucleotide insertions in three regions (TCCATATCCGTGT, AAAAAA, and A, respectively) and one deletion (AA) within L2 pX poly(A) region. All the insertions and deletions were located in non-coding regions (NCR). The insertions of "TCCATATCCGTGT" were located at the upstream of E1A poly(A) region, whereas the insertions of "AAAAAA" were located within IX poly(A) region, and the insertion of "A" were located within L2 pX poly(A) region (**Table 5**).

DISCUSSION

Human adenoviruses were traditionally classified primarily according to their serological profile and hemagglutination

TABLE 3 | Amino acid percent identities of select HAdV-55 strain BJ01 proteins with representative HAdVs from all species, including all species B adenoviruses.

Protein	E1A	E1B	E2B	L1	L2	L3	E2A	L4	E3	L5	E4
	29.1 kDa	**20 kDa**	**DNA polymerase**	**pIIIa**	**Penton base**	**Hexon**	**DBP**	**pVIII**	**11.7 kDa**	**Fiber**	**ORF6**
HAdV-B35	95.8	98.3	93.2	99.5	98.6	94.4	62.9	99.1	**99.1**	62.1	97.7
HAdV-B34	97.7	99.4	98.7	99.3	95.3	91.3	99.4	99.1	98.1	62.2	97.7
HAdV-B14	**97.7**	**100.0**	**99.7**	**99.8**	**99.5**	92.2	**99.8**	**99.6**	**99.1**	**99.1**	**99.3**
HAdV-B11	96.6	98.3	93.0	99.3	98.4	**98.4**	99.2	99.1	98.1	92.3	98.0
HAdV-B50	79.4	88.9	90.8	91.2	91.8	90.7	83.4	94.7	89.6	61.5	96.0
HAdV-B21	79.4	89.0	90.6	90.3	92.0	92.4	83.4	94.3	89.6	61.5	96.0
HAdV-B16	79.8	88.9	91.0	92.9	85.2	85.3	83.4	94.7	89.6	51.4	89.0
HAdV-B7	79.4	87.8	89.9	92.7	85.3	86.6	82.6	94.3	90.6	91.1	96.7
HAdV-B3	79.0	87.2	89.9	93.0	85.5	86.3	83.8	94.3	89.6	56.7	97.3
SAdV-B21	79.8	87.9	91.5	92.0	91.5	90.5	89.0	95.2	89.6	55.2	84.1
HAdV-B66	79.4	87.8	90.7	92.9	85.5	86.3	82.4	94.7	90.6	56.1	97.0
HAdV-B68	69.5	88.9	90.7	92.9	85.2	85.7	83.2	94.7	89.6	51.4	89.0
HAdV-A12	42.4	42.2	70.2	71.0	72.2	76.8	47.1	77.4	61.0	16.8	49.5
HAdV-C1	36.3	49.2	74.0	74.5	68.4	76.6	55.3	79.7	51.4	17.5	9.3
HAdV-D9	41.6	53.0	74.3	79.0	76.3	81.2	59.8	80.6	65.1	26.3	64.6
HAdV-E4	54.7	60.0	84.7	86.7	82.7	82.3	72.7	89.9	74.5	23.0	70.0
HAdV-F40	38.1	46.1	70.1	70.4	72.5	78.6	45.0	79.0	14.8	20.6	45.3
HAdV-G52	37.7	46.6	72.4	70.5	72.7	78.7	48.5	77.7	57.1	24.6	48.0

The proteins above span the whole genome. The highest values from each selected protein are in bold.

TABLE 4 | Nucleotide substitution rate and selection pressures for the HAdV-55 major capsid protein genes.

Gene	Length(bp)	No. of sequences	Mean Non-synonymous Substations/site	Mean Synonymous Substitutions/site	dN/dS
Hexon	2839	23	0.00004	0.00064	0.06254
Penton base	1674	17	0.00048	0.00059	0.81874
Fiber	978	43	0.00037	0.00039	0.96781

The mean numbers of non-synonymous (dN) and synonymous(dS) substitutions per site from between sequences were noted and dN/dS were calculated. This selection pressure analysis was conducted using the maximum-composite-likelihood model, and included nucleotide sequences from 23 hexon, 43 fiber, and 17 penton base genes of HAdV-55 available from GenBank. All positions containing gaps were eliminated automatically. Evolutionary analyses were performed with MEGA 5.05 version.

properties (Hierholzer et al., 1991), and these methods are mainly based on the interaction between antibodies and the major capsid proteins. Presently, 51 HAdV serotypes have been recognized. However, serological methods seem not appropriate to characterize adenoviruses just by the epitopes. As an example, HAdV-D15, HAdV-D29, and HAdV-D56 were found to share the same virus neutralization (VN) epitopes (Stevens et al., 1967; Wigand, 1987; Robinson et al., 2011, 2013a), but all three viruses contain divergent genomes and biological properties (Robinson et al., 2011, 2013a). Currently, more and more traditional techniques have been replaced by genomic criteria. The genome data were proposed to be used to type HAdVs (Seto et al., 2011), *i.e.*, HAdVs should be identified, typed, and characterized based on the complete genome sequences instead of serological methods (Zhang et al., 2006, 2012a; Robinson et al., 2009; Walsh et al., 2010; Zhou et al., 2012; Zhang Q. et al., 2016).

HAdV-B55 was first isolated from an ARD outbreak in a military training base in 1969, then it was named HAdV-B11a by partial characterization of its hexon and fiber genes (Hierholzer et al., 1974), as well as restriction enzyme patterns (Zhang Q. et al., 2016). Until 2006, along with several HAdV-B55-associated ARD outbreaks (Hierholzer et al., 1974; Chmielewicz et al., 2005; Yang et al., 2009; Kajon et al., 2010), it was ultimately revised as HAdV-B55 by Walsh et al. (2010) after bioinformatic analysis of the complete genome of strain QS-DLL. In 2011, 5 years after the emergence of the first HAdV-B55 strain QS-DLL in China (Walsh et al., 2010), HAdV-B55 re-emerged and caused a CAP outbreak in China (Gu et al., 2012; Zhang et al., 2012a; Cao et al., 2014). Since then, there have been more than 10 HAdV-B55-associated ARD outbreaks in China, for example, in Shanxi province, Chongqing, Beijing, Jiangsu province, Hebei province, Jinan, Tianjin, and Guangdong province (Yang et al., 2009; Walsh et al., 2010; Zhang et al., 2012a; Li et al., 2014; Chen et al., 2016; Gao et al., 2016; Tan et al., 2016; Yi et al., 2017), with severe and fatal cases (Zhu et al., 2009; Cao et al., 2014; Tan et al., 2016; Zhang S.Y. et al., 2016). Similar ARD outbreaks were also reported in other countries (Geng et al., 2013; Lafolie et al., 2016; Salama et al., 2016; Park et al., 2017).

Here presented is the detailed comparative genomic analysis of the re-emergent HAdV-B55 strain BJ01 with the first isolate QS-DLL. The genomic nucleotide identity between the two strains was 99.87%, along with 26 mutations, including 11 synonymous and 10 non-synonymous substitutions, 3 insertions, one deletion and one G to A mutation in L2 NCR (**Table 5**).

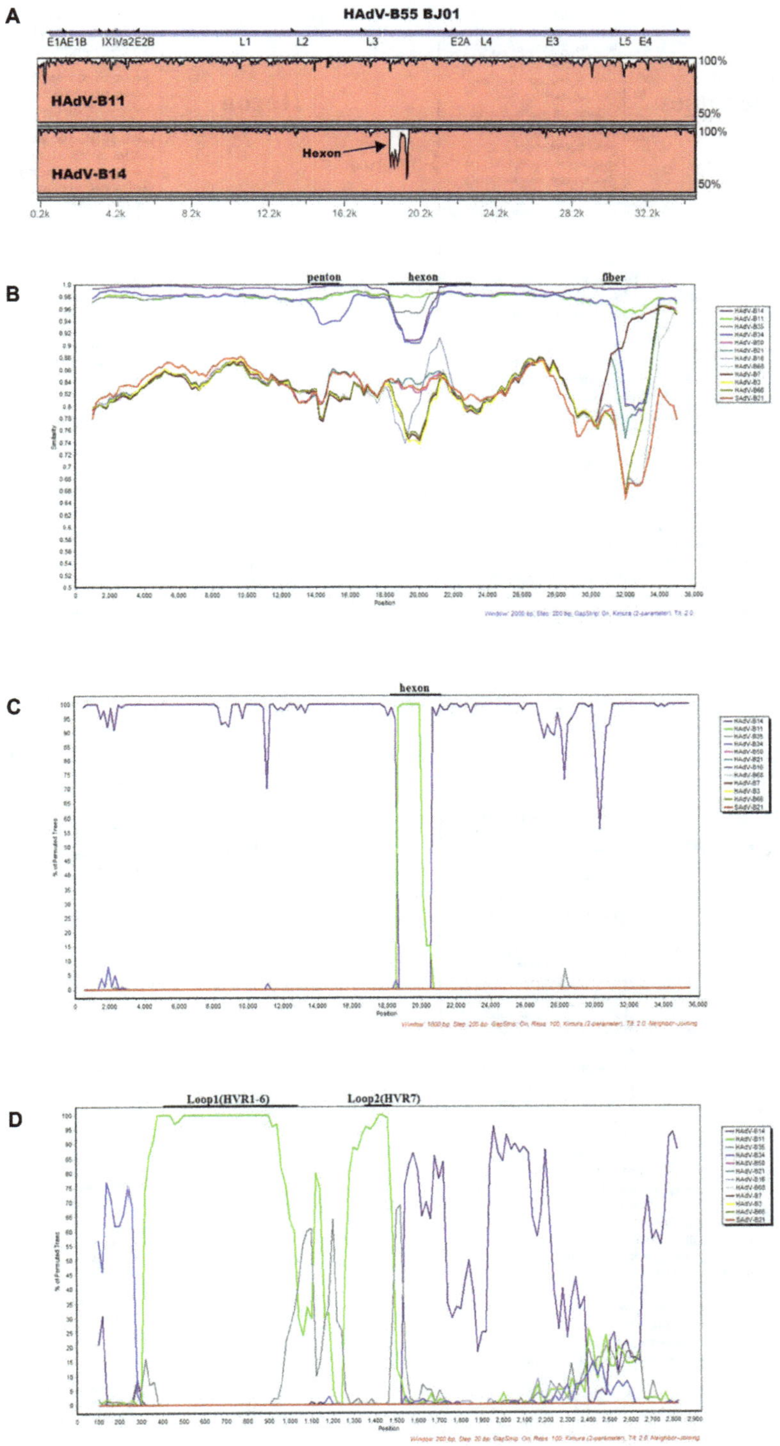

FIGURE 2 | Genome and recombination analysis of HAdV-B55 Strain BJ01. **(A)** Global pairwise alignment of HAdV-B55 (BJ01) with HAdV-B11 and HAdV-B14 using mVISTA LAGAN. Transcription units are shown above the graph by black arrows relative to their position and orientation in the HAdV genome. The y-axis represents the sequence similarity and the genome positions are indicated on the x-axis. **(B)** Simplot and **(C)** Bootscan analysis of the complete genomes of strain BJ01 compared to other species B adenoviruses. **(D)** Bootscan analysis of the hexon genes compared with other HAdV-B types. Parameters are as follows: 100 repetitions; Kimura distance model; neighbor-joining tree model; **(B)** 2,000-bp window, 200-bp step; **(C)** 1,000-bp window, 200-bp step; **(D)** 200-bp window, 20-bp step. Genome nucleotide positions are noted along the x-axis, and the sequence similarities are indicated along the y-axis. The landmarks above each graph demonstrate the approximate positions of the major capsid protein genes. **(B)/(C)/(D)**: Main genomes used were marked in the graph. Colors: violet, HAdV-B14; bright green, HAdV-B11; dark gray, HAdV-B35; blue, HAdV-B34; pink, HAdV-B50; blue green, HAdV-B21; gray-violet, HAdV-B16; light gray, HAdV-B68; dull-red, HAdV-B7; yellow, HAdV-B3, brown, HAdV-B66; bright red, SAdV-B21.

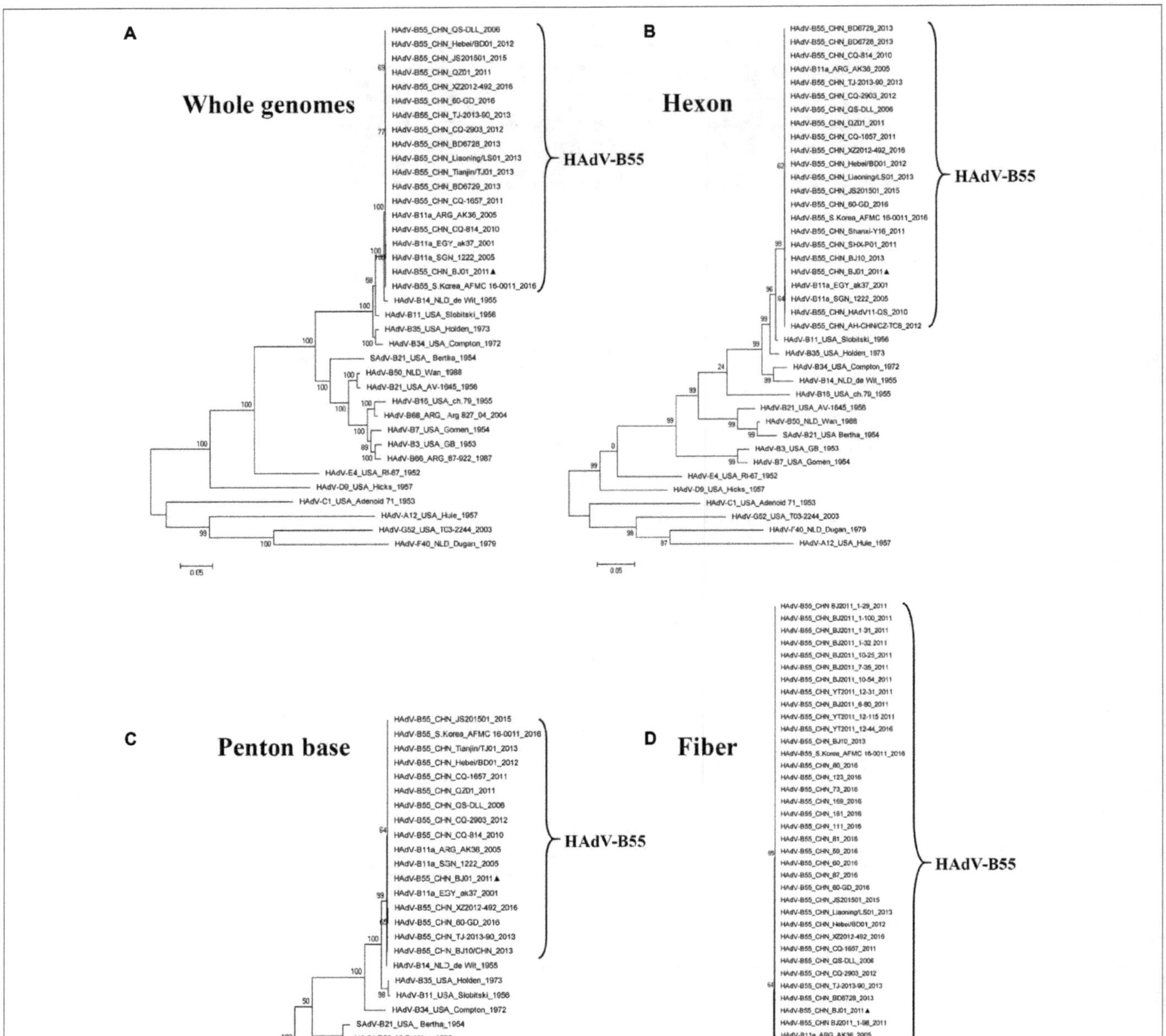

FIGURE 3 | Phylogenetic analysis of HAdV-B55 strain BJ01. The HAdV nucleotide sequences of the whole genome **(A)**, hexon **(B)**, penton base **(C)**, and fiber **(D)** genes, were analyzed for their phylogenetic relationships. For reference, taxon names include the corresponding GenBank accession number, country of isolation, strain name, year of isolation, and genome type. Bootstrapped, maximum likelihood trees with 1,000 replicates were constructed using the MEGA 5.05 software (see Footnote 5). and by applying default parameters, with a maximum-composite-likelihood method. Bootstrap numbers shown at the nodes indicate the percentages of 1,000 replications producing the clade. The scale bar indicates units of nucleotide substitutions per site. The sequences used for phylogenic analyses are retrieved from GenBank and summarized in **Table 1**. Sequences from strain BJ01 are noted for reference (▲).

Compared with other HAdV types, such as HAdV-B3, -C5, -B7, -B14, -D36, of which the genomes are usually conserved and stable (Mahadevan et al., 2010; Seto et al., 2010b; Nam et al., 2014; Alkhalaf et al., 2015; Yu et al., 2016; Zhang et al., 2017), HAdV-B55 showed similarly conserved genomes when looking at the two strains isolated five years apart (2006 vs 2011). However, the major population distribution of HAdV-B55 associated disease has been changed from juveniles to adults, whereas the disease severity remains similar. The major gene mutations between the two isolates are located in the L3 pVI protein, one of the structural proteins of HAdVs, in which six single-nucleotide non-synonymous substitutions and one synonymous substitution were identified (**Figure 4**). pVI and its processed form protein VI are special proteins because they have different functions at various stages of HAdV infections. For example, during adenoviral infection, protein VI aids the virion particle to escape from the endosome by inducing a pH-independent disruption of the membrane (Wiethoff et al., 2005). The N-terminal domain in pVI with predicted amphipathic α-helical structure is required for membrane

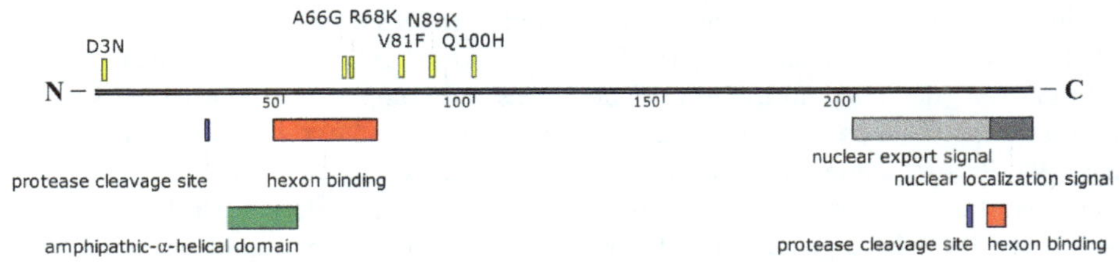

FIGURE 4 | Schematic representation of HAdV-B55 protein VI. The amino acid mutations between HAdV-B55 strains BJ01 and QS-DLL are indicated in yellow. Sites for cleavage by the protease, nuclear export signal, and nuclear localization signal are also indicated in different colors. The hexon binding domains are located between amino acid residues 48 to 74 and 235 to 239. A predicted amphipathic-α-helical domain is also shown. The location of these domains was estimated from the previous report by Wiethoff et al. (2005).

TABLE 5 | Comparative genomics analysis of twc HAdV-B55 strains: QS-DLL and BJ01.

Region	Product	Position	Mutation in DNA	Substitution in protein	
				Non-synonymous	Synonymous
E1A	NCR	1463	▼TCCATATCCGTGT	–	–
E1B	20kDa	1721	A→T	I→L	–
		1885	T→C	–	A→A
	55kDa	2170	T→C	S→P	–
		2823	A→G	–	K→K
IX	NCR	3910	▼AAAAAA	–	–
E2B	DNA polymerase	8352	A→G	–	I→I
	pTP	10309	G→A	P→S	–
L1	43kDa	11293	G→A	–	A→A
L2	pV	16892	C→T	–	R→R
	NCR	17310-17311	▲AA	–	–
	NCR	17328	▼A	–	–
	NCR	17374	G→A	–	–
L3	pVI	17383	G→A	*D→N*	–
		17573	CG	*A→G*	–
		17579	GA	*R→K*	–
		17598	GA	–	Q→Q
		17617	GT	*V→F*	–
		17643	TG	*N→K*	–
		17676	GC	*Q→H*	–
	Hexon	19861	T→C	–	L→L
E2A	DNA Binding Protein	22846	A→C	–	L→L
L4	Hexon-assembly Associated Protein	25509	A→G	–	L→L
E3	11.7kDa	27198	T→C	–	H→H
	20.1kDa	28827	G→A	–	K→K
	14.9kDa	30017	G→T	A→S	–

Nucleic acid and amino acid sequence changes are noted, along with their genome locations and coding consequences. The reference genome is HAdV-B55 strain QS-DLL. NCR, non-coding region; ▼, insertion; ▲, deletion; –, no change or not applicable. The major non-synonymous substitutions in pVI are italicized.

lytic activity (Wiethoff et al., 2005). Additionally, it binds the hexon protein and facilitate nuclear import of hexon (Matthews and Russell, 1995). Two regions, between amino acid residues 48–74 and 233–239 of pVI, were required for the interaction with the hexon protein, where two non-synonymous substitutions were identified (**Figure 4**). Whether the non-synonymous substitutions in pVI can speed up the adenoviral maturation and further change the population distribution of HAdV-B55 infection remains unknown. Further wet-bench confirmation is necessary.

Phylogenetic analysis of genome sequences, as well as individual genes, showed a subclade composed of HAdV-B55 isolates (BJ01 included) with high bootstrap values (**Figures 3A–D**). HAdV-B55 was closely related to HAdV-B11 (Slobitski) and HAdV-B14 (de Wit), forming a clade (**Figures 3A–D**), which was consistent with the global pairwise alignment data (**Figure 2A**). Recombination analysis further revealed the mechanism that the two loops of the HAdV-B11 hexon were embedded in the whole genome of HAdV-B14 (**Figures 2B–D**), giving evidence that the hexon gene, particularly hypervariable regions, acts as an important hotspot for genome recombination. Although the penton base and shaft/knob boundary of the fiber gene were also known to be two recombination sites (Robinson et al., 2009; Liu et al., 2011), no recombination in these regions was identified in HAdV-B55 genomes. The neutralizing and protective antibodies in human are induced primarily by the hexon protein, partially by the fiber and penton base proteins (Gahery-Segard et al., 1998; Hong et al., 2003; Sumida et al., 2005). The lack of non-synonymous substitutions in the three capsid proteins of HAdV-B55 strains make the HAdV-B55 vaccine development easier when compared with other respiratory viruses, such as influenza viruses.

Genome recombination is an important strategy driving HAdV evolution (Robinson et al., 2009, 2011; Kajon et al., 2010; Walsh et al., 2010, 2011; Liu et al., 2011, 2012; Matsushima et al., 2012), and results in the changes in pathogenicity (Walsh et al., 2009; Singh et al., 2012; Zhou et al., 2012). For HAdVs, to some extent, recombination can be defined as an adaptive change resulting from environmental pressures. In the example of HAdV-B55, the initial HAdV-B14 infection may induce neutralizing antibodies against this type. Meanwhile the co-infection and co-replication of HAdV-B11 and HAdV-B14 in the intestine may lead to the recombination between HAdV-B11 and HAdV-B14 hexon genes, *i.e.*, the resulting HAdV-B55 can escape from pre-existing immunity against HAdV-B14 from the host due to its acquisition of HAdV-B11 loops. The previous study has confirmed that the neutralizing and protective antibodies in human are induced primarily by the two hexon loops. The acquisition both loops of HAdV-B11 is beneficial to the survival and spreading of the recombinant HAdV-B55, because the previous absence of circulating HAdV-B11 in China (Han et al., 2013; Chen et al., 2016; Yu et al., 2016) led to a corresponding low level of herd immunity, which might be associated with the subsequent more and more ARD outbreaks caused by HAdV-B55 (Yang et al., 2009; Zhu et al., 2009; Walsh et al., 2010; Zhang et al., 2012a; Zhang S.Y. et al., 2016; Cao et al., 2014; Li et al., 2014; Chen et al., 2016; Gao et al., 2016; Tan et al., 2016; Yi et al., 2017). This is one of the immune escape capabilities of HAdVs. The detailed recombination mechanism of HAdV-B55 might be illustrated by *in vitro* co-infection and replication of the two types of adenoviruses, HAdV-B11 and -B14. In addition, we also infected A549, Hela, HEp-2, Hep-G2, and Vero cells with HAdV-B55, -B11, and -B14, respectively (data not shown). The replication efficiency of different types in the cells was compared. The three types of HAdVs replicated most efficiently in A549 cells. Unfortunately, no significant difference of replication efficiency among the three types of HAdVs was identified in all the tested cell clines. The prevalence and outbreak of HAdV-B55 might be not associated with the virus replication efficiency.

In summary, comparative genomic analysis of re-emergent HAdV-B55 pathogens revealed conserved capsid proteins and low non-synonymous substitutions per site of HAdV-B55, which provides the foundation for the development of effective vaccines against this pathogen. It also facilitates the further studies of the adenovirus epidemiology, molecular evolution, patterns of pathogen emergence and re-emergence (Zhang et al., 2017), and the predication of genome recombination between adenoviruses, as well as the development of public health strategies, including surveillance.

AUTHOR CONTRIBUTIONS

QZ, XW, and BC conceived and designed the study. ZC, YY, SJ, W-GL, W-WC, JZ, ML, ShZ, NC, JO, and SuZ performed the computational analyses and made the figures and tables. ZC, YY, and QZ wrote the manuscript. All authors reviewed the manuscript.

ACKNOWLEDGMENTS

This work was supported by the National Natural Science Foundation of China (31570155, 31370199, 81471961) and "Young Top-notch Talents" of the Guangdong Province Special Support Program (2014), as well as the Excellent Young Teacher Training Plan of Guangdong Province (Yq2013039) and Guangzhou Healthcare Collaborative Innovation Major Project (201803040004, 201803040007).

REFERENCES

Alissa Alkhalaf, M., Al Qurashi, Y. M., Guiver, M., and Cooper, R. J. (2014). Genome sequences of three species d adenoviruses isolated from AIDS patients. *Genome Announc.* 2:e01267-13. doi: 10.1128/genomeA.01267-13

Alkhalaf, M. A., Guiver, M., and Cooper, R. J. (2015). Genome stability of adenovirus types 3 and 7 during a simultaneous outbreak in Greater Manchester. UK. *J. Med. Virol.* 87, 117–124. doi: 10.1002/jmv.23969

Brudno, M., Do, C. B., Cooper, G. M., Kim, M. F., Davydov, E., Green, E. D., et al. (2003). LAGAN and Multi-LAGAN: efficient tools for large-scale multiple alignment of genomic DNA. *Genome Res.* 13, 721–731. doi: 10.1101/gr.926603

Cao, B., Huang, G. H., Pu, Z. H., Qu, J. X., Yu, X. M., Zhu, Z., et al. (2014). Emergence of community-acquired adenovirus type 55 as a cause of community-onset pneumonia. *Chest* 145, 79–86. doi: 10.1378/chest.13-1186

Chen, Y., Liu, F., Wang, C., Zhao, M., Deng, L., Zhong, J., et al. (2016). Molecular identification and epidemiological features of human adenoviruses associated with acute respiratory infections in hospitalized children in Southern China, 2012-2013. *PLOS One* 11:e0155412. doi: 10.1371/journal.pone.0155412

Chmielewicz, B., Benzler, J., Pauli, G., Krause, G., Bergmann, F., and Schweiger, B. (2005). Respiratory disease caused by a species B2 adenovirus in a military camp in Turkey. *J. Med. Virol.* 77, 232–237. doi: 10.1002/jmv.20441

Chu, W., and Pavan-Langston, D. (1979). Ocular surface manifestations of the major viruses. *Int. Ophthalmol. Clin.* 19, 135–167. doi: 10.1097/00004397-197919020-00010

Dehghan, S., Liu, E. B., Seto, J., Torres, S. F., Hudson, N. R., Kajon, A. E., et al. (2012). Five genome sequences of subspecies B1 human adenoviruses associated with acute respiratory disease. *J. Virol.* 86, 635–636. doi: 10.1128/JVI.06593-11

Dhurandhar, N. V., Kulkarni, P., Ajinkya, S. M., and Sherikar, A. (1992). Effect of adenovirus infection on adiposity in chicken. *Vet. Microbiol.* 31, 101–107. doi: 10.1016/0378-1135(92)90068-5

Dingle, J. H., and Langmuir, A. D. (1968). Epidemiology of acute, respiratory disease in military recruits. *Am. Rev. Respir. Dis.* 97(Suppl.), 1–65.

Echavarria, M. (2008). Adenoviruses in immunocompromised hosts. *Clin. Microbiol. Rev.* 21, 704–715. doi: 10.1128/CMR.00052-07

Gahery-Segard, H., Farace, F., Godfrin, D., Gaston, J., Lengagne, R., Tursz, T., et al. (1998). Immune response to recombinant capsid proteins of adenovirus in humans: antifiber and anti-penton base antibodies have a synergistic effect on neutralizing activity. *J. Virol.* 72, 2388–2397.

Gao, H. W., Wei, M. T., Fan, H. J., Ding, H., Wei, W., Liu, Z. Q., et al. (2016).). Dynamic changes in clinical characteristics during an outbreak of human adenovirus Serotype 55 in China. *Disaster Med. Public Health Prep.* [Epub ahead of print].

Geng, X., Zhang, J., and Yang, G. (2013). Investigation of an adenovirus-induced respiratory disease outbreak. *Adv. Infect. Dis.* 3, 257–262. doi: 10.4236/aid.2013.34039

Gu, L., Liu, Z., Li, X., Qu, J., Guan, W., Liu, Y., et al. (2012). Severe community-acquired pneumonia caused by adenovirus type 11 in immunocompetent adults in Beijing. *J. Clin. Virol.* 54, 295–301. doi: 10.1016/j.jcv.2012.04.018

Hage, E., Liebert, U. G., Bergs, S., Ganzenmueller, T., and Heim, A. (2015). Human Adenovirus type 70: a novel, multiple recombinant species D adenovirus isolated from diarrheal faeces of a haematopoietic stem cell transplantation recipient. *J. Gen. Virol.* 96, 2734–2742. doi: 10.1099/vir.0.000196

Hakim, F. A., and Tleyjeh, I. M. (2008). Severe adenovirus pneumonia in immunocompetent adults: a case report and review of the literature. *Eur. J. Clin. Microbiol. Infect. Dis.* 27, 153–158. doi: 10.1007/s10096-007-0416-z

Han, G., Niu, H., Zhao, S., Zhu, B., Wang, C., Liu, Y., et al. (2013). Identification and typing of respiratory adenoviruses in Guangzhou, Southern China using a rapid and simple method. *Virol. Sin.* 28, 103–108. doi: 10.1007/s12250-013-3308-7

Hashimoto, S., Gonzalez, G., Harada, S., Oosako, H., Hanaoka, N., Hinokuma, R., et al. (2018). Recombinant type Human mastadenovirus D85 associated with epidemic keratoconjunctivitis since 2015 in Japan. *J. Med. Virol.* 90, 881–889. doi: 10.1002/jmv.25041

Hierholzer, J. C., Pumarola, A., Rodriguez-Torres, A., and Beltran, M. (1974). Occurrence of respiratory illness due to an atypical strain of adenovirus type 11 during a large outbreak in Spanish military recruits. *Am. J. Epidemiol.* 99, 434–442. doi: 10.1093/oxfordjournals.aje.a121632

Hierholzer, J. C., Stone, Y. O., and Broderson, J. R. (1991). Antigenic relationships among the 47 human adenoviruses determined in reference horse antisera. *Arch. Virol.* 121, 179–197. doi: 10.1007/BF01316753

Hilleman, M. R., Werner, J. H., and Gauld, R. L. (1953). Influenza antibodies in the population of the USA; an epidemiological investigation. *Bull. World Health Organ.* 8, 613–631.

Hong, S. S., Habib, N. A., Franqueville, L., Jensen, S., and Boulanger, P. A. (2003). Identification of adenovirus (ad) penton base neutralizing epitopes by use of sera from patients who had received conditionally replicative ad (addl1520) for treatment of liver tumors. *J. Virol.* 77, 10366–10375. doi: 10.1128/JVI.77.19.10366-10375.2003

Ishiko, H., Shimada, Y., Konno, T., Hayashi, A., Ohguchi, T., Tagawa, Y., et al. (2008). Novel human adenovirus causing nosocomial epidemic keratoconjunctivitis. *J. Clin. Microbiol.* 46, 2002–2008. doi: 10.1128/JCM.01835-07

Jones, M. S. II, Harrach, B., Ganac, R. D., Gozum, M. M., Dela Cruz, W. P., Riedel, B., et al. (2007). New adenovirus species found in a patient presenting with gastroenteritis. *J. Virol.* 81, 5978–5984. doi: 10.1128/JVI.02650-06

Kajon, A. E., Dickson, L. M., Metzgar, D., Houng, H. S., Lee, V., and Tan, B. H. (2010). Outbreak of febrile respiratory illness associated with adenovirus 11a infection in a Singapore military training cAMP. *J. Clin. Microbiol.* 48, 1438–1441. doi: 10.1128/JCM.01928-09

Kojaoghlanian, T., Flomenberg, P., and Horwitz, M. S. (2003). The impact of adenovirus infection on the immunocompromised host. *Rev. Med. Virol.* 13, 155–171. doi: 10.1002/rmv.386

Lafolie, J., Mirand, A., Salmona, M., Lautrette, A., Archimbaud, C., Brebion, A., et al. (2016). Severe pneumonia associated with adenovirus type 55 infection, France, 2014. *Emerg. Infect. Dis.* 22, 2012–2014. doi: 10.3201/eid2211.160728

Le, C. T., Gray, G. C., and Poddar, S. K. (2001). A modified rapid method of nucleic acid isolation from suspension of matured virus: applied in restriction analysis of DNA from an adenovirus prototype strain and a patient isolate. *J. Med. Microbiol.* 50, 571–574. doi: 10.1099/0022-1317-50-6-571

Li, X., Kong, M., Su, X., Zou, M., Guo, L., Dong, X., et al. (2014). An outbreak of acute respiratory disease in China caused by human adenovirus type B55 in a physical training facility. *Int. J. Infect. Dis.* 28, 117–122. doi: 10.1016/j.ijid.2014.06.019

Liu, E. B., Ferreyra, L., Fischer, S. L., Pavan, J. V., Nates, S. V., Hudson, N. R., et al. (2011). Genetic analysis of a novel human adenovirus with a serologically unique hexon and a recombinant fiber gene. *PLOS One* 6:e24491. doi: 10.1371/journal.pone.0024491

Liu, E. B., Wadford, D. A., Seto, J., Vu, M., Hudson, N. R., Thrasher, L., et al. (2012). Computational and serologic analysis of novel and known viruses in species human adenovirus D in which serology and genomics do not correlate. *PLOS One* 7:e33212. doi: 10.1371/journal.pone.0033212

Lole, K. S., Bollinger, R. C., Paranjape, R. S., Gadkari, D., Kulkarni, S. S., Novak, N. G., et al. (1999). Full-length human immunodeficiency virus type 1 genomes from subtype C-infected seroconverters in India, with evidence of intersubtype recombination. *J. Virol.* 73, 152–160.

Lu, Q. B., Tong, Y. G., Wo, Y., Wang, H. Y., Liu, E. M., Gray, G. C., et al. (2014). Epidemiology of human adenovirus and molecular characterization of human adenovirus 55 in China, 2009-2012. *Influenza Other Respir. Viruses* 8, 302–308. doi: 10.1111/irv.12232

Mahadevan, P., Seto, J., Tibbetts, C., and Seto, D. (2010). Natural variants of human adenovirus type 3 provide evidence for relative genome stability across time and geographic space. *Virology* 397, 113–118. doi: 10.1016/j.virol.2009.10.052

Matsushima, Y., Shimizu, H., Kano, A., Nakajima, E., Ishimaru, Y., Dey, S. K., et al. (2012). Novel human adenovirus strain, Bangladesh. *Emerg. Infect. Dis.* 18, 846–848. doi: 10.3201/eid1805.111584

Matsushima, Y., Shimizu, H., Kano, A., Nakajima, E., Ishimaru, Y., Dey, S. K., et al. (2013). Genome sequence of a novel virus of the species human adenovirus d associated with acute gastroenteritis. *Genome Announc.* 1:e00068-12. doi: 10.1128/genomeA.00068-12

Matsushima, Y., Shimizu, H., Phan, T. G., and Ushijima, H. (2011). Genomic characterization of a novel human adenovirus type 31 recombinant in the hexon gene. *J. Gen. Virol.* 92, 2770–2775. doi: 10.1099/vir.0.034744-0

Matthews, D. A., and Russell, W. C. (1995). Adenovirus protein-protein interactions: molecular parameters governing the binding of protein VI to hexon and the activation of the adenovirus 23K protease. *J. Gen. Virol.* 76(Pt 8), 1959–1969. doi: 10.1099/0022-1317-76-8-1959

Nam, J. H., Na, H. N., Atkinson, R. L., and Dhurandhar, N. V. (2014). Genomic stability of adipogenic human adenovirus 36. *Int. J. Obes.* 38, 321–324. doi: 10.1038/ijo.2013.67

Nei, M., and Gojobori, T. (1986). Simple methods for estimating the numbers of synonymous and nonsynonymous nucleotide substitutions. *Mol. Biol. Evol.* 3, 418–426.

Park, J. Y., Kim, B. J., Lee, E. J., Park, K. S., Park, H. S., Jung, S. S., et al. (2017). Clinical Features and Courses of adenovirus pneumonia in healthy young adults during an outbreak among Korean military personnel. *PLOS One* 12:e0170592. doi: 10.1371/journal.pone.0170592

Robinson, C. M., Rajaiya, J., Walsh, M. P., Seto, D., Dyer, D. W., Jones, M. S., et al. (2009). Computational analysis of human adenovirus type 22 provides evidence for recombination among species D human adenoviruses in the penton base gene. *J. Virol.* 83, 8980–8985. doi: 10.1128/JVI.00786-09

Robinson, C. M., Singh, G., Henquell, C., Walsh, M. P., Peigue-Lafeuille, H., Seto, D., et al. (2011). Computational analysis and identification of an emergent human adenovirus pathogen implicated in a respiratory fatality. *Virology* 409, 141–147. doi: 10.1016/j.virol.2010.10.020

Robinson, C. M., Singh, G., Lee, J. Y., Dehghan, S., Rajaiya, J., Liu, E. B., et al. (2013a). Molecular evolution of human adenoviruses. *Sci. Rep.* 3:1812. doi: 10.1038/srep01812

Robinson, C. M., Zhou, X., Rajaiya, J., Yousuf, M. A., Singh, G., Deserres, J. J., et al. (2013b). Predicting the next eye pathogen: analysis of a novel adenovirus. *mBio* 4:e00595-12. doi: 10.1128/mBio.00595-12

Rowe, W. P., Huebner, R. J., Gilmore, L. K., Parrott, R. H., and Ward, T. G. (1953). Isolation of a cytopathogenic agent from human adenoids undergoing spontaneous degeneration in tissue culture. *Proc. Soc. Exp. Biol. Med.* 84, 570–573. doi: 10.3181/00379727-84-20714

Salama, M., Amitai, Z., Amir, N., Gottesman-Yekutieli, T., Sherbany, H., Drori, Y., et al. (2016). Outbreak of adenovirus type 55 infection in Israel. *J. Clin. Virol.* 78, 31–35. doi: 10.1016/j.jcv.2016.03.002

Seto, D., Chodosh, J., Brister, J. R., Jones, M. S., and Members of the Adenovirus Research Community (2011). Using the whole-genome sequence to characterize and name human adenoviruses. *J. Virol.* 85, 5701–5702. doi: 10.1128/JVI.00354-11

Seto, J., Walsh, M. P., Mahadevan, P., Zhang, Q., and Seto, D. (2010a). Applying genomic and bioinformatic resources to human adenovirus genomes for use in vaccine development and for applications in vector development for gene delivery. *Viruses* 2, 1–26. doi: 10.3390/v2010001

Seto, J., Walsh, M. P., Metzgar, D., and Seto, D. (2010b). Computational analysis of adenovirus serotype 5 (HAdV-C5) from an HAdV coinfection shows genome stability after 45 years of circulation. *Virology* 404, 180–186. doi: 10.1016/j.virol.2010.05.010

Singh, G., Robinson, C. M., Dehghan, S., Jones, M. S., Dyer, D. W., Seto, D., et al. (2013). Homologous recombination in E3 genes of human adenovirus species D. *J. Virol.* 87, 12481–12488. doi: 10.1128/JVI.01927-13

Singh, G., Robinson, C. M., Dehghan, S., Schmidt, T., Seto, D., Jones, M. S., et al. (2012). Overreliance on the hexon gene, leading to misclassification of human adenoviruses. *J. Virol.* 86, 4693–4695. doi: 10.1128/JVI.06969-11

Stevens, D. A., Schaeffer, M., Fox, J. P., Brandt, C. D., and Romano, M. (1967). Standardization and certification of reference antigens and antisera for 30 human adenovirus serotypes. *Am. J. Epidemiol.* 86, 617–633. doi: 10.1093/oxfordjournals.aje.a120771

Sumida, S. M., Truitt, D. M., Lemckert, A. A., Vogels, R., Custers, J. H., Addo, M. M., et al. (2005). Neutralizing antibodies to adenovirus serotype 5 vaccine vectors are directed primarily against the adenovirus hexon protein. *J. Immunol.* 174, 7179–7185. doi: 10.4049/jimmunol.174.11.7179

Tamura, K., Dudley, J., Nei, M., and Kumar, S. (2007). MEGA4: molecular Evolutionary Genetics Analysis (MEGA) software version 4.0. *Mol. Biol. Evol.* 24, 1596–1599. doi: 10.1093/molbev/msm092

Tamura, K., Peterson, D., Peterson, N., Stecher, G., Nei, M., and Kumar, S. (2011). MEGA5: molecular evolutionary genetics analysis using maximum likelihood, evolutionary distance, and maximum parsimony methods. *Mol. Biol. Evol.* 28, 2731–2739. doi: 10.1093/molbev/msr121

Tan, D., Zhu, H., Fu, Y., Tong, F., Yao, D., Walline, J., et al. (2016). Severe community-acquired pneumonia caused by human adenovirus in immunocompetent adults: a multicenter case series. *PLOS One* 11:e0151199. doi: 10.1371/journal.pone.0151199

Wadell, G., Hammarskjold, M. L., Winberg, G., Varsanyi, T. M., and Sundell, G. (1980). Genetic variability of adenoviruses. *Ann. N. Y. Acad. Sci.* 354, 16–42. doi: 10.1111/j.1749-6632.1980.tb27955.x

Walsh, M. P., Chintakuntlawar, A., Robinson, C. M., Madisch, I., Harrach, B., Hudson, N. R., et al. (2009). Evidence of molecular evolution driven by recombination events influencing tropism in a novel human adenovirus that causes epidemic keratoconjunctivitis. *PLOS One* 4:e5635. doi: 10.1371/journal.pone.0005635

Walsh, M. P., Seto, J., Jones, M. S., Chodosh, J., Xu, W., and Seto, D. (2010). Computational analysis identifies human adenovirus type 55 as a re-emergent acute respiratory disease pathogen. *J. Clin. Microbiol.* 48, 991–993. doi: 10.1128/JCM.01694-09

Walsh, M. P., Seto, J., Liu, E. B., Dehghan, S., Hudson, N. R., Lukashev, A. N., et al. (2011). Computational analysis of two species C human adenoviruses provides evidence of a novel virus. *J. Clin. Microbiol.* 49, 3482–3490. doi: 10.1128/JCM.00156-11

Wiethoff, C. M., Wodrich, H., Gerace, L., and Nemerow, G. R. (2005). Adenovirus protein VI mediates membrane disruption following capsid disassembly. *J. Virol.* 79, 1992–2000. doi: 10.1128/JVI.79.4.1992-2000.2005

Wigand, R. (1987). Pitfalls in the identification of adenoviruses. *J. Virol. Methods* 16, 161–169. doi: 10.1016/0166-0934(87)90001-2

Wood, D. J. (1988). Adenovirus gastroenteritis. *Br. Med. J. Clin. Res.* 296, 229–230. doi: 10.1136/bmj.296.6617.229-a

Yang, Z., Zhu, Z., Tang, L., Wang, L., Tan, X., Yu, P., et al. (2009). Genomic analyses of recombinant adenovirus type 11a in China. *J. Clin. Microbiol.* 47, 3082–3090. doi: 10.1128/JCM.00282-09

Yi, L., Zou, L., Lu, J., Kang, M., Song, Y., Su, J., et al. (2017). A cluster of adenovirus type B55 infection in a neurosurgical inpatient department of a general hospital in Guangdong, China. *Influenza Other Respir. Viruses* 11, 328–336. doi: 10.1111/irv.12457

Yu, Z., Zeng, Z., Zhang, J., Pan, Y., Chen, M., Guo, Y., et al. (2016). Fatal community-acquired pneumonia in children caused by re-emergent human adenovirus 7d associated with higher severity of illness and fatality rate. *Sci. Rep.* 6:37216. doi: 10.1038/srep37216

Zhang, S. Y., Luo, Y. P., Huang, D. D., Fan, H., Lu, Q. B., Wo, Y., et al. (2016). Fatal pneumonia cases caused by human adenovirus 55 in immunocompetent adults. *Infect. Dis.* 48, 40–47. doi: 10.3109/23744235.2015.1055585

Zhang, Q., Dehghan, S., and Seto, D. (2016). Pitfalls of restriction enzyme analysis in identifying, characterizing, typing, and naming viral pathogens in the era of whole genome data, as illustrated by HAdV type 55. *Virologica Sinica* 31, 448–453. doi: 10.1007/s12250-016-3862-x

Zhang, Q., Jing, S., Cheng, Z., Yu, Z., Dehghan, S., Shamsaddini, A., et al. (2017). Comparative genomic analysis of two emergent human adenovirus type 14 respiratory pathogen isolates in China reveals similar yet divergent genomes. *Emerg. Microbes Infect.* 6:e92. doi: 10.1038/emi.2017.78

Zhang, Q., Seto, D., Cao, B., Zhao, S., and Wan, C. (2012a). Genome sequence of human adenovirus type 55, a re-emergent acute respiratory disease pathogen in China. *J. Virol.* 86, 12441–12442. doi: 10.1128/JVI.02225-12

Zhang, Q., Seto, D., Zhao, S., Zhu, L., Zhao, W., and Wan, C. (2012b). Genome sequence of the first human adenovirus type 14 isolated in China. *J. Virol.* 86, 7019–7020. doi: 10.1128/JVI.00814-12

Zhang, Q., Su, X., Gong, S., Zeng, Q., Zhu, B., Wu, Z., et al. (2006). Comparative genomic analysis of two strains of human adenovirus type 3 isolated from children with acute respiratory infection in southern China. *J. Gen. Virol.* 87, 1531–1541. doi: 10.1099/vir.0.81515-0

Zhao, S., Wan, C., Ke, C., Seto, J., Dehghan, S., Zou, L., et al. (2014). Re-emergent human adenovirus genome type 7d caused an acute respiratory disease outbreak in Southern China after a twenty-one year absence. *Sci. Rep.* 4:7365. doi: 10.1038/srep07365

Zhou, X., Robinson, C. M., Rajaiya, J., Dehghan, S., Seto, D., Jones, M. S., et al. (2012). Analysis of human adenovirus type 19 associated with epidemic keratoconjunctivitis and its reclassification as adenovirus type 64. *Invest. Ophthalmol. Vis. Sci.* 53, 2804–2811. doi: 10.1167/iovs.12-9656

Zhu, Z., Zhang, Y., Xu, S., Yu, P., Tian, X., Wang, L., et al. (2009). Outbreak of acute respiratory disease in China caused by B2 species of adenovirus type 11. *J. Clin. Microbiol.* 47, 697–703. doi: 10.1128/JCM.01769-08

5

Andrographolide Prevents EV-D68 Replication by Inhibiting the Acidification of Virus-Containing Endocytic Vesicles

Dongyin Wang[1,2], Haoran Guo[2], Junliang Chang[2,3], Dong Wang[1,2], Bin Liu[4], Pujun Gao[1]* and Wei Wei[2]**

[1] Department of Hepatology, The First Hospital of Jilin University, Jilin University, Changchun, China, [2] Institute of Virology and AIDS Research, The First Hospital of Jilin University, Changchun, China, [3] Changchun Institute of Biological Products, Changchun, China, [4] Department of Hand Surgery, The First Hospital of Jilin University, Changchun, China

***Correspondence:**
Bin Liu
kjkliubin@126.com
Pujun Gao
gpj0411@163.com
Wei Wei
wwei6@jlu.edu.cn

Enterovirus D68 (EV-D68) has emerged as a significant respiratory pathogen that can cause severe respiratory disease and acute neurologic disease. At present, there are no approved antiviral agents or vaccines for EV-D68. In this study, we demonstrate that andrographolide (ADO), an active component of *Andrographis paniculata*, exerts substantial antiviral activity against EV-D68 infection. ADO treatment dramatically inhibited EV-D68 RNA replication (EC_{50} = 3.45 μM) and protein synthesis without producing significant cytotoxicity at virucidal concentrations. ADO-treated cells did not show any changes in host immune activation, EV-D68 attachment, or viral 5′ UTR activity. Using a pH-sensitive fluorescent indicator system for endocytosis in living cells, we found that ADO prevented the acidification of endocytic vesicles after receptor-mediated endocytosis. Finally, we showed that ADO inhibited the viral replication of circulating isolated EV-D68 strains. In summary, our results demonstrate that ADO suppresses EV-D68 replication by targeting the maturation of virus-containing endosomes of EV-D68. This mechanism represents a promising strategy for drug development.

Keywords: enterovirus D68, andrographolide, endocytosis, acidification, drug development

INTRODUCTION

The genus Enterovirus (EV) of the family Picornaviridae includes several medically important pathogens such as poliovirus, echoviruses, coxsackieviruses, numbered enteroviruses, and rhinoviruses (Baggen et al., 2018). In past decades, several enteroviruses have emerged as serious public health concerns. Recently, enterovirus D68 (EV-D68; originally classified as human rhinovirus 87) (Ishiko et al., 2002), caused a large outbreak of severe lower respiratory tract disease in North America. EV-D68 was first isolated in California from patients with pneumonia and bronchiolitis in 1962 (Schieble et al., 1967) and has since been infrequently reported in association with a wide range of clinical manifestations including mild-to-severe respiratory disease (Kaida et al., 2011; Huang et al., 2017). In 2014, the largest outbreak of EV-D68 infection occurred in the United States (Midgley et al., 2014, 2015). Most patients were children with severe respiratory conditions that necessitated intensive care. Patients with a history (Baggen et al., 2018) of asthma or reactive airway disease were more likely to require ventilator support (Midgley et al., 2015). Since the 2014 outbreak, an increasing number of clusters of EV-D68 infection have been reported in Europe, Asia, and Oceania (Messacar et al., 2015, 2016; Oermann et al., 2015; Reiche et al., 2015; Wei et al., 2016). EV-D68 has also been implicated in polio-like neurological disorders such as acute flaccid myelitis (Greninger et al., 2015; Maloney et al., 2015).

EV-D68 differs from other enteroviruses in that it is most often detected in cases of respiratory illness and has biological similarity to rhinovirus (Blomqvist et al., 2002; Oberste et al., 2004; Mertz et al., 2015). EV-D68 is a small, icosahedral virus with a single, positive-stranded RNA genome. The viral genome contains only 1 open reading frame (ORF) that encodes viral polyprotein, which is self-digested by viral proteins 2A and 3C to yield four structural proteins (VP1, VP2, VP3, and VP4) and seven non-structural proteins (2A, 2B, 2C, 3A, 3B, 3C, and 3D) (Baggen et al., 2018). The viral crystal structure of EV-D68 also shows similarity to that of human rhinovirus (Oberste et al., 2004). The EV-D68 capsid consists of 60 copies of each of the subunit proteins VP1, VP2, VP3, and VP4 and has a deep surface depression (canyon) circling each of the 12 pentameric vertices, which is thought to be responsible for viral receptor recognition (Liu et al., 2015b). Previous studies have suggested that cell surface sialic acid is required for host cell infection by EV-D68 (Liu et al., 2015a; Baggen et al., 2016). We recently identified neuro-specific intercellular adhesion molecule 5 (ICAM-5/telencephalin) as a functional entry receptor for sialic acid-dependent and -independent EV-D68 viruses (Wei et al., 2016).

Despite the spread of EV-D68 viruses, there are no effective vaccines or antiviral agents available for clinical use. It was recently reported that three antiviral drugs in clinical trials for enteroviral infections (pleconaril, pocapavir, and vapendavir) failed to inhibit EV-D68 infection (Liu et al., 2015b; Rhoden et al., 2015; Sun et al., 2015).

Andrographis paniculata Nees has been traditionally used for centuries in Asia to treat various diseases such as respiratory infection, fever, diarrhea, and bacterial dysentery (Panraksa et al., 2017). Andrographolide (ADO) is a bicyclic diterpenoid lactone and is thought to be the major bioactive component of *A. paniculata*, exerting anti-inflammatory, anti-cancer, and antiviral activities (Wintachai et al., 2015; Panraksa et al., 2017). Previous studies have shown that ADO has activity against several viruses including the human immunodeficiency virus (Calabrese et al., 2000), hepatitis B virus (Chen et al., 2014), hepatitis C virus (Lee et al., 2014), dengue virus (Panraksa et al., 2017), chikungunya virus (Wintachai et al., 2015), and herpes simplex virus (Aromdee et al., 2011). In this study, we evaluated the activity of ADO against the EV-D68 virus. Our results reveal the antiviral activity of ADO and shed light on its utility for the treatment of EV-D68 infections.

MATERIALS AND METHODS

Cells and Viruses

Human rhabdomyosarcoma RD cells (ATCC, CCL-136) were cultured in Dulbecco's modified Eagle medium (DMEM; Hyclone^{TM}, cat no: SH30022.01) supplemented with 10% fetal bovine serum (Biological Industries, REF: 04-001-1) and 1% penicillin/streptomycin solution. EV-D68 prototype Fermon (ATCC, VR-1826) and EV-D68 circulating strains from the 2014 United States outbreak, US/MO/14-18947 (ATCC, VR-1823D) and US/KY/14-18953 (ATCC, VR-1825D), were propagated in RD cells. A mixture of cell and supernatant was collected at approximately 5 days post-infection and subjected to multiple cycles of freezing and thawing. Then, the mixture was clarified by low-speed centrifugation and passed through a 0.22-mm filter, and viral particles were pelleted through a 20% sucrose cushion in a SW28 rotor by centrifugation at 28,000 rpm for 90 min. Purified virions were stored at −80°C until use.

Cell Viability Assay

RD cells were cultured in 96-well plates with complete medium until they reached 90% confluence. Then, cell culture medium was removed and replaced with complete medium containing 0.4% dimethyl sulfoxide (DMSO) or various concentrations of ADO (MCE, HY-N0191) (0, 1.25, 2.5, 5, 10, 20, and 40 μM). Negative control (only media) and positive control wells (0.4% DMSO) were included on each plate. The cells were incubated for 24 h and then 30 μl MTS was added to each well. Three hours later, the color intensity of each well was detected at 490 nm using a 550 Bio-Rad plate reader. Each data point represents the average of three replicates in cell culture.

Viral Attachment Assays

For virus attachment experiments, the cells were first washed with cold DMEM, and then EV-D68 viruses were added to the cells. After incubation at 4°C for 2 h, treated cells were washed with cold DMEM to remove unbound viruses. Total RNAs were extracted using an RNeasy Mini Kit (Qiagen). The bound virus RNA was determined by using qRT-PCR.

Virus Titer Assay

Virus titers were determined by endpoint dilution assay (EPDA). Briefly, RD cells were cultured under standard conditions in 96-well plates at a density of 10,000 cells per well. EV-D68 was serially diluted (10-fold) with DMEM containing 1% FBS and added to cells. Virus titers were determined by the appearance of cytopathic effects (CPEs) in RD cells using a microtitration analysis in accordance with the Reed-Muench method (Reed and Muench, 1938).

RNA Quantitation by qRT-PCR

Total RNA from cells was isolated using Trizol (Life Technologies) according to the manufacturer's instructions, including the DNase I digestion step. Samples were incubated in 10 μl of diethyl pyrocarbonate (DEPC)-treated water with 1x RQ1 RNase-Free DNase buffer, 1 μl of RQ1 RNase-free DNase (Promega), and 4 U of RNase inhibitor (New England Biolabs) for 30 min at 37°C. The DNase activity was inactivated by the addition of 1 μl RQ1 DNase stop solution and incubation at 65°C for 10 min. The RNA was reverse-transcribed by using random primers and Multiscribe reverse transcriptase from the High-Capacity cDNA Archive Kit (Applied Biosystems, Carlsbad, CA,

United States), according to the manufacturer's instructions. The cDNA was either used undiluted or serially diluted in DEPC-treated water before the real-time PCR reaction to ensure that the amplification was within the linear range of detection. The StepOne Real-Time PCR system (Applied Biosystems) was used for qRT-PCR amplification. The reactions were performed under the following conditions: 50°C for 2 min and 95°C for 10 min, followed by 40 cycles of 95°C for 15 s and 60°C for 1 min, followed by a dissociation protocol. Single peaks in the melting curve analysis indicated specific amplicons. qRT-PCR was performed with the following primer sequence: GAPDH forward primer 5′-GCAAATTCCATGGCACCGT-3′; GAPDH reverse primer 5′-TCGCCCCACTTGATTTTGG-3′; EV-D68 forward primer 5′-TGTTCCCACGGTTGAAAACAA-3′; and -EV-D68 reverse primer 5′-TGTCTAGCGTCTCATGGTTTTCAC-3′. IFN-β: 5′-TTGTGCTTCTCCACTACAGC-3′ (forward) and 5′-CTGTAAGTCTGTTAATGAAG-3′ (reverse); ISG56: 5′-CAACCAAGCAAATGTGAGGA-3′ (forward) and 5′-AGGGGAAGCAAAGAAAATGG-3′ (reverse). The relative levels of EV-D68 RNA in different samples were determined using a comparative $2^{-\Delta\Delta CT}$ method with normalization against the GAPDH gene (Wei et al., 2016).

Immunoblotting

Cells were harvested at various time points post-infection, washed twice with cold phosphate-buffered saline (PBS), and lysed in lysis buffer (150 mM Tris [pH 7.5] containing 150 mM NaCl, 1% Triton X-100, and complete protease inhibitor cocktail [Roche]) and loading buffer (0.08 M Tris [pH 6.8] containing 2.0% SDS,10% glycerol, 0.1 M DTT, and 0.2% bromphenol blue). The solutions were boiled and vortexed for 10 min and then centrifuged at 14000 × *g* for 10 min. Supernatant proteins were separated by SDS-PAGE and transferred to nitrocellulose membranes using a semidry apparatus (Bio-Rad). The membranes were probed with primary antibodies (anti-EV-D68 VP1 polyclonal antibody [Genetex, GTX132312] and anti-β-actin monoclonal antibody [Sigma, A3853]) at 4°C overnight, followed by incubation with secondary antibodies (alkaline phosphatase-conjugated goat anti-rabbit IgG [Jackson ImmunoResearch Laboratories, code:115-005-045] and goat anti-mouse IgG [Jackson ImmunoResearch Laboratories, code: 115-055-062]) for 1 h at 25°C. The membranes were stained with 5-bromo-4-chloro-3-indolyl phosphate and nitrotetrazolium blue chloride (Sigma-Aldrich) and visualized for band quantification.

Immunofluorescence and Confocal Microscopy

Cells were grown on glass plates (Nest, cat no.: 801001) in the presence of 10 μM ADO or 0.1% DMSO vehicle overnight until they reached subconfluence. EV-D68 was bound to cells for 45 min at 4°C in DMEM containing 1% FBS. Then, the cells were washed with PBS and incubated at 37°C in 1% DMEM. At various time points, the cells were fixed with 4% paraformaldehyde (PFA) for 15 min, permeabilized with 0.3% Triton X-100 for 5 min, blocked with goat serum (ZSGB-BIO, ZLI-9022) for 1 h 25°C, and finally stained with EV-D68 VP1 antibody (1:250) at 4°C overnight. The next day, the cells were washed five times with PBS and then incubated with Alexa Fluro® 488 conjugated goat anti-rabbit IgG antibody (Life Technologies, A11088) for 1 h at room temperature. DAPI stain (1:100 dilution, Biotopped, top0221) was added 10 min prior to visualization under fluorescence microscopy (Olympus, IX5 or Olympus Fluo-View-1000 with a 100X objective lens) with Fluo View software v. 1.7. Representative cells were selected and photographed.

Intraendosomal pH Determination

We used amine-reactive pHrodo dyes (Life technologies, cat no.: P35368) to detect changes in the pH of virus-containing endosomes. EV-D68 fermon was purified and dissolved in PBS and incubated with amine-reactive pHrodo dyes for 40 min at room temperature in the dark before infection. RD cells were then seeded on glass plates in the presence of 10 μM ADO or 0.1% DMSO vehicle overnight. Then, the cells were infected with dye-conjugated EV-D68 virus at 4°C for 30 min, washed with PBS and incubated in 37°C, and observed at different time points (1, 2, and 3 h) with a confocal microscope.

Luciferase Assay

To evaluate the effect of ADO on the viral transcriptional activity of EV-D68, we constructed a promoter-driven firefly luciferase plasmid pT7-5′UTR-pGL3 and expression plasmid p3D-VR_{1012}. p5′UTR-Luc (200 ng) was transfected or co-transfected with pEV-D68-3D (800 ng) into cells pre-treated with ADO or 0.1% DMSO vehicle. Luciferase activity was assessed 24 h after transfection. Briefly, the cells were harvested and lysed with passive lysis buffer and then centrifuged at 12000 × *g* for 10 min. Supernatants and luciferase substrate (Promega, E190) were mixed in a 96-well plate and fluorescence was quantified with a Fluoroskan Ascent™ FL instrument (Thermo Fisher, 5210450).

Statistical Analysis

All data are shown as the mean value and standard deviation of biological replicates (details are explained in figure legends). Statistically significant differences between groups were estimated using two-tailed unpaired Student's *t*-test with GraphPad Prism (version 6.0) software. P-value < 0.05 was considered statistically significant.

RESULTS

ADO Inhibits EV-D68 Replication

Andrographolide is a labdane diterpenoid with broad-spectrum antiviral properties (**Figure 1A**). To investigate the anti-EV-D68 activity of ADO, permissive RD cells were pretreated with 10 μM ADO or 0.1% DMSO vehicle for 16 h, followed by challenge with an EV-D68 prototype Fermon virus (MOI of 0.1). CPEs were detected at 48 h post-infection in vehicle-treated cells; in contrast, ADO-treated cells showed obvious resistance to CPEs (**Figure 1B**). qRT-PCR data indicated that ADO treatment decreased viral RNA replication by 98-fold at

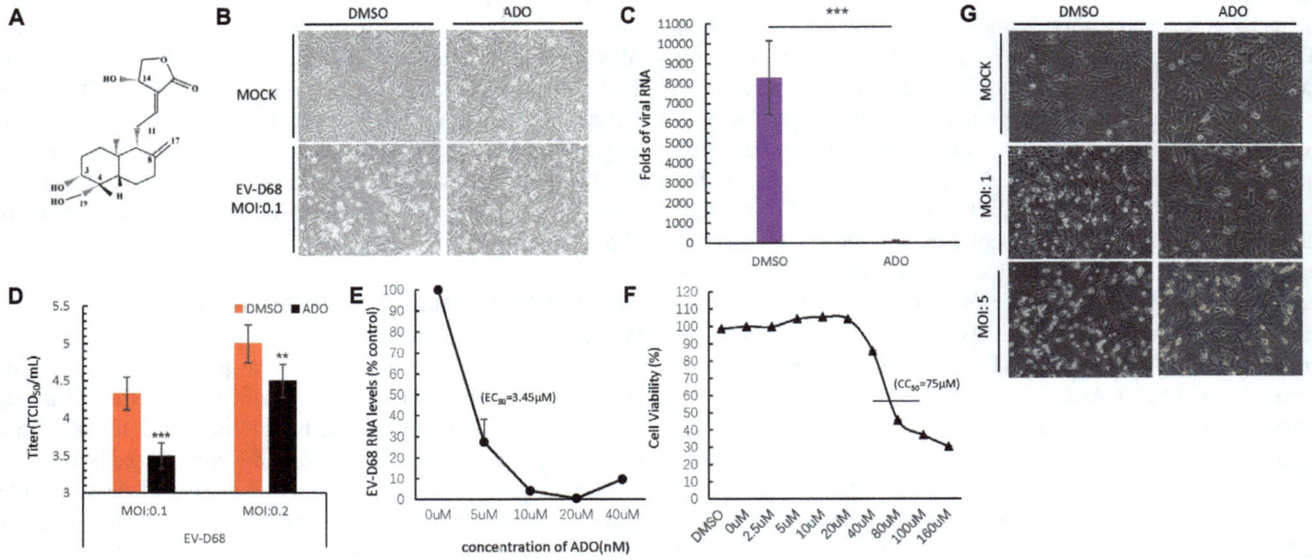

FIGURE 1 | Andrographolide inhibits EV-D68 replication. **(A)** Structure of andrographolide (ADO; molecular formula: $C_{20}H_{30}O_5$). **(B)** RD cells were pre-treated with ADO or DMSO vehicle before infection or mock-infection with EV-D68 virus. The cells were incubated under standard conditions. Cytopathic effects (CPEs) were observed 48 h post-infection. **(C)** qRT-PCR assessment of EV-D68 RNA replication. **(D)** Determination of progeny viron production. Supernatants were collected 48 h post-infection and viral titers were determined by standard plaque assay. **(E)** Effect of ADO on EV-D68 RNA replication (EC_{50} = ~3.45 μM). **(F)** Cell viability assay. Cellular toxicity was evaluated by MTS assay and is expressed as the percentage relative to DMSO vehicle-treated control cells. Experiments were performed in triplicate. **(G)** RD cells were pretreated the same way as cells in **(B)**, then the cells were infected or mock-infected with EV-D68 virus at an MOI of 1 and 5. CPEs were observed 24 h post-infection. Error bars indicate the standard deviation (*$P < 0.05$; **$P < 0.01$; ***$P < 0.001$).

48 h post-infection (**Figure 1C**). Additionally, ADO treatment significantly decreased titers of EV-D68 progeny virus compared to vehicle treatment (**Figure 1D**), suggesting that ADO inhibits the proliferation of EV-D68. In addition, we confirmed that ADO exhibited powerful inhibitory effect on EV-D68 at higher MOI of 1 and 5 (**Figure 1G**). The EC_{50} value of ADO against EV-D68 replication was approximately 3.45 μM (**Figure 1E**). We also measured ADO cytotoxicity using the MTS assay and determined that the median lethal concentration of ADO was 75 μM (**Figure 1F**), which was much higher than the EC_{50} of antiviral activity.

ADO Inhibits EV-D68 RNA Replication and VP1 Synthesis

We next sought to determine the part of EV-D68 life cycle that was inhibited by ADO treatment. We analyzed EV-D68 growth curves during infection of RD cells (MOI of 10) in the presence of 10 μM ADO or 0.1% DMSO vehicle (**Figure 2A**). Viral RNA was quantified using qRT-PCR at 0, 2, 4, 8, 12, and 24 h post-infection. ADO treatment decreased the amount of intracellular EV-D68 RNA by more than 80% compared to vehicle at 8 h post-infection (**Figure 2A**). At 24 h post-infection, the amount of EV-D68 RNA in vehicle-treated cells was 19-fold higher than that in ADO-treated cells (**Figure 2A**). Consistent with this result, there was an observable reduction in EV-D68 VP1 protein expression in ADO-treated cells compared to vehicle-treated cells on immunoblotting (**Figures 2B,C**) and immunofluorescence assays (**Figure 2D**). To clarify the dynamics of ADO against EV-D68, a time-of-addition analysis was undertaken, with ADO treatment at 16 and 3 h prior to infection and 0, 2, and 6 h post-infection. VP1 expression was evaluated by immunoblotting. The results indicated that ADO treatment post-infection had no obvious effect on EV-D68 (**Figure 2E**). All these data suggested that ADO treatment impeded the early stage of EV-D68 infection.

ADO Does Not Influence EV-D68 3D-5′ UTR Activity or Innate Immune Responses

The 5′ UTR region of enteroviruses is a determinant for viral translation and RNA replication, and the activity of this region can be enhanced by viral polymerase 3D protein. To assess viral 3D protein-dependent 5′ UTR activation, we next established a firefly luciferase reporter assay (**Figure 3A**) and found that ADO treatment had no influence on 5′ UTR activity regardless of 3D expression (**Figure 3B**).

Previous studies have characterized ADO as a strong plant-derived immunomodulator that affects the NF-κB and JAK-STAT signaling pathways, which are involved in host innate immune responses (Ding et al., 2017). Therefore, we next measured endogenous mRNA levels of interferon-β (IFN-β) and an interferon-stimulated gene ISG56 at 0, 2, 4, 8, and 12 h post-infection (**Figures 4A,B**). IFN-β mRNA was increased at 12 h post-infection, suggesting that EV-D68 infection produced innate immune activation in permissive cells (**Figure 4A**). ADO treatment at a concentration of 10 μM did not have a significant effect on IFN-β or ISG56 mRNA expression during EV-D68 infection in RD cells (**Figures 4A,B**), indicating that ADO did not

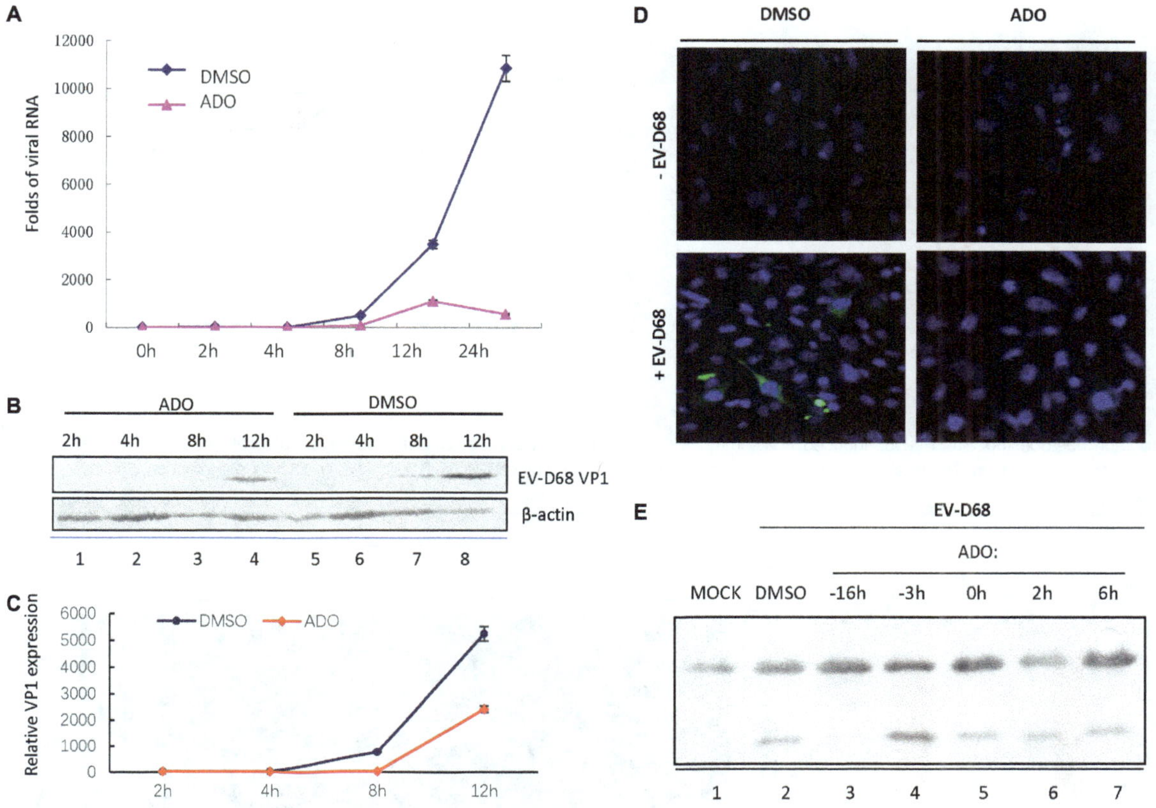

FIGURE 2 | Andrographolide inhibits EV-D68 RNA replication and VP1 synthesis. RD cells were pretreated with andrographolide or DMSO vehicle overnight and subsequently infected with EV-D68. Viral RNA **(A)** and VP1 **(B–D)** were measured at several specific time points. **(A)** Growth curves of EV-D68 in infected cells. **(B,C)** Immunoblotting of VP1 expression at 8 h post-infection. **(D)** Immunofluorescence of VP1 expression at 10 h post-infection. **(E)** RD cells were incubated with 10 μM ADO or vehicle only at the indicated time points before and after infection or mock infection with EV-D68 virus. VP1 was analyzed by western blotting 24 h post-infection, with actin as a control. Experiments were performed in triplicate. Data represent the mean and standard deviation.

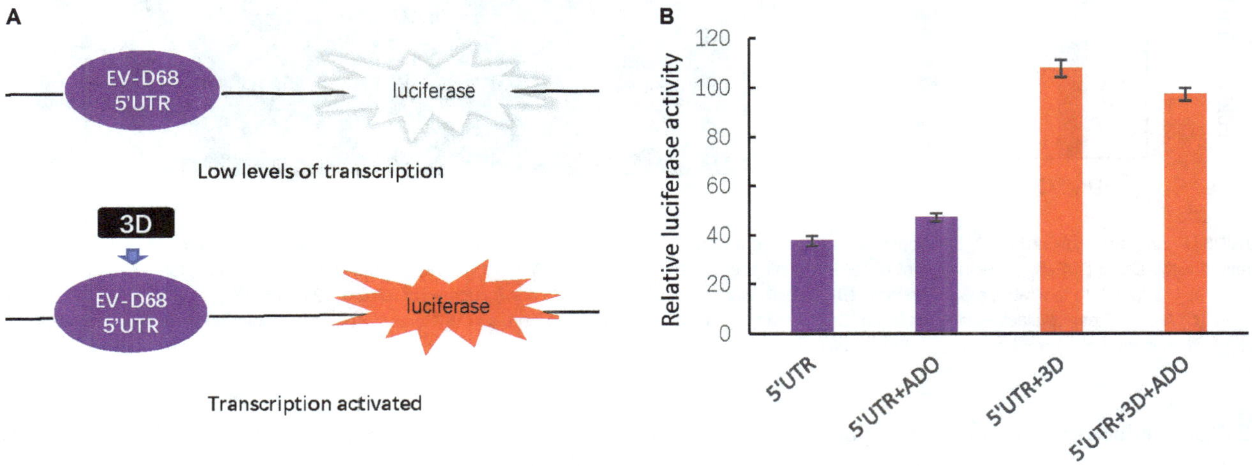

FIGURE 3 | Andrographolide does not influence EV-D68 3D-dependent 5′ UTR transcriptional activity or the cellular innate immune response. **(A)** To assess the effect of andrographolide on EV-D68 transcription, we generated a firefly luciferase reporter assay of 5′ UTR activity. **(B)** Assay of 3D-dependent 5′ UTR activation. p5′UTR-luc (200 ng) was transfected or co-transfected with pEV-D68-3D (800 ng) into HEK293T cells pretreated with ADO or DMSO vehicle in a 12-well plate. Luciferase activity was detected 24 h post-transfection.

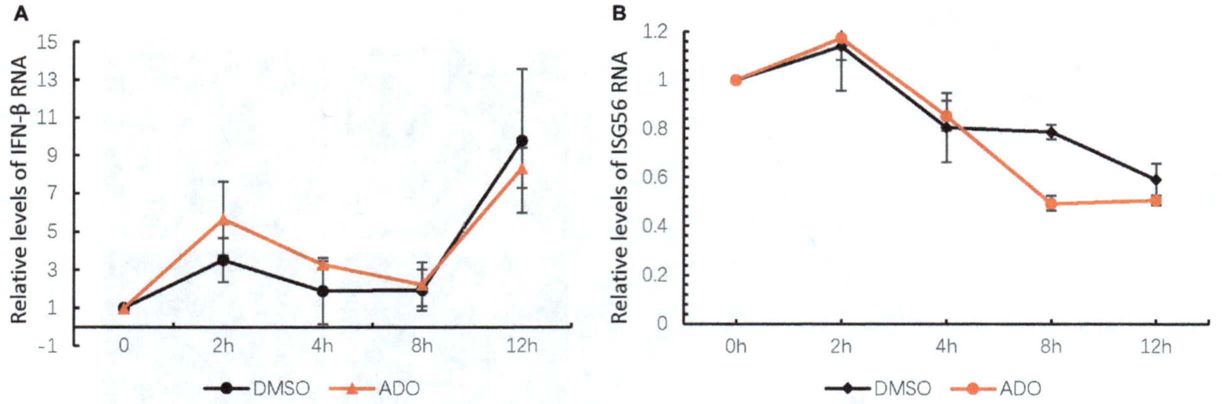

FIGURE 4 | Andrographolide does not alter EV-D68-induced innate immune responses at the cellular level. Gene expression of IFN-β **(A)** and ISG-56 **(B)**, respectively, as indicators of virus-stimulated innate immune response. mRNA was quantified by qRT-PCR at 0, 2, 4, 8, and 12 h post-infection. Error bars indicate the standard deviation.

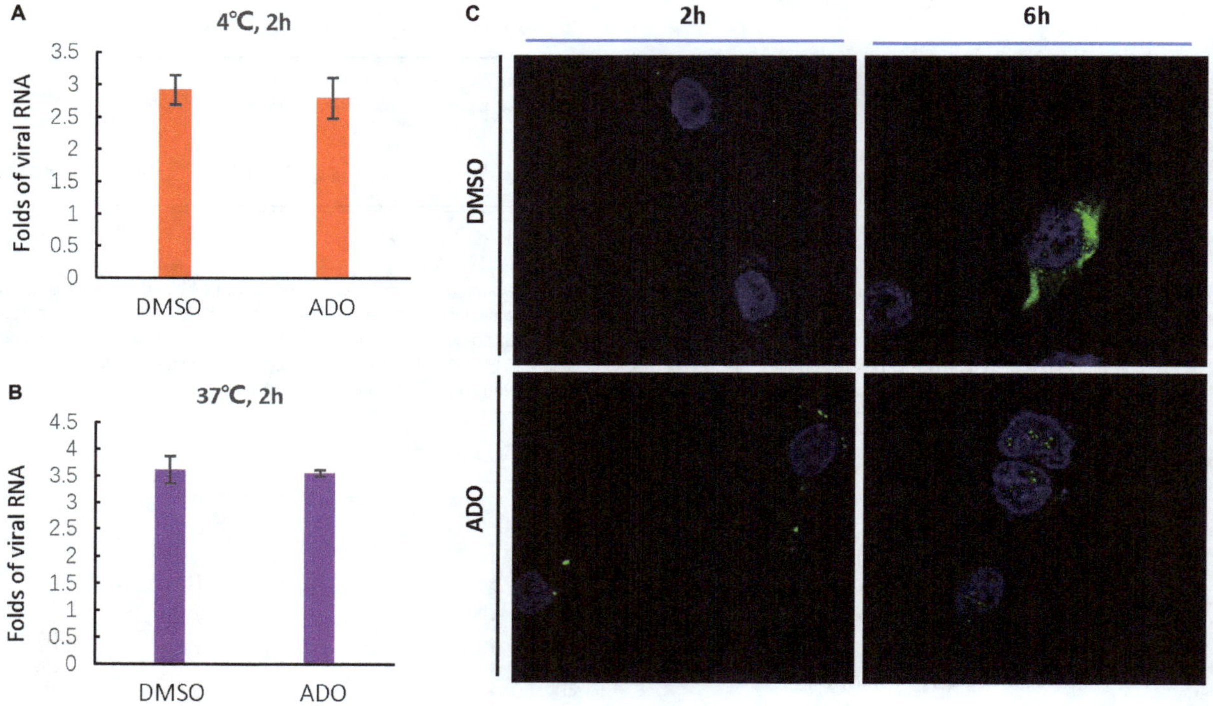

FIGURE 5 | Andrographolide inhibits EV-D68 replication in a post-entry step. Andrographolide had no effect on EV-D68 attachment or entry into cells. Cells were pre-treated with ADO or DMSO vehicle in 12-well plates for 16 h under standard conditions. **(A)** Cells were incubated at 4°C for 30 min before infection and then incubated at 4°C for 2 h to facilitate virus attachment. **(B)** RD cells were infected with EV-D68 and incubated at 37°C for 2 h. qRT-PCR was performed to quantify viral RNA. **(C)** Assay of intracellular VP1 accumulation. Cells were fixed at 2 and 6 h post-infection, and VP1 was observed by confocal microscopy. Experiments were performed in triplicate. Error bars indicate the standard deviation.

alter EV-D68-induced innate immune responses at the cellular level.

ADO Does Not Influence EV-D68 Entry Into Cells

Based on the above studies, we determined that ADO likely inhibited a step in the EV-D68 lifecycle occurring prior to viral RNA replication and protein expression. Therefore, we next investigated whether ADO inhibited EV-D68 replication at the entry step. Viral attachment and entry experiments were performed in the presence of 10 μM ADO or 0.1% DMSO vehicle. Virus attachment and entry were assessed by quantification of intracellular EV-D68 RNA at 2 h post-infection. Repeated experiments demonstrated that pre-treatment of cells with ADO had no detectable effect on viral attachment (**Figure 5A**) or entry (**Figure 5B**). Next, we detected intracellular

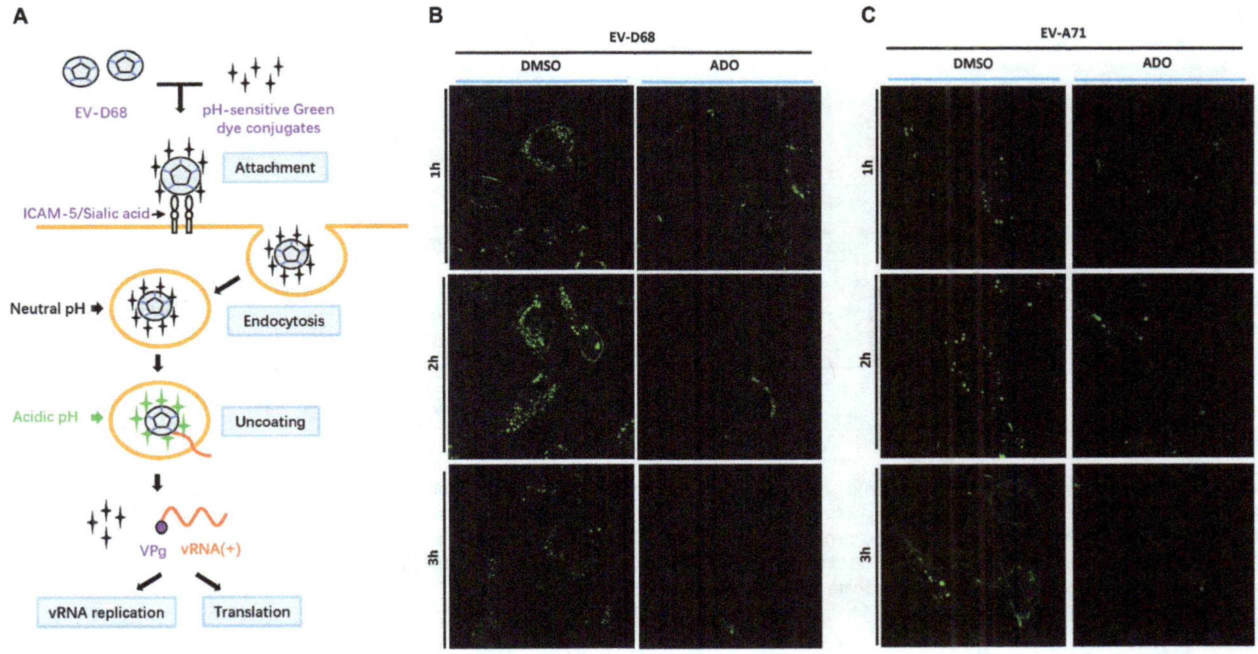

FIGURE 6 | Andrographolide interferes with endosome maturation. **(A)** Viruses are endocytosed at the cell surface before trafficking toward the nucleus. Gradual acidification occurs alongside endosome maturation. Viral proteins require low pH to undergo conformational changes or protease activation that permit disruption of the endosome membrane and the release of viral particles into the cytoplasm. **(B,C)** Assay of endosome acidification. EV-D68 and EV-A71 were incubated with pH-sensitive green dye and then infected into pre-treated RD cells. Fluorescence was detected in live cells using Alexa Fluor 488 filters and confocal microscopy at specific time points (1, 2, and 3 h post-infection). Fluorescence increased with acidity of the surrounding environment.

VP1 protein expression using immunofluorescence at 2 and 6 h post-infection. Consistent with previous result, there was no effect of ADO treatment at 2 h post-infection; however, ADO treatment significantly decreased EV-D68 VP1 protein expression at 6 h post-infection (**Figure 5C**). These results collectively demonstrated that ADO inhibited EV-D68 RNA replication and protein accumulation in a post-entry step.

ADO Inhibits the Acidification of EV-D68-Containing Endosomes

Enteroviruses share a common mechanism in the early steps of viral infection that involves specific receptor binding, viral entry through an endocytic pathway, and subsequent travel through the cytoplasm encased in an endosomal compartment. In most cases, endosomes that contain pathogens undergo maturation to lysosomes to degrade the pathogens. Therefore, the virus must exit the endosome to escape degradation. Viruses use the low pH of endosomes to activate penetration proteins or undergo conformational changes that facilitate escape (Lagache et al., 2012). To track the process of EV-D68 endocytosis in the presence or absence of ADO treatment, we established a pH-sensitive reporter system during EV-D68 infection by using an acidic pH-sensitive green dye. The dye has a pH-sensitive fluorescence emission that increases in intensity with increasing acidity, with peak fluorescence in the range pH 5–8 (i.e., the known range of endosome vesicle acidification; **Figure 6A**). Fluorescence intensity peaked at around 2 h post-infection and was quickly quenched by 3 h post-infection in vehicle-treated RD cells (**Figure 6B**). In contrast, ADO-treated cells exhibited limited fluorescence, suggesting that ADO inhibited the maturation process of EV-D68 endocytosis. Furthermore, we demonstrated that ADO treatment can inhibit the acidification of virus-containing endosome of an enteric enterovirus EV-A71 (**Figure 6C**). Thus, applying a broadly antiviral activity of ADO against diverse viruses via inhibiting endosome acidification.

ADO Inhibits Isolated Circulating Strains of EV-D68

Recent studies presented by our lab and others have demonstrated that the EV-D68 prototype virus and circulating strains have different sensitivities for sialic acid-mediated viral replication. Therefore, we examined the antiviral activity of ADO against viral infection by primary EV-D68 isolates (US/MO/14-18947 [MO] and US/KY/14-18953 [KY]). The cells were harvested at 24 h post-infection for immunoblotting of EV-D68 VP1, and CPEs were observed 48 h post-infection. The results indicated that ADO protected RD cells against both circulating strains of EV-D68 as evidenced by decreases in related CPEs (**Figure 7A**). Further, ADO treatment significantly decreased intracellular amounts of viral RNA after infection with the MO (**Figure 7B**) and KY strains (**Figure 7C**) compared to vehicle treatment. Finally, ADO treatment significantly decreased VP1 protein expression after infection with the MO

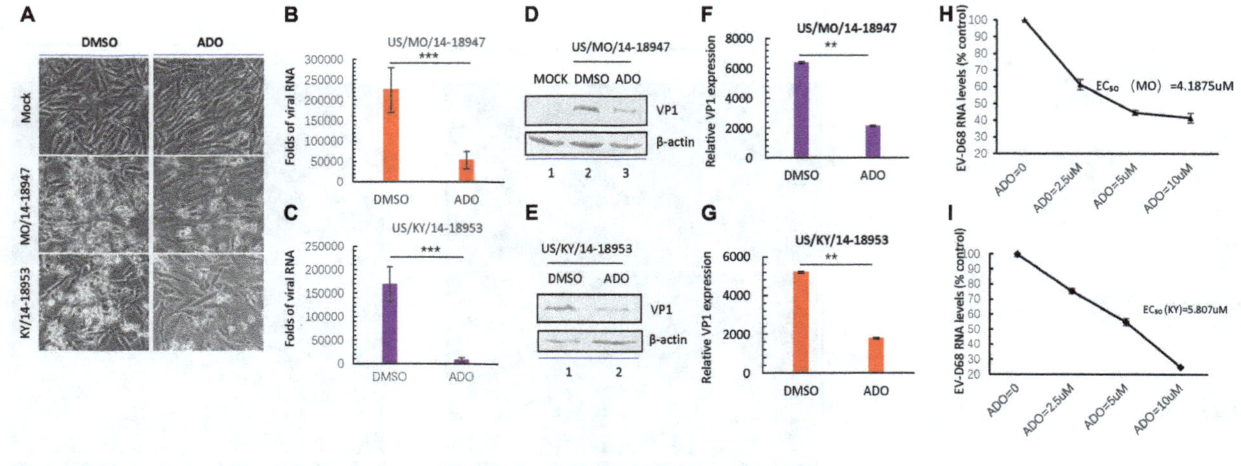

FIGURE 7 | Andrographolide inhibits isolated circulating strains of EV-D68. **(A)** RD cells were pre-treated with 10 μM andrographolide or DMSO vehicle and then infected with US/MO/14-18947 or US/KY/14-18953. Cells were incubated under standard conditions. Cytopathic effects (CPEs) were observed 48 h post-infection. **(B,C)** qRT-PCR analysis of viral RNA. **(D–G)** Immunoblotting of VP1 expression at 24 h post-infection with the US/MO/14-18947 **(D,F)** and US/KY/14-18953 strains **(E,G)**. **(H,I)** Effect of ADO on RNA replication of EV-D68 circulating strains. US/MO/14-18947:EC_{50} = ~4.1875 μM **(H)**; US/KY/14-18953: EC_{50} = ~5.807 μM. The experiment was performed three times. Error bars indicate the standard deviation (*$P < 0.05$; **$P < 0.01$; ***$P < 0.001$).

(**Figures 7D,F**) and KY strains (**Figures 7E,G**) compared to vehicle treatment. The EC_{50} values of ADO against MO and KY replication were approximately 4.19 μM (**Figure 7H**) and 5.807 μM (**Figure 7I**), which was close to that of AOD against EV-D68 prototype Fermon. In summary, ADO exerted broad antiviral effects against both prototype and circulating EV-D68 viruses.

DISCUSSION

To our knowledge, this is the first study to report the inhibition of viral endocytosis by ADO, a major bioactive constituent of *A. paniculata*. ADO treatment conferred significant antiviral activity against EV-D68 virus without producing significant toxicity in RD cells. ADO treatment was associated with significant decreases in viral RNA replication and protein synthesis. Notably, ADO had no influence on viral attachment, viral endocytosis processes, or innate immune activation in infected cells. By using a pH-sensitive fluorescent dye conjugate to track virus endocytosis in live cells, we revealed that ADO interfered with viral cytoplasmic traffic by preventing vesicle acidification.

Andrographis paniculata has long been an important constituent of traditional herbal medicine in Asia (Kumar et al., 2004) and Scandinavia (Jayakumar et al., 2013), with several studies demonstrating the antiviral, antimicrobial, anti-parasitic, and anti-inflammatory effects of ADO as a principal active component. Research has demonstrated the therapeutic utility of ADO in respiratory infection by influenza A virus (IAV) by inhibition of IAV-induced RIG-I like receptor signaling pathway in human bronchial epithelial cells (Yu et al., 2014). However, the mechanisms by which ADO exerts broad-spectrum antiviral activity have been poorly defined in previous studies. In our experiments, ADO treatment did not influence EV-D68 infection-mediated innate immune activation as represented by the induction of IFN-β and ISG56.

In this study, we analyzed the growth curves of EV-D68 RNA replication and VP1 synthesis during infection and found that ADO dramatically decreased intracellular viral RNA copy numbers and VP1 expression. This finding was consistent with previous studies demonstrating the ability of ADO to prevent the infection of diverse viruses by inhibiting viral protein expression (HSV-1, HCV, HPV, and CHIKV) and viral genome replication (HBV, HSV-1, and CHIKV). The 5′ UTR activity of enteroviruses including poliovirus, EV71, CV-A16, and rhinovirus is crucial for viral RNA replication and protein translation (Gamarnik and Andino, 2000). In this study, we found that ADO did not affect the 5′ UTR activity of EV-D68 in a viral RNA polymerase 3D-dependent 5′ UTR reporter assay, indicating that ADO targeted a step prior to the initiation of viral RNA and protein syntheses.

A previous study of the antiviral activity of ADO and its analogs showed that ADO prevented the entry of HSV-1 into cells (Aromdee et al., 2011). The life cycle of an enterovirus starts with binding of a cell surface receptor. Previous studies have demonstrated that sialic acid is required for the cellular entry of certain EV-D68 viruses (Liu et al., 2015a). To this end, our lab identified ICAM-5 as a functional receptor for both sialic acid-sensitive and insensitive EV-D68 strains (Wei et al., 2016). In this study, we found that ADO did not influence the entry of EV-D68 into RD cells.

Enterovirus binds its specific receptor on the cell surface and then enters the host cell through receptor-mediated endocytosis. Subsequently, receptor binding or changes in pH in the virus-containing endosome trigger virus uncoating. Notably, EV-D68 is a unique respiratory enterovirus that is sensitive to acidic conditions and prefers lower culture temperatures (Oberste et al., 2004). Consistent with these properties, we found that acidification of the virus-containing endocytic vesicle was a critical step inhibited by ADO that ultimately inhibited EV-D68 infection. Consistent with this observation, previous studies have indicated that drugs inhibiting endosome acidification (Bafilomycin A1 and concanamycin A) prevented EV71 multiplication. Therefore, disrupting endosome acidification may represent an important antiviral strategy for therapeutic development against EV-D68. Furthermore, ADO has been shown to inhibit autophagosome–lysosome fusion and suspended autophagy processes (Zhou et al., 2012). Future studies are needed to identify the cellular targets of ADO that inhibit endosome/autophagosome maturation.

The work described herein provides compelling evidence that ADO inhibits EV-D68 replication by preventing endosome acidification as a novel antiviral property. Our results show virus–host interactions and highlight the potential therapeutic utility of ADO as a clinical therapeutic against EV-D68 infection.

AUTHOR CONTRIBUTIONS

DyW, HG, JC, and DW performed the experiments. DyW, HG, PG, and WW analyzed the data. WW, DyW, PG, and BL wrote the paper with help from all authors. WW, PG, and BL directed the project.

FUNDING

This work was supported in part by funding from the National Natural Science Foundation of China (Grant Nos. 81772183, 31600132, and 31800150), the Chinese Ministry of Science and Technology (Grant No. 2018ZX10731101-001-016), the Department of Science and Technology of Jilin Province (Grant No. 20180101127JC), the Program for JLU Science and Technology Innovative Research Team (Grant No. 2017TD-08), and the Fundamental Research Funds for the Central Universities.

ACKNOWLEDGMENTS

We thank Jiaxin Yang, Yuanyuan Li, Guoqiang Zhou, and Chuanyan Dai for technical assistance and Editage for editorial assistance.

REFERENCES

Aromdee, C., Suebsasana, S., Ekalaksananan, T., Pientong, C., and Thongchai, S. (2011). Stage of action of naturally occurring andrographolides and their semisynthetic analogues against herpes simplex virus type 1 in vitro. *Planta Med.* 77, 915–921. doi: 10.1055/s-0030-1250659

Baggen, J., Thibaut, H. J., Staring, J., Jae, L. T., Liu, Y., Guo, H., et al. (2016). Enterovirus D68 receptor requirements unveiled by haploid genetics. *Proc. Natl. Acad. Sci. U.S.A.* 113, 1399–1404. doi: 10.1073/pnas.1524498113

Baggen, J., Thibaut, H. J., Strating, J. R. P. M., and Van Kuppeveld, F. J. M. (2018). The life cycle of non-polio enteroviruses and how to target it. *Nat. Rev. Microbiol.* 16, 368–381. doi: 10.1038/s41579-018-0005-4

Blomqvist, S., Savolainen, C., Raman, L., Roivainen, M., and Hovi, T. (2002). Human rhinovirus 87 and enterovirus 68 represent a unique serotype with rhinovirus and enterovirus features. *J. Clin. Microbiol.* 40, 4218–4223. doi: 10.1128/JCM.40.11.4218-4223.2002

Calabrese, C., Berman, S. H., Babish, J. G., Ma, X., Shinto, L., Dorr, M., et al. (2000). A phase I trial of andrographolide in HIV positive patients and normal volunteers. *Phytother. Res.* 14, 333–338. doi: 10.1002/1099-1573(200008)14:5<333::AID-PTR584>3.0.CO;2-D

Chen, H., Ma, Y. B., Huang, X. Y., Geng, C. A., Zhao, Y., Wang, L. J., et al. (2014). Synthesis, structure-activity relationships and biological evaluation of dehydroandrographolide and andrographolide derivatives as novel anti-hepatitis B virus agents. *Bioorg. Med. Chem. Lett.* 24, 2353–2359. doi: 10.1016/j.bmcl.2014.03.060

Ding, Y., Chen, L., Wu, W., Yang, J., Yang, Z., and Liu, S. (2017). Andrographolide inhibits influenza A virus-induced inflammation in a murine model through NF-kappaB and JAK-STAT signaling pathway. *Microbes Infect.* 19, 605–615. doi: 10.1016/j.micinf.2017.08.009

Gamarnik, A. V., and Andino, R. (2000). Interactions of viral protein 3CD and poly(rC) binding protein with the 5' untranslated region of the poliovirus genome. *J. Virol.* 74, 2219–2226. doi: 10.1128/JVI.74.5.2219-2226.2000

Greninger, A. L., Naccache, S. N., Messacar, K., Clayton, A., Yu, G., Somasekar, S., et al. (2015). A novel outbreak enterovirus D68 strain associated with acute flaccid myelitis cases in the USA (2012-14): a retrospective cohort study. *Lancet Infect. Dis.* 15, 671–682. doi: 10.1016/S1473-3099(15)70093-9

Huang, Y. P., Lin, T. L., Lin, T. H., and Wu, H. S. (2017). Molecular and epidemiological study of enterovirus D68 in Taiwan. *J. Microbiol. Immunol. Infect.* 50, 411–417. doi: 10.1016/j.jmii.2015.07.015

Ishiko, H., Miura, R., Shimada, Y., Hayashi, A., Nakajima, H., Yamazaki, S., et al. (2002). Human rhinovirus 87 identified as human enterovirus 68 by VP4-based molecular diagnosis. *Intervirology* 45, 136–141. doi: 10.1159/000065866

Jayakumar, T., Hsieh, C. Y., Lee, J. J., and Sheu, J. R. (2013). Experimental and clinical pharmacology of andrographis paniculata and its major bioactive phytoconstituent andrographolide. *Evid. Based Complement. Alternat. Med.* 2013:846740. doi: 10.1155/2013/846740

Kaida, A., Kubo, H., Sekiguchi, J., Kohdera, U., Togawa, M., Shiomi, M., et al. (2011). Enterovirus 68 in children with acute respiratory tract infections. Osaka Japan. *Emerg. Infect. Dis.* 17, 1494–1497. doi: 10.3201/eid1708.110028

Kumar, R. A., Sridevi, K., Kumar, N. V., Nanduri, S., and Rajagopal, S. (2004). Anticancer and immunostimulatory compounds from *Andrographis paniculata*. *J. Ethnopharmacol.* 92, 291–295. doi: 10.1016/j.jep.2004.03.004

Lagache, T., Danos, O., and Holcman, D. (2012). Modeling the step of endosomal escape during cell infection by a nonenveloped virus. *Biophys. J.* 102, 980–989. doi: 10.1016/j.bpj.2011.12.037

Lee, J. C., Tseng, C. K., Young, K. C., Sun, H. Y., Wang, S. W., Chen, W. C., et al. (2014). Andrographolide exerts anti-hepatitis C virus activity by up-regulating haeme oxygenase-1 via the p38 MAPK/Nrf2 pathway in human hepatoma cells. *Br. J. Pharmacol.* 171, 237–252. doi: 10.1111/bph.12440

Liu, Y., Sheng, J., Baggen, J., Meng, G., Xiao, C., Thibaut, H. J., et al. (2015a). Sialic acid-dependent cell entry of human enterovirus D68. *Nat. Commun.* 6:8865. doi: 10.1038/ncomms9865

Liu, Y., Sheng, J., Fokine, A., Meng, G., Shin, W. H., Long, F., et al. (2015b). Structure and inhibition of EV-D68, a virus that causes respiratory illness in children. *Science* 347, 71–74. doi: 10.1126/science.1261962

Maloney, J. A., Mirsky, D. M., Messacar, K., Dominguez, S. R., Schreiner, T., and Stence, N. V. (2015). MRI findings in children with acute flaccid paralysis and cranial nerve dysfunction occurring during the 2014 enterovirus D68 outbreak. *AJNR Am. J. Neuroradiol.* 36, 245–250. doi: 10.3174/ajnr.A4188

Mertz, D., Alawfi, A., Pernica, J. M., Rutherford, C., Luinstra, K., and Smieja, M. (2015). Clinical severity of pediatric respiratory illness with enterovirus D68 compared with rhinovirus or other enterovirus genotypes. *CMAJ* 187, 1279–1284. doi: 10.1503/cmaj.150619

Messacar, K., Abzug, M. J., and Dominguez, S. R. (2015). 2014 outbreak of enterovirus D68 in North America. *J. Med. Virol.* 88, 739–745. doi: 10.1002/jmv.24410

Messacar, K., Hawkins, S. M., Baker, J., Pearce, K., Tong, S., Dominguez, S. R., et al. (2016). Resource burden during the 2014 enterovirus D68 respiratory disease outbreak at children's hospital colorado: an unexpected strain. *JAMA Pediatr.* 170, 294–297. doi: 10.1001/jamapediatrics.2015.3879

Midgley, C. M., Jackson, M. A., Selvarangan, R., Turabelidze, G., Obringer, E., Johnson, D., et al. (2014). Severe respiratory illness associated with enterovirus D68 - Missouri and Illinois, 2014. *MMWR Morb. Mortal. Wkly. Rep.* 63, 798–799.

Midgley, C. M., Watson, J. T., Nix, W. A., Curns, A. T., Rogers, S. L., Brown, B. A., et al. (2015). Severe respiratory illness associated with a nationwide outbreak of enterovirus D68 in the USA (2014): a descriptive epidemiological investigation. *Lancet Respir. Med.* 3, 879–887. doi: 10.1016/S2213-2600(15)00335-5

Oberste, M. S., Maher, K., Schnurr, D., Flemister, M. R., Lovchik, J. C., Peters, H., et al. (2004). Enterovirus 68 is associated with respiratory illness and shares biological features with both the enteroviruses and the rhinoviruses. *J. Gen. Virol.* 85, 2577–2584. doi: 10.1099/vir.0.79925-0

Oermann, C. M., Schuster, J. E., Conners, G. P., Newland, J. G., Selvarangan, R., and Jackson, M. A. (2015). Enterovirus d68. *A focused review and clinical highlights from the* 2014 U.S. Outbreak. *Ann. Am. Thorac. Soc.* 12, 775–781. doi: 10.1513/AnnalsATS.201412-592FR

Panraksa, P., Ramphan, S., Khongwichit, S., and Smith, D. R. (2017). Activity of andrographolide against dengue virus. *Antiviral Res.* 139, 69–78. doi: 10.1016/j.antiviral.2016.12.014

Reed, L. J., and Muench, H. (1938). A simple method of estimating fifty per cent endpoints. *Am. J. Hyg.* 27, 493–497.

Reiche, J., Bottcher, S., Diedrich, S., Buchholz, U., Buda, S., Haas, W., et al. (2015). Low-level circulation of enterovirus D68-associated acute respiratory infections. Germany, 2014. *Emerg. Infect. Dis.* 21, 837–841. doi: 10.3201/eid2105.141900

Rhoden, E., Zhang, M., Nix, W. A., and Oberste, M. S. (2015). *In vitro* efficacy of antiviral compounds against enterovirus D68. *Antimicrob. Agents Chemother.* 59, 7779–7781. doi: 10.1128/AAC.00766-15

Schieble, J. H., Fox, V. L., and Lennette, E. H. (1967). A probable new human picornavirus associated with respiratory diseases. *Am. J. Epidemiol.* 85, 297–310. doi: 10.1093/oxfordjournals.aje.a120693

Sun, L., Meijer, A., Froeyen, M., Zhang, L., Thibaut, H. J., Baggen, J., et al. (2015). Antiviral activity of broad-spectrum and enterovirus-specific inhibitors against clinical isolates of enterovirus D68. *Antimicrob. Agents Chemother.* 59, 7782–7785. doi: 10.1128/AAC.01375-15

Wei, W., Guo, H., Chang, J., Yu, Y., Liu, G., Zhang, N., et al. (2016). ICAM-5/telencephalin is a functional entry receptor for enterovirus D68. *Cell Host Microbe* 20, 631–641. doi: 10.1016/j.chom.2016.09.013

Wintachai, P., Kaur, P., Lee, R. C., Ramphan, S., Kuadkitkan, A., Wikan, N., et al. (2015). Activity of andrographolide against chikungunya virus infection. *Sci. Rep.* 5:14179. doi: 10.1038/srep14179

Yu, B., Dai, C. Q., Jiang, Z. Y., Li, E. Q., Chen, C., Wu, X. L., et al. (2014). Andrographolide as an anti-H1N1 drug and the mechanism related to retinoic acid-inducible gene-I-like receptors signaling pathway. *Chin. J. Integr. Med.* 20, 540–545. doi: 10.1007/s11655-014-1860-0

Zhou, J., Hu, S. E., Tan, S. H., Cao, R., Chen, Y., Xia, D., et al. (2012). Andrographolide sensitizes cisplatin-induced apoptosis via suppression of autophagosome-lysosome fusion in human cancer cells. *Autophagy* 8, 338–349. doi: 10.4161/auto.18721

6

Topical Application of a Vitamin A Derivative and its Combination with Non-Ablative Fractional Laser Potentiates Cutaneous Influenza Vaccination

Peiyu Li[1,2,3†], Ji Wang[2,4†], Miao Cao[1], Qiwen Deng[3], Shibo Jiang[1,5], Mei X. Wu[2,6*] and Lu Lu[1*]*

[1] Key Laboratory of Medical Molecular Virology of MOE/MOH, School of Basic Medical Sciences & Shanghai Public Health Clinical Center, Fudan University, Shanghai, China, [2] Wellman Center for Photomedicine, Massachusetts General Hospital, Department of Dermatology, Harvard Medical School, Boston, MA, United States, [3] Department of Infectious Diseases and the Key Lab of Endogenous Infection, Shenzhen Nanshan People's Hospital, Guangdong Medical University, Shenzhen, China, [4] The First Affiliated Hospital of Sun Yat-sen University, Sun Yat-sen University, Guangzhou, China, [5] Lindsley F. Kimball Research Institute, New York Blood Center, New York, NY, United States, [6] Harvard-MIT Division of Health Sciences and Technology, Cambridge, MA, United States

***Correspondence:**
Shibo Jiang
shibojiang@fudan.edu.cn
Mei X. Wu
mwu5@mgh.harvard.edu
Lu Lu
lul@fudan.edu.cn

† These authors have contributed equally to this work

Skin contains a large number of antigen presenting cells, making intradermal (ID) injection one of the most effective ways for vaccine administration. However, although current adjuvants may cause severe local reactions and inflammations in the skin, no adjuvant has been approved for ID vaccination so far. Here, we report that topical application of all-*trans* retinoic acid (ATRA), a vitamin A derivative produced in the human body, augmented cutaneous influenza vaccination. The adjuvant effects were evaluated in a murine vaccination/challenge model by using A/California/07/2009 pandemic vaccine (09V) or a seasonal influenza vaccine (SIV). ATRA drove a Th2-biased immune response, as demonstrated by profoundly elevated IgG1 titer rather than IgG2 titer. Combining ATRA with a non-ablative fractional laser (NAFL), which represents a new category of vaccine adjuvant utilizing physical stimuli to induce self-immune stimulators, further enhanced the efficacy of influenza vaccines with a more balanced Th1/Th2 immune response. The dual adjuvant strengthened cross-reactive immune responses against both homogenous and heterogeneous influenza viral strains. Analysis of gene expression profile showed that ATRA/NAFL stimulated upregulation of cytosolic nucleic acid sensors and their downstream factors, leading to a synergistic elevation of type I interferon expression. Consistent with this finding, knocking out IRF3 or IRF7, two key downstream regulatory factors in most nucleic acid sensing pathways, resulted in a significant decrease in the adjuvant effect of ATRA/NAFL. Thus, our study demonstrates that the self molecule ATRA could boost cutaneous influenza vaccination either alone or ideally in combination with NAFL.

Keywords: all-*trans* retinoic acid, cutaneous adjuvant, influenza vaccine, interferon regulatory factor 3, interferon regulatory factor 7, non-ablative fractional laser, type I interferon

INTRODUCTION

Vaccination is the most effective way to prevent pathogen infections, such as influenza viruses which can cause worldwide circulation and infection with an annual infection rate estimated at 5–10% in adults and 20–30% in children[1], resulting in severe morbidity and mortality (Iuliano et al., 2018). Owing to their expansive genetic diversity, rapid antigenic drift and shift across subtypes, influenza viruses are prone to generate new subtypes continuously, a phenomenon which poses a substantial biological threat to public health (Lu et al., 2012; Uyeki et al., 2017; Petrova and Russell, 2018). Wider vaccination has been suggested to mitigate the burden of influenza-related morbidity and mortality (Monto et al., 2009; Pawelec and McElhaney, 2018; Sullivan, 2018); therefore, continuous updating is required to keep pace with the evolution of the circulating and mutated viruses (Paules et al., 2017; Xu et al., 2017). Moreover, many existing vaccines initiate weak immune responses that do not offer adequate protection against viral infections. This requires the use of safer and more effective adjuvants (McKee et al., 2007; Reed et al., 2013; He et al., 2016), especially for those influenza vaccines with low immunogenicity (Petrovsky and Aguilar, 2004; Di Pasquale et al., 2015). Most current vaccines are administered via intramuscular injection (IM). In fact, skin comprises a network of immune cells, and such network plays an important role in host defense against pathogenic invaders (Pasparakis et al., 2014). Vaccines delivered by intradermal injection (ID) are more effective than those administered by intramuscular injection (IM) based on minimizing the doses of vaccine used (dose-sparing), the significance of which is notable in the case of unanticipated vaccine shortages during influenza pandemics (Kenney et al., 2004; Hung et al., 2012; Williams, 2013). However, most adjuvants are not compatible with ID immunization strategies because they are prone to cause severe local reactions at the injection site, including erythema, swelling, and even ulcers for several weeks (Andrianov et al., 2009; Wang et al., 2016b). To date, no adjuvant has been approved for cutaneous vaccination, calling for the development of new and safe adjuvants to accompany a growing number of vaccines using novel intradermal immunization technologies like microneedle arrays (McAllister et al., 2014; Galvez-Cancino et al., 2018; Golombek et al., 2018).

All-*trans* retinoic acid (ATRA), also known as retinoic acid (RA) or vitamin A acid, is a ligand for both the retinoic acid receptor (RAR) and the retinoid X receptor (RXR), and it is the active metabolic intermediate of vitamin A in animals (Hall et al., 2011). Vitamin A and its metabolite RA are known to play important roles in the mucosal immune system, mainly in regulating T-cell homing (Johansson-Lindbom and Agace, 2004; Svensson et al., 2008; Zeng et al., 2013), priming T cell migration into the epidermis (Sigmundsdottir and Butcher, 2008) and regulating intestinal and skin dendritic cells (Raverdeau and Mills, 2014; Bakdash et al., 2015; Zeng et al., 2016). Moreover, vitamin A was shown to synergize with catechin as a vaccine adjuvant to enhance immunity (Patel et al., 2016), and RA also has an adjuvant role in a broad spectrum of biological functions, including induction of Th1 and Th2 effector T cells (Erkelens and Mebius, 2017). Additionally, vitamin A has been recognized as an essential nutrient for immune responses for nearly 100 years (Green and Mellanby, 1928; Hashimoto-Hill et al., 2017), and ATRA (Tretinoin), a medication used for the treatment of acne and photodamaged wound of skin (Cho et al., 2005), has been approved by the U.S. Food and Drug Administration (FDA) for application to the skin in the form of a cream[2]. It is easy to obtain and has been proven to be extremely safe after years of validation and application. Moreover, the RA inducible gene I (RIG- I), which can be activated and induced by ATRA, plays an important role in innate immune defense against viral infections as a sensor of viral nucleic acids (Errett and Gale, 2015). These evidences suggest that ATRA has the potential to be used as a promising cutaneous adjuvant and its adjuvant efficiency should be determined.

The laser has been recently developed as a new category of vaccine adjuvant that activates the immune system without introducing non-self molecules into human body (Chen et al., 2010, 2012, 2013; Wang et al., 2014, 2015, 2016a,b; Kashiwagi et al., 2016; Kim et al., 2016; Lopes et al., 2018). Of these vaccine adjuvants, the non-ablative fractional laser (NAFL) is very promising. The micro-sterile inflammation-induced array of self-renewable microthermal zones (MTZs) generated by NAFL will attract a large number of antigen-presenting cells at the vaccination site (Wang et al., 2014). Meanwhile, dead cells in MTZs release nucleic acid, such as dsDNA, and activated nucleic acid sensing pathways, such as the cGAS/STING pathway, to induce type I interferons (Roers et al., 2016). Although the use of NAFL adjuvant alone has significant advantages owing to its super safety, efficacy can still be improved. Therefore, it is necessary to explore a natural biological or chemical-free substance that can enhance its adjuvanticity. ATRA treatment is well known to induce many genes involving nucleic acid sensing which is the major mechanism underlying the adjuvant effect of NAFL, suggesting a possible synergy between NAFL and ATRA.

Given the safety and immune-stimulatory effects, we here evaluate the potential of topical ATRA and its combination with NAFL as a safe and effective adjuvant for cutaneous influenza vaccination. The murine vaccination/challenge model is enrolled to demonstrate the adjuvant effect of ATRA/NAFL for both pandemic and seasonal influenza vaccines (SIVs). Furthermore, the underlying molecular mechanism of ATRA/NAFL is explored by an extensive screening of related pathways. The ATRA/NAFL is demonstrated to be safe and effective with a clear mechanism involving nucleic acid-sensing pathways and type I interferons.

MATERIALS AND METHODS

Animals

Inbred C57BL/6 mice and outbred Swiss Webster female mice at 6–8 weeks of age were purchased from Charles River or

[1]http://www.who.int/mediacentre/factsheets/fs211/en/

[2]https://www.accessdata.fda.gov/scripts/cder/daf/index.cfm?event=overview.process&applno=075264

Jackson Laboratories. IRF3$^{-/-}$ and IRF7$^{-/-}$ mice on the C57BL/6J background were a kind gift of Dr. T. Taniguchi, Tokyo University (Honda et al., 2005). All mice were maintained under specific pathogen-free conditions at the animal facilities of Fudan University and Massachusetts General Hospital (MGH). All studies were approved and monitored by Fudan University and MGH Institutional Animal Care and Use Committee (IACUC).

Influenza Vaccines and Viruses

A/California/7/2009 H1N1, A/New Caledonia/20/1999 H1N1, and A/Puerto Rico/8/1934 H1N1 influenza viruses were obtained from American Type Culture Collection (ATCC) and BEI Resources. They were propagated in 10-day-old embryonated chicken eggs (Charles River Laboratories, Boston; Beijing Merial Vital Laboratory Animal Technology Co., Ltd.) at 35°C for 3 days, harvested, purified by sucrose gradient ultracentrifugation, and stored at −80°C until use. A/California/7/2009 H1N1 influenza vaccine was currently obtained from influenza viruses collected as described above after inactivation with 0.025% formalin and dialysis with PBS. Seasonal influenza vaccine (2011–2012 formulation) was purchased from GlaxoSmithKline (Research Triangle Park, NC), containing three strains, A/California/07/2009, A/Victoria/210/2009, and B/Brisbane/60/2008.

Laser Device and Adjuvants

The powder and cream of ATRA were purchased from Sigma (R2625) and Perrigo (NDC 45802-361-02), respectively. An FDA-approved, home-use, hand-held NAFL (PaloVia Skin Renewing Laser, Palomar Medical Technologies) was used as adjuvant via skin in mice. The device emits laser light in the wavelength of 1410 nm, and 2 hits at high power were used at the inoculation site in the skin before vaccination to create an array of self-healing microthermal zones (MTZs).

Mice Immunization and Challenge Procedures

6–8-week-old C57BL/6, Swiss Webster, IRF3$^{-/-}$ and IRF7$^{-/-}$ knockout mice were anesthetized intraperitoneally (IP) with 100 mg/kg ketamine and 10 mg/kg xylazine. The hair on the back of mice was removed and illuminated with NAFL on the lower back of the skin on the next day before the vaccine was ID immunized with a 20 μl dose, including 300 ng A/California/7/2009 H1N1 vaccine or 5 μl SIV at 6–8 weeks. After ID immunization, the inoculation site was either left alone or topically applied with ATRA cream (Perrigo), and then the site was covered with Tegaderm film (3M) for 4 h. Mice were challenged with a dose of 20 μl 10 × LD50 A/California/7/2009 H1N1 virus 2 weeks post-immunization of A/California/7/2009 H1N1 vaccine, and the survival rate was monitored for 2 weeks.

Blood Collection and ELISA Assays

Blood was collected by retro-orbital sinus 2 weeks post-immunization, and serum was separated by centrifuge after clotting for 1–2 h at room temperature. Influenza virus-specific antibodies were determined by ELISA. Briefly, A/California/7/2009 H1N1 vaccine or influenza seasonal vaccine was coated on 96-well plates and blocked by 5% skimmed milk. Serum was diluted by 1:100 and then diluted by fourfold, incubated for 2 h at room temperature. After washing, anti-mouse IgG (NA931V, GE Healthcare, dilution 1:6000), IgG1 (1073-05, Southern Biotech, 1:4000), IgG2a (61-0220, Life Technologies, dilution 1:2000), IgG2c (1079-05, Southern Biotech, 1:5000) were added with HRP-conjugated Streptavidin into plates for 1 h. One SIGMAFAST^{TM} OPD (o-Phenylenediamine dihydrochloride) tablet and one urea hydrogen peroxide/buffer tablet (P9187-50set, Sigma) were dissolved in 20 ml of water to prepare the reaction buffer, and 50 μl buffer was added into each well for reaction. Fifteen minutes later, the reaction was stopped by 50 μl 2M H_2SO_4. The optical density is A490.

Hemagglutination Inhibition (HAI) Assay

Hemagglutination is the process by which influenza virus (and other viruses) causes red blood cells to agglutinate. In short, serum samples were treated with receptor-destroying enzyme (RDE) (Denka Seiken) for 18–24 h at 37°C, followed by treatment at 56°C for 30 min to remove complement and inactivate RDE. The resultant serum samples were serially diluted and incubated with 4 hemagglutination units (HAU) of influenza virus A/California/7/2009 H1N1, A/New Caledonia/20/1999 H1N1 or A/Puerto Rico/8/34 H1N1 for 30 min at room temperature. Then the mixture was incubated with 0.5% chicken red blood cells (Lampire Biological Laboratories) at room temperature for 30 min. The HAI titer was defined as the reciprocal of the highest serum dilution that inhibited 4 HAU.

Histological Examination

Mice were treated with ATRA, NAFL, ATRA/NAFL for 24 h. The inoculation sites were photographed after 24 h treatment. The skin at the inoculation site was dissected 24 h after treatment, fixed, and stained by a standard H&E procedure.

mRNA Expression Level at Skin Inoculation Site

The lower dorsal skin of C57BL/6 mice was treated by ATRA adjuvant, NAFL adjuvant, and ATRA/NAFL adjuvant, respectively. Twenty-four hours later, the skin at the inoculation site was isolated, excised, and total RNA was extracted by the RNeasy Mini Kit (Qiagen). The cDNA was synthesized by using the High Capacity RNA-to-cDNA Kit (Applied Biosystems). The mRNA expression level was amplified and determined by real-time PCR using an SYBR Green PCR Kit (Roche). Glyceraldehyde 3-phosphate dehydrogenase (GAPDH) was used as an internal control. A heat map diagram of the genes of interest was illustrated with HemI software. See **Table 1** for primer sequences of all genes.

TABLE 1 | Primers for qPCR analysis.

Gene	Forward primer	Reverse primer
Aim2	ACGTTGTTAAGAGAGCCAGGG	AGCACCAACACCTCCATTGT
Cgas	GGAAGCCCTGCTGTAACACT	CCAGCCAGCCTTGAATAGGT
Cxcl-10	CCAAGTGCTGCCGTCATTTTC	TCCCTATGGCCCTCATTCTCA
Ddx41	CTCTCGCTTGGAGAAAGGCA	CCTACCATTCTGTCCGGTCG
Dhx9	TTGAAATTGTGCCCCCACCT	GTGACCAAGGAACCACTCCC
Gapdh	*ATCAAGAAGGTGGTGAAGCA*	AGACAACCTGGTCCTCAGTGT
Ifnb1	CAGCTCCAAGAAAGGACGAAC	GGCAGTGTAACTCTTCTGCAT
Irf1	CCAGCTCTTGCTTTCGGACG	TCGAGTGATTGGCATGGTGG
Irf3	AACCGGAAAGAAGTGTTGCG	CCCTGGAGTCACAAACTCATAC
Irf7	TCCAGTTGATCCGCATAAGGT	CTTCCCTATTTTCCGTGGCTG
Ku70	CACCAAGCGGTCTCTGACTT	AGAGAGGGCCTCAGGTAGTG
Mavs	CTGCCTCACAGCTAGTGACC	CCGGCGCTGGAGATTATTG
Mre11	CGGTCAATGTCGGTGGAGAA	CCTAAGCCGTACAGAGCGAG
Myd88	AGGACAAACGCCGGAACTTTT	GCCGATAGTCTGTCTGTTCTAT
Pol III	TGGCTTGCGACTTGGAGAAA	GTAGTGGCACCAGCCAGAAT
Rig-I	CCACCTACATCCTCAGCTACATGA	TGGGCCCTTGTTGTTCTTCT
Sting	TCTCCTGTCTAACCCCTCCC	GGATTTCCAGAGGCCCCAAA
Tbk1	*GTACGGCACAGAAGAGTACCT*	ATGGTAGAATGTCACTCCAACAC
Tnf-α	CCTGTAGCCCACGTCGTAG	GGGAGTAGACAAGGTACAACCC
Traf3	CGTGCCGACTGCAAAGAAAA	TTGATCATGGGCACTTGGCT
Zbp1	TACCGCCTGAAGAAGGAGGA	TTCTCAGGGATTGCAGGAGC

Statistical Analysis

A two-tailed *t*-test (*t*-test) was used to analyze the difference between two groups. One-way ANOVA was used among multiple groups involving one factor, and two-way ANOVA was used to analyze experiments involving two factors each with multiple groups. Percentages of survival were analyzed by log-rank test. *P*-value was calculated by PRISM software (GraphPad), and the difference was considered significant if the *p*-value was less than 0.05.

RESULTS

The Adjuvant Effect of ATRA/NAFL for Pandemic Influenza Vaccine

To determine the individual effect of ATRA and NAFL, respectively, and the synergistic effect of ATRA/NAFL in augmenting the efficacy of influenza vaccines, C57BL/6 mice were first treated with or without NAFL following by injection of A/California/7/2009 H1N1 pandemic influenza vaccine and topical application of ATRA ointment or PBS at the inoculation site (**Figure 1A**). As shown in the figures (**Figures 1B–D**), influenza vaccine with ATRA alone significantly elevated the vaccine-specific IgG and IgG1 titers, which is roughly equal to the titers lifted by NAFL alone, but not IgG2c, suggesting that ATRA chiefly induces Th2-dominated immune responses. NAFL significantly enhanced the efficacy of 2009 vaccine with both influenza-specific IgG1 and IgG2c antibody titers elevated (**Figures 1C,D**), consistent with our previous report (Wang et al., 2014). Although ATRA or NAFL alone can promote vaccine immunization, the promotion needs to be further strengthened. Surprisingly, ATRA/NAFL combination augmented influenza-specific IgG, IgG1, and IgG2c antibody titers. Particularly, ATRA/NAFL combination significantly enhanced the higher IgG2c antibody titers than either ATRA or NAFL alone, being considered as promoting Th1 immune response (**Figure 1D**).

Next, the immunized mice were challenged by a mouse-adapted A/California/7/2009 H1N1 viruses 2 weeks post-vaccination. The survival curve (**Figure 1E**) displayed that all mice in 2009 vaccine alone group died. While vaccination with ATRA or NAFL alone slightly elevated the survival rate, only ATRA/NAFL combination achieved significant protection (**Figure 1E**). These results proved that the combination of ATRA and NAFL synergistically enhanced immune responses induced by the pandemic influenza vaccine.

The Safety of ATRA/NAFL in Mice

The safety of ATRA/NAFL in cutaneous vaccination was next evaluated. ATRA, NAFL, ATRA/NAFL were applied onto the skin for 24 h. As shown in **Figure 2A**, NAFL treatment only induced slight skin swelling which quickly dissipated in 10 min without causing any erythema or other obverse local reactions. On the other hand, ATRA treatment did not induce any observable skin irritations either. Encouragingly, the combination of ATRA and NAFL was comparable with NAFL treatment alone in terms of local reactogenicity. The safety of the combination was further confirmed by histological examination, in which neither infiltration of inflammatory cells nor morphology change of epidermis and dermis was found in the skin 24 h after adjuvants treatment (**Figure 2B**).

The Adjuvant Effect of ATRA/NAFL for Seasonal Influenza Vaccine

Next, the adjuvant effect of ATRA and ATRA/NAFL was also explored in SIVs. As shown in **Figure 3A**, although both ATRA and NAFL slightly increased IgG titers by twofold, only the ATRA/NAFL combination showed a significant adjuvant effect and elevated IgG titers by tenfold. Consistent with the result of pandemic influenza vaccine, ATRA mainly enhanced Th2 immune responses, but not Th1, as indicated by elevated IgG1 titers (**Figures 3B,C**). On the other hand, the ATRA/NAFL combination greatly enhanced both Th1 and Th2 immune responses by sixfold or eightfold, respectively, compared to vaccine alone (**Figures 3B,C**), but also significantly enhanced the higher IgG1 titer over NAFL adjuvant (**Figure 3B**). Sera were next measured for hemagglutination inhibition (HAI) titer, a standard criterion of influenza vaccination, in which a serum HAI titer greater than, or equal to, 1:40 is considered protective. The protective immune responses were subsequently assessed by measuring HAI titer against both homogeneous and heterogeneous H1N1 strains. Strikingly, ATRA/NAFL greatly elevated HAI titers in an immunization condition (**Figure 3D**). Moreover, antibodies induced by vaccination in the presence of ATRA/NAFL significantly inhibited the binding of not only a homogeneous viral stain contained in

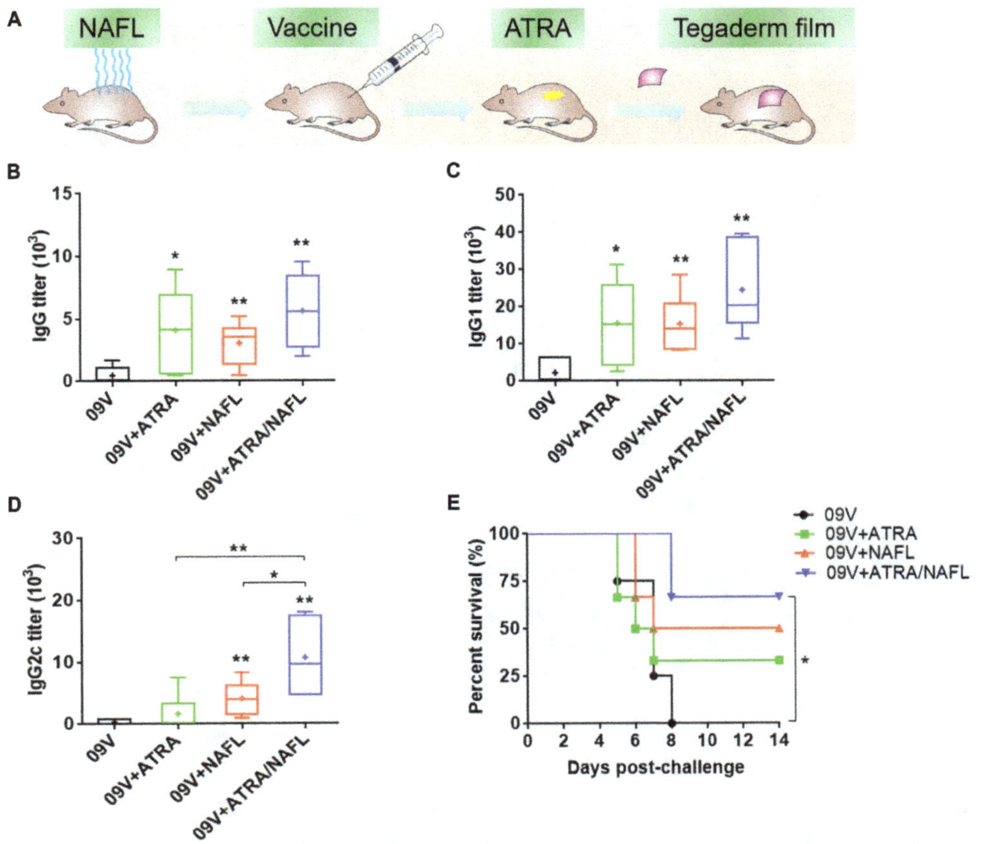

FIGURE 1 | NAFL and ATRA enhanced protective immunity on pandemic 2009 H1N1 vaccine in C57BL/6 mice. 300 ng A/California/7/2009 H1N1 vaccine (HA content) was immunized i.d. alone or with adjuvant ATRA, NAFL (2 hits, high) or ATRA/NAFL (2 hits, high) as illustrated in **(A)**, and then vaccine-specific antibody titer for **(B)** IgG, **(C)** IgG1 and **(D)** IgG2c was determined 2 weeks post-immunization. Data are presented as box and whiskers plots, in which whiskers are min-to-max. Three lines of the box are the 25th percentile, the median, and the 75th percentile, respectively. Mean is shown as " + ". The immunized mice alone or with different adjuvants were intranasally challenged with 10 × LD50 of A/California/7/2009 H1N1 virus 2 weeks post- immunization, and **(E)** survival rate of the challenged mice was monitored every day for 2 weeks. $N = 6$. $^*P < 0.05$ or $^{**}P < 0.01$, respectively.

the vaccine formulation, A/California/7/2009 H1N1, but also heterogeneous viral strains, A/New Caledonia/20/1999 H1N1 and A/Puerto Rico/8/1934 H1N1 (**Figures 3E,F**). These results further confirmed the synergistic adjuvant effect of ATRA and NAFL.

The Mechanism Underlying Synergistic Adjuvant Effects of ATRA and NAFL

To investigate the underlying mechanisms of synergistic adjuvant effects of ATRA/NAFL, we determined the expression level of genes like dsDNA sensors and downstream genes at the skin inoculation site. The expression level of a cluster of genes was detected, including nucleic acid sensing signal system and cytokines possibly associated with ATRA and NAFL. The gene expression profile was summarized as a heat map and histograms (**Figure 4**). ATRA/NAFL synergistically upregulated two key adaptors for innate immunity signaling: MyD88 (**Figures 4A,B**) and IRF3/IRF7 (**Figures 4A,C,D**). However, a profound upregulation of IFN-β, but not TNF-α (**Figures 4A,E**), indicates that IRF3/IRF7 is the key pathway involved in the adjuvant effect of ATRA/NAFL. ATRA treatment alone did not contribute to the induction of IFN-β but upregulated a number of nucleic acid sensors, including cGAS, MRE11, Pol III, and DDX41 (**Figures 4A,F,G**). On the other hand, NAFL treatment contributed directly to the activation of IFN-β induction pathways (**Figures 4A,C,D**). As a result, the combination of NAFL and ATRA synergistically upregulated cGAS, MRE11, DDX41, STING, TRAF3, TBK1, IRF3, and IRF7, leading to a profound elevation of IFN-β (**Figures 4A,C–I**).

To further confirm the crucial role of the nucleic acid sensing pathway in the adjuvant of ATRA/NAFL, IRF3 and IRF7 knockout mice were enrolled since they are common downstream adaptors in nearly all known type I interferon-producing nucleic acid sensing pathways. The SIV, including adjuvants, was immunized under the same conditions as those described above in wild-type C57BL/6 mice, IRF3$^{-/-}$ and IRF7$^{-/-}$ mice. Vaccine-specific antibody IgG (**Figure 5A**), IgG1 (**Figure 5B**) and IgG2c (**Figure 5C**) titers were determined 2 weeks post-immunization. In wild-type C57BL/6 mice, the NAFL group enhanced the titers of vaccine-specific antibodies IgG, IgG1 and IgG2c compared to the vaccine group, while the

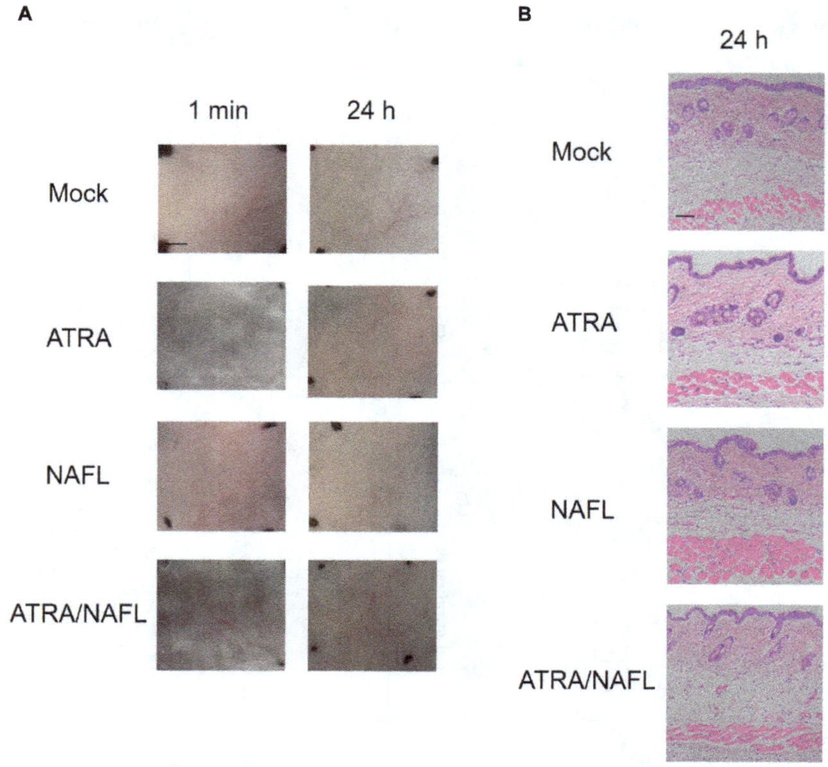

FIGURE 2 | Histology examination of NAFL/ATRA treated skin. Mice were treated with ATRA, NAFL, ATRA/NAFL, respectively. Then the ATRA-treated site was covered with Tegaderm film (3 M) for 4 h. **(A)** Photos were taken at indicated time points, and representative photos are shown with four mice in each group. Scale bar, 0.5 cm. **(B)** Representative hematoxylin and eosin-stained sections of the inoculation site 24 h post-treatment. Scale bar, 200 μm.

ATRA/NAFL group further elevated the titer of all antibodies in agreement with previous results. A significant decrease of total IgG generated by NAFL and NAFL/ATRA vaccination was noticed in both knockout mice **(Figure 5A)**. Furthermore, the adjuvant effects of ATRA/NAFL on Th1 and Th2 immune responses were significantly reduced when the nucleic acid sensing pathway was not intact, as indicated by the inability of ATRA/NAFL to augment IgG1 and IgG2c titers **(Figures 5B,C)**.

DISCUSSION

Influenza virus has a high mutation rate, and the emergence of a novel pandemic is unpredictable (Xu et al., 2013; Medina, 2018; Xie et al., 2018). Once a pandemic occurs, it will pose a great threat to human life and health. For example, in March 2009, a new swine-origin influenza, A (H1N1) pdm09, emerged in the United States, which then spread worldwide to 30 countries by human-to-human transmission in just 2 months, causing large numbers of deaths (Smith et al., 2009). During pandemics, it is common to see vaccine supplies dwindle, and developed countries receive vaccines much earlier than less developed countries (Kumar et al., 2012). We know that dose-sparing of influenza vaccine can be achieved by ID injection, calling for an adjuvant able to work for a pandemic vaccine via ID immunization (Kenney et al., 2004; Hung et al., 2012). In this study, we found that the topical application of ATRA primarily enhanced cutaneous influenza vaccination, especially via a Th2-biased immune response compared to the predominantly Th1 immune response initiated by NAFL. The combination of ATRA and NAFL synergistically balanced the Th1/Th2 immune responses and significantly strengthened the efficacy of both pandemic and SIVs.

Safety is the most important factor in vaccine development, and it cannot be ignored in the development of adjuvants, especially for intradermal immunization with higher adjuvant safety requirements. ATRA cream has been used clinically for many years, and NAFL has also been approved by the FDA for commercial use; thus, the safety of each has been widely recognized. Vitamin A has a reparative effect on skin wound caused by light damage. Therefore, it can provide a layer of bio-natural protective film for rapid protection of the laser-induced sterile inflammation microenvironment. Accordingly, the ATRA/NAFL combination does not introduce foreign chemicals to the body or cause damage to the outer surface of the skin. Furthermore, ATRA/NAFL activates the immune system without introducing any non-self molecules into the skin, and as such, it could be considered as an "all-natural" vaccine adjuvant, warranting a high level of safety.

Non-ablative fractional laser has been previously demonstrated to enhance vaccination efficacy by inducing

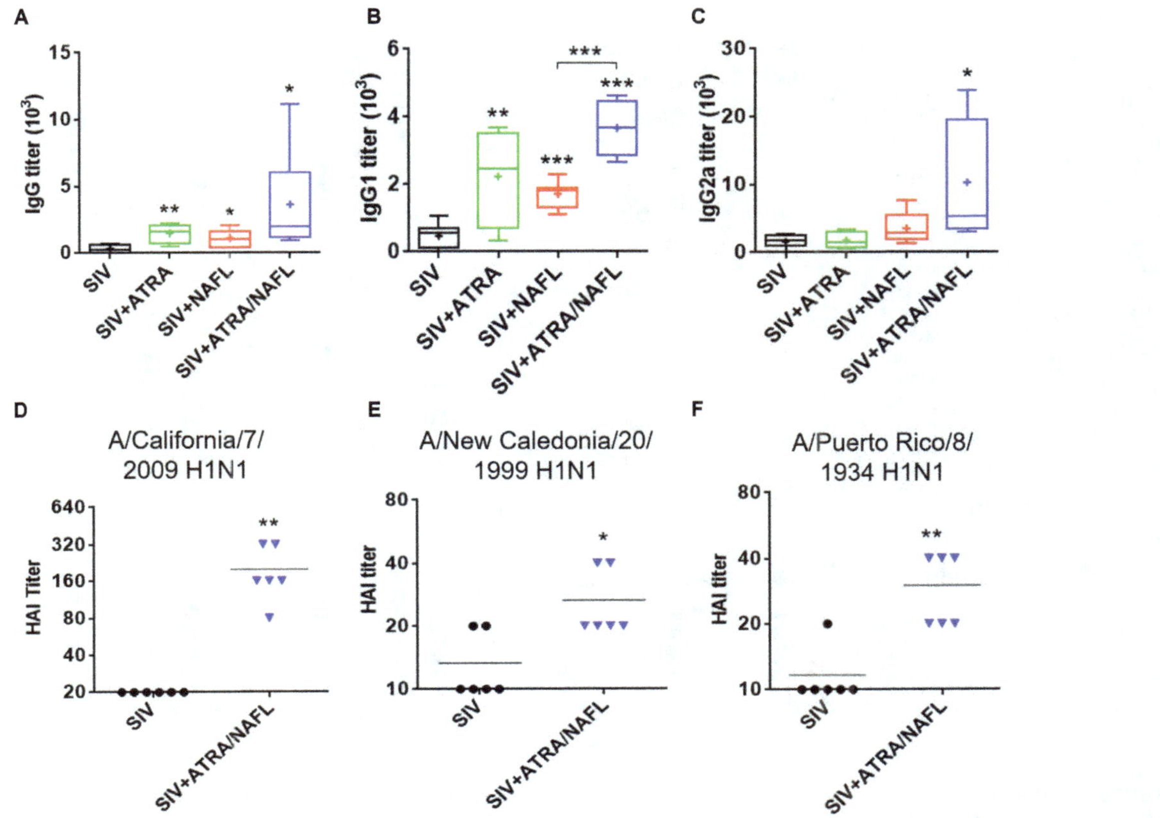

FIGURE 3 | ATRA and NAFL enhanced immune responses of seasonal influenza vaccine (SIV). 5 μl SIV was immunized i.d. alone or with adjuvant ATRA, NAFL (2 hits, high) or ATRA/NAFL (2 hits, high) in 6- to 8-week-old female Swiss Webster (SW) mice, and vaccine-specific antibody titer for **(A)** IgG, **(B)** IgG1 and **(C)** IgG2a was determined 2 weeks post-immunization. $N = 7$, except for the SIV + ATRA group ($N = 4$). Data are presented as box and whiskers plots, in which whiskers are min-to-max. Three lines of the box are the 25th percentile, the median, and the 75th percentile, respectively. Mean is shown as " + ". HAI titers of sera were determined by HAI assays against **(D)** A/California/7/2009 H1N1, **(E)** A/New Caledonia/20/1999 H1N1 and **(F)** A/Puerto Rico/8/1934 H1N1 influenza viruses 2 weeks post-immunization. Data are represented as mean. $N = 6$. Each symbol represents data from individual mice, and horizontal bars indicate mean. $^{*}P < 0.05$, $^{**}P < 0.01$ or $^{***}P < 0.001$, respectively.

cell death and damage-associated molecular patterns (DAMPs), as noted above, particularly dsDNA (Wang et al., 2014, 2015). In the current study, we found that ATRA treatment synergistically strengthened dsDNA sensing and promoted the production of type I interferon in the skin. DAMPs are components of host cells released during cell damage or death. DAMPs initiate innate immune responses in the absence of infection, also called sterile inflammation. Sensing of cytosolic nucleic acids is a major mechanism by which the innate immune system detects foreign pathogens and cellular damage (Cai et al., 2014; Vance, 2016). To date, many cytosolic receptors of nucleic acids have been identified, and these are depicted in **Figure 6**. Among these receptors, cyclic GMP-AMP (cGAMP) synthase (cGAS) is a major cytosolic dsDNA sensor which triggers innate immune responses via the synthesis of the second messenger cGAMP. Subsequently, cGAMP binds to STING and recruits the downstream IFN-inducing proteins TBK1 and IRF3 (Burdette and Vance, 2013; Tsuchiya et al., 2016). Initial IFN-β signaling could trigger an autocrine loop that upregulates IRF7 and produces more type I interferons. Indeed, the adjuvant effect of NAFL depends on STING, IRF3, and IRF7, as further confirmed by the current study. ATRA is well known to induce the expression of RIG-I (Liu et al., 2000) which is responsible for dsRNA sensing involving TANK binding kinase-1 (TBK1) and IκB kinase epsilon (IKKε) to promote the expression of type I and type III interferons through phosphorylation of IRF3 and IRF7 (Belgnaoui et al., 2011). Our study revealed that ATRA treatment not only induce RIG-I, which is in accordance with the previous studies (Balmer and Blomhoff, 2002) but also induce other nucleic acid sensors, especially cGAS, which upregulates the expression of STING, TBK1, TRAF3, IRF3, and IRF7, resulting in elevated IFN-β expression (**Figure 6**). Based on these results, we proposed a working mechanism of ATRA/NAFL such that NAFL provides the initial source, or dsDNA, to trigger nucleic acid sensing pathways, and ATRA treatment, or the combination, increases the number of key sensors and downstream factors to support a vigorous activation and production of type I interferons. ATRA/NAFL stimulates the induction and activation of pathways associated with RIG-I and STING, as discussed in many other reports in the literature, confirming that these two

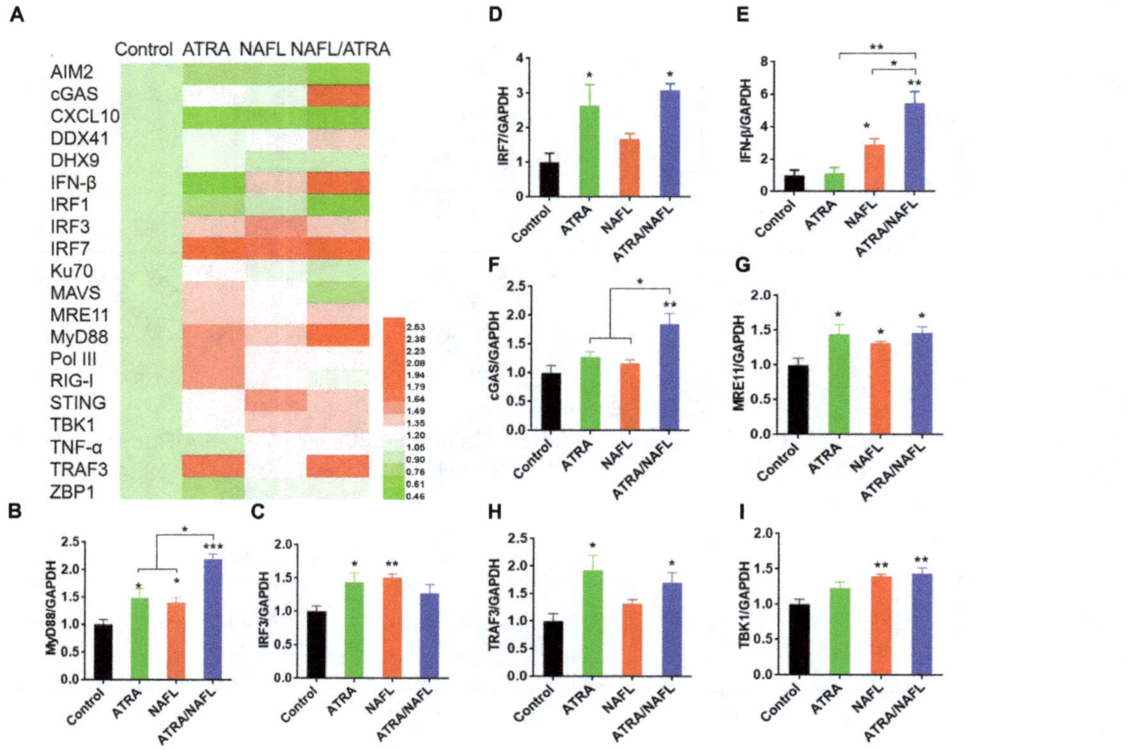

FIGURE 4 | RNA expression level of skin at the inoculation site post-treatment of adjuvants. The lower dorsal back skin of C57BL/6 mice was exposed with ATRA, NAFL (high, 2 hits) and ATRA/NAFL for 24 h; then the skin was isolated, and RNA was extracted for qRT-PCR. **(A)** Heat map diagram of gene expression level of skin inoculation site. Changes in expression levels are displayed from green (downregulation) to red (upregulation), as shown in the color gradient at the bottom right corner. Rows indicate different genes and the columns represent samples post-treatment of ATRA, NAFL, ATRA/NAFL. Averages of replicates of different groups were shown. The heat map was illustrated using Heml 1.0 software. The mRNA expression level of **(B)** MyD88, **(C)** IRF3, **(D)** IRF7, **(E)** IFN-β, **(F)** cGAS, **(G)** MRE11, **(H)**, TRAF3 and **(I)** TBK1. $N = 4$. Data are presented as mean ± s.e.m. $^*P < 0.05$; $^{**}P < 0.01$ or $^{***}P < 0.001$, respectively.

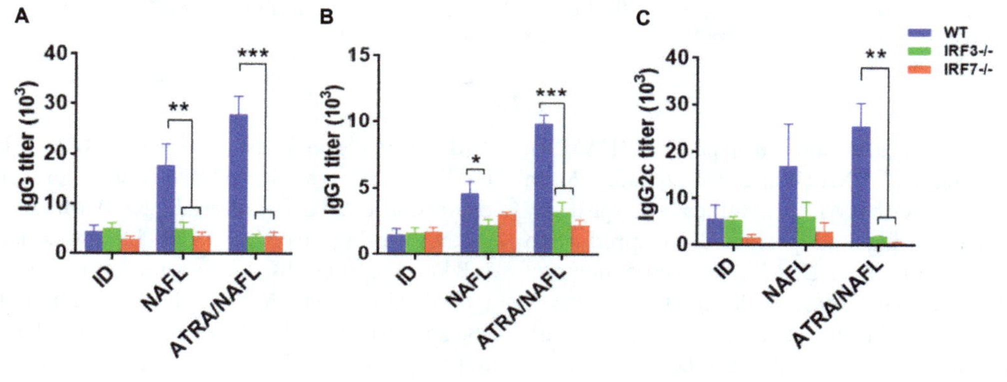

FIGURE 5 | IRF3 and IRF7 play an important role in enhancing the humoral immunity of ATRA and NAFL. 5 μl SIV were immunized i.d. alone or with adjuvant ATRA or combined with NAFL (2 hits, high) in wild-type C57BL/6 mice, $IRF3^{-/-}$ and $IRF7^{-/-}$ knockout mice, and vaccine-specific antibody titer for **(A)** IgG, **(B)** IgG1 and **(C)** IgG2c were determined 2 weeks post-immunization. $N = 4$. Data are presented as mean ± s.e.m. $^*P < 0.05$; $^{**}P < 0.01$ or $^{***}P < 0.001$, respectively.

pathways are, to a certain extent, interrelated and may play an important role in immunity (Fischer et al., 2017; Zevini et al., 2017).

Our immunization experiments with IRF3 and IRF7 knockout mice also supported the conclusion that ATRA/NAFL's adjuvanticity depends on the generation of type I interferon. Type I interferons can serve as molecular adjuvants by driving the maturation and migration of antigen presenting cells and supporting T- and B-cell survival, activation and differentiation (Tailor et al., 2006; Xu et al., 2014). Given the clear mode of action, our study raises the possibility that ATRA/NAFL could serve as a safe and effective adjuvant for skin vaccination for different types of influenza vaccines, including pandemic and SIVs. These studies shed light on the contribution of ATRA in

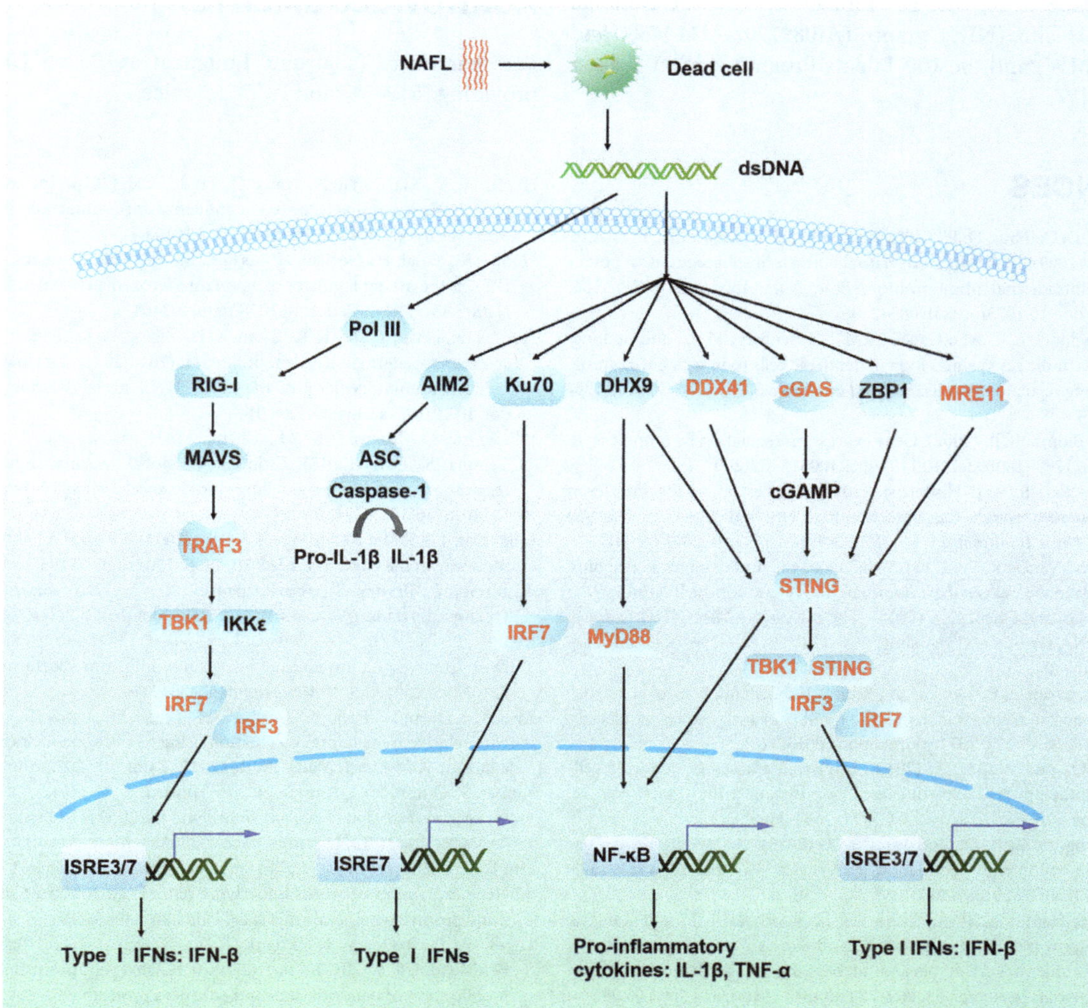

FIGURE 6 | Schematic illustration of nucleic acid recognition and interferon production mechanism of ATRA/NAFL. Dead cells generated by NAFL or ATRA/NAFL released nucleic acid-like dsDNA in the cytoplasm which is sensed by many sensors leading to the production of type I IFNs via adaptors MAVS, STING, and transcriptional factors IRF3 and IRF7. Most DNA sensors like DHX9, DDX41, cGAS, ZBP1, and MRE11 are believed to activate STING, recruit TBK1 to phosphorylate IRF3/IRF7, and then dimerize and enter the nucleus, resulting in the production of type I IFNs. Pol III transcribes dsDNA to synthesize RNA, which is sensed by RIG-I, while RIG-I can be induced and activated by ATRA. RIG-I recruits TRAF3 via MAVS to trigger the activation of the downstream kinases TBK1 and IKKε and then phosphorylates IRF3 and IRF7, which homodimerize and enter the nucleus to induce the production of type I IFNs. Genes upregulated by ATRA/NAFL are shown in the bold red font. Abbreviations: AIM2, absent in melanoma 2; ASC, PYD and CARD domain containing (PYCARD); cGAMP, 2′3′ guanosine–adenosine monophosphate; cGAS, cyclic GMP–AMP synthase; DDX41, DEAD-box helicase 41; DHX9, DExH-box helicase 9; IFN-β, interferon beta; IKKε, IkB kinase epsilon; IL-1β, interleukin 1 beta; IRF3, interferon regulatory factor 3; IRF7, interferon regulatory factor 7; ISRE, interferon-sensitive response element; Ku70, Lupus Ku autoantigen protein p70; MAVS, mitochondrial antiviral-signaling protein; MRE11, meiotic recombination 11 homolog A; MyD88, myeloid differentiation primary response 88; NF-κB, nuclear factor kappa light chain enhancer of activated B cells; Pol III, RNA polymerase III; RIG-I, RA inducible gene-I; STING, stimulator of interferon genes; TBK1, TANK binding kinase 1; TNF-α, Tumor necrosis factor alpha; TRAF3, TNF receptor associated factor 3; ZBP1, Z-DNA binding protein 1.

strengthening the nucleic acid sensing pathway, inspiring the combinatorial use of ATRA with other immune stimulatory molecules which activate this pathway. As a micro-sterile inflammation array-based adjuvant, ATRA/NAFL merits further studies as a cutaneous adjuvant for various vaccines.

AUTHOR CONTRIBUTIONS

MW, LL, and SJ conceived and designed the experiments. PL, JW, and MC performed the experiments. PL, JW, QD, LL, MW, and SJ analyzed the data and wrote the manuscript.

FUNDING

This work was supported by the National Megaprojects of China for Major Infectious Diseases (2018ZX10301403 to LL), National Natural Science Foundation of China (81630090 to SJ and 81661128041, 81672019 to LL), the National Key Research and Development Program of China (2016YFC1201000 and

2016YFC1200405 to SJ, 2016YFC1202901 to LL), the National Institutes of Health (NIH) grants (AI089779, AI114458, and AI135233 to MW) and the 100 Talents Program of Sun Yat-sen University to JW.

ACKNOWLEDGMENTS

We thank Dr. Tadatsugu Taniguchi at Tokyo University for providing IRF3$^{-/-}$ and IRF7$^{-/-}$ mice.

REFERENCES

Andrianov, A. K., DeCollibus, D. P., Gillis, H. A., Kha, H. H., Marin, A., Prausnitz, M. R., et al. (2009). Poly[di(carboxylatophenoxy)phosphazene] is a potent adjuvant for intradermal immunization. *Proc. Natl. Acad. Sci. U.S.A.* 106, 18936–18941. doi: 10.1073/pnas.0908842106

Bakdash, G., Vogelpoel, L. T., van Capel, T. M., Kapsenberg, M. L., and de Jong, E. C. (2015). Retinoic acid primes human dendritic cells to induce gut-homing, IL-10-producing regulatory T cells. *Mucosal Immunol.* 8, 265–278. doi: 10.1038/mi.2014.64

Balmer, J. E., and Blomhoff, R. (2002). Gene expression regulation by retinoic acid. *J. Lipid Res.* 43, 1773–1808. doi: 10.1194/jlr.R100015-JLR200

Belgnaoui, S. M., Paz, S., and Hiscott, J. (2011). Orchestrating the interferon antiviral response through the mitochondrial antiviral signaling (MAVS) adapter. *Curr. Opin. Immunol.* 23, 564–572. doi: 10.1016/j.coi.2011.08.001

Burdette, D. L., and Vance, R. E. (2013). STING and the innate immune response to nucleic acids in the cytosol. *Nat. Immunol.* 14, 19–26. doi: 10.1038/ni.2491

Cai, X., Chiu, Y. H., and Chen, Z. J. (2014). The cGAS-cGAMP-STING pathway of cytosolic DNA sensing and signaling. *Mol. Cell.* 54, 289–296. doi: 10.1016/j.molcel.2014.03.040

Chen, X., Kim, P., Farinelli, B., Doukas, A., Yun, S. H., Gelfand, J. A., et al. (2010). A novel laser vaccine adjuvant increases the motility of antigen presenting cells. *PLoS One* 5:e13776. doi: 10.1371/journal.pone.0013776

Chen, X., Zeng, Q., and Wu, M. X. (2012). Improved efficacy of dendritic cell-based immunotherapy by cutaneous laser illumination. *Clin. Cancer Res.* 18, 2240–2249. doi: 10.1158/1078-0432.CCR-11-2654

Chen, X. Y., Wang, J., Shah, D., and Wu, M. X. (2013). An update on the use of laser technology in skin vaccination. *Expert Rev. Vaccines* 12, 1313–1323. doi: 10.1586/14760584.2013.844070

Cho, S., Lowe, L., Hamilton, T. A., Fisher, G. J., Voorhees, J. J., and Kang, S. (2005). Long-term treatment of photoaged human skin with topical retinoic acid improves epidermal cell atypia and thickens the collagen band in papillary dermis. *J. Am. Acad. Dermatol.* 53, 769–774. doi: 10.1016/j.jaad.2005.06.052

Di Pasquale, A., Preiss, S., Tavares Da Silva, F., and Garcon, N. (2015). Vaccine adjuvants: from 1920 to 2015 and beyond. *Vaccines* 3, 320–343. doi: 10.3390/vaccines3020320

Erkelens, M. N., and Mebius, R. E. (2017). Retinoic acid and immune homeostasis: a balancing act. *Trends Immunol.* 38, 168–180. doi: 10.1016/j.it.2016.12.006

Errett, J. S., and Gale, M. (2015). Emerging complexity and new roles for the RIG-I-like receptors in innate antiviral immunity. *Virol. Sin.* 30, 163–173. doi: 10.1007/s12250-015-3604-5

Fischer, J. C., Bscheider, M., Eisenkolb, G., Lin, C. C., Wintges, A., Otten, V., et al. (2017). RIG-I/MAVS and STING signaling promote gut integrity during irradiation- and immune-mediated tissue injury. *Sci. Transl. Med.* 9:eaag2513. doi: 10.1126/scitranslmed.aag2513

Galvez-Cancino, F., Lopez, E., Menares, E., Diaz, X., Flores, C., Caceres, P., et al. (2018). Vaccination-induced skin-resident memory CD8 + T cells mediate strong protection against cutaneous melanoma. *Oncoimmunology* 7:e1442163. doi: 10.1080/2162402X.2018.1442163

Golombek, S., Pilz, M., Steinle, H., Kochba, E., Levin, Y., Lunter, D., et al. (2018). Intradermal delivery of synthetic mRNA using hollow microneedles for efficient and rapid production of exogenous proteins in skin. *Mol. Ther. Nucl. Acids* 11, 382–392. doi: 10.1016/j.omtn.2018.03.005

Green, H. N., and Mellanby, E. (1928). Vitamin A as an anti-infective agent. *Br. Med. J.* 2, 691–696. doi: 10.1136/bmj.2.3537.691

Hall, J. A., Grainger, J. R., Spencer, S. P., and Belkaid, Y. (2011). The role of retinoic acid in tolerance and immunity. *Immunity* 35, 13–22. doi: 10.1016/j.immuni.2011.07.002

Hashimoto-Hill, S., Friesen, L., Kim, M., and Kim, C. H. (2017). Contraction of intestinal effector T cells by retinoic acid-induced purinergic receptor P2X7. *Mucosal Immunol.* 10, 912–923. doi: 10.1038/mi.2016.109

He, B., Fu, Y., Xia, S., Yu, F., Wang, Q., Lu, L., et al. (2016). Intranasal application of polyethyleneimine suppresses influenza virus infection in mice. *Emerg. Microbes Infect.* 5:e41. doi: 10.1038/emi.2016.64

Honda, K., Yanai, H., Negishi, H., Asagiri, M., Sato, M., Mizutani, T., et al. (2005). IRF-7 is the master regulator of type-I interferon-dependent immune responses. *Nature* 434, 772–777. doi: 10.1038/nature03464

Hung, I. F., Levin, Y., To, K. K., Chan, K. H., Zhang, A. J., Li, P., et al. (2012). Dose sparing intradermal trivalent influenza (2010/2011) vaccination overcomes reduced immunogenicity of the 2009 H1N1 strain. *Vaccine* 30, 6427–6435. doi: 10.1016/j.vaccine.2012.08.014

Iuliano, A. D., Roguski, K. M., Chang, H. H., Muscatello, D. J., Palekar, R., Tempia, S., et al. (2018). Estimates of global seasonal influenza-associated respiratory mortality: a modelling study. *Lancet* 391, 1285–1300. doi: 10.1016/S0140-6736(17)33293-2

Johansson-Lindbom, B., and Agace, W. W. (2004). Vitamin A helps gut T cells find their way in the dark. *Nat. Med.* 10, 1300–1301. doi: 10.1038/nm1204-1300

Kashiwagi, S., Brauns, T., and Poznansky, M. C. (2016). Classification of laser vaccine adjuvants. *J Vaccines Vaccin.* 7:307. doi: 10.4172/2157-7560.1000307

Kenney, R. T., Frech, S. A., Muenz, L. R., Villar, C. P., and Glenn, G. M. (2004). Dose sparing with intradermal injection of influenza vaccine. *N. Engl. J. Med.* 351, 2295–2301. doi: 10.1056/Nejmoa043540

Kim, K. S., Kim, H., Park, Y., Kong, W. H., Lee, S. W., Kwok, S. J. J., et al. (2016). Noninvasive transdermal vaccination using hyaluronan nanocarriers and laser adjuvant. *Adv. Funct. Mater.* 26, 2512–2522. doi: 10.1002/adfm.201504879

Kumar, S., Quinn, S. C., Kim, K. H., and Hilyard, K. M. (2012). US public support for vaccine donation to poorer countries in the 2009 H1N1 pandemic. *PLoS One* 7:e33025. doi: 10.1371/journal.pone.0033025

Liu, T. X., Zhang, J. W., Tao, J., Zhang, R. B., Zhang, Q. H., Zhao, C. J., et al. (2000). Gene expression networks underlying retinoic acid-induced differentiation of acute promyelocytic leukemia cells. *Blood* 96, 1496–1504.

Lopes, P. P., Todorov, G., Pham, T. T., Nesburn, A. B., Bahraoui, E., and BenMohamed, L. (2018). Laser adjuvant-assisted peptide vaccine promotes skin mobilization of dendritic cells and enhances protective CD8 + TEM and TRM cell responses against herpesvirus infection and disease. *J. Virol.* 92:e2156-17. doi: 10.1128/JVI.02156-17

Lu, L., Liu, Q., and Jiang, S. (2012). Biosecurity and biosafety in research on emerging pathogens. *Emerg. Microbes Infect.* 1:e44. doi: 10.1038/emi.2012.39

McAllister, L., Anderson, J., Werth, K., Cho, I., Copeland, K., Le Cam Bouveret, N., et al. (2014). Needle-free jet injection for administration of influenza vaccine: a randomised non-inferiority trial. *Lancet* 384, 674–681. doi: 10.1016/S0140-6736(14)60524-9

McKee, A. S., Munks, M. W., and Marrack, P. (2007). How do adjuvants work? Important considerations for new generation adjuvants. *Immunity* 27, 687–690. doi: 10.1016/j.immuni.2007.11.003

Medina, R. A. (2018). 1918 influenza virus: 100 years on, are we prepared against the next influenza pandemic? *Nat. Rev. Microbiol.* 16, 61–62. doi: 10.1038/nrmicro.2017.174

Monto, A. S., Ohmit, S. E., Petrie, J. G., Johnson, E., Truscon, R., Teich, E., et al. (2009). Comparative efficacy of inactivated and live attenuated influenza vaccines. *N. Engl. J. Med.* 361, 1260–1267. doi: 10.1056/NEJMoa0808652

Pasparakis, M., Haase, I., and Nestle, F. O. (2014). Mechanisms regulating skin immunity and inflammation. *Nat. Rev. Immunol.* 14, 289–301. doi: 10.1038/nri3646

Patel, S., Akalkotkar, A., Bivona, J. J. III, Lee, J. Y., Park, Y. K., Yu, M., et al. (2016). Vitamin A or E and a catechin synergize as vaccine adjuvant to enhance immune responses in mice by induction of early interleukin-15 but not interleukin-1beta responses. *Immunology* 148, 352–362. doi: 10.1111/imm.12614

Paules, C. I., Marston, H. D., Eisinger, R. W., Baltimore, D., and Fauci, A. S. (2017). The pathway to a universal influenza vaccine. *Immunity* 47, 599–603. doi: 10.1016/j.immuni.2017.09.007

Pawelec, G., and McElhaney, J. (2018). Vaccines for improved cellular immunity to influenza. *EBioMedicine* 30, 12–13. doi: 10.1016/j.ebiom.2018.03.001

Petrova, V. N., and Russell, C. A. (2018). The evolution of seasonal influenza viruses. *Nat. Rev. Microbiol.* 16, 47–60. doi: 10.1038/nrmicro.2017.118

Petrovsky, N., and Aguilar, J. C. (2004). Vaccine adjuvants: current state and future trends. *Immunol. Cell Biol.* 82, 488–496. doi: 10.1111/j.0818-9641.2004.01272.x

Raverdeau, M., and Mills, K. H. (2014). Modulation of T cell and innate immune responses by retinoic Acid. *J. Immunol.* 192, 2953–2958. doi: 10.4049/jimmunol.1303245

Reed, S. G., Orr, M. T., and Fox, C. B. (2013). Key roles of adjuvants in modern vaccines. *Nat. Med.* 19, 1597–1608. doi: 10.1038/nm.3409

Roers, A., Hiller, B., and Hornung, V. (2016). Recognition of endogenous nucleic acids by the innate immune system. *Immunity* 44, 739–754. doi: 10.1016/j.immuni.2016.04.002

Sigmundsdottir, H., and Butcher, E. C. (2008). Environmental cues, dendritic cells and the programming of tissue-selective lymphocyte trafficking. *Nat. Immunol.* 9, 981–987. doi: 10.1038/ni.f.208

Smith, G. J., Vijaykrishna, D., Bahl, J., Lycett, S. J., Worobey, M., Pybus, O. G., et al. (2009). Origins and evolutionary genomics of the 2009 swine-origin H1N1 influenza A epidemic. *Nature* 459, 1122–1125. doi: 10.1038/nature08182

Sullivan, S. (2018). Challenges in reducing influenza-associated mortality. *Lancet* 391, 1242–1244. doi: 10.1016/S0140-6736(17)33292-0

Svensson, M., Johansson-Lindbom, B., Zapata, F., Jaensson, E., Austenaa, L. M., Blomhoff, R., et al. (2008). Retinoic acid receptor signaling levels and antigen dose regulate gut homing receptor expression on CD8 + T cells. *Mucosal Immunol.* 1, 38–48. doi: 10.1038/mi.2007.4

Tailor, P., Tamura, T., and Ozato, K. (2006). IRF family proteins and type I interferon induction in dendritic cells. *Cell Res.* 16, 134–140. doi: 10.1038/sj.cr.7310018

Tsuchiya, Y., Jounai, N., Takeshita, F., Ishii, K. J., and Mizuguchi, K. (2016). Ligand-induced ordering of the C-terminal tail primes STING for phosphorylation by TBK1. *EBioMedicine* 9, 87–96. doi: 10.1016/j.ebiom.2016.05.039

Uyeki, T. M., Katz, J. M., and Jernigan, D. B. (2017). Novel influenza A viruses and pandemic threats. *Lancet* 389, 2172–2174. doi: 10.1016/S0140-6736(17)31274-6

Vance, R. E. (2016). Cytosolic DNA sensing: the field narrows. *Immunity* 45, 227–228. doi: 10.1016/j.immuni.2016.08.006

Wang, J., Li, B., and Wu, M. X. (2015). Effective and lesion-free cutaneous influenza vaccination. *Proc. Natl. Acad. Sci. U.S.A.* 112, 5005–5010. doi: 10.1073/pnas.1500408112

Wang, J., Li, P. Y., Chen, X. Y., and Wu, M. X. (2016a). Laser facilitates vaccination. *J. Innov. Opt. Heal. Sci.* 9:1630003. doi: 10.1142/S1793545816300032

Wang, J., Li, P. Y., and Wu, M. X. (2016b). Natural STING agonist as an "Ideal" adjuvant for cutaneous vaccination. *J. Invest. Dermatol.* 136, 2183–2191. doi: 10.1016/j.jid.2016.05.105

Wang, J., Shah, D., Chen, X. Y., Anderson, R. R., and Wu, M. X. (2014). A micro-sterile inflammation array as an adjuvant for influenza vaccines. *Nat. Commun.* 5:4447. doi: 10.1038/ncomms5447

Williams, S. C. (2013). Under the skin of intradermal vaccines. *Proc. Natl. Acad. Sci. U.S.A.* 110, 10049–10051. doi: 10.1073/pnas.1309653110

Xie, J. F., Zhang, Y. H., Zhao, L., Xiu, W. Q., Chen, H. B., Lin, Q., et al. (2018). Emergence of Eurasian avian-like swine influenza A (H1N1) virus from an adult case in Fujian Province, China. *Virol. Sin.* 33, 282–286. doi: 10.1007/s12250-018-0034-1

Xu, H. C., Grusdat, M., Pandyra, A. A., Polz, R., Huang, J., Sharma, P., et al. (2014). Type I interferon protects antiviral CD8 + T cells from NK cell cytotoxicity. *Immunity* 40, 949–960. doi: 10.1016/j.immuni.2014.05.004

Xu, W., Dai, Y., Hua, C., Wang, Q., Zou, P., Deng, Q., et al. (2017). Genomic signature analysis of the recently emerged highly pathogenic A(H5N8) avian influenza virus: implying an evolutionary trend for bird-to-human transmission. *Microbes Infect.* 19, 597–604. doi: 10.1016/j.micinf.2017.08.006

Xu, W., Lu, L., Shen, B., Li, J., Xu, J. Q., and Jiang, S. B. (2013). Serological investigation of subclinical influenza A (H7H9) infection among healthcare and non-healthcare workers in Zhejiang Province, China. *Clin. Infect. Dis.* 57, 919–921. doi: 10.1093/cid/cit396

Zeng, R., Bscheider, M., Lahl, K., Lee, M., and Butcher, E. C. (2016). Generation and transcriptional programming of intestinal dendritic cells: essential role of retinoic acid. *Mucosal Immunol.* 9, 183–193. doi: 10.1038/mi.2015.50

Zeng, R., Oderup, C., Yuan, R., Lee, M., Habtezion, A., Hadeiba, H., et al. (2013). Retinoic acid regulates the development of a gut-homing precursor for intestinal dendritic cells. *Mucosal Immunol.* 6, 847–856. doi: 10.1038/mi.2012.123

Zevini, A., Olagnier, D., and Hiscottt, J. (2017). Crosstalk between cytoplasmic RIG-I and STING sensing pathways. *Trends Immunol.* 38, 194–205. doi: 10.1016/j.it.2016.12.004

7

Can Machines Learn Respiratory Virus Epidemiology?: A Comparative Study of Likelihood-Free Methods for the Estimation of Epidemiological Dynamics

Heidi L. Tessmer[1†], Kimihito Ito[1] and Ryosuke Omori[1,2†]*

[1] Division of Bioinformatics, Research Center for Zoonosis Control, Hokkaido University, Sapporo, Japan, [2] Precursory Research for Embryonic Science and Technology (PRESTO), Japan Science and Technology Agency, Saitama, Japan

***Correspondence:**
Ryosuke Omori
omori@czc.hokudai.ac.jp*

[†] These authors have contributed equally to this work.

To estimate and predict the transmission dynamics of respiratory viruses, the estimation of the basic reproduction number, R_0, is essential. Recently, approximate Bayesian computation methods have been used as likelihood free methods to estimate epidemiological model parameters, particularly R_0. In this paper, we explore various machine learning approaches, the multi-layer perceptron, convolutional neural network, and long-short term memory, to learn and estimate the parameters. Further, we compare the accuracy of the estimates and time requirements for machine learning and the approximate Bayesian computation methods on both simulated and real-world epidemiological data from outbreaks of influenza A(H1N1)pdm09, mumps, and measles. We find that the machine learning approaches can be verified and tested faster than the approximate Bayesian computation method, but that the approximate Bayesian computation method is more robust across different datasets.

Keywords: respiratory virus, infectious disease epidemiology, machine learning, approximate Bayesian computation, basic reproduction number, mathematical model

INTRODUCTION

Prediction of infectious disease epidemics is essential to their control, but also a difficult process. This is because the epidemiological dynamics, i.e., the time evolution of the number of infected individuals, are non-linear, with the probability of a susceptible individual acquiring infection depending on the number of infected individuals. Previous studies have constructed mathematical models describing the transmission dynamics of infectious disease, known as the Susceptible-Infectious-Removed (SIR) model, and fit the model to the time series data of the number of infected individuals (Bjrnstad et al., 2002). Conventional statistical methods, e.g., maximum likelihood estimation, require explicit solution of the time series data of the number of infected individuals from the SIR model. However, an explicit solution is difficult to obtain due to the nonlinearity of the model. Therefore several approximations are required to fit the SIR model with the epidemiological data of infectious diseases. Furthermore, the transmission of infectious disease is a stochastic event. A mathematical model taking into account stochasticity is required to estimate parameters.

One common property of transmission dynamics is the threshold for outbreak: an outbreak occurs only if the basic reproduction number, R_0, exceeds unity. In a biological sense, R_0 is the expected number of secondary infections by an infected individual when a population is fully susceptible (Diekmann et al., 1990). Estimation of R_0 helps to predict the outbreak potential, final epidemic size, timing of the epidemic peak, and vaccination coverage required to prevent an outbreak. To estimate R_0, a common method is to fit the SIR model to epidemiological data. The simplest SIR model has only this one parameter, R_0, by scaling the unit time in the SIR model. In this paper, we use a Susceptible Exposed Infectious Removed (SEIR) model, a variation of the SIR model. The SEIR model is comprised of additional parameters and follows more complex epidemiological dynamics, which reflect realistic disease dynamics.

Due to the importance of estimating R_0, numerous methods have been developed (Magal and Ruan, 2014). The accuracy of the estimates depends on both the estimation method and the data. For example, in one approach R_0 can be estimated from the slope of the time series data of infected individuals at the initial phase of an epidemic (Nishiura et al., 2009). This method approximates the epidemiological dynamics at the initial phase as an exponential growth. The accuracy of this method is sensitive to the period of epidemiological data available. An alternative approach estimates R_0 from the final epidemic size, i.e., the total number of infected individuals (Vynnycky et al., 2007). Because the relationship between the final epidemic size and R_0 cannot be described explicitly, the likelihood function of R_0 with an arbitrary final epidemic size cannot be described in an explicit form. Consequently numerical solutions or approximations are required to construct the likelihood function.

Recently a likelihood-free method has been proposed: approximate Bayesian computation (ABC) (Sunnåker et al., 2013; Saulnier et al., 2017). This method approximates the posterior distribution using a rejection algorithm with the numerical integration of the SEIR model. This method is easy to implement, however several limitations remain. Some issues include (a) parameter estimation takes a long time, particularly as the epidemiological model complexity increases and (b) the ABC method accuracy is dependent on both the summary statistic and the accept/reject decision threshold, but there are no fixed rules for the selection of either.

A second likelihood-free approach has recently emerged in the form of machine learning (ML). The field of machine learning has grown rapidly with a large expansion of theories, applications, and algorithms. Problems can be categorized as either supervised or unsupervised and as classification or regression (Bishop, 2006). A supervised learning problem has a dataset and an answer, for example the pixels making up a photograph of a number can be a dataset and the numerical representation of the number is the answer (e.g., the number "7"). These two pieces of information are passed to the ML model during training so the model learns to recognize pixels of the type given as the answers it receives. Once the model is trained, a separate, new dataset is given which contains only the pixel information. The model is then asked to predict the answer based on the data it had previously seen. This example of supervised learning is also an example of a classification problem. The number problem can be split into 10 discrete categories (the whole numbers "0"–"9"), and the machine learns to classify the results into these categories. A regression problem, on the other hand, seeks to find a continuous value answer to the input it receives. Predicting housing prices is a common example of a regression problem, where, given a set of information about properties, the ML model can predict a continuous, numerical value estimate for the cost of the property.

Supervised ML models combine linear regression, gradient descent, maximum likelihood, and least squares functions to develop weight matrices and comparison functions to predict and estimate parameter outputs based on the historical knowledge of input/output pairs (Bishop, 2006). With the expansion of the field of ML, new models continue to be developed and improved, connecting the building blocks of ML in new ways to uncover hidden connections in data. Some methods, such as convolutional neural networks (CNN) are well suited for two-dimensional image analysis (Krizhevsky et al., 2012), while other methods, like long-short term memory models (LSTM), specialize in handling time series data (Hochreiter and Schmidhuber, 1997).

In this study, we propose a ML approach to estimate the R_0 of a respiratory virus from a time series of incidences of the disease as a supervised regression problem. Additionally, we seek to estimate other parameters associated with the SEIR model and time series generation. As mentioned above, R_0 is highly dependent on the mathematical model. Our final goal is a likelihood-free estimation of R_0, as well as other model parameters. The ML methods used in this study are two separate multi-layer perceptrons (MLP), a CNN, and a LSTM model. For reference and comparison, we also use the ABC approach to estimate the same values using the same datasets. We compare not only the accuracy of the two methods, with credible and confidence intervals, but also the time required by each approach to reach its answer. Of the four ML methods tested, the MLP with time model was the most robust as well as being significantly faster than the more complex CNN and LSTM models.

MATERIALS AND METHODS

This study can be broken into five main parts. The first is the development of an individual-based (IBM) SEIR epidemiological model for generating data; the second is the ABC method used for estimating parameters; the third is the learning by MLP, CNN, and LSTM machine learning models, again to estimate parameters; the fourth is the dataset creation and bootstrapping of the real-world and test data to create confidence intervals on the machine learning solutions; and finally calculation of the time it took for each method to obtain its estimates.

The ML models were trained on 100,000 datasets, validated on 1,000 datasets, and tested on 1,000 datasets. ABC was run on 1,000 sample datasets and compared against a total of 100,000 comparison datasets. The ABC sample and ML test datasets were the same and the ABC comparison and ML training datasets were the same. An explanation of these datasets is in the following section. We evaluate the accuracy of estimation by two measurements, the average error and the width of the credible interval for ABC and confidence intervals for ML. Each parameter range was divided into 10 subranges. The errors among parameters in each subrange were then averaged to create the "average error." The average width of credible/confidence intervals is the average difference between the lower and upper bound of the interval.

Terminology

As the different likelihood-free methods used in this paper (ABC and ML) each have their own standard vocabularies, we first clarify terminology in this paper to make a direct comparison of methods possible.

ML typically uses three datasets. The "training" set is a large dataset which is given to the ML model during the learning phase. The "test" set is a completely new and unseen dataset which the ML method passes through the trained model to estimate the posterior parameter values. The "validation" or "development" dataset, like the "test" set is a new and unseen dataset used as an interim test. That is, this dataset is used to verify the model is learning, check accuracy of estimates, and when running trials of different hyperparameter sets. In ABC there is no dataset equivalent to ML's validation set.

According to the notation used by Sunnåker et al. (2013) we use the symbols D for the data in question, either real-world observed data or generated "test" data, and $\hat{D}$ for comparison data. In ABC, $\hat{D}$ would normally be the Markov chain Monte Carlo generated data presented to the rejection algorithm. The rejection algorithm takes a set of generated data and compares it to the data in question, D. In ABC, the summary statistic is used to calculate the distance between $\hat{D}$ and D, and the parameters are accepted or rejected if the estimated distance falls beneath an accept/reject threshold. Our summary statistic for ABC is the Euclidean distance between the dataset D and the simulated dataset $\hat{D}$:

$$\sqrt{\sum(D-\hat{D})^2}$$

Comparing the ML and ABC terminology, datasets comprising D would be the test set in ML, while a dataset comprising $\hat{D}$ is given to an ML algorithm as a training set. To compare the ABC and ML methods we use the same pre-generated datasets for both methods.

SEIR Epidemiological Model

The SEIR model is an expansion of the SIR model, which describes the time evolution of the number of infected individuals during a disease outbreak. The host population is classified by their health status, susceptible (S), exposed (E), infectious (I), and removed (R) (recovered or deceased). Transmission events happen via contact of S and E with constant rate β. The SEIR model can be expressed mathematically through the following simple equations (Bjrnstad et al., 2002; Diekmann et al., 2009; Magal and Ruan, 2014):

$$\begin{aligned}
N &= S(t) + E(t) + I(t) + R(t),\\
\frac{dS}{dt} &= -\beta S\frac{I}{N},\\
\frac{dE}{dt} &= \beta S\frac{I}{N} - \epsilon E,\\
\frac{dI}{dt} &= \epsilon E - \gamma I,\\
\frac{dR}{dt} &= \gamma I.
\end{aligned}$$

Here N describes the total host population size. In this model, R_0 is given by:

$$R_0 = \frac{\beta}{\gamma}.$$

This is a deterministic model and S, E, I, and R are continuous. To fit the model with the data, it is required to expand this model to a stochastic one with discrete S, E, I, and R. An individual-based SEIR model describes the stochastic process of transmission dynamics at the individual level. Let H_x be the health state of the x-th individual.

$$H_x \in \{S, E, I, R\}$$

The probability of transition between each health state can be written by:

$$\begin{aligned}
Pr(H_x(t) = S &\rightarrow H_x(t+\Delta t) = E) = \beta I(t)\Delta t,\\
Pr(H_x(t) = E &\rightarrow H_x(t+\Delta t) = I) = \epsilon\Delta t,\\
Pr(H_x(t) = I &\rightarrow H_x(t+\Delta t) = R) = \gamma\Delta t.
\end{aligned}$$

We simulate this model to create data which can be used to learn the different parameter sets of R_0, ϵ, and γ. ϵ is the latent period, or the rate at which exposed individuals become infectious. γ is the recovery rate, the rate individuals move from state I to state R. The host population size for the general study, $N = 2225$. For the real-world comparisons, $N = 500$ for mumps (Sullivan et al., 1985), $N = 343$ for measles (Mossong and Muller, 2000), and $N = 2{,}225$ for influenza A(H1N1)pdm09 (Lessler et al., 2009). We set $S(0) = N - I(0)$, $E(0) = 0$, $I(0) = 22$, and $R(0) = 0$ as the initial conditions, which were parameterized based on the epidemiological data of Lessler et al. (2009). Time series data of incidence were created by IBM model with randomly chosen parameter sets to consist of 100,000 training, 1,000 validation, and 1,000 test samples. Throughout this study we set $\Delta t = 1/10$ day, meaning the SEIR model parameters were updated 10 times each day, with each change in time (Δt) equal to 1/10 day.

Approximate Bayesian Computation

We use ABC to estimate the parameters R_0, ϵ, and γ, the parameter values associated with the SEIR epidemiological model. For our ABC calculations, we used simulated datasets for $\hat{D}$, calculating the distances between each D dataset and $\hat{D}$ datasets. The Euclidean distance was used as the summary statistic to calculate distances between datasets, and multiple acceptance thresholds were established. An acceptance threshold of 60 was used for the **Figures 1**, **3**, **4**, here as it was large enough to produce accepted posterior parameter sets for each of the D datasets and have enough samples to create credible intervals, but small enough to generally discriminate between similar and dissimilar datasets.

The Euclidean distance between the dataset D and simulated dataset $\hat{D}$ is:

$$\sqrt{\sum(D - \hat{D})^2}$$

Machine Learning

Three separate machine learning models and one variation were implemented and run with early-stopping manually executed by comparing the loss at each epoch, stopping when the loss no longer decreased (for 10 or 20 epochs), and using the weights from the best epoch, i.e., the epoch with the smallest loss. The learning rate for all models was 0.0001. The ML models in this study were implemented in Python using Lasagne and Theano (Bergstra et al., 2010) libraries. For all ML models, numerous hyperparameters for the number of hidden layers, number of hidden units, learning rate, activation functions, and number of training samples were explored and the hyperparameters which routinely yielded the best results were selected. For example, we ran an MLP model with 2, 3, 4, 5, 6, and 7 hidden layers and found that there was little benefit in models deeper than three hidden layers, yet two hidden layers learned poorly. For this reason, three hidden layers were used in the final model.

Multi-Layer Perceptron

The first model selected for this paper was a simple MLP where the entire time series dataset was passed in as a single input array and the parameters were estimated from learned relationships in that dataset. Small changes in parameter values have a large impact on the shape and behavior of the time series graph, so it was important for the MLP to see all of the data with equal importance, which is why the time series was passed in as a single input.

The MLP model accepted the time series information for the number of incidences of infection per day as created by the IBM model as input for learning. This input was given to the model as a single entity consisting of the number of newly infected individuals at each timestep. It also received the "answers" of the R_0, γ, and ϵ model parameters which were used to generate the time series data. The model was asked to learn these answer parameters in a supervised manner given the time series of incidences. The MLP model was created with three hidden layers having 400 hidden units per layer. The hidden layers used rectified linear units (Maas et al., 2013) for their activation functions, with a linear activation function in the final output layer.

Multi-Layer Perceptron With Time

A second MLP model was constructed to incorporate the concept of "time" into the time series information. In a standard MLP, the sequence of values passed in has no connection and there is no concept of order in the analysis and training. This second model added a time element by creating a tuple consisting of the day and the number of new incidences that day. This simple method created a model which understands time as an individual value, though unlike LSTM described later, it does not have any kind of memory mechanism to compare previous and future datapoints.

This MLP also had three hidden layers, though with 400, 200, and 100 hidden units per layer, in that order. Again, the hidden layers used rectified linear units for their activation functions with a linear activation function in the final output layer. The addition of the time element changed the input to the model from a one-dimensional array to a two-dimensional matrix.

Convolutional Neural Network

While the CNN is not a traditional choice for problems involving time series data, it was selected in this case due to the complex nature of the SEIR modeling data. The mathematical models being simulated are highly non-linear, nearly chaotic at times. As CNNs are known to be capable of modeling very complex behavior (Krizhevsky et al., 2012), they were tested in this problem space for comparison.

The CNN model was constructed of two one-dimensional convolutional layers and two pooling layers, with a single dense hidden layer prior to the output. The convolutional and hidden layers all used rectified linear units for their activation functions, while the output layer again used a linear activation function.

Long-Short Term Memory

A recurrent neural network (RNN) approach, LSTM models are designed for analysis of time series data (Hochreiter and

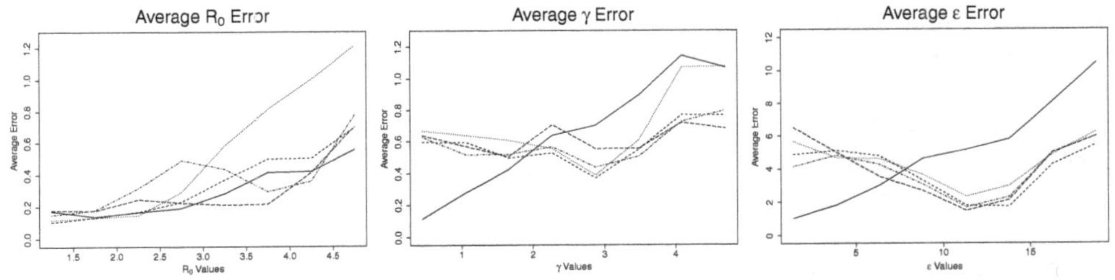

FIGURE 1 | Average error for ABC (solid line), CNN (long dashed line), MLP (dotted line), MLP with time (dashed line), and LSTM (dashed and dotted) estimates against actual parameter values for an SEIR mocel with three parameters, on 100,000 training datasets.

Schmidhuber, 1997), like that found in this study. The memory aspect is built into the model using a memory cell and gates (input, output, and forget) to control the data in the model. These components ensure continuity in the data of the LSTM model and accept the time order as an important feature of the data.

The LSTM model implemented for this study consists of two LSTM layers with 16 hidden units and gradient clipping at 100 (to prevent exploding gradients). No activation function is applied in the LSTM layers, however a linear activation function is applied on the output layer.

Datasets

The datasets for this study come from two sources. The first, generated data, is a set of SEIR epidemiological model datasets generated using individual-based, Monte Carlo simulations, as described in the Epidemiological Model section. The second source comes from time series sets of incidences from published papers by Lessler et al. (2009), Sullivan et al. (1985), and Mossong and Muller (2000). We estimate R_0 for these time series datasets and compare our estimates against the general or estimated value from the papers.

The data in these datasets are comprised of two parts. The first part is a time series of the number of newly infected individuals per day over the course of an outbreak. The second piece of information is the parameter set of R_0, γ, and ϵ used in the simulation to generate the time series. The time series is the information the ML model trains on, while the parameter set is the answer it is trying to achieve. In ABC, the time series is the dataset $\hat{D}$, and the parameter set is the answer it is estimating.

Bootstrap Resampling

To date, machine learning has most often been used in classification problems with discrete correct answers and myriad ways to determine the performance of any given model, such as accuracy, precision/recall, F-score, and receiver operator characteristic (ROC) (Sokolova et al., 2006). Regression problems, by contrast, have few methods to explore the quality of the output. To address this issue, we created a novel method to build confidence intervals for the outputs of the ML model.

We started by creating a standard machine learning test set of 1,000 datasets. Running this time series dataset through the trained model gives estimates for the parameter values, but there is no indication on the quality of the estimates—no certainty or confidence associated with the values. Next, we created 1,000 bootstrap-resampled datasets for each test dataset, for a total of one million tests. For bootstrap resampling of the time series data of incidence, the time series data of incidence can be interpreted as the set of emergence times. For example, the data when incidence at $t = 1$ is 1 and incidence at $t = 2$ is 2 is equivalent to a set of emergence times, $\{t = 1, t = 2, t = 2\}$. We resampled the emergence times by bootstrap resampling from this set of times, and converted them back into time series data of incidence.

For the estimates returned for the 1,000 resamples of each dataset, we calculated the mean, median, mode, and 95% confidence intervals. This method provides a measure of credibility for each estimated output parameter.

Time Calculations

The ABC computations were conducted on a server with 2.80 GHz processors and 1 TB of memory. The computations were run across multiple CPUs and the time calculated is the combined time to run all scripts. The ML computations were conducted on a server with 3.50 GHz processors, 64 GB memory, and a GeForce GTX 1080 Ti® graphics card for GPU processing. Typically between four and eight processes were run simultaneously on the graphics card.

The time to complete each method is shown in **Table 1**. For ABC, the time to verify its results by comparison of the distances between 1,000 D datasets with 100,000 $\hat{D}$ datasets was measured, including time to split by thresholds and create credible intervals for accepted datasets. The time for a single comparison against 100,000 $\hat{D}$ datasets was then measured for the test comparison. For the ML models, the time included the bootstrapping of the test dataset, training of the learning model, and computation of the confidence intervals. The test was then run by obtaining the estimates for a single bootstrapped sample, that is, running 1,000 samples from one set of parameters through a trained ML model and collating the results.

Experiments on Real-World Datasets

For experiments, we used an SEIR model dataset with three parameters: R_0, γ, ϵ, calculating distances with ABC and comparing at various acceptance thresholds, and training CNN, LSTM, and two MLP models, then running a test dataset through the trained model. Finally, we tested our trained and verified models against three real-world datasets: (1) an outbreak of mumps (Sullivan et al., 1985), (2) an outbreak of measles (Mossong and Muller, 2000), and (3) an outbreak of influenza A(H1N1)pdm09 (Lessler et al., 2009) to see if we could accurately estimate the parameter R_0 with both our ABC and ML models.

For ABC, the time series of infectives is set as D and compared against the $\hat{D}$ generated data used throughout this paper. The required accept/reject threshold was 300, 20, and 20 for the influenza, measles, and mumps datasets, respectively. The accept/reject thresholds were selected where there were enough accepted datasets for the calculation of credible intervals. The parameters were then estimated from the accepted datasets. To construct confidence intervals of the estimates by ML, the real-world time series of incidence was resampled using the bootstrap resampling method discussed in the Bootstrap Resampling section. The set containing the original and bootstrap resampled time series are given to the model, the parameters are estimated,

TABLE 1 | The time required to train 100,000 samples and test on a single sample for the ABC, MLP, CNN, and LSTM methods.

Method	Train (min)	Test (min)
ABC	410	0.65
MLP	68	0.03
MLP with time	71	0.03
CNN	184	0.05
LSTM	364	0.06

and finally the confidence intervals are calculated from the ML model outputs.

RESULTS

Comparisons of Average Errors

Figure 1 shows the average errors compared to the actual parameter values associated with each method. The average errors of estimates made with ABC and ML are most similar for R_0. ABC and MLP with time show nearly identical patterns, consisting of low errors when R_0 is <3.0 and then increasing with increasing values of R_0. ABC has slightly lower average error than MLP with time for all values of R_0. For R_0 below 2.25, MLP performs as well as ABC and MLP with time. For R_0 >2.25 the average error from MLP estimates increases greatly, until R_0 reaches 5.0, at which point the error from MLP is approximately twice the error from ABC. CNN has a nearly constant average error of 0.2 for $R_0 < 3.8$. For $R_0 > 3.8$, the average error on CNN estimates increases linearly to approximately 0.7 at $R_0 =$ 5.0. Finally, LSTM shows erratic behavior in R_0 estimation. Until R_0 reaches 3.0, LSTM has the worst estimates among the methods tested, with an error reaching nearly 0.6. From 2.8 to 3.8, the average error by LSTM decreases, becoming smaller than all but CNN. From $R_0 = 3.8$ to 5.0, the error by LSTM increases again, with behavior similar to ABC, CNN, and MLP with time for this range of R_0.

The patterns for average error for the parameters γ and ϵ are similar to one another. ABC follows one pattern while the ML solutions follow a different pattern. For ABC, the average error increases with increasing values of the parameters, γ and ϵ. For $\gamma < 2.0$ days^{-1} and ϵ less than about 7.5 days^{-1}, the ABC average error is smaller than the average error for all ML estimates. For γ more than 2.0 days^{-1} and ϵ more than 7.5 days^{-1}, the average error for ABC is larger than the average error of all ML estimates. When the number of training samples is increased to one million, the point at which ML becomes more accurate than ABC is 1.6 days^{-1} for γ and approximately 6.5 days^{-1} for ϵ (see **Figure 2**). The ML approaches maintained a nearly consistent average error for all γ of 0.6 days^{-1} until $\gamma = 3.9$ days^{-1}, when they increased to average errors of approximately 0.6 days^{-1}. From $\gamma = 3.9$ to 5.0 days^{-1}, MLP increased much more quickly to approximately 1.1 days^{-1}, the same as ABC. All four ML models behaved the same for ϵ, with average errors decreasing with increasing ϵ until $\epsilon = 11$ days^{-1}, at which point they increased with increasing ϵ at a rate similar to ABC, but approximately 3 days^{-1} smaller.

Comparisons of Credible/Confidence Intervals

The credible intervals for the estimates for ABC and confidence intervals for ML are shown in **Figure 3**. CNN has a constant size confidence interval for R_0. MLP and MLP with time have a confidence interval similar in shape to ABC's credible intervals for R_0, though their confidence intervals are larger. These three methods start with small credible/confidence intervals for small R_0, increasing with R_0 until $R_0 = 2.6$–4.0 and then decreasing slightly. LSTM's confidence interval increases until R_0 reaches approximately 2.25, then decreases with increasing R_0. The credible/confidence intervals for both the ABC and ML models decrease as γ increases. CNN has the smallest confidence interval for γ, followed by LSTM, MLP with time, ABC, and MLP.

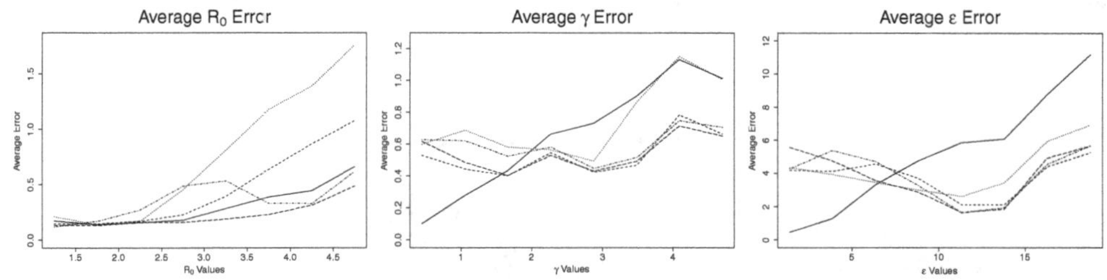

FIGURE 2 | Average error for ABC (solid line), CNN (long dashed line), MLP (dotted line), MLP with time (dashed line), and LSTM (dashed and dotted) estimates against actual parameter values for an SEIR model with three parameters, for one million training datasets.

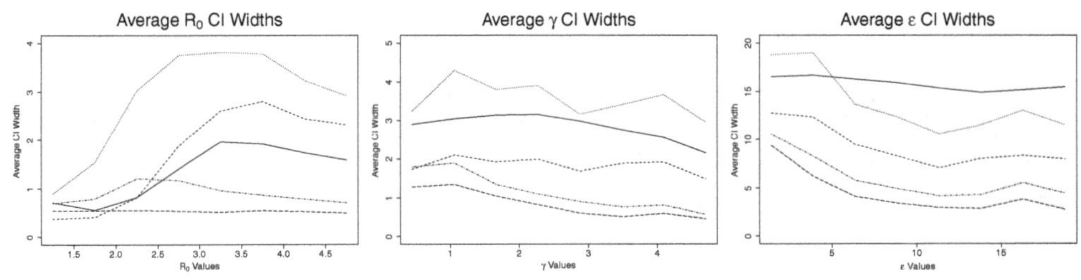

FIGURE 3 | Average credible/confidence interval width for ABC (solid line), CNN (long dashed line), MLP (dotted line), MLP with time (dashed line), and LSTM (dashed and dotted) estimates against actual parameter values for an SEIR model with three parameters, on 100,000 training datasets.

In ABC, the credible intervals for ϵ remain mostly constant at about 16.0 day^{-1} for all values of ϵ. For the ML models, the confidence intervals decrease with increasing ϵ, increasing slightly around $\epsilon = 15.0$ days^{-1} and then decreasing again. Again, CNN has the smallest confidence interval for ϵ, followed by LSTM, MLP with time, MLP (for $\epsilon > 5$ days^{-1}), and ABC.

Comparisons of Estimated and Actual Values

Figure 4 shows the estimated parameter values compared to the actual values for each method. ABC estimates agree closely with the actual values for $R_0 < 3.0$, with increasing error as R_0 grows beyond 3.0. MLP also estimates R_0 close to the actual values

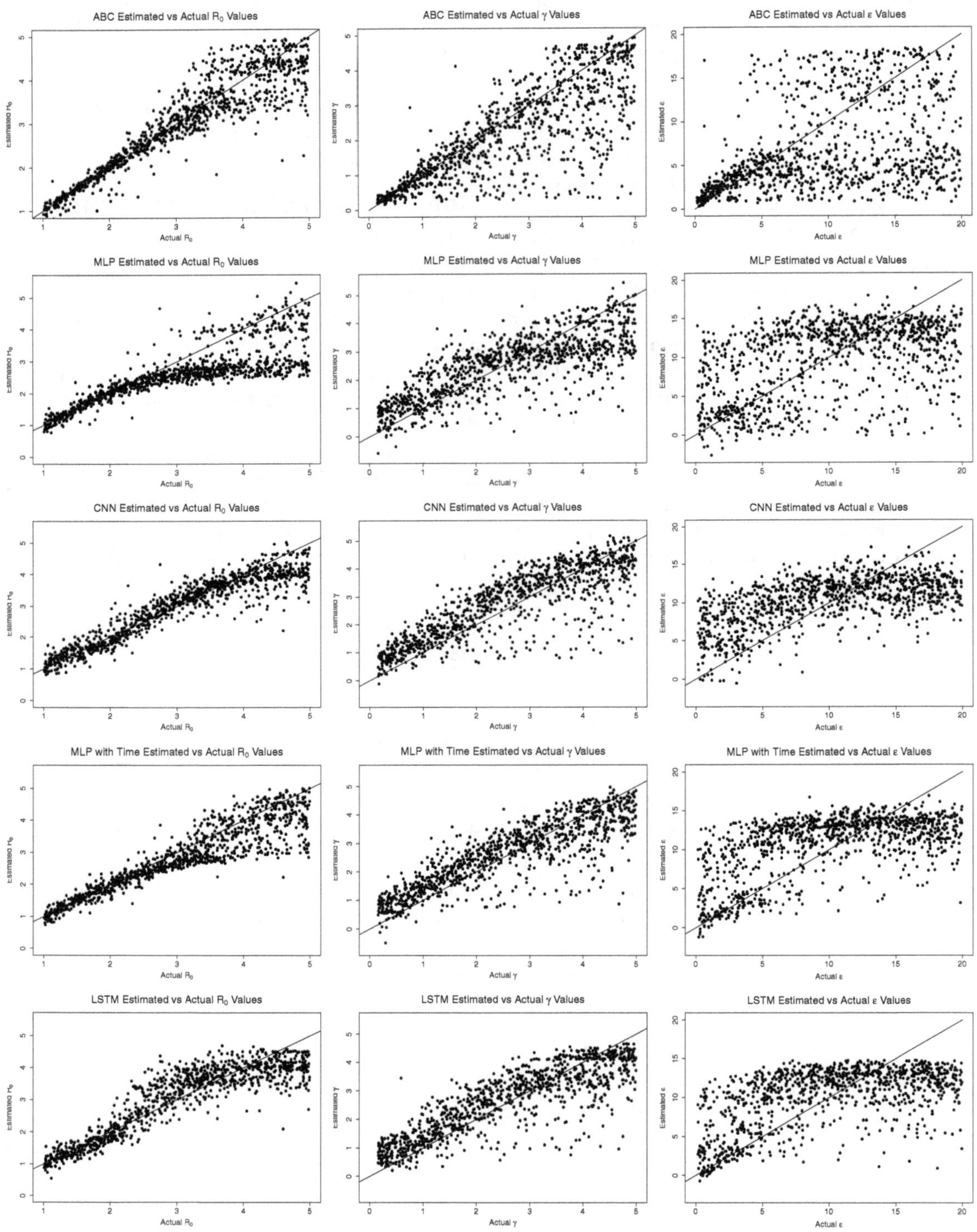

FIGURE 4 | The estimated and actual parameter values from ABC, MLP, CNN, MLP with time, and LSTM.

for $R_0 < 3.0$. After $R_0 = 3.0$, however, the estimate by MLP is nearly constant at a little <3.0. CNN estimates R_0 close to the actual values while R_0 is <4.0. MLP with time's trend is similar to ABC, with estimates near actual values for $R_0 < 3.0$. LSTM shows close estimation for $R_0 < 2.0$, then overestimates from 2.0 to 4.0, then underestimates for $R_0 > 4.0$. Overall, the ML methods appear to underestimate R_0 values, whereas ABC shows equal over- and underestimates. The ML methods show larger over- and underestimation than ABC for low R_0.

All ML methods generally overestimate all values for γ. LSTM, MLP with time, and CNN estimates were close for all γ, while MLP again began estimating a constant, approximately 3.0 days^{-1} for $\gamma > 3.0$ days^{-1}. ABC closely estimates γ values <2.0 days^{-1} and ϵ values <5.0 days^{-1}. ABC, and to a lesser extent MLP with time and LSTM, appear to estimate ϵ somewhat closely for ϵ <5.0 days^{-1}, but for values >5.0 days^{-1} the results for all methods are nearly random.

Run Times

The time to complete each method is shown in **Table 1**. The ABC method took 410 min to calculate the distances and accept/reject 1,000 test datasets from 100,000 training datasets. The time for a single dataset to be compared against 100,000 training datasets was 0.65 min. The fastest ML model, MLP, took 68 min to train while the slowest, LSTM, took 364 min. MLP with time and CNN took 71 and 184 min to train, respectively. This makes training of the ML models between 1.1 and 6.0 times faster than the time to verify a similar ABC method on 100,000 training datasets. Testing on a single dataset for the ML models took 0.03, 0.03, 0.05, and 0.06 min for MLP, MLP with time, CNN, and LSTM, respectively. These times are between 10.8 and 21.7 times faster than the estimate calculation for a single sample via ABC. When the size of the training set is increased from 100,000 to one million, the time required to estimate the parameters for a single ABC test set scales linearly with the number of comparisons, however the estimation via machine learning remains constant regardless of the number of samples used to train the data (**Table 2**).

Application to Real-World Epidemiological Data

We also compared ABC and ML with epidemiological data for mumps, measles and influenza.

R_0 for mumps has been estimated between 3.6 and 4.5 (Edmunds et al., 2000). **Table 3** shows the comparison of ML and ABC estimations of R_0 with the typical real-world values. MLP, MLP with time, and CNN estimated R_0 at approximately 4.0 using the data from Sullivan et al. (1985) for an outbreak in Centerville, OH, USA. ABC estimated R_0 as slightly lower at 3.74, while LSTM greatly underestimated R_0 at 2.71. These values were created based on an estimation of the effective reproductive number and the vaccine coverage of students within the school of 72.7%.

For an outbreak of measles at Wincrange, Luxembourg (Mossong and Muller, 2000), the effective reproductive number was estimated as 1.5 (95% CI: 0.9, 2.2). **Table 4** shows the comparison of ML and ABC estimations with the effective reproductive number estimated for the outbreak. All five of our methods underestimated the effective reproductive number of measles, but their estimates fell within the 95% CI estimated by the previous study.

The estimated R_0 of an outbreak of influenza at a high school in New York during the 2009 influenza pandemic was 1.23 (Lessler et al., 2009). **Table 5** shows the comparison of ML and ABC estimations of R_0 with the effective reproductive number estimated for the outbreak. ABC estimated R_0 nearly exactly at 1.24. MLP with time slightly underestimated the value at 1.06 (95% CI: 0.86, 1.30). Standard MLP greatly underestimated R_0 at 0.40, while CNN and LSTM greatly overestimated the R_0 at 2.84 and 1.84, respectively.

Based on the general analysis for various R_0 values shown in **Figures 1–3**, most of the results above agree. For the mumps outbreak, the effective reproductive numbers were estimated around 1.0–1.2. At this low range of R_0, based on **Figure 1**, the

TABLE 2 | The time required to train one million samples and test on a single sample for the ABC, MLP, CNN, and LSTM methods.

Method	Train (min)	Test (min)
ABC	3,962	4.75
MLP	420	0.03
MLP with time	531	0.03
CNN	747	0.05
LSTM	784	0.06

TABLE 3 | The estimation results for R_0 from previous published research on mumps and ABC, two MLP, CNN, and LSTM models.

Methods	R_0 for mumps
Previous study	3.6–4.5 (Edmunds et al., 2000)
ABC	3.74 (1.21, 12.09)
MLP	4.07 (1.10, 9.08)
MLP with time	3.92 (3.41, 4.25)
CNN	4.21 (2.53, 4.76)
LSTM	2.71 (1.83, 4.54)

Estimates shown include the 95% credible/confidence intervals.

TABLE 4 | The estimation results for effective reproduction number from previous published research on measles and ABC, two MLP, CNN, and LSTM models.

Methods	Effective reproduction number of measles
Previous study	1.5 (Mossong and Muller, 2000)
ABC	1.16 (0.59, 4.88)
MLP	1.00 (0.63, 1.88)
MLP with time	0.91 (0.69, 1.07)
CNN	0.96 (0.19, 1.26)
LSTM	1.08 (0.80, 1.52)

Estimates shown include the 95% credible/confidence intervals.

TABLE 5 | The estimation results for R_0 from previous published research on influenza and ABC, two MLP, CNN, and LSTM models.

Methods	R_0 for influenza
Previous study	1.23 (Lessler et al., 2009)
ABC	1.24 (0.96, 1.74)
MLP	0.40 (0.00, 0.79)
MLP with time	1.06 (0.86, 1.30)
CNN	2.84 (2.08, 3.35)
LSTM	1.84 (1.38, 3.54)

Estimates shown include the 95% credible/confidence intervals.

average error for all methods is relatively low, though LSTM and ABC have higher average errors than the other methods and also exhibit a small tendency to underestimate R_0 for values near 1.0. All five methods also underestimated the effective reproduction number for measles, which was estimated at 1.5. With the exception of MLP with time, the methods contained 1.5 in their 95% CI intervals. However, the estimates for all five methods were within the 95% CI of the previous study. Finally, for the flu estimates, CNN and LSTM greatly overestimate R_0 as 2.84 and 1.84, respectively. LSTM both over- and underestimates values around $R_0 = 1.2$. The estimation of 2.84 by CNN is not robust with expected values, as though CNN does tend to overestimate more than underestimate at $R_0 = 1.2$, an R_0 of 2.84 is outside its average error window.

DISCUSSION

In this study we applied ML methods to estimate the epidemiological parameters of infectious diseases, and compared their accuracy and speed with ABC. In general, the width of confidence intervals estimated by ML are smaller than the credible intervals estimated by ABC. The average error of ML estimates are similar to ABC for R_0, and larger for small values, but smaller for large values of γ and ϵ. Furthermore, the ML models were faster to train than ABC.

ABC was more robust to changes in the data, as shown in **Tables 3–5**. MLP with time was the most robust of the ML methods, with a tendency to underestimate R_0. Given the difference in calculation times between ABC and MLP with time (410 min for ABC compared to 71 min for MLP to train 100,000 samples and 3,962 min for ABC compared to 531 min for MLP on one million samples), it is worth exploring methods which can reduce the underestimation of R_0 in the MLP with time solution. Possibilities include increasing the amount of training data, hyperparameter tuning, increasing the depth of the model, and other general ML tuning methods which may be applied (Bishop, 2006). The ML methods estimated γ well, but with an obvious overestimation bias which can be observed in **Figure 4**, which may also be corrected by applying the previously mentioned approaches.

Interestingly, the point at which ABC is better than ML shifts with increasing sample size for γ and ϵ. When trained on one million datasets, this point decreased from <2.0 to 1.6 days^{-1} for γ and from <7.5 to 6.5 days^{-1} for ϵ. CNN and MLP with time showed similar estimation capability with ABC for R_0, with average errors around 0.2 for $R_0 < 3.0$ and increasing with increasing R_0. The MLP and LSTM approaches showed poor estimation ability for R_0.

While the ML models were faster to train than ABC was to verify, it should be noted that ABC verification of varying parameter values is not required, but ML training on all parameter values is necessary (Palmer and Chakravarty, 2014). That is, an ABC test estimate can be made in approximately <1 min without thorough verification of the general efficacy of the method, while the ML models must be fully trained before calculating a test estimate. However, once trained, the ML models do not need to be retrained unless there is a large amount of new data or some other reason arises to retrain the model (Bishop, 2006).

The problem of parameter estimation explored in this paper can be classified as a ML regression problem where the values of the estimates are continuous. The vast majority of ML research is on classification problems with discrete solutions and therefore "right" and "wrong" answers (Dreiseitl and Ohno-Machado, 2002). In bioinformatics and medicine, another characteristic of a large amount of ML solutions is the use of 2-dimensional images, again typically for classification, for example identifying breast cancer or analyzing MRIs (Sahiner et al., 1996; Chaplot et al., 2006; Krizhevsky et al., 2012). One example of ML being used for regression comes from the European Space Agency (ESA) (Verrelst et al., 2012; Caicedo et al., 2014), where neural networks and regression methods were explored for use in analyzing the large quantity of data being returned by the Sentinal-2 and Sentinel-3 satellites searching for life on far planets. Overall, the application of ML methods on regression problems requires further analysis to improve accuracy.

Note that the R_0 value of 1.2 cited from the paper by Lessler et al. (2009) is the estimate made over the entire course of the outbreak. This value agrees with existing genetic analysis of the virus, as well as additional epidemiological studies which estimated the R_0 value of influenza A(H1N1)pdm09 between 1.4 and 1.6 (Fraser et al., 2009).

Several disadvantages of ML for estimation of epidemiological parameters were found. First, ML approaches are highly sensitive to the size of parameter ranges (Ma et al., 1994). As parameter ranges increase, accuracy of the estimates decreases. In additional tests, we used normalization and standardization to try to reduce the impact of range size on model estimatibility, with limited success (Ioffe and Szegedy, 2015). Moreover, ML is not robust to changes in the initial condition of the model (Kolen and Pollack, 1991), even outside the parameters of interest, though ABC, too, showed sensitivity to initial conditions. This sensitivity may be reducible with larger datasets, deeper models, or the introduction of pruning algorithms and may be explored in later papers (Berthold and Hand, 2003).

In this paper, we have explored a single set of continuous time data, capturing parameters as constant values in a mathematical model. The transmission process of infectious disease does not strictly follow mathematical models and parameters can change values over time. Two approaches for future work which would partially address these issues are (1) a "discrete time analysis" to observe changes in parameter values over time and (2) testing the robustness of our estimates by checking values from different epidemiological models. "Discrete time analysis" is a discretization of the time component of our model with the assumption that the parameter values are constant between time intervals to observe changes in parameter values over time. To check the robustness of our estimates, but still using simulated data, we could create multiple datasets from the Susceptible-Exposed-Infectious-Removed-Susceptible (SEIRS) (Cooke and van den Driessche, 1996) epidemiological model and use this much more complex data to test a model trained from simpler SIR or SEIR model data. This would check the robustness of the systems to changes in unknown parameters and allow us to observe and estimate the sensitivity of our systems. Furthermore, using an SEIRS data model for data generation would allow for analysis of longer and recurring epidemics (Cooke and van den Driessche, 1996) and the efficacy of ML and ABC in estimating more complex disease dynamics.

In conclusion, we have confirmed that both ABC and ML can estimate SEIR model parameters, with ABC and MLP with time being the most robust methods for different SEIR models and parameters. ML models learn more quickly than ABC can be verified, however ABC verification is highly parallelizable, i.e., the problem can be broken into several processes and estimated concurrently, while the learning time for ML models is more difficult to reduce. A key benefit of ML is the speed with which new datasets can be analyzed. A single, new sample can be analyzed in a few seconds, compared to several minutes by ABC, and is constant regardless of the number of datasets used for training. This means a trained ML model would be helpful when estimating large batches of new data.

AUTHOR CONTRIBUTIONS

RO and HT conceived the experiments; HT, RO, and KI participated in discussions; HT and RO conducted the experiments; RO and HT analyzed the results; HT, RO, and KI wrote the manuscript. All authors reviewed the manuscript.

REFERENCES

Bergstra, J., Breuleux, O., Bastien, F., Lamblin, P., Pascanu, R., Desjardins, G., et al. (2010). "Theano: A cpu and gpu math compiler in python," in *Proceedings of the 9th Python in Science Conference*, (Austin, TX), 1–7.

Berthold, M., and Hand, D. J. (2003). *Intelligent Data Analysis: An Introduction.* Verlag: Springer Science & Business Media.

Bishop, C. M. (2006). *Pattern Recognition and Machine Learning.* New York, NY: Springer.

Bjrnstad, O. N., Finkenstdt, B. F., and Grenfell, B. T. (2002). Dynamics of measles epidemics: estimating scaling of transmission rates using a time series sir model. *Ecol. Monogr.* 72, 169–184. doi: 10.1890/0012-9615(2002)072[0169:DOMEES]2.0.CO;2

Caicedo, J. P. R., Verrelst, J., Muoz-Mar, J., Moreno, J., and Camps-Valls, G. (2014). Toward a semiautomatic machine learning retrieval of biophysical parameters. *IEEE J. Sel. Top. Appl. Earth Obs. Remote Sens.* 7, 1249–1259. doi: 10.1109/JSTARS.2014.2298752

Chaplot, S., Patnaik, L., and Jagannathan, N. (2006). Classification of magnetic resonance brain images using wavelets as input to support vector machine and neural network. *Biomed. Signal Proc. Control* 1, 86–92. doi: 10.1016/j.bspc.2006.05.002

Cooke, K. L., and van den Driessche, P. (1996). Analysis of an seirs epidemic model with two delays. *J. Math. Biol.* 35, 240–260. doi: 10.1007/s002850050051

Diekmann, O., Heesterbeek, J., and Roberts, M. (2009). The construction of next-generation matrices for compartmental epidemic models. *J. R. Soc. Interface* 7, 873–885. doi: 10.1098/rsif.2009.0386

Diekmann, O., Heesterbeek, J. A. P., and Metz, J. A. (1990). On the definition and the computation of the basic reproduction ratio r0 in models for infectious diseases in heterogeneous populations. *J. Math. Biol.* 28, 365–382. doi: 10.1007/BF00178324

Dreiseitl, S., and Ohno-Machado, L. (2002). Logistic regression and artificial neural network classification models: a methodology review. *J. Biomed. Inform.* 35, 352–359. doi: 10.1016/S1532-0464(03)00034-0

Edmunds, W. J., Gay, N. J., Kretzschmar, M., Pebody, R. G., and Wachmann, H. (2000). The pre-vaccination epidemiology of measles, mumps and rubella in europe: implications for modelling studies. *Epidemiol. Infect.* 125, 635–650. doi: 10.1017/S0950268800004672

Fraser, C., Donnelly, C. A., Cauchemez, S., Hanage, W. P., Van Kerkhove, M. D., Hollingsworth, T. D., et al. (2009). Pandemic potential of a strain of influenza a (h1n1): early findings. *Science* 324, 1557–1561. doi: 10.1126/science.1176062

Hochreiter, S., and Schmidhuber, J. (1997). Long short-term memory. *Neural Comput.* 9, 1735–1780. doi: 10.1162/neco.1997.9.8.1735

Ioffe, S., and Szegedy, C. (2015). "Batch normalization: Accelerating deep network training by reducing internal covariate shift," in *Proceedings of the 32nd International Conference on Machine Learning*, Vol. 37, eds F. Bach and D. Blei, *Proceedings of Machine Learning Research*, (Lille: PMLR), 448–456.

Kolen, J. F., and Pollack, J. B. (1991). "Back propagation is sensitive to initial conditions," in *Advances in Neural Information Processing Systems* (Cambridge, MA), 860–867.

Krizhevsky, A., Sutskever, I., and Hinton, G. E. (2012). "Imagenet classification with deep convolutional neural networks," in *Advances in Neural Information Processing Systems 25*, eds F. Pereira, C. J. C. Burges, L. Bottou and K. Q. Weinberger (Cambridge, MA: Curran Associates, Inc.), 1097–1105.

Lessler, J., Reich, N. G., Cummings, D. A., the New York City Department of Health, and Team, M. H. S. I. I. (2009). Outbreak of 2009 pandemic influenza a (h1n1) at a new york city school. *N. Engl. J. Med.* 361, 2628–2636. doi: 10.1056/NEJMoa0906089

Ma, H., El-Keib, A. A., and Ma, X. (1994). "Training data sensitivity problem of artificial neural network-based power system load forecasting," in *Proceedings of 26th Southeastern Symposium on System Theory* (New York, NY), 650–652.

Maas, A. L., Hannun, A. Y., and Ng, A. Y. (2013). "Rectifier nonlinearities improve neural network acoustic models," in *Proceedings of 30th International Conference on Machine Learning*, Vol. 30. New York, NY.

Magal, P., and Ruan, S. (2014). Susceptible-infectious-recovered models revisited: from the individual level to the population level. *Math. Biosci.* 250, 26–40. doi: 10.1016/j.mbs.2014.02.001

Mossong, J., and Muller, C. (2000). Estimation of the basic reproduction number of measles during an outbreak in a partially vaccinated population. *Epidemiol. Infect.* 124, 273–278. doi: 10.1017/S0950268899003672

Nishiura, H., Castillo-Chavez, C., Safan, M., and Chowell, G. (2009). Transmission potential of the new influenza a (h1n1) virus and its age-specificity in japan. *Euro Surveill* 14:19227. doi: 10.2807/ese.14.22.19227-en

Palmer, J., and Chakravarty, A. (2014). "Supervised machine learning," in *An Introduction To High Content Screening: Imaging Technology, Assay*

Development, and Data Analysis in Biology and Drug Discovery, eds S. A. Haney, D. Bowman, and A. Chakravarty (Hoboken, NJ: John Wiley & Sons, Inc.), 231.

Sahiner, B., Chan, H.-P., Petrick, N., Wei, D., Helvie, M. A., Adler, D. D., et al. (1996). Classification of mass and normal breast tissue: a convolution neural network classifier with spatial domain and texture images. *IEEE Trans. Med. Imaging* 15, 598–610. doi: 10.1109/42.538937

Saulnier, E., Gascuel, O., and Alizon, S. (2017). Inferring epidemiological parameters from phylogenies using regression-abc: a comparative study. *PLOS Comput. Biol.* 13:e1005416. doi: 10.1371/journal.pcbi.1005416

Sokolova, M., Japkowicz, N., and Szpakowicz, S. (2006). *Beyond Accuracy, F-Score and ROC: A Family of Discriminant Measures for Performance Evaluation.* Berlin; Heidelberg: Springer Berlin Heidelberg, 1015–1021.

Sullivan, K. M., Halpin, T. J., Marks, J. S., and Kim-Farley, R. (1985). Effectiveness of mumps vaccine in a school outbreak. *Am. J. Dis. Child.* 139, 909–912. doi: 10.1001/archpedi.1985.02140110063030

Sunnåker, M., Busetto, A. G., Numminen, E., Corander, J., Foll, M., and Dessimoz, C. (2013). Approximate bayesian computation. *PLOS Comput. Biol.* 9:e1002803. doi: 10.1371/journal.pcbi.1002803

Verrelst, J., Muñoz, J., Alonso, L., Delegido, J., Rivera, J. P., Camps-Valls, G., et al. (2012). Machine learning regression algorithms for biophysical parameter retrieval: Opportunities for sentinel-2 and -3. *Remote Sens. Environ.* 118, 127–139. doi: 10.1016/j.rse.2011.11.002

Vynnycky, E., Trindall, A., and Mangtani, P. (2007). Estimates of the reproduction numbers of spanish influenza using morbidity data. *Int. J. Epidemiol.* 36, 881–889. doi: 10.1093/ije/dym071

8

Seroprevalence of Neutralizing Antibodies to Human Adenovirus Type 4 and 7 in Healthy Populations from Southern China

Xianmiao Ye[1,2†], Lijun Xiao[3†], Xuehua Zheng[1†], Jinlin Wang[1,2], Tao Shu[1,2], Ying Feng[4], Xinglong Liu[1], Wan Su[1,5], Qian Wang[1,2], Chufang Li[4], Ling Chen[1,4] and Liqiang Feng[1*]*

[1] State Key Laboratories of Respiratory Diseases, Guangzhou Institutes of Biomedicine and Health, Chinese Academy of Sciences, Guangzhou, China, [2] University of Chinese Academy of Sciences, Beijing, China, [3] Center for Disease Control and Prevention of Chenzhou, Chenzhou, China, [4] The First Affiliated Hospital of Guangzhou Medical University, Guangzhou, China, [5] School of Biomedical Sciences, Huaqiao University, Quanzhou, China

***Correspondence:**
Ling Chen
chen_ling@gibh.ac.cn
Liqiang Feng
feng_liqiang@gibh.ac.cn

†These authors have contributed equally to this work

Human adenoviruses type 4 (HAdV4) and 7 (HAdV7) are two major respiratory pathogens and sporadically cause outbreaks of acute respiratory diseases. The neutralizing antibody (nAb) response to these two adenoviruses in civilian populations, which is important for dissecting previous circulations and predicting potential outbreaks, remains largely unknown. In this study, we generated replication-competent HAdV4 and HAdV7 reporter viruses expressing secreted-alkaline-phosphatase (SEAP), and established neutralization assays to investigate the seroprevalence of pre-existing nAb in healthy volunteers from Hunan Province, southern China. The seropositivity rates are 58.4 and 63.8% for anti-HAdV4 nAb and anti-HAdV7 nAb, respectively. High nAb titers (> 1000) were frequently detected in HAdV4-seropositive individuals, whereas most HAdV7-seropositive volunteers had moderate nAb titers (201–1000). The seropositivity rates of anti-HAdV4 nAb and anti-HAdV7 nAb increase with age, with individuals younger than 20 exhibiting the lowest seropositivity rates. Both seropositivity rates and nAb titers are comparable between different sex groups. Notably, HAdV4-seropositive individuals tend to be HAdV7-seropositive and *vice versa*. Because HAdV4 antisera showed no neutralizing activity to HAdV7 whereas HAdV7 antisera cannot neutralize HAdV4, a subgroup of individuals might be susceptible to infection by HAdV4 and HAdV7 and thus generate nAb to both of them. These results revealed the continuous circulation of HAdV4 and HAdV7 and the lack of protective immunity in more than 35% of people, which emphasized the surveillance of these two HAdVs and the development of prophylactic vaccines.

Keywords: human adenovirus type 4, human adenovirus type 7, neutralizing antibody, seroprevalence, Southern China

INTRODUCTION

Human adenoviruses (HAdVs) are non-enveloped, double-stranded DNA viruses belonging to *Adenoviridae*. To date, more than 85 genotypes of HAdVs have been identified and classified into seven species (A-G) on the basis of biological characteristics and genomic homology (Kajan et al., 2017; Hashimoto et al., 2018). HAdVs are common pathogens responsible for a variety of diseases, including acute respiratory disease (ARD), conjunctivitis, gastroenteritis, urinary infection and meningoencephalitis (Ghebremedhin, 2014; Radke and Cook, 2018). HAdV infection in immuno-competent healthy adults is usually asymptomatic (Berciaud et al., 2012). However, in particular populations such as immuno-compromised individuals, infants, and children, HAdV infections may lead to severe and even fatal diseases (Ghebremedhin, 2014; Radke and Cook, 2018). Outbreaks of HAdV infection are frequently reported in crowded populations such as school students and military recruits (Ghebremedhin, 2014).

HAdV4 and HAdV7, two members belonging to species E and B respectively, are major causative pathogens of ARD and acute conjunctivitis (Hong et al., 2001; Erdin et al., 2015). Outbreaks of ARD or conjunctivitis caused by HAdV4 have been reported in the United States, Australia, and Japan (McNeill et al., 2000; Aoki and Tagawa, 2002; Zhang et al., 2016), whereas HAdV7-associated epidemics have also been documented in the United States, China, Japan and the Philippines (Tang et al., 2011; Yamamoto et al., 2014; Scott et al., 2016; Yang et al., 2017). These endemics and epidemics have rendered significant economic and healthy burdens in both military and civilian populations (Hoke and Snyder , 2013). The application of live-oral vaccines against HAdV4 and HAdV7 greatly reduced HAdV-associated ARDs in United States military trainees (Hoke and Snyder , 2013). During the cessation of vaccination between 1999 and 2011, HAdV infections sharply increased to pre-vaccine level (Erdman et al., 2002; Kajon et al., 2007). A retrospective survey revealed that low level of neutralizing antibody (nAb) to HAdV4 and HAdV7 in unimmunized military recruits facilitated the return of HAdV infections (Barraza et al., 1999). Although the new live-oral HAdV4 and HAdV7 vaccines were approved and re-introduced in 2011, vaccination was restricted to military recruits but was not applicable for general populations due to safety concerns (Radin et al., 2014; Choudhry et al., 2016). There is still no adenovirus vaccine for civilian populations worldwide. Besides, the knowledge about the seroprevalence of anti-HAdV4 nAb and anti-HAdV7 nAb in civilian populations is quite limited. We proposed that an investigation of pre-existing nAb could help to understand previous circulations of these two HAdVs and to predict potential outbreaks.

Recently, replication competent and incompetent genetic vectors based on HAdV4 and HAdV7 have been developed (Weaver, 2014; Peng et al., 2016). These vectors have great potency for oral administration (Deal et al., 2013). Several vaccine candidates against human immunodeficiency virus, hepatitis B virus, respiratory syncytial virus, and influenza A H5N1 virus based on HAdV4 or HAdV7 vectors have been undergoing preclinical and clinical trials, and exhibited good safety and immunogenicity (Hung et al., 1990; Hsu et al., 1992; Alexander et al., 2012; Weaver, 2014; Khurana et al., 2015). However, pre-existing nAb to HAdV4 and HAdV7 may limit the efficacy of these vaccines (Dharmapuri et al., 2009; Lanzi et al., 2011). Therefore, investigating the seroprevalence of anti-HAdV4 nAb and anti-HAdV7 nAb can also help to select subpopulations suitable for the application of these vaccines.

In this study, we constructed replication-competent HAdV4 and HAdV7 expressing secreted-alkaline-phosphatase (SEAP), and established convenient neutralization assays based on these reporter viruses. Using these neutralization assays, we investigated the seroprevalence of anti-HAdV4 nAb and anti-HAdV7 nAb in a civilian cohort from Hunan Province, southern China. We also analyzed the distributions of seropositivity rates and nAb titers in different age and sex groups.

MATERIALS AND METHODS

Recombinant HAdV4 and HAdV7 Reporter Viruses

HAdV4 (GenBank NO. KF006344.1) and HAdV7 (GenBank No. HQ659699), two clinical isolates, were kindly provided by Prof. Rong Zhou (Guangzhou Medical University). Recombinant HAdV4 and HAdV7 expressing SEAP were constructed according to previously described methods (Zheng et al., 2017). In brief, viral genomic DNA was extracted by sodium-dodecyl-sulfonate lysis (Sigma-Aldrich, St Louis, MO, United States) followed by phenol-chloroform extraction. The terminal regions of HAdV4 and HAdV7 genome, which were used as homology arms, were amplified by PCR and subcloned into pMD19T-Simple vectors (TaKaRa, Dalian, China) to obtain shuttle plasmids pT-Ad4(L+R) and pT-Ad7(L+R), respectively. A unique restriction site for BamHI was introduced between the two arms, and two restriction sites for AsiSI were introduced at the 5′ terminal of the left arm and the 3′ terminal of the right arm. After digestion with BamHI (Thermo Fisher Scientific, Waltham, MA, United States), linearized pT-Ad4(L+R) and pT-Ad7(L+R) were subjected to homologous recombination with viral genomes in E. coli BJ5183 competent cells (Agilent Technologies, Santa Clara, CA, United States) to obtain genomic plasmids pAd4 and pAd7, respectively. Subsequently, the homology arms for E3 deletion, which contain 500 base pairs (bp) upstream of HAdV4 E3 region, or 520 bp upstream of HAdV7 E3 region, or 710 bp downstream of HAdV4 E3 region, or 660 bp downstream of HAdV7 E3 region, were amplified by PCR. Two shuttle plasmids, p4E3LR and p7E3LR, were constructed by inserting the respective homology arms into pVAX1 plasmids (Thermo Fisher Scientific, Waltham, MA, United States). The ligated homology arms were released from p4E3LR and p7E3LR by digestion with BstZ17I and SgrAI (Thermo Fisher Scientific, Waltham, MA, United States). Meanwhile, pAd4 and pAd7 were linearized by digestion with BclI and EcoRI (Thermo Fisher Scientific, Waltham, MA, United States), respectively. The E3 regions were then deleted by homologous recombination between E3LR fragments and linearized pAd4 and pAd7 to obtain pAd4ΔE3 and pAd7ΔE3, respectively. To construct recombinant HAdV4 and HAdV7 reporter viruses, the coding sequences for SEAP flanked by a CMV promoter and a BGH poly(A) signal were amplified by PCR using pGA1-SEAP as the template (Zheng et al., 2017), and inserted into p4E3LR and p7E3LR to obtain shuttle reporter plasmids pGK43-SEAP and pGK73-SAEP, respectively. Finally, pGK43-SEAP and pGK73-SAEP were linearized by digestion with BstZ17I and SgrAI, whereas genomic plasmids pAd4ΔE3 or pAd7ΔE3 were linearized by digestion with SwaI (Thermo Fisher Scientific, Waltham, MA, United States), and pAd4-SEAP and pAd7-SEAP were constructed by homologous recombination between linearized shuttle reporter plasmids and genomic plasmids. To rescue HAdV4-SEAP and HAdV7-SEAP, pAd4-SEAP and pAd7-SEAP were linearized by digestion with AsiSI (Thermo Fisher Scientific, Waltham, MA, United States) and transfected into HEK293 cells (ATCC). After successfully rescued, HAdV4-SEAP and HAdV7-SEAP were propagated in HEK293 cells and purified using cesium chloride gradient centrifugation. The infectious virus titers were determined as described previously (Aste-Amezaga et al., 2004).

Human Serum Samples

A total of 1302 healthy blood donors were included in this study. The serum samples were collected in the medical examination center of Center for Disease Control and Prevention of Chenzhou, Hunan Province, China, from January 1, 2017 to July 20, 2017. The volunteers ranged from 7 to 70 years old. The percentages of male and female were 54.1 and 45.9%, respectively. The demographic information of serum samples was summarized in **Supplementary Table S1**. Fresh blood samples were collected into serum tubes and let stand for 30 min at room temperature. Serum samples were then isolated by centrifugation at 3000 rpm for 10 min. 1302 serum samples were obtained, heat-inactivated for 90 min at 56°C and preserved at −80°C. The research with human samples was approved by the Ethics Committee of Guangzhou Institutes of Biomedical and Health (GIBH). Informed consents from each volunteer were signed.

Mouse Antisera

Six-week-old female BALB/c mice were purchased from Beijing Vital River Laboratory Animal Technology Co., Ltd., and housed in the Animal Experimental Center of GIBH. Animal experiments were approved by Institutional Animal Care and Use Committee of GIBH (IACUC, No. 2015014). HAdV4 antisera and HAdV7 antisera were prepared according to previously described methods (Feng et al., 2018). In brief, HAdV4 and HAdV7 were treated with 0.2% of β-propiolactone (BPL) (Tokyo Chemical Industry, Japan) overnight at 4°C followed by incubation for 2 h at 37°C. In this condition, HAdVs were completely inactivated. Mice were then intramuscularly inoculated with inactivated HAdV4 or HAdV7 at 1.0×10^9 viral particles (vp) per mouse. At 4 weeks after the first immunization, the mice were boosted with similar formulations. At 2 weeks post the final immunization, the mice were bled and euthanized. Serum samples were then collected, inactivated and preserved at −80°C.

HAdV4 and HAdV7 Neutralization Assays

The nAb titers against HAdV4 and HAdV7 were determined using neutralization assays based on HAdV4-SEAP and HAdV7-SEAP, respectively. In brief, HEK293 cells were seeded into 96-well plates at 3×10^4 cells per well. One day later, HAdV4-SEAP or HAdV7-SEAP at 4×10^6 vp per well (~100 vp/cell) were incubated for 1 h at 37°C either alone (virus infection alone) or together with serial dilutions of human sera or mouse antisera. Subsequently, each sample was added to the 96-well plates and incubated for 24 h at 37°C. Finally, the supernatants were harvested and the SEAP activity was assessed using the chemiluminescent substrate CSPD according to the manufacturer's protocols (Thermo Fisher Scientific, Waltham, MA, United States). The relative light units (RLU) were recorded using a luminometer (MlX Microtiter, Dynex Technologies, Inc., United States) and the titers were calculated as the dilutions that inhibited 50% of RLU values.

Statistical Analysis

Comparisons of the seropositivity rates in different groups were conducted using Chi-square test or Chi-square test for trend. Comparisons of the nAb titers among groups were performed using the Mann-Whitney test or the Kruskal-Wallis test. SPSS version 13.0 (SPSS Inc., Chicago, IL) was used for statistical analyses, and *p*-values less than 0.05 were considered statistically significant. The graphs were generated with GraphPad Prism version 6 (GraphPad Software, La Jolla, CA, United States).

RESULTS

Establishment of Neutralization Assays With HAdV4-SEAP and HAdV7-SEAP

To establish a new neutralization assay alternative for traditional cytopathic effect based neutralization assays, we constructed recombinant HAdV4 and HAdV7 reporter viruses expressing SEAP (**Figure 1A**). HAdV4-SEAP and HAdV7-SEAP were successfully rescued and propagated. The SEAP activity was linearly correlated with the infection dosage of HAdV4-SEAP and HAdV7-SEAP from 0.01 vp/cell to 100 vp/cell (**Figure 1B**). We chose an infection dosage of 100 vp/cell for assessing the titers of nAb in the serum samples.

We established the neutralization assays using mice antisera generated by immunizing BALB/c mice with inactivated HAdV4 or HAdV7 viral particles. The neutralization curve of antisera to HAdV4-SEAP and HAdV7-SEAP were shown (**Figures 1C,D**). SEAP activity in the culture supernatants sharply decreased at certain dilutions of serum samples, reflecting the neutralization of antisera to HAdV4 and HAdV7. Notably, SEAP expression in cells infected with HAdV4-SEAP was only suppressed by HAdV4 antisera but not significantly influenced by HAdV7 antisera, whereas SEAP expression in HAdV7-SEAP infected cells was only inhibited by HAdV7 antisera but not HAdV4 antisera. This result suggested that HAdV4 specific nAb have minimal, if any, cross-neutralizing activity to HAdV7, and *vice versa*.

Overall Seroprevalence of Anti-HAdV4 nAb and Anti-HAdV7 nAb in Healthy Populations From Hunan Province, Southern China

Using reporter virus based neutralization assays, we investigated the seroprevalence of anti-HAdV4 nAb and anti-HAdV7 nAb in a cohort of 1302 healthy volunteers from Human Province, China (**Supplementary Table S1**). The overall seropositivity

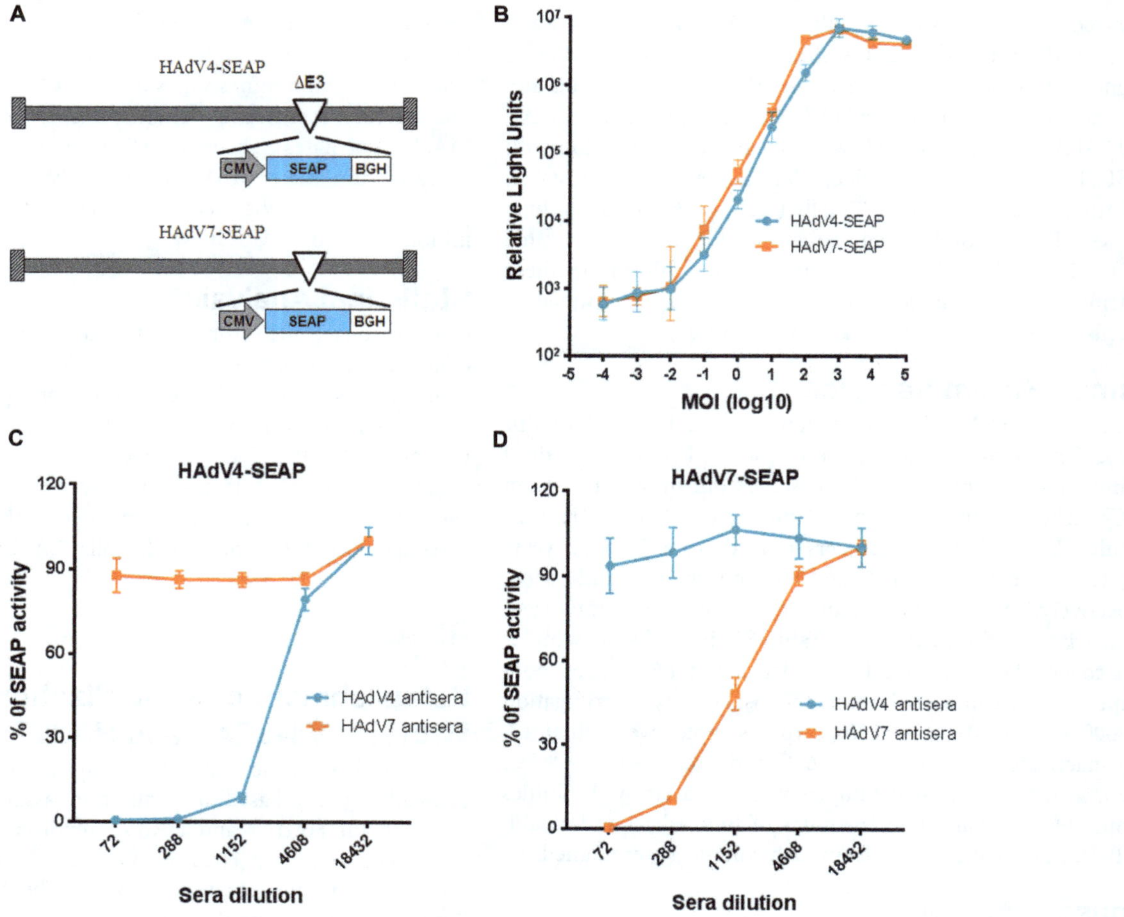

FIGURE 1 | Establishment of neutralization assays based on HAdV4-SEAP and HAdV7-SEAP. **(A)** The schematic diagram of HAdV4-SEAP and HAdV7-SEAP. **(B)** Detection of SEAP activity in the culture supernatants of HAdV4-SEAP or HAdV7-SEAP infected cells. HEK293 cells were infected with HAdV4-SEAP or HAdV7-SEAP at serially increasing doses. At 24 h after infection, the culture supernatants were collected and the SEAP activity was assessed. Shown are the representative data of three independent experiments. **(C,D)** Neutralization curves of HAdV4 antisera and HAdV7 antisera to HAdV4-SEAP **(C)** and HAdV7-SEAP **(D)**. Mouse antisera were serially diluted and incubated with HAdV4-SEAP **(C)** or HAdV7-SEAP **(D)**. After incubation for 1 h, the mixtures were added to HEK293 cells. One day later, the SEAP activity in the culture supernatants were examined. Cells infected with HAdV4-SEAP or HAdV7-SEAP in the absence of antisera were used as viral infection alone controls. Shown are the percentages of SEAP activity in the presence of antisera versus viral infection alone. The data were representative of two independent experiments. Error bars stand for mean ± standard deviation (SD).

rate of anti-HAdV4 nAb was 58.4% (95% Confidence Interval, CI, 55.7–61.1%), which was significantly lower than that of anti-HAdV7 nAb (63.8%, 95% CI 61.2–66.4%) (Chi-square test, $P < 0.01$; **Supplementary Tables S2, S3**). In the whole cohort, HAdV4-seropositive individuals had significantly higher nAb titers than HAdV7-seropositive ones (Mann-Whitney test, $P < 0.001$, **Figure 2A**). According to nAb titers, the serum samples were categorized into four subgroups: negative, < 72; low, 72–200; moderate, 201–1000; and high, > 1000. The distributions of different nAb titers were analyzed (**Figure 2B**). 34.0% of serum samples (95% CI 32.6–38.0%) contained high nAb titers to HAdV4, whereas only 22.9% (95% CI 21.9–26.9%) of serum samples had high nAb titers to HAdV7 (Chi-square test, $P < 0.001$). Significantly more serum samples contained moderate nAb titers to HAdV7 (26.8%; 95% CI 24.4–29.2%) than to HAdV4 (16.3%; 95% CI 14.3–18.3%) (Chi-square test, $P < 0.001$, **Figure 2B**). These results suggested that although the seropositivity rate of anti-HAdV4 nAb was lower than that of anti-HAdV7 nAb, HAdV4-seropositive individuals tended to have higher nAb titers in comparison with HAdV7-seropositive individuals.

Seropositivity Rates but Not Titers of Anti-HAdV4 nAb and Anti-HAdV7 nAb Increased With Age

We analyzed the trends of seroprevalence in different age groups. The overall seropositivity rates of anti-HAdV4 nAb and anti-HAdV7 nAb increased with age (Chi-square test for trend, HAdV4: $P < 0.001$; HAdV7: $P < 0.001$; **Figure 3A**). The frequency of serum samples with moderate and high anti-HAdV4 nAb and anti-HAdV7 nAb titers also progressively increased with age (**Figures 3B,C**). However, the frequency of serum samples with low anti-HAdV4 nAb and anti-HAdV7 nAb titers increased

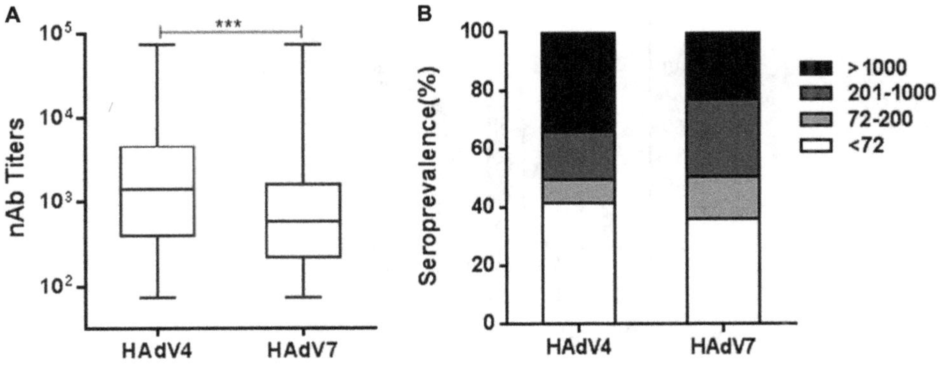

FIGURE 2 | The overall seroprevalence of anti-HAdV4 nAb and anti-HAdV7 nAb. **(A)** The nAb titers against HAdV4 and HAdV7 in seropositive individuals. The data was analyzed with the Mann-Whitney test. ***$P < 0.001$. **(B)** The distributions of anti-HAdV4 nAb and anti-HAdV7 nAb titers. nAb titers were classified into four subgroups: negative, < 72; low, 72–200; moderate, 201–1000; and high, > 1000. The percentages of individuals with negative, low, moderate, and high nAb titers were shown.

with age before 50 but decreased thereafter (**Figures 3B,C**). Notably, in each age group, the percentage of individuals with high anti-HAdV4 nAb titers was higher than that with moderate and low anti-HAdV4 nAb titers (**Figure 3B**), whereas individuals with moderate anti-HAdV7 nAb titers dominated in HAdV7-seropositive ones (**Figure 3C**). The titers of anti-HAdV4 nAb was higher in the age group younger than 20 than the other age groups (Kruskal-Wallis test, $P < 0.001$; **Figure 3D**). However, no difference was observed for the titers of anti-HAdV7 nAbs among age groups (Kruskal-Wallis test, $P = 0.399$; **Figure 3E**). These results revealed a different distribution of seropositivity rates as well as nAb titers for HAdV4 and HAdV7, and implied that individuals younger than 20 may be more susceptible to HAdV4 and HAdV7 infection than older individuals because of relatively lower nAb seropositivity rates.

Seropositivity Rates and Titers of Anti-HAdV4 nAb and Anti-HAdV7 nAb Were Not Affected by Sex

We next analyzed the seroprevalence and titer distributions of anti-HAdV4 nAb and anti-HAdV7 nAb in sex groups. The seropositivity rates of anti-HAdV4 nAb in males was slightly higher than that in females, but this difference did not reach statistical significance (**Figure 4A**). Similarly, no significant differences were observed for the seroprevalence of anti-HAdV7 nAb between males and females (**Figure 4B**). The titers of anti-HAdV4 nAb and anti-HAdV7 nAb in seropositive males were also comparable to those in seronegative females (**Figures 4C,D**). Therefore, the seroprevalence of anti-HAdV4 nAb and anti-HAdV7 nAb were associated with age, but not with sex.

Analysis of the Seroprevalence and nAb Titers in Double-Positive and Single-Positive Individuals

We also analyzed the seropositivity rates of anti-HAdV4 nAb in HAdV7-seropositive or -seronegative individuals. Significantly more HAdV4-seropositive samples were detected in HAdV7-seropositive individuals than in HAdV7-seronegative ones (Chi-square test, $P < 0.001$; **Figure 5A**). The percentages of sera with low, moderate and high anti-HAdV4 nAb titers in HAdV7-seropositive individuals were similar to those in HAdV7-seronegative ones (**Figure 5B**). Similarly, the seropositivity rate of anti-HAdV7 nAb in HAdV4-seropositive individuals was significantly higher than that in HAdV4-seronegative ones (chi-square test, $P < 0.001$; **Figure 5A**). The percentages of sera with low, moderate and high anti-HAdV7 nAb titers in HAdV4-seropositive individuals were also comparable to those in HAdV4-seronegative ones (**Figure 5C**). Moreover, the titers of anti-HAdV4 nAb and anti-HAdV7 nAb in double-positive sera were comparable to that in single-positive sera (**Figures 5D,E**). These results revealed that HAdV7-seropositive individuals tend to be HAdV4-seropositive, and *vice versa*, but the nAb titers to these two HAdVs were comparable in single- and double-positive individuals.

DISCUSSION

HAdV4 and HAdV7 represent two major respiratory pathogens in civilian populations and military trainees worldwide (Top, 1975; Tang et al., 2011; Yamamoto et al., 2014). However, surveillances of nAb to these two HAdVs in large civilian cohorts are extremely rare, possibly due to the lack of convenient neutralization assays. Here, we developed neutralization assays using HAdV4-SEAP and HAdV7-SEAP (**Figure 1**). These assays have been shown to be more sensitive, convenient, and objective than traditional cytopathic effect based methods (Aste-Amezaga et al., 2004; Zheng et al., 2017), and thus enabled the surveillance of pre-exiting anti-HAdV4 nAb and anti-HAdV7 nAb in large cohorts. To our knowledge, we are the first to report the seroprevalence of nAb to HAdV4 and HAdV7 in civilian population. We found that, the seropositivity rates of anti-HAdV4 nAb and anti-HAdV7 nAb were 58.4 and 63.8% (**Figure 2**), respectively, which were lower than that of anti-HAdV5 nAb but higher than that of anti-HAdV14 nAb and

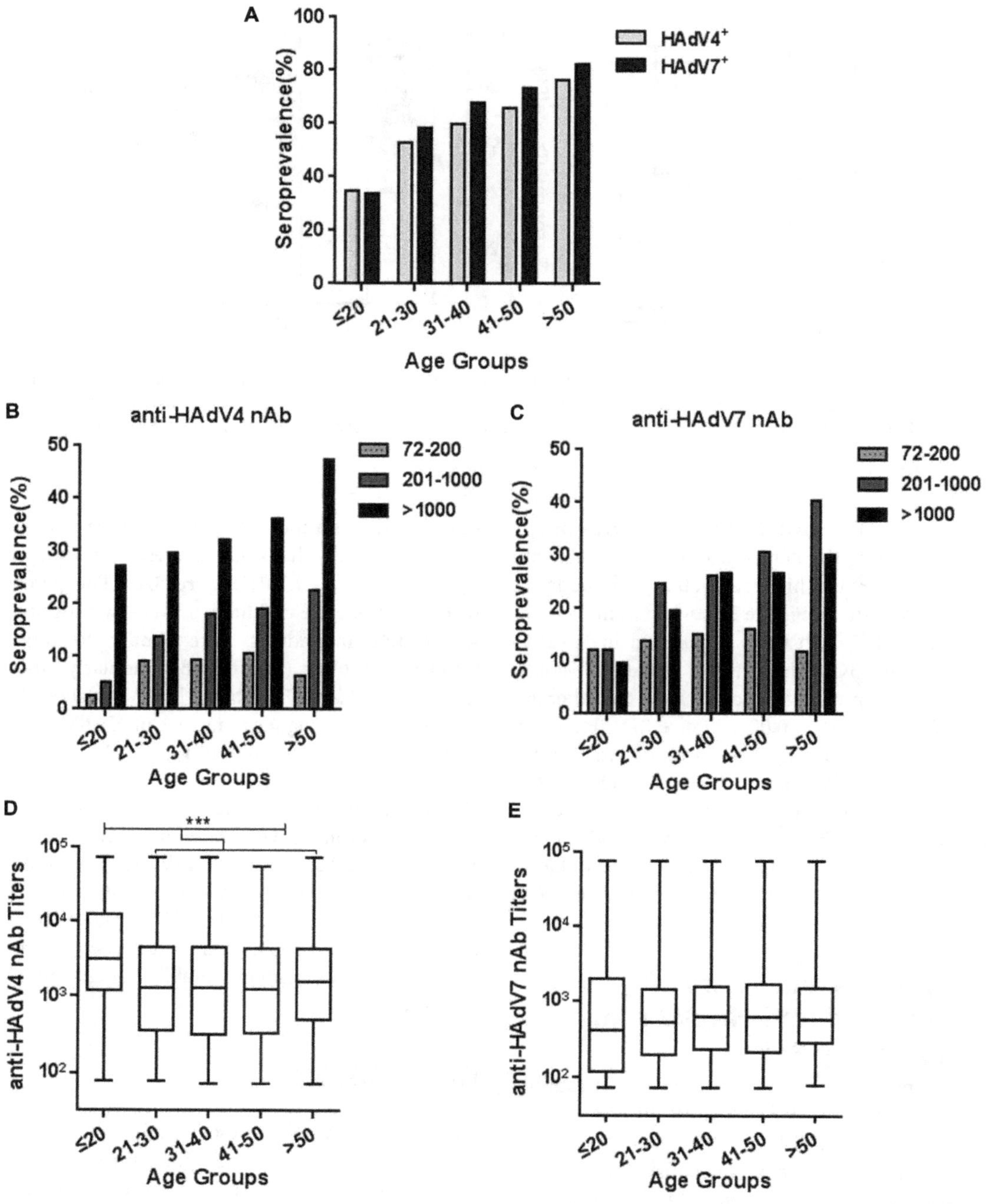

FIGURE 3 | Seroprevalence and titer distribution of anti-HAdV4 nAb and anti-HAdV7 nAb in different age groups. **(A)** The seropositivity rates of anti-HAdV4 nAb and anti-HAdV7 nAb in different age groups. The data were analyzed with Chi-square test for trend. **(B,C)** The distributions of the low (72–200), moderate (201–1000), and high (> 1000) titers of anti-HAdV4 nAb **(B)** and anti-HAdV7 nAb **(C)** in different age groups. **(D,E)** The titers of nAb to HAdV4 **(D)** and HAdV7 **(E)** in different age groups. The data was analyzed with the Kruskal-Wallis test. $^{***}P < 0.001$.

anti-HAdV55 nAb (Hong et al., 2001; Sun et al., 2011; Zheng et al., 2017). At least 41.6 and 36.2% of individuals in this population are still susceptible for HAdV4 and HAdV7 infection respectively, due to the absence of protective nAb (Barraza et al., 1999; Clemmons et al., 2017). Our results reinforced that HAdV4 and HAdV7 should be considered when ARD outbreaks. A prophylactic vaccine may be necessary for the prevention of HAdV4 and HAdV7 infection.

Recently, the pre-existing nAb to a variety of HAdVs including HAdV2, 5, 14, 26, 35, and 55 have been investigated (Barouch et al., 2004; Abbink et al., 2007; Zheng et al., 2017). However, Investigations of anti-HAdV4 nAb and anti-HAdV7 nAb were mainly conducted in military recruits (Ludwig et al., 1998; Kolavic-Gray et al., 2002; Choudhry et al., 2016). Results from United States military trainees revealed that the overall seroprevalence of anti-HAdV4 nAb was significantly lower than

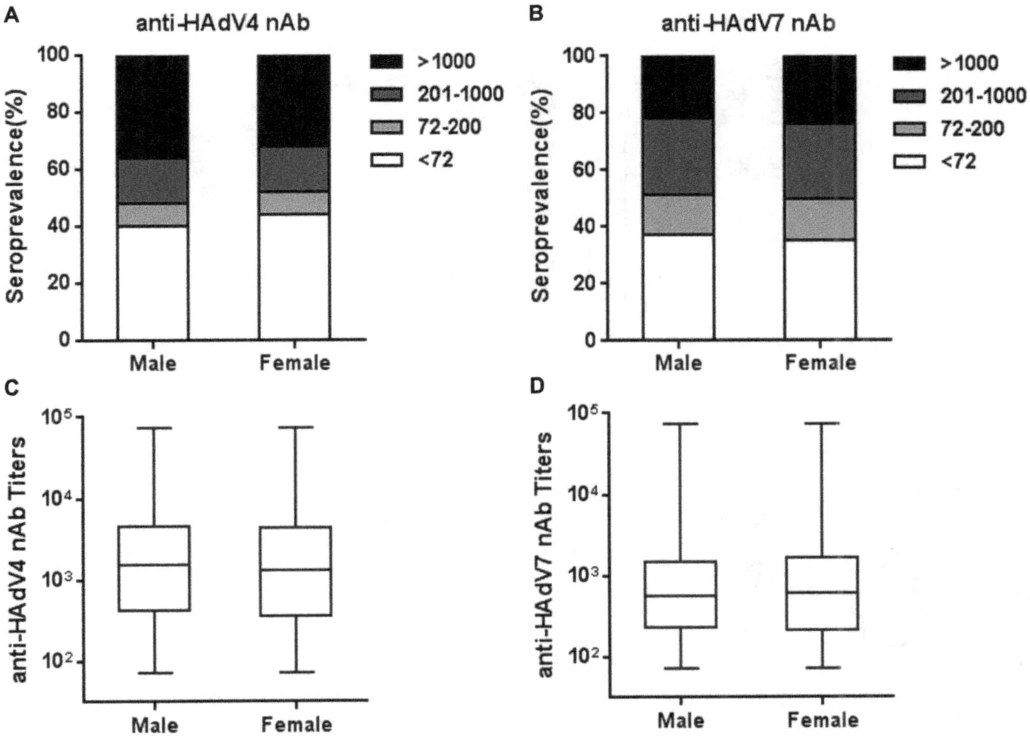

FIGURE 4 | Seroprevalence and titer distribution of anti-HAdV4 nAb and anti-HAdV7 nAb in sex groups. **(A,B)** The distributions of anti-HAdV4 nAb **(A)** and anti-HAdV7 nAb **(B)** titers in sex groups. **(C,D)** The titers of nAb to HAdV4 **(C)** and HAdV7 **(D)** in seropositive males and females. The data were analyzed using the Mann-Whitney test.

that of anti-HAdV7 nAb, whereas individuals with high titers of anti-HAdV4 nAb were much more than those with high titers of anti-HAdV7 nAb (Ludwig et al., 1998). Our results in civilian populations showed a similar trend. That is, the frequency of HAdV4-seropositive individuals is lower than that of HAdV7-seropositive ones, but the titers of anti-HAdV4 nAb were significantly higher than that of anti-HAdV7 nAb (**Figure 2**). The similar results from two different populations imply that HAdV4 circulation in these populations may be more recent than HAdV7, or HAdV4 infection may induce stronger nAb responses than HAdV7 infection.

Several studies have shown that the seroprevalence of nAb to other HAdVs such as HAdV5 increased with age (Sun et al., 2011; Yu et al., 2012), but the nAb titers would decrease gradually in years post infection due to cumulative saturation of infection in adults (Yang et al., 2016). However, we found that both HAdV4 and HAdV7 seropositivity rates gradually increased with age (**Figure 3**), consistent to previous results from army trainees (Ludwig et al., 1998), suggesting that infection rates of HAdV4 and HAdV7 would not be saturated in adults. The sporadic appearance of adult patients with HAdV4- or HAdV7-associated severe pneumonia also supported the absence of protective immunity in a proportion of individuals (Barraza et al., 1999; Clemmons et al., 2017). Thus, close attention should be paid to HAdV4- and HAdV7-associated ARDs not only for children, but also for adults. Similar to HAdV14 and HAdV55 seroprevalence (Zheng et al., 2017), sex is not an important factor influencing either seropositivity rates or nAb titers of HAdV4 and HAdV7 (**Figure 4**). Intriguingly, we found that HAdV4-seropositive individuals tend to be HAdV7-seropositive, and *vice versa* (**Figure 5**). Given that HAdV4 antisera and HAdV7 antisera showed no significant cross-neutralizing activity to HAdV4 and HAdV7 (**Figure 1**), this result implied that a proportion of individuals might be more susceptible to HAdV infection. These individuals may be successively or simultaneously infected by HAdV4 and HAdV7 and thereby generated nAb responses to both of them. However, the mechanisms underlying this phenomenon need to be elucidated in future studies.

Recombinant adenoviral vectors based on HAdV4 and HAdV7 have been explored as vaccine vectors for a variety of pathogenic viruses (Hung et al., 1990; Hsu et al., 1992; Alexander et al., 2012; Weaver, 2014; Khurana et al., 2015). A potential limitation of recombinant adenoviral vectors is the pre-existing nAb resulted from natural exposure (Lanzi et al., 2011). The sensitive neutralization assays established in this study can potentially facilitate the screening of HAdV4- and HAdV7-seronegative individuals, which may be important for the clinical evaluation of vaccines based on recombinant HAdV4 or HAdV7 vectors. In this particular cohort, 41.6 and 36.2% of participants were seronegative for anti-HAdV4 nAb and anti-HAdV7 nAb, respectively, and thereby could be included in the clinical trials for HAdV4- or HAdV7-vectored vaccines.

HAdV4 has been shown to originate from a recombinant event between HAdV16 and simian adenovirus type 26 (SAdV26)

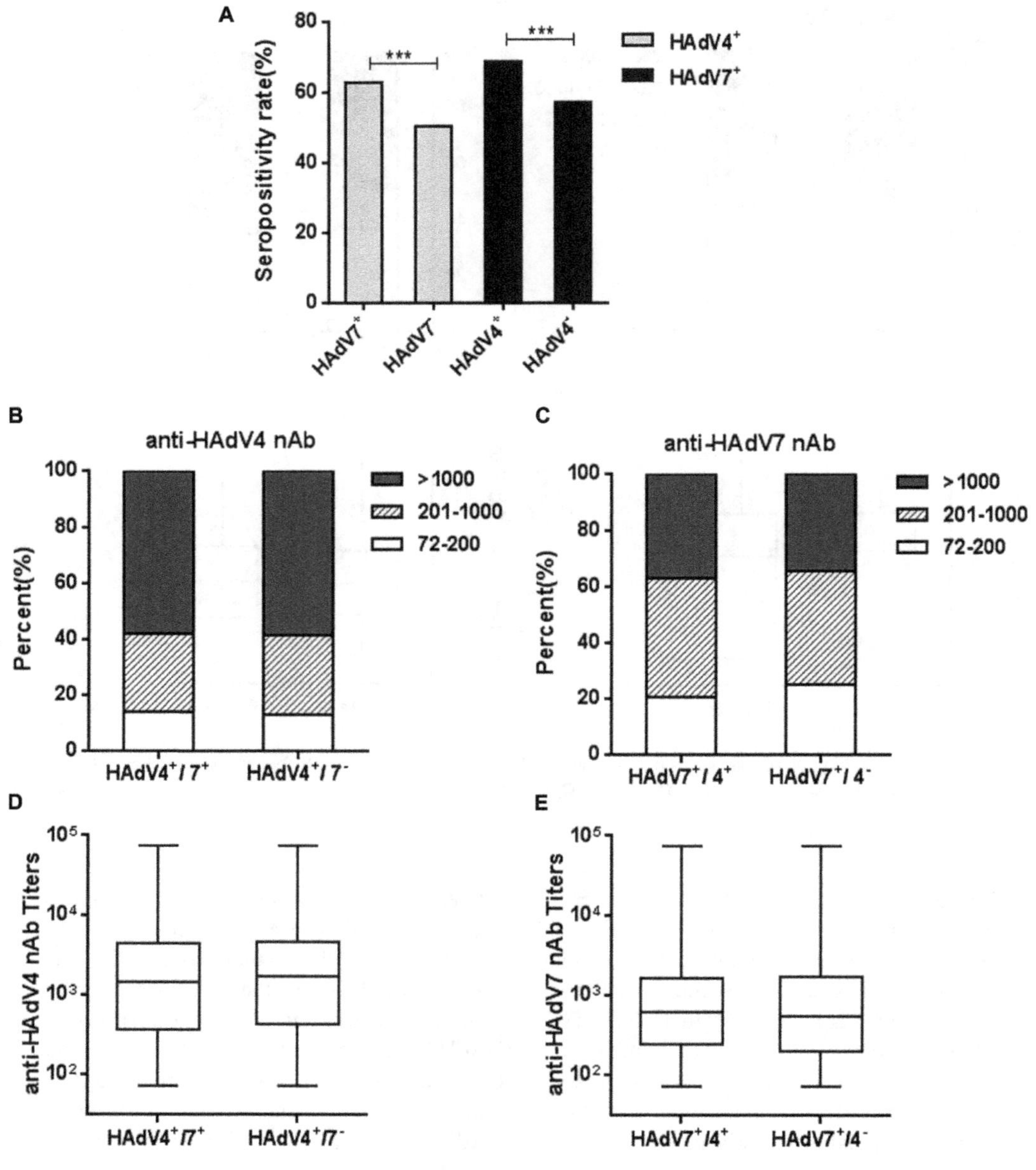

FIGURE 5 | Seropositivity rates and titers of anti-HAdV4 nAb and anti-HAdV7 nAbs in single- and double-positive samples. **(A)** The seropositivity rates of anti-HAdV4 nAb and anti-HAdV7 nAb in single-positive and double-positive serum samples. The data were analyzed with Chi-square test. $^{***}P < 0.001$. **(B,C)** The distributions of anti-HAdV4 nAb **(B)** and anti-HAdV7 nAb **(C)** titers in single-positive and double-positive serum samples. **(D,E)** Overall titers of anti-HAdV4 nAb **(D)** and anti-HAdV7 nAb **(E)** in single-positive and double-positive serum samples. The data were analyzed using the Mann-Whitney test.

(Dehghan et al., 2013), and comprises loop 1 and loop 2 of HAdV16 hexon in the genome chassis of SAdV26. Because hexon loop 1 and loop2 contain the major targets of anti-HAdV nAb (Pichla-Gollon et al., 2007; Yuan et al., 2009; Feng et al., 2018), screening of anti-HAdV4 nAb with HAdV4-SEAP cannot discriminate the nAb induced by HAdV16 infection. However, dissecting the seroprevalence of anti-HAdV4 nAb, resulted no matter from HAdV4 infection or from HAdV16 infection, could help to understand the herd immunity to HAdV4. Moreover, to our best knowledge, no outbreaks of HAdV16 infection have ever been reported in Hunan province, China. The circulation of HAdV16 in this district is not dominant and even rare. Therefore, the pre-existing anti-HAdV4 nAb in the investigated cohorts was most likely resulted from HAdV4 infection but not HAdV16 infection. Future studies, such as detection of fiber-specific nAb and surveillance of the circulating HAdV strains may help to clarify the real seroprevalence of anti-HAdV4 nAb induced by HAdV4 infection.

In summary, we developed reporter virus based neutralization assays for HAdV4 and HAdV7, and investigated the pre-existing nAb responses in a civilian population. HAdV4 and HAdV7 can be potential causative pathogens for ARDs in civilian populations in southern China. Our results provided insightful information not only for understanding the herd immunity to these two

HAdVs but also for the development of vaccines against HAdV infection.

AUTHOR CONTRIBUTIONS

XY, LX, and XZ collected the samples, performed the neutralization assays and analyzed the results. JW, TS, YF, XL, WS, and QW contributed to the data analysis. CL reviewed the manuscript. LC and LF conceived and designed the study, wrote the manuscript, and approved the submission.

REFERENCES

Abbink, P., Lemckert, A. A., Ewald, B. A., Lynch, D. M., Denholtz, M., Smits, S., et al. (2007). Comparative seroprevalence and immunogenicity of six rare serotype recombinant adenovirus vaccine vectors from subgroups B and D. *J. Virol.* 81, 4654–4663. doi: 10.1128/JVI.02696-06

Alexander, J., Ward, S., Mendy, J., Manayani, D. J., Farness, P., Avanzini, J. B., et al. (2012). Pre-clinical evaluation of a replication-competent recombinant adenovirus serotype 4 vaccine expressing influenza H5 hemagglutinin. *PLoS One* 7:e31177. doi: 10.1371/journal.pone.0031177

Aoki, K., and Tagawa, Y. (2002). A twenty-one year surveillance of adenoviral conjunctivitis in Sapporo. Japan. *Int. Ophthalmol. Clin.* 42, 49–54. doi: 10.1097/00004397-200201000-00008

Aste-Amezaga, M., Bett, A. J., Wang, F., Casimiro, D. R., Antonello, J. M., Patel, D. K., et al. (2004). Quantitative adenovirus neutralization assays based on the secreted alkaline phosphatase reporter gene: application in epidemiologic studies and in the design of adenovector vaccines. *Hum. Gene Ther.* 15, 293–304. doi: 10.1089/104303404322886147

Barouch, D. H., Pau, M. G., Custers, J. H., Koudstaal, W., Kostense, S., Havenga, M. J., et al. (2004). Immunogenicity of recombinant adenovirus serotype 35 vaccine in the presence of pre-existing anti-Ad5 immunity. *J. Immunol.* 172, 6290–6297. doi: 10.4049/jimmunol.172.10.6290

Barraza, E. M., Ludwig, S. L., Gaydos, J. C., and Brundage, J. F. (1999). Reemergence of adenovirus type 4 acute respiratory disease in military trainees: report of an outbreak during a lapse in vaccination. *J. Infect. Dis.* 179, 1531–1533. doi: 10.1086/314772

Berciaud, S., Rayne, F., Kassab, S., Jubert, C., Faure-Della Corte, M., Salin, F., et al. (2012). Adenovirus infections in Bordeaux University Hospital 2008-2010: clinical and virological features. *J. Clin. Virol.* 54, 302–307. doi: 10.1016/j.jcv.2012.04.009

Choudhry, A., Mathena, J., Albano, J. D., Yacovone, M., and Collins, L. (2016). Safety evaluation of adenovirus type 4 and type 7 vaccine live, oral in military recruits. *Vaccine* 34, 4558–4564. doi: 10.1016/j.vaccine.2016.07.033

Clemmons, N. S., McCormic, Z. D., Gaydos, J. C., Hawksworth, A. W., and Jordan, N. N. (2017). Acute respiratory disease in US Army Trainees 3 years after reintroduction of adenovirus vaccine (1). *Emerg. Infect. Dis.* 23, 95–98. doi: 10.3201/eid2301.161297

Deal, C., Pekosz, A., and Ketner, G. (2013). Prospects for oral replicating adenovirus-vectored vaccines. *Vaccine* 31, 3236–3243. doi: 10.1016/j.vaccine.2013.05.016

Dehghan, S., Seto, J., Liu, E. B., Walsh, M. P., Dyer, D. W., Chodosh, J., et al. (2013). Computational analysis of four human adenovirus type 4 genomes reveals molecular evolution through two interspecies recombination events. *Virology* 443, 197–207. doi: 10.1016/j.virol.2013.05.014

Dharmapuri, S., Peruzzi, D., and Aurisicchio, L. (2009). Engineered adenovirus serotypes for overcoming anti-vector immunity. *Expert. Opin. Biol. Ther.* 9, 1279–1287. doi: 10.1517/14712590903187053

Erdin, B. N., Pas S. D., Durak, I., Schutten, M., and Sayiner, A. A. (2015). A 5-year study of adenoviruses causing conjunctivitis in Izmir. Turkey. *J. Med. Virol.* 87, 472–477. doi: 10.1002/jmv.24071

Erdman, D. D., Xu, W., Gerber, S. I., Gray, G. C., Schnurr, D., Kajon, A. E., et al. (2002). Molecular epidemiology of adenovirus type 7 in the United States, 1966-2000. *Emerg. Infect. Dis.* 8, 269–277. doi: 10.3201/eid0803.010190

Feng, Y., Sun, X., Ye, X., Feng, Y., Wang, J., Zheng, X., et al. (2018). Hexon and fiber of adenovirus type 14 and 55 are major targets of neutralizing antibody but only fiber-specific antibody contributes to cross-neutralizing activity. *Virology* 518, 272–283. doi: 10.1016/j.virol.2018.03.002

Ghebremedhin, B. (2014). Human adenovirus: viral pathogen with increasing importance. *Eur. J. Microbiol. Immunol.* 4, 26–33. doi: 10.1556/EuJMI.4.2014.1.2

Hashimoto, S., Gonzalez, G., Harada, S., Oosako, H., Hanaoka, N., Hinokuma, R., et al. (2018). Recombinant type Human mastadenovirus D85 associated with epidemic keratoconjunctivitis since 2015 in Japan. *J. Med. Virol.* 90, 881–889. doi: 10.1002/jmv.25041

Hoke, C. H. Jr., and Snyder, C. E. Jr. (2013). History of the restoration of adenovirus type 4 and type 7 vaccine, live oral (Adenovirus Vaccine) in the context of the department of defense acquisition system. *Vaccine* 31, 1623–1632. doi: 10.1016/j.vaccine.2012.12.029

Hong, J. Y., Lee, H. J., Piedra, P. A., Choi, E. H., Park, K. H., Koh, Y. Y., et al. (2001). Lower respiratory tract infections due to adenovirus in hospitalized Korean children: epidemiology, clinical features, and prognosis. *Clin. Infect. Dis.* 32, 1423–1429. doi: 10.1086/320146

Hsu, K. H. L., Lubeck, M. D., Davis, A. R., Bhat, R. A., Selling, B. H., Bhat, B. M., et al. (1992). Immunogenicity of recombinant adenovirus-respiratory syncytial virus-vaccines with adenovirus type-4. type-5, and type-7 vectors in dogs and a chimpanzee. *J. Infect. Dis.* 166, 769–775. doi: 10.1093/infdis/166.4.769

Hung, P. P., Chanda, P. K., Natuk, R. J., Mason, B. B., Chengalvala, M., Bhat, B. M., et al. (1990). Adenovirus vaccine strains genetically engineered to express Hiv-1 or Hbv antigens for use as live recombinant vaccines. *Nat. Immun. Cell. Growth. Regul.* 9, 160–164.

Kajan, G. L., Kajon, A. E., Pinto, A. C., Bartha, D., and Arnberg, N. (2017). The complete genome sequence of human adenovirus 84, a highly recombinant new human mastadenovirus D type with a unique fiber gene. *Virus Res.* 242, 79–84. doi: 10.1016/j.virusres.2017.09.012

Kajon, A. E., Moseley, J. M., Metzgar, D., Huong, H. S., Wadleigh, A., Ryan, M. A., et al. (2007). Molecular epidemiology of adenovirus type 4 infections in US military recruits in the postvaccination era (1997-2003). *J. Infect. Dis.* 196, 67–75. doi: 10.1086/518442

Khurana, S., Coyle, E. M., Manischewitz, J., King, L. R., Ishioka, G., Alexander, J., et al. (2015). Oral priming with replicating adenovirus serotype 4 followed by subunit H5N1 vaccine boost promotes antibody affinity maturation and expands H5N1 cross-clade neutralization. *PLoS One* 10:e0115476. doi: 10.1371/journal.pone.0115476

Kolavic-Gray, S. A., Binn, L. N., Sanchez, J. L., Cersovsky, S. B., Polyak, C. S., Mitchell-Raymundo, F., et al. (2002). Large epidemic of adenovirus type 4 infection among military trainees: epidemiological, clinical, and laboratory studies. *Clin. Infect. Dis.* 35, 808–818. doi: 10.1086/342573

Lanzi, A., Ben Youssef, G., Perricaudet, M., and Benihoud, K. (2011). Anti-adenovirus humoral responses influence on the efficacy of vaccines based on epitope display on adenovirus capsid. *Vaccine* 29, 1463–1471. doi: 10.1016/j.vaccine.2010.12.025

Ludwig, S. L., Brundage, J. F., Kelley, P. W., Nang, R., Towle, C., Schnurr, D. P., et al. (1998). Prevalence of antibodies to adenovirus serotypes 4 and 7 among unimmunized US Army trainees: results of a retrospective nationwide seroprevalence survey. *J. Infect. Dis.* 178, 1776–1778. doi: 10.1086/314498

McNeill, K. M., Benton, F. R., Monteith, S. C., Tuchscherer, M. A., and Gaydos, J. C. (2000). Epidemic spread of adenovirus type 4-associated acute respiratory disease between US army installations. *Emerg. Infect. Dis.* 6, 415–419. doi: 10.3201/eid0604.000419

Peng, Y., Lai, M. M., Lou, Y. Y., Liu, Y. Q., Wang, H. Y., and Zheng, X. Q. (2016). Efficient induction of cross-presentating human B cell by transduction with human adenovirus type 7 vector. *Immunol. Lett.* 169, 41–51. doi: 10.1016/j.imlet.2015.11.011

Pichla-Gollon, S. L., Drinker, M., Zhou, X. Y., Xue, F., Rux, J. J., Gao, G. P., et al. (2007). Structure-based identification of a major neutralizing site in an adenovirus hexon. *J. Virol.* 81, 1680–1689. doi: 10.1128/Jvi.02023-06

Radin, J. M., Hawksworth, A. W., Blair, P. J., Faix, D. J., Raman, R., Russell, K. L., et al. (2014). Dramatic decline of respiratory illness among US military recruits after the renewed use of adenovirus vaccines. *Clin. Infect. Dis.* 59, 962–968. doi: 10.1093/cid/ciu507

Radke, J. R., and Cook, J. L. (2018). Human adenovirus infections: update and consideration of mechanisms of viral persistence. *Curr. Opin. Infect. Dis.* 31, 251–256. doi: 10.1097/Qco.0000000000000451

Scott, M. K., Chommanard, C., Lu, X., Appelgate, D., Grenz, L., Schneider, E., et al. (2016). Human adenovirus associated with severe respiratory infection. Oregon, USA, 2013-2014. *Emerg. Infect. Dis.* 22, 1044–1051. doi: 10.3201/eid2206.151898

Sun, C., Zhang, Y., Feng, L., Pan, W., Zhang, M., Hong, Z., et al. (2011). Epidemiology of adenovirus type 5 neutralizing antibodies in healthy people and AIDS patients in Guangzhou, southern China. *Vaccine* 29, 3837–3841. doi: 10.1016/j.vaccine.2011.03.042

Tang, L., Wang, L., Tan, X., and Xu, W. (2011). Adenovirus serotype 7 associated with a severe lower respiratory tract disease outbreak in infants in Shaanxi province. China. *Virol. J.* 8:23. doi: 10.1186/1743-422X-8-23

Top, F. H. Jr. (1975). Control of adenovirus acute respiratory disease in U.S. Army trainees. *J. Biol. Med.* 48, 185–195.

Weaver, E. A. (2014). Vaccines within vaccines the use of adenovirus types 4 and 7 as influenza vaccine vectors. *Hum. Vaccin. Immunother.* 10, 544–556. doi: 10.4161/hv.27238

Yamamoto, D., Okamoto, M., Lupisan, S., Suzuki, A., Saito, M., Tamaki, R., et al. (2014). Impact of human adenovirus serotype 7 in hospitalized children with severe fatal pneumonia in the Philippines. *Jpn. J. Infect. Dis.* 67, 105–110. doi: 10.7883/yoken.67.105

Yang, W. X., Zou, X. H., Jiang, S. Y., Lu, N. N., Han, M., Zhao, J. H., et al. (2016). Prevalence of serum neutralizing antibodies to adenovirus type 5 (Ad5) and 41 (Ad41) in children is associated with age and sanitary conditions. *Vaccine* 34, 5579–5586. doi: 10.1016/j.vaccine.2016.09.043

Yang, X. X., Wang, Q. S., Liang, B. B., Wu, F. L., Li, H., Liu, H. B., et al. (2017). An outbreak of acute respiratory disease caused by a virus associated RNA II gene mutation strain of human adenovirus 7 in China, 2015. *PLoS One* 12:e0172519. doi: 10.1371/journal.pone.0172519

Yu, B., Zhou, Y., Wu, H., Wang, Z., Zhan, Y., Feng, X., et al. (2012). Seroprevalence of neutralizing antibodies to human adenovirus type 5 in healthy adults in China. *J. Med. Virol.* 84, 1408–1414. doi: 10.1002/jmv.23325

Yuan, X. H., Qu, Z. Y., Wu, X. M., Wang, Y. C., Liu, L., Wei, F. X., et al. (2009). Molecular modeling and epitopes mapping of human adenovirus type 3 hexon protein. *Vaccine* 27, 5103–5110. doi: 10.1016/j.vaccine.2009.06.041

Zhang, L., Zhao, N., Sha, J., Wang, C., Jin, X., Amer, S., et al. (2016). Virology and epidemiology analyses of global adenovirus-associated conjunctivitis outbreaks, 1953-2013. *Epidemiol. Infect.* 144, 1661–1672. doi: 10.1017/S0950268815003246

Zheng, X., Rong, X., Feng, Y., Sun, X., Li, L., Wang, Q., et al. (2017). Seroprevalence of neutralizing antibodies against adenovirus type 14 and 55 in healthy adults in Southern China. *Emerg. Microbes. Infect.* 6:e43. doi: 10.1038/emi.2017.29

9

Asprellcosides B of *Ilex asprella* Inhibits Influenza A Virus Infection by Blocking the Hemagglutinin-Mediated Membrane Fusion

Wen Zhang[1], Si-Tai Chen[1], Qiu-Yan He[1], Li-Quan Huang[2], Xiong Li[3], Xiao-Ping Lai[1,4], Shao-Feng Zhan[5], Hui-Ting Huang[5], Xiao-Hong Liu[1], Jianguo Wu[6,7*] and Geng Li[1*]*

[1] Laboratory Animal Center, Guangzhou University of Chinese Medicine, Guangzhou, China, [2] The First Affiliated Hospital of Zhejiang Chinese Medical University, Hangzhou, China, [3] Guangdong Provincial Academy of Chinese Medical Sciences, Guangzhou, China, [4] Dongguan Mathematical Engineering Academy of Chinese Medicine, Guangzhou University of Traditional Chinese Medicine, Dongguan, China, [5] The First Affiliated Hospital of Guangzhou University of Chinese Medicine, Guangzhou, China, [6] Key Laboratory of Virology, Institute of Medical Microbiology, Jinan University, Guangzhou, China, [7] Guangdong Longfan Biological Science and Technology Company, Ltd., Foshan, China

***Correspondence:**
Xiao-Hong Liu
rsclxh@gzucm.edu.cn
Jianguo Wu
wu9988@vip.sina.com
Geng Li
lg@gzucm.edu.cn

Ilex asprella is routinely used in China as a traditional medicinal herb to treat influenza (Flu). However, its specific antiviral activity and underlying molecular mechanism have not yet been determined. In this study, we sought to determine the antiviral activity and mechanism of Asprellcosides B, an active component extracted from *Ilex asprella,* and used against the influenza A virus cell culture. We also performed a computer-assisted structural modeling analysis and carried out surface plasmon resonance (SPR) experiments in the hope of determining the viral target of Asprellcosides B. Results from our studies show that Asprellcosides B reduced virus replication by up to 63% with an IC50 of about 9 μM. It also decreased the low pH-induced and virus-mediated hemolysis by 71% *in vitro*. Molecular docking simulation analysis suggested a possible binding of Asprellcosides B to the hemagglutinin (HA), which was confirmed by a surface plasmon resonance (SPR) assay. Altogether, our findings demonstrate that Asprellcosides B inhibits the influenza A virus, through a specific binding to the HA, resulting in the blockade of the HA-mediated membrane fusion.

Keywords: triterpenoid saponins sulfate, *Ilex asprella*, anti-influenza activity, hemagglutinin (HA) protein, competitive inhibition, inhibition of membrane fusion

INTRODUCTION

The Influenza A virus infects hundreds of millions of people worldwide every year, posing a great threat to global health. Belonging to the *Orthomyxoviridae* family, the Influenza A virus contains a segmented and single-stranded RNA genome of negative polarity (International Committee on Taxonomy of Viruses, 2012). Historically, amantadine (Davies et al., 1964; Hay et al., 1985) and rimantadine (Dolin et al., 1982; Wintermeyer and Nahata, 1995) were used to treat influenza. However, the rapid emergence of drug-resistant mutants have limited their use in clinics (Dong et al., 2015). Currently, neuraminidase (NA) inhibitors such as Zanamivir (Woods et al., 1993) and Oseltamivir (Eisenberg et al., 1997) are mainly used as antiviral drugs for the treatment of influenza. The drug-resistance to NA inhibitors represents a new challenge for antiviral therapies treating influenza (Huang et al., 2018), even though Peramivir (Babu et al., 2010) and Laninamivir (Yamashita et al., 2009) are effective against Zanamivir- and/or Oseltamivir-resistant influenza viruses. Therefore, there is an unmet medical need to discover and develop new classes of antiviral drugs to control influenza (Hayden, 2006; Król et al., 2014). Traditional Chinese medicine may serve as an alternative to identify novel antiviral drugs (Wang et al., 2006; Chattopadhyay et al., 2009; Ge et al., 2010).

Ilex asprella is comprised of a variety of Aquifoliaceae, found in different regions across China (Du et al., 2017). It has been routinely used in China as a Chinese herbal medicine to treat the "common cold". Previous studies found that its main components include triterpenoid saponins, phenolic acids, and alkaloids (Huang et al., 2012; Lei et al., 2014). Several recent studies demonstrated the anti-influenza activity of triterpenoid saponin (Li et al., 2007; Song et al., 2016; Gong et al., 2017). The antiviral activity of *Ilex asprella* extracts was also demonstrated in an animal model of influenza A virus infection (Peng et al., 2016).

In this study, we have extracted pure Asprellcosides B from *Ilex asprella,* using phytochemistry and chromatographic methodologies (Porath and Flodin, 1959; Lerman, 1987) and evaluated its anti-influenza virus activity. We have also determined the HA as the viral target of Asprellcosides B, based on findings from a molecular docking simulation (Wang et al., 2015, 2016; Makau et al., 2017) and surface plasmon resonance (SPR) analysis (Giannetti, 2011). These results suggest that Asprellcosides B blocks the HA-mediated cell entry of the influenza A virus.

MATERIALS AND METHODS

Plant Material

The radix and stems of a selection of *Ilex asprella* (Hook. Et Arn.) Champ. Ex Benth (Eisenberg et al., 1997) was taken from a commercial plantation situated in Longyan city in Fujian Province, China. The plant material was dried without delay in a vacuum decompression drying oven at 60°C for 3 h, to a moisture content of less than 13% and then pulverized by a muller (YoN GLI).

Preparation of Asprellcosides B

Plant material (20 kg) was extracted four times with 70% Ethyl alcohol (EtOH) (4 × 40 L/12 h, 25°C) under reflux, and evaporated under reduced pressure to obtain a residue (638g). The residue was resuspended with water (4 L) and extracted three times with Ethyl acetate (EtOAc) (3 × 638 mL, 25°C), and incubated each time at room temperature for 1 h. The EtOAc-soluble fraction (185 g) was subjected to AB-8 macroporous resin with distilled water, until the eluent was colorless. It was then washed with a gradient elution with EtOH (0.74 L) (20, 50, 70, and 95%) to afford four fractions. Fraction 2 (elution with 50% EtOH) was evaporated under reduced pressure to obtain a residue (86 g). The residue was dissolved in (Methanol, MeOH) and subjected to column chromatography on a Sephadex LH-20 column (MeOH, 100%, 0.43 L) with isocratic elution. The elution was then identified by TLC (Waksmundzka-Hajnos et al., 2008) and the eluent was visualized with a 10% ethanol sulfate solution. Fraction 3, which was visible purplish red by the results of TLC, was collected and enriched, and the product was dried.

The product was fractionated by C18 reversed-phase column chromatography (Shinoda et al., 2002) with MeOH (20, 30, 40, 50, 60, 70, and 80%). The fractions were then concentrated and identified by TLC with a 10% ethanol sulfate solution. The fractions that were visible purplish red by TLC were collected and enriched. The fractions (MeOH 50%) were then purified by silica gel column chromatography (20% MeOH to 70% MeOH) to obtain subfractions 1 and 2. The 60% MeOH fraction was purified by (High-performance liquid chromatography, HPLC) (Huang et al., 2018) (MeOH-H_2O, 75:25) to yield subfractions 3, 4, and 5; subfraction 2 was purified by recrystallization to obtain compound 2 (19.3 mg). Compound 2 was named Asprellcosides B. The flow diagram of extraction and isolation is shown in **Figure 1**.

Virus and Cell

A/FM/1/47(H1N1), A/PuertoRico/8/34(H1N1), A/Chicken/Guangdong/1996(H9N2) and A/HongKong/498/97(H3N2) were propagated in an embryonated hen egg. The Zika virus (GenBank accession number, KU955589.1), DENV-2 (TSV01, GenBank accession AY037116) and HSV-1 (Shuwen Wu, Wuhan University, Wuhan, China) were propagated in Vero cells. The viruses were aliquoted and stored at −80°C. Cells (China Center for type culture collection, China) were grown in Dulbecco's modified Eagle's medium (DMEM), supplemented with 10% fetal bovine serum, 100 U/mL penicillin, and 100 U/mL streptomycin. Infection medium applied in anti-influenza assays were DMEM, containing 2 μg/mL tosyl phenylalanylchloromethyl ketone (TPCK)-treated trypsin and 1% bovine serum albumin, BSA.

Anti-influenza Virus Activities of Asprellcosides B

Virus Infection

The influenza virus A/FM/1/47 (H1N1) was used in the antiviral assays. A549 Cells were seeded at a density of 2 $\times 10^4$ cells per well, in the 96-well plates and were maintained at 37°C, 5% v/v CO_2 in a humidified incubator. Dissolved Asprellcosides B in Dimethylsulfoxide (DMSO) was diluted with serum-free Dulbecco's Modified Eagle Medium (DMEM), and the final concentration of DMSO was 1%. The viral group and control group received different treatments. The viral group was infected with the influenza virus (50$TCID_{50}$) on confluent monolayers in 100 μL of the infection medium, while the control group was infected on confluent monolayers with 100 μL of the infection medium. Both groups were then incubated at 37°C for 1 h.

The Methods of Adding the Drugs

After the virus infection, the media was removed and cells were washed twice with 100 μL of a phosphate buffer saline (PBS) solution at pH7.4. Following that, a twofold gradient of Asprellcosides B and a positive control medicine (Oseltamivir phosphate) were diluted by the infection medium containing 1% DMSO, at an initial concentration of 200 μM in a total of nine

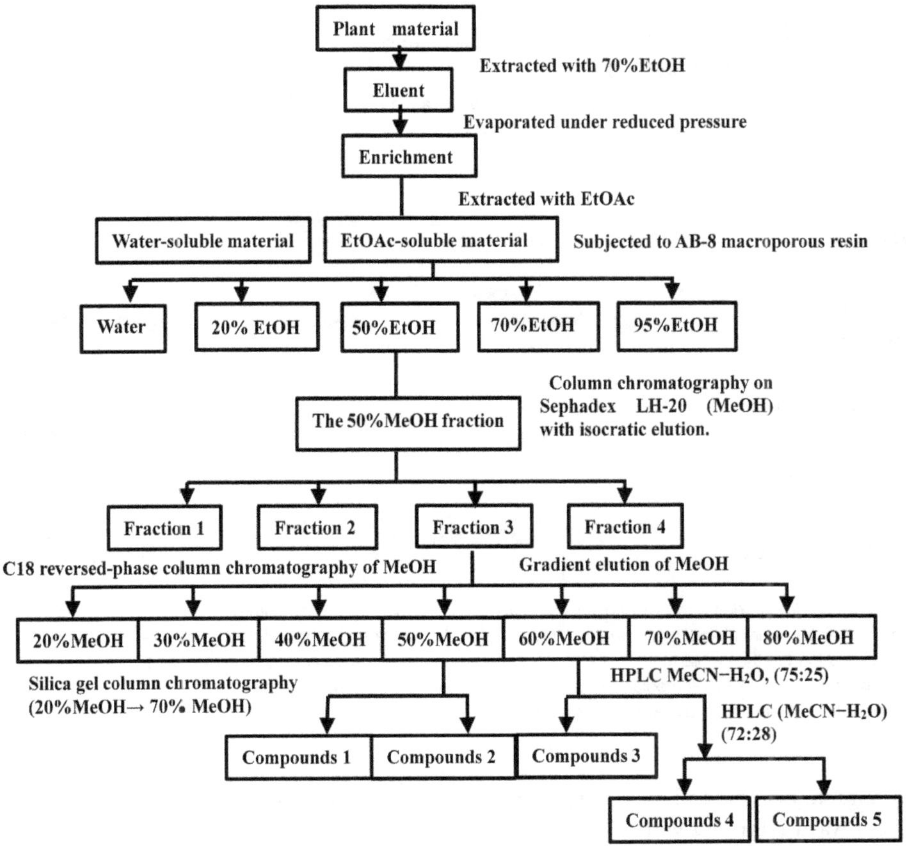

FIGURE 1 | Flow chart of the extraction and isolation of Asprellcosides B.

gradients. The first row of a 96-well plate was a blank control with normal cells, in 100 μL of the infection medium containing 1% DMSO, while the last row of the plate was a negative control of the cells infected by the virus in 100 μL of the infection medium containing 1% DMSO.

Columns 2–10 of the 96-well plate received dilutions with different concentrations of Asprellcosides B and Oseltamivir. The first column was the initial concentration; and the concentrations subsequently decreased, with the tenth column as the blank control. Asprellcosides B was added to rows 2–4 of the 96-well plate, and Oseltamivir was added to rows 5–8. Each concentration of drugs was repeated three times and then incubated for 48 h at 37°C, 5% v/v CO_2 in a humidified incubator. The method of adding the drugs are shown in **Figure 2**.

WST-8 Assay

The viability of A549 cells was quantified by the Total Superoxide Dismutase Assay Kit with WST-8 (WST-8 assay) (Tahara et al., 2017) using a Cell Counting Kit-8 (Dojindo). Cells were incubated in 10% of WST-8 reagent in a volume of 100 μL at 37°C and 5% v/v CO_2 for 30min. The absorbance was measured at 450 nm by a multimode microplate reader (PerkinElmer).

The cytotoxicity of Asprellcosides B was assessed by the WST-8 assay using a Cell Counting Kit-8 (Dojindo). A549 cells were grown in 96-well plates at 37°C and 5% v/v CO_2 for 24 h and then incubated with different concentrations of Asprellcosides B for 48 h. The absorbance was then measured at 450 nm using a Multimode Microplate Reader.

Neuraminidase Assay

The inhibitory effects of Asprellcosides B on the influenza virus neuraminidase activity, were measured by a fluorescence assay (Sidwell and Smee, 2000). The reaction mixture, containing 50 μL of NA-Fluor^{TM} Substrate, 50 μL of the supernatant of cell and virus cultures, was incubated at 37°C for 1 h in 96-well microtiter plates. The reaction was terminated by adding 100 μL of NA-Fluor^{TM} Stop Solution to each well. The absorbance was then measured at 365/450 nm by the multimode microplate reader showing the content of neuraminidase.

RT-PCR Assay

The MDCK and Vero cells were grown to approximately 90% confluence, infected with 50 $TCID_{50}$ of the influenza A and Zika virus, DEVN. The drugs were then continuously added. At 48 h post-infection, cells were collected and centrifuged (12,000 g for 5 min). The extraction of the total RNA from cells was carried out using the Ultrapure RNA kit (CoWin Biotech, Beijing, China), and cDNA was then synthesized from the total RNA using the M-MLV Reverse Transcriptase kit (Promega, Madison,

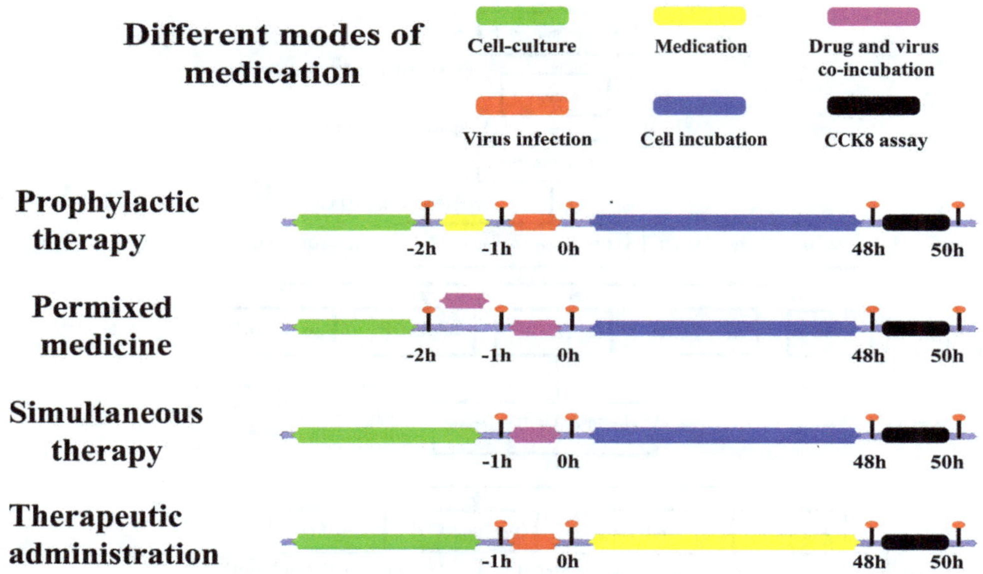

FIGURE 2 | Sketch of different medication modes. Prophylactic administration: drugs added to the cell culture before the infectious virus was added to A549 cells. Premixed administration: drugs and virus were mixed, incubated at 4°C for 1 h, and then added to the cell culture mixture. Simultaneous administration: Drugs and virus were mixed and immediately added to the cell culture. Therapeutic administration: drugs were added after infection by the virus to A549 cells. Green: the period of cell culture; Yellow: in this time, the drug was in the medium; Red: the time of the virus infection; Magenta: drugs and the virus in the medium at the same time; Blue: there was cell culture without drugs and virus; Black: this was the period of detection.

WI, United States) with random primers and oligo (dT) primers. The PCR reactions system was performed with 25 μL reaction buffer (17 μL of RNA template, 5 μL of M-MLV 5× reaction buffer, 50 pmol of the primers, 0.1 mM dNTPs, 25units of ribonuclease inhibitor, and 200 units of M-MLV RT polymerase). The amplification conditions of RT-PCR analysis were 1 cycle at 95°C for 3 min; 39 cycles at 95°C for 10 s, 60°C for 10 s, and 72°C for 20 s; and 1 cycle at 95°C for 10 s.

The specific primers for HA mRNA and NP mRNA of A/FM/1/47(H1N1) to detect viral RNA were: 5′-CCCAGGAG ATTTCGCCGACTATG-3′ and 5′-TGCCGTTACTCCTCT GGTTATGTTG-3′; 5′-CATCTTTCTGGCACGGTCTG-3′ and 5′-GGCTACTGCAGGTCCATACA-3′, while for GAPDH, which was used as an internal control, the primer sequences (Nogales et al., 2014) were 5′-AACATCATCCCTGCTTCCAC-3′ and 5′-GACCACCTGGTCCTCAGTGT-3′. The primers of the dengue virus were: 5′-CATTCCAAGTGAGAATCTCTTTGTCA-3′ and 5′-CAGATCTCTGATGAATAACCAACG-3′. The primers for the Zika virus were: 5′-GGTCAGCGTCCTCTCTAATAAACG-3′ and 5′-GCACCCTAGTGTCCACTTTTTCC-3′.

Plaque Reduction Assay

The MDCK cells were grown to approximately 90% confluence12-well plates, infected with supernatants for 2 h at 37°C. The supernatants collected from the cells were infected with 50 $TCID_{50}$ of the influenza A/PuertoRico/8/34(H1N1) virus, then added to different concentrations of Asprellcosides B and incubated for 48 h at 37°C. The infected substance was then removed and cell was washed with PBS. The cell monolayers were overlaid with agar containing supplemented MEM (1% low melting point agarose, 1% bovine serum albumin and 1 μg/ml TPCK-treated trypsin) and incubated at 37°C for 2–3 days. The sample was fixed with 4% paraformaldehyde for 2 h and removed with an agarose overlay. Cells were then stained with 2% (w/v) crystal violet.

Pharmacodynamic Mechanism Research

Time of Addition Experiments

The cells infected with the influenza virus were medicated at different time-points. After virus infection (50$TCID_{50}$), cells were washed twice with 100 μL of (Phosphate Buffer Solution, PBS) (pH7.4) and added to a twofold gradient of Asprellcosides B, diluted with the infection medium containing 1% DMSO. The initial concentration was 300 μM and a total of four gradients were used. Dilutions of 100 μL were added at different time-points (−2−−1 h, −1–0 h, 0–2 h, 2–4 h, 4–6 h, and 4–48 h), and the negative control was 100 μL of the infection medium, containing 1% DMSO. Cells were then incubated for 48 h at 37°C, 5% v/v CO_2 in a humidified incubator.

Hemagglutinin Inhibiting Assay

Samples were diluted twofold in a phosphate-buffered saline (PBS, pH7.4), in a V shape, in 96-well-plates. The samples had different concentrations of drugs, and the initial concentration was 500 μM. A total of 25 μL of the specimen and then 25 μL of the influenza virus was added to each sample (Inouye and Kono, 1972). After 30 min of incubation at 4°C, 50 μL of 1% suspension of chick erythrocytes was added to each well. The virus titer was $TCID_{50} = 10^{-2.5}/0.1$ mL. Plates were incubated for 20 min at 37°C, and the agglutination could be observed with the naked eye.

Hemolysis Inhibiting Assay

The compound was diluted in PBS with the final concentration of 100 μM/mL, and 100 μL of the specimen dilution was added to the long well 96-well-plates. The blank control was a PBS solution. 100 μL of the undiluted virus stock was then added to the sample wells and the negative control wells, and the virus titer was $TCID_{50} = 10^{-2.5}/0.1$ mL. The wells with samples were completely mixed, and the entire plate was incubated for 30 min at room temperature. 200 μL 2% suspension of chick erythrocytes was then added, which was preheated in a water bath at 37°C. The plates were then shaken for 60 s and were incubated at 37°C for 30 min. After the incubation, 100 μL of prepared solutions of acetic acid-sodium acetate at different pH values (4.6, 4.8, 5.0, 5.2, 5.4, 5.6, 5.8, and 6.0) were added and sufficiently mixed. Plates were then incubated in an incubator at 37°C for 30 min. After centrifugation at 1200 rpm for 6 min, the absorbance of the supernatant at 540 nm (Optical density at 540 nm, OD_{540}) was detected.

Docking Simulation Analyses

The primary 3D structure of Asprellcosides B was drawn using Chemoffice 2015 software. Its conformation was optimized by the RDkit (Ebejer et al., 2012), and several low-energy conformers were selected for molecular dynamics simulation (MD) by AutoDockTools (Morris et al., 2009). The crystal structure of HA of A/WSN/33 H1N1 strains was analogous to the structure of A/Puerto Rico/8/1934 H1N1, and it was downloaded from the Protein Data Bank (PDB ID:1RU7 and 1RVX) (Gamblin et al., 2004).

Coordinate files were prepared using AutoDockTools. Docking of Asprellcosides B was performed using the HA1 sialic acid binding pocket by AutoDock 4.26. The docking areas were within 3 Å from the crystallization of the ligand and the 90-Helex, 130-Loop, 220-Loop sites (PD ID: 1RVX). Prediction of the binding site of Asprellcosides B and HA2 by Autoligand was performed (Russell et al., 2008; Song et al., 2016), and the terminal binding site was confirmed by molecular docking (PDB ID: 1RU7, 3EYM). Docking results were analyzed with AutoDockTools.

SPR Analyses

Kinetic information of the binding of Asprellcosides B and HA protein was obtained using a Biacore T100 instrument (GE Healthcare, Uppsala, Sweden). Hemagglutinin (HA) protein (Sino Biological INC., Beijing, China), influenza (A/WSN/33 H1N1 with His Tag) was immobilized on a CM7 sensor chip (GE Healthcare, Uppsala, Sweden) in 10 mM sodium acetate at pH4.5, using the amine coupling method. The chip density was 20,000 (Resonance Units, RU). The reference flow cell was used as a control for non-specific binding. Compounds of Asprellcosides B were gradually diluted in a Phosphate buffer solution and Polyoxyethylenesorbitan 20 (PBS-P: 10 mM phosphate buffers with 2.7 mM Potassium Chloride, KCl and 137 mM Sodium Chloride, NaCl, 0.05% surfactant P20, pH7.4) and 1% DMSO. The specimens were prepared by twofold dilution, with their concentrations ranging from 312.5 nM to 20 μM. Samples were injected for 180 s and the flow rate was 30 μL/min. The dissociation followed for 240 s and surface regeneration was with 50 mM NaOH for 30 s. Data were fit using a 1:1 binding model by Biacore T100 Evaluation software Version 2.0.3.

RESULTS

Asprellcosides B Is an Ursane Type Triterpenoid Saponin With 3-*O*-Xyl, 28-*O*-β-D-Glucopyranoside

Asprellcosides B was a colorless tabular crystal (MeOH). Its molecular formula was $C_{41}H_{66}O_{16}S$ as a basis for (Electrospray Ionization Mass Spectrometry, ESI-MS) (m/z845 $[M-H]^-$), ^{13}C (Nuclear Magnetic Resonance, NMR) (100 MHz, Pyridine-d5), and ^1H NMR (400 MHz, Pyridine-d5). The Infrared Radiation (IR) Potassium Bromide Tablet (KBr) spectral absorption peak of the compound was [3421 cm^{-1} (hydroxyl)], [2941, 2875, 1457, and 1387 cm^{-1} (methyl)], [1735 and 1646 cm^{-1} (ester group)], [1250 and 1072 cm^{-1} (sulfonic)], [876 and 586 cm^{-1} (Double bond hydrogen)], and the Under Voltage (UV) (MeOH) spectral absorption peak was approximately 206 nm; according to the elemental analysis, the sulfur content was 3.655%.

The ^1H NMR and ^{13}C NMR spectra showed that there were seven methyl groups [δ_H 1.41, 0.98, 0.88, 1.18, 1.73, 1.29, and 1.0 (3H, S, 7 × CH_3); δ_C 28.1 (C−23), 16.5(C−24), 15.3(C−25), 17.1(C−26), 15.8(C−27), 29.4(C−29), and 24.0(C−30)], seven quaternary carbons [δ_C 39.1(C−4), 40.1(C−8), 36.6(C−10), 138.5(C−13), 42.5(C−14), 48.0(C−17), and 41.78(C−19)], one ester carbonyl (δ_C 176.7), and two alkenyl groups [δ_C 127.25(C−12) and 138.5(C−13)]. The analysis of $[M-H]^-$ ion in the negative ion HRESIMS (m/z 845, m/z 683), ^1H NMR and ^{13}C NMR spectra displayed that they were 3-*O*-xyl [δ_H 4.60, d (7.2), 6.35, d (7.6), (α:4.77, β:3.76,(dd)); δ_C 106.6(C−1′), 73.3(C−2′), 73.7(C−3′), 67.8(C−4′), 66.4(C−5′)], and 28-*O*-β-D-glucopyranoside [δ_C 95.49(C−1″), 73.0(C−2″), 78.7(C−3″), 70.7(C−4″), 78.9(C−5″), 61.8 (C−6″); δ_H 6.35, d (7.6), 4.24, t (8.5), 4.32, t (8.5), 4.45 (m), 4.21 (dd), (α:0.79, β:1.43)]. Thus, the structure of the compound was established as an Ursane type triterpenoid saponin with 3-*O*-xyl, 28-*O*-β-D-glucopyranoside (Zhou et al., 2008, 2012; Yao et al., 2009) (**Figure 3A**).

Asprellcosides B Represses Influenza A Virus Infection in A549 Cells

The cytotoxicity and antiviral activity of Asprellcosides B in the regulation of the influenza virus H1N1 A/FM/1/47(H1N1) in A549 cells, were determined by Neuraminidase (NA) inhibition assays and WST-8 cell proliferation and cytotoxicity assays. There was a low toxicity of Asprellcosides B in confluent A549 cells, monolayers with concentrations of 1.03–250 μM, and the TC_{50} was >250 μM. With different modes of medication, Asprellcosides B displayed anti-influenza virus activity (**Table 1** and **Figure 3**). The cytopathic effect (CPE) was observed at 48 h post-infection. At the same time the determination of cell viability (CPE inhibition) was employed to represent the inhibition rate by using the WST-8 assay (**Figures 3B–E**). According to the data, the inhibitory effect of Asprellcosides B in

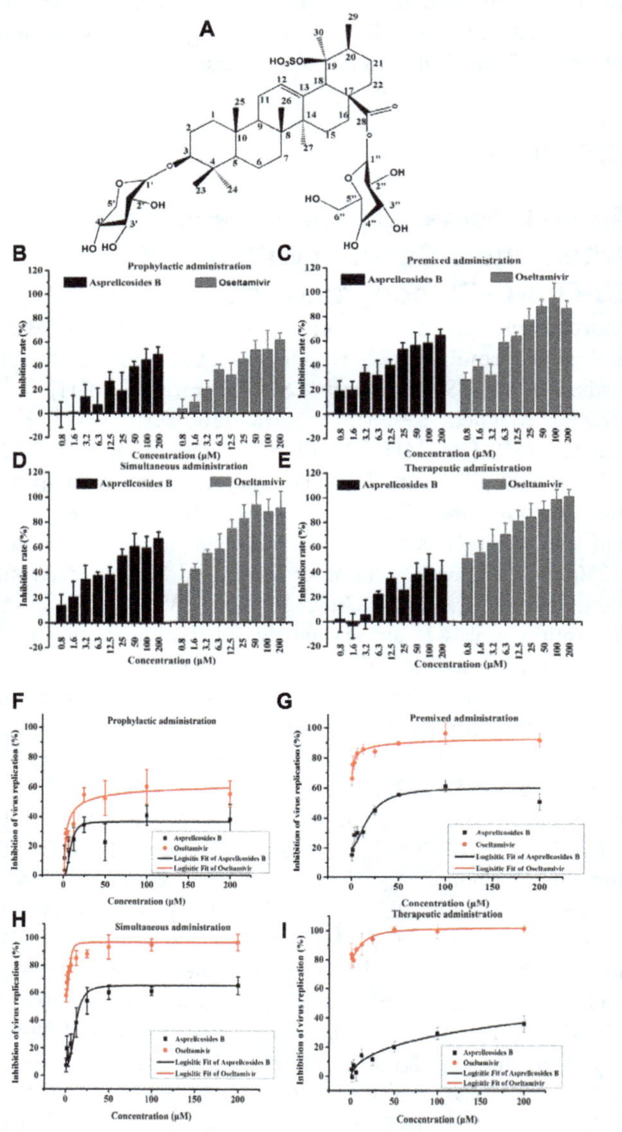

FIGURE 3 | Asprellcosides B inhibited influenza A virus infection in A549 cells. **(A)** The structure of Asprellcosides B. **(B–E)** Different modes of medication. The cell survival rates of Asprellcosides B and Oseltamivir on influenza A/FM/1/47(H1N1) were determined by WST-8 assay at 48 h post-infection ($n = 3$, each concentration conducted in triplicate). **(F–I)** Different modes of medication. The inhibitory effects of Asprellcosides B and Oseltamivir on the neuraminidase activity of influenza A/FM/1/47(H1N1) were determined by fluorescence assay at 48 h post-infection. $n = 3$, each concentration conducted in triplicate.

Premixed administration and Simultaneous administration were superior in terms of dose-dependence. The inhibitory effect of 25 μM Asprellcosides B was over 50%.

With an intention to identify the inhibitory effect of Asprellcosides B on influenza virus infection, Asprellcosides B mediated inhibition of viral protein synthesis in A549 cells was examined through Neuraminidase assay. We analyzed virus neuraminidase activity using NA-Fluor Substrate at 48 h post-infection. In Premixed administration and Simultaneous administration, the inhibitory effect of Asprellcosides B displayed higher dose-dependence (**Figures 3D,E**). In Prophylactic therapy, Neuraminidase assay featured Asprellcosides B inhibited cell viability with IC50 above 8.87 μM (**Figures 3F–I** and **Table 1**); hence, the selection index (SI) exceeded 28.18, indicating that Asprellcosides B may possess a promising safety profile. The solubility of Asprellcosides B in water was only 1.66 μg/mL. Consequently, it did not reach a complete inhibition even at 200 μM as Oseltamivir did. This result might be attributed to its low solubility.

Asprellcosides B Attenuates Influenza A Virus mRNA Transcription in MDCK Cells

We conducted a quantitative real-time PCR to determine how the synthesis of viral mRNA in MDCK cells was inhibited by Asprellcosides B. Isolated from the infected cells, the total RNA was investigated by quantitative real-time PCR using primers of the viral HA mRNA and NP mRNA at 48 h post-infection. Upon the results, HA mRNA and NP mRNA transcription declined as a result of adding Asprellcosides B to influenza-virus-infected cells in a dose-dependent manner (**Figures 4A,B**). We found that Asprellcosides B had a significant effect in the inhibiting infection by A/PuertoRico/8/34 (H1N1), A/Chicken/Guangdong/1996 (H9N2) and, HSV virus, but less inhibition on the A/HongKong/498/97(H3N2) (**Figure 4C**), respectively, while it had no inhibition on the infection by ursane type triterpenoid the Dengue virus (DENV) and Zika virus (ZIKV) (**Figure 4D**). The results demonstrate that Asprellcosides B specifically represses the mRNA transcription of influenza A virus. The plaque reduction assay showed that Asprellcosides B can reduce the plaque numbers in a dose-dependent manner (**Figure 4E**).

Asprellcosides B Represses Influenza A Virus Replication at the Early Stage of Its Lifecycle

Time-of-addition and time course studies concerning the inhibitory effects of Asprellcosides B were carried out to recognize the steps of Asprellcosides B inhibiting the influenza lifecycle. It has been reported that at least 6 h are required to detect a progeny virus after inoculation of the influenza A/PR/8/34 virus (Li et al., 2009). There were six intervals (−2-−1 h, −1-0 h, 0-2 h, 2-4 h, 4-6 h, and 4-48 h) selected for the inhibition time course, which determined the expression of the NA protein. The addition of Asprellcosides B to the cells within −1-0 h of viral infection in A549 cells presented an evident inhibition of virus replication (**Figure 5**). Asprellcosides B failed to demonstrate its antiviral activity when it was added more than 2 h after the infection (**Figure 5**), implying that Asprellcosides B is effective during the early stages, viral binding and the fusion and entry of the viral lifecycle. In summary, the above-mentioned results provides evidence that Asprellcosides B exerts an inhibitory effect on the early stages of the influenza virus lifecycle. It is worth mentioning that the inhibitory effect of Asprellcosides B on viral replication may be performed by targeting the hemagglutinin protein, because the Premixed

TABLE 1 | *In vitro* anti-viral activity against H1N1 A/FM/1/47 by Asprellcosides B and *Ilex asprella* (Hook. Et Arn.) Champ. *Ex Benth* isolated from the radix and stems, with different medication modes.

Virus	Therapy	Asprellcosides B TC50 > 250 μM		Oseltamivir TC50 > 250 μM	
		IC50 (μM)	SI (μM)	IC50 (μM)	SI (μM)
H1N1	Therapeutic administration	796.46	0.31	13.21	18.92
	Simultaneous administration	11.21	22.30	4.26×10^{-5}	5.87×10^{6}
	Premixed administration	18.39	13.59	1.64×10^{-5}	1.52×10^{7}
	Prophylactic administration	8.87	28.18	6.10	40.98

The TC50 and IC50 values were determined by WST-8 assay and neuraminidase assay. n = 3, each concentration in triplicate.

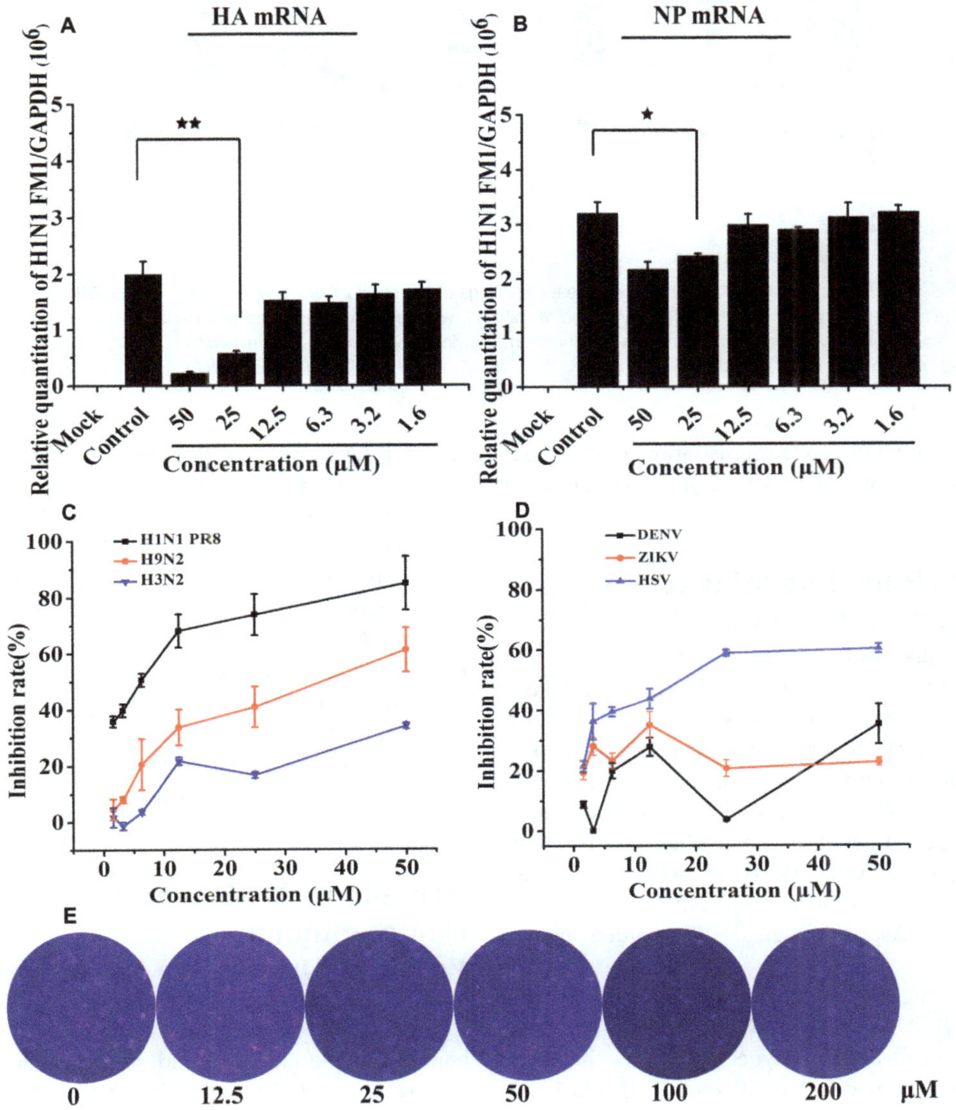

FIGURE 4 | Asprellcosides B attenuates influenza A virus mRNA transcription in MDCK cells. **(A,B)** The inhibitory effect of Asprellcosides B on the expression of influenza A/FM/1/47(H1N1) HA mRNA and NA mRNA were detected by quantitative real-time PCR at 48 h post-infection. $^{**}p < 0.01$, $^{*}p < 0.05$. Assessed the antiviral activity of other influenza virus. **(C)** The antiviral activity of H1N1 PR8, H9N2, H3N2, and HSV virus were assessed through CPE inhibition by using WST-8 assay, and **(D)** the antiviral activity of ZIKA and DEVN virus was determined by quantitative real-time PCR. **(E)** The plaque was fixed and stained at 48 h post infection, and the experimental method was detailed in the Section "Materials and Methods."

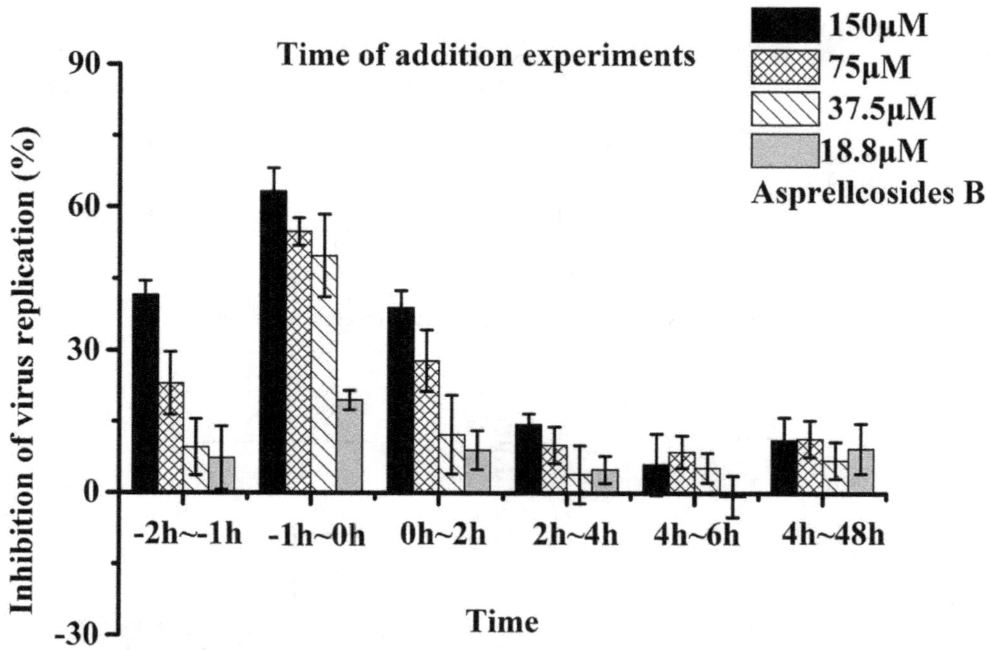

FIGURE 5 | Asprellcosides B represses influenza A virus replication at the early stage of its lifecycle. Cells were inoculated with $50TCID_{50}$: 0.1 mL of the influenza virus A/FM/1/47(H1N1) in a time-of-addition assay. 18.8–150 μM of Asprellcosides B was added at the designated times and was removed after each incubation period. The cells were then incubated with fresh media until 48 h post infection. The virus replication was determined through Neuraminidase assay. $n = 3$, each concentration performed in triplicate.

administration and Simultaneous administration of the A549 cells with Asprellcosides B markedly impair the infection of the influenza virus.

Asprellcosides B Inhibits Influenza A Virus HA-Mediated Hemolysis

For the purpose of disclosing the exact domain targeted by Asprellcosides B, a hemagglutinin inhibition assay was devised to observe whether the interaction between HA and cellular receptors could be interfered by ursane type triterpenoid of Asprellcosides B, after which virus attachment to the cell could be blocked (**Figure 6A**). The data showed that Asprellcosides B did not inhibit viral attachment to the cell, which was primarily intervened by the HA subunit. Moreover, whether viral-cell membrane fusion, which was mediated by HA2 subunit, could be interfered with by Asprellcosides B still requires further study.

Therefore, we designed the hemolysis assay with the influenza virus H1N1 A/FM/1/47(H1N1) to identify the effect of Asprellcosides B on fusion. To trigger hemolysis, the virus-cell suspension was briefly acidified to different pH (pH4.85–6.0) to initiate HA conformational changes that lyse chicken red blood cells (cRBCs). Wells absent in the virus were used as controls to determine the effect of compounds on cRBCs. The results revealed that in the virus control group, OD value increased rapidly when pH < 5.2, while OD value remained steady when pH < 4.94; when pH < 5.2, OD value in the blank control group and Asprellcosides B group raised progressively as PH declined; when pH < 4.94, OD value stayed stable, but its growth level in the blank control group and Asprellcosides B group was lower than that in the virus control group, while the Asprellcosides B group was similar to that of the blank control group (**Figures 6B,C**). While experimenting with the inhibition ratio of hemolysis by Asprellcosides, it was found that the virus content reached its highest level at a pH of 5.05, and the drug's inhibition ratio arrived at 70.83%. Considering the results, Asprellcosides B could have an inhibitory influence on influenza-virus-HA mediated hemolysis, which suggests that the membrane fusion process was targeted by Asprellcosides B through virus entry.

Asprellcosides B Directly Interacts With Hemagglutinin

Molecular docking simulation displayed the highest probability of the binding between Asprellcosides B and HA. Asprellcosides B was bound to the HA2 main structure with multiple non-polar bonds, and the glycoside and sulfate groups of Asprellcosides B were hydrogen-bound to lysine (L:568), glutamine (L:562), lysine (K:308), and aspartic acid (L:585). The L peptide chain and K peptide chain were split from the same HA2 protein (**Figures 7B–D**). The binding sites were similar to tert-butyl hydroquinone (TBHQ) (Yao et al., 2009), which is an inhibitor that binds to the hydrophobic pocket of HA.

It has been hypothesized that a binding affinity between HA protein and Asprellcosides B is present, and we confirmed

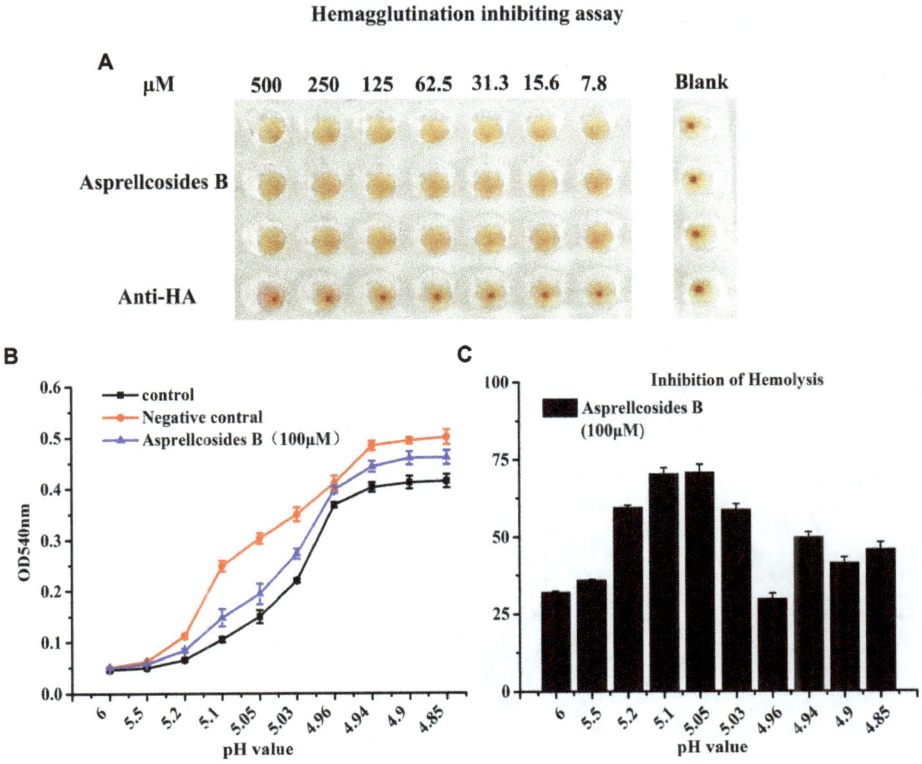

FIGURE 6 | Asprellcosides B inhibits influenza A virus HA-mediated hemolysis. **(A)** 25 μL influenza A/FM/1/47(H1N1) virus was incubated at room temperature with a twofold gradient of diluted Asprellcosides B for 30 min. Added with dilutions of 100 μL at different time-points, the virus was subsequently incubated at room temperature for 48 h. The blank control was a PBS solution. Note the inhibition on hemagglutinin of Asprellcosides B. **(B)** Hemolysis inhibition assay of Asprellcosides B against the influenza A/FM/1/47(H1N1) virus strain. Asprellcosides B was diluted by PBS and was mixed in a 96-well-plate with an equal volume of the influenza virus A/FM/1/47(H1N1). 1% suspension of chicken erythrocytes was added after incubation at room temperature for 30 min. The plates were incubated for 20 min at 37°C. Then, sodium acetate at different pH values (4.6, 4.8, 5.0, 5.2, 5.4, 5.6, 5.8, and 6.0) was added and incubated at 37°C for 30 min to bring about hemolysis. At the end of incubation, the plates were centrifuged at 12,000 rpm for 6 min, and the supernatants were detected. A microtiter plate reader was used to read the $OD_{540\ nm}$. $n = 3$, each pH value in triplicate. **(C)** The inhibition ratios (%) of hemolysis of influenza virus H1N1 A/FM/1/47 with different pH values by Asprellcosides B.

it by a surface plasmon resonance (SPR) assay designed to determine the binding between two molecules. SPR analyses showed that there was a good kinetic affinity between Asprellcosides B and the HA protein, and the resonance units of the drug were present at concentration dependence. A 1:1 binding model was used, and the dissociation constant (KD) was calculated from the curve (**Figure 7A**). The association rate constant K_a was 583.5(1/Ms), and the dissociation rate constant K_d was 0.004343(1/s). Then, the affinity constant KD value (ratio K_d/K_a) was calculated to be 7.44 μM.

DISCUSSION AND CONCLUSION

Influenza A virus infection is a major contributor to yearly mortality worldwide. It poses a grave concern for loss of life in influenza pandemics, exemplified by the 1918 Spanish flu that killed around 50 million people. Current antiviral therapies using NA inhibitors are inadequate to control the spread of the influenza virus caused by the rapid emergence of drug-resistant mutations. There is an urgent need to discover and develop more efficacious antiviral drugs that target various viral proteins essential for infection and replication. The HA is essential for mediating virus attachment to cells and inducing membrane fusion between viral and cellular membranes and therefore is an ideal antiviral target.

In this study, we have demonstrated that Asprellcosides B greatly inhibited influenza A virus infection in cell cultures with an EC50 of about 9 μM. It was not toxic to cells up to 250 μM with a selective index of greater than 28. The time-of-addition experiments suggested that Asprellcosides B acted on an early step of virus infection, possibly at the membrane fusion step (Ackermann and Maassab, 1954). The HA is essential for virus attachment and membrane fusion between viral and cellular membranes upon the low pH-induced conformational change (Du et al., 2013). Several previous studies have identified inhibitors of the receptor binding or membrane fusion activities of HA (Deshpande et al., 2001; Yao et al., 2009). Our results also suggest that the HA is the molecular target of Asprellcosides B. Asprellcosides B did not affect hemagglutination *in vitro* but significantly inhibited the virus-mediated and low pH-induced hemolysis. This conclusion is

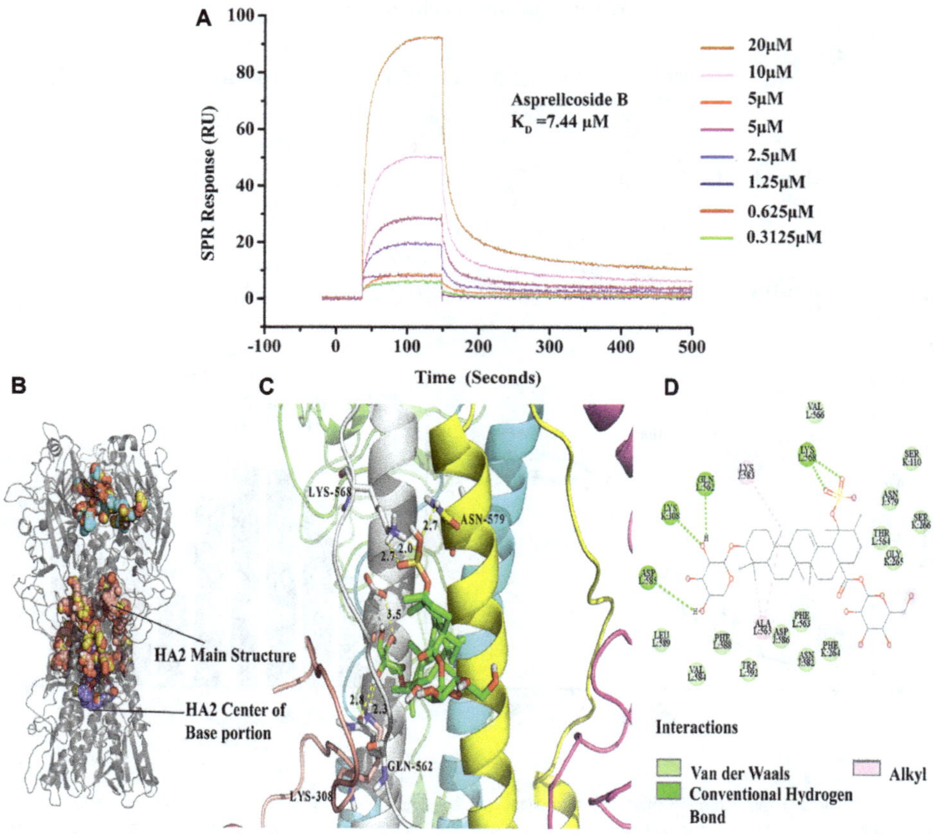

FIGURE 7 | Asprellcosides B directly interacts with hemagglutinin. **(A)** The binding curve of Asprellcosides B with HA protein in SPR assay. **(B,C)** The 3D drawing of the estimated domain of the HA2 protein bound to Asprellcosides B. **(D)** The 2D drawing of the calculated domain of the insertion of Asprellcosides B in the HA2 protein-binding site.

also supported by the molecular docking suggesting a multi-hydrogen-bound interaction between the glycoside and sulfate groups of Asprellcosides B and the HA2. Similarly, the interaction between Asprellcosides B and the HA2 was confirmed by a surface Plasmon resonance analysis, demonstrating high affinity binding. In summary, Asprellcosides B inhibited the influenza A virus infection in cell cultures, through a specific interaction with the HA2, resulting in a blockade of the HA-mediated membrane fusion.

AUTHOR CONTRIBUTIONS

GL conceived and designed the experiments. WZ, S-TC, Q-YH, L-QH, XL, S-FZ, H-TH, and X-HL analyzed the data. X-PL and JW contributed reagents, materials, and analysis tools. WZ wrote the manuscript. All authors participated in the work and read and approved the final manuscript.

FUNDING

This work was funded by the National Natural Science Foundation of China (Nos. 81803813 and 81730061), the Major Program of Guangdong Natural Science Foundation of China (Nos. S2012030006598 and S2012010011143), the Science & Technology Planning Project of Guangdong Province of China (No. 2013B020224005), the Science & Technology Planning Project of Guangzhou (No. 201804010029), the Innovative Program of State Key Laboratory of Virology (No. 2016IOV003), Science & Technology Planning Project of Guangdong Province Office of Education (No. 2014GKXM032), and the State Major Research Program for Innovation Team of Guangdong Province (No. E1-KFD015151K02).

ACKNOWLEDGMENTS

We want to thank the Institutes of Tropical Medicine, Guangzhou Respiratory Disease Research Institute and South China Agricultural University Veterinary Science and Technology Center for providing the influenza virus (A/FM/1/47[H1N1]), (A/PuertoRico/8/34[H1N1]) and (A/Chicken/Guangdong/1996[H9N2]). We also thank the Center for Diseases Control and Prevention of Guangdong Province and Wuhan Institute of Virology, Chinese Academy of Sciences for providing the A/HongKong/498/97(H3N2), HSV-1, Zika virus and the DENV virus.

REFERENCES

Ackermann, W. W., and Maassab, H. F. (1954). Growth characteristics of influenza virus: the influence of a sulfonic acid. *J. Exp. Med.* 99, 105–117. doi: 10.1084/jem.99.2.105

Babu, Y. S., Chand, P., Bantia, S., Kotian, P., Dehghani, A., El-Kattan, Y., et al. (2010). BCX-1812 (RWJ-270201): discovery of a novel, highly potent, orally active, and selective influenza neuraminidase inhibitor through structure-based drug design. *J. Med. Chem.* 7, 3482–3486.

Chattopadhyay, D., Sarkar, M. C., Chatterjee, T., Sharma Dey, R., Bag, P., Chakraborti, S., et al. (2009). Recent advancements for the evaluation of antiviral activities of natural products. *N. Biotechnol.* 25, 347–368. doi: 10.1016/j.nbt.2009.03.007

Davies, W. L., Grunert, R. R., Haff, R. F., Mcgahen, J. W., Neumayer, E. M., Paulshock, M., et al. (1964). Antiviral activity of 1-adamantanamine (Amantadine). *Science* 144, 862–863. doi: 10.1126/science.144.3620.862

Deshpande, M. S., Wei, J., Luo, G., Cianci, C., Danetz, S., Torri, A., et al. (2001). An approach to the identification of potent inhibitors of influenza virus fusion using parallel synthesis methodology. *Bioorg. Med. Chem. Lett.* 11, 2393–2396. doi: 10.1016/S0960-894X(01)00459-0

Dolin, R., Reichman, R. C., Madore, H. P., Maynard, R., Linton, P. N., and Webber-Jones, J. (1982). A controlled trial of amantadine and rimantadine in the prophylaxis of influenza a infection. *N. Engl. J. Med.* 307, 580–584. doi: 10.1056/NEJM198209023071002

Dong, G., Peng, C., Luo, J., Wang, C., Han, L., Wu, B., et al. (2015). Adamantane-resistant influenza a viruses in the world (1902-2013): frequency and distribution of m2 gene mutations. *PLoS One* 10:e0119115. doi: 10.1371/journal.pone.0119115

Du, B.-Z., Yang, X.-Y., Feng, X., Yin, X., Zhang, H.-X., Zhao, F., et al. (2017). A phytochemical and pharmacological advance on *Ilex asprella*. *Zhongguo Zhong Yao Za Zhi* 42, 20–28. doi: 10.19540/j.cnki.cjcmm.20161222.025

Du, L., Jin, L., Zhao, G., Sun, S., Li, J., Yu, H., et al. (2013). Identification and structural characterization of a broadly neutralizing antibody targeting a novel conserved epitope on the influenza virus H5N1 hemagglutinin. *J. Virol.* 87, 2215–2225. doi: 10.1128/JVI.02344-12

Ebejer, J. P., Morris, G. M., and Deane, C. M. (2012). Freely available conformer generation methods: how good are they? *J. Chem. Inf. Model.* 52, 1146–1158. doi: 10.1021/ci2004658

Eisenberg, E. J., Bidgood, A., and Cundy, K. C. (1997). Penetration of GS4071, a novel influenza neuraminidase inhibitor, into rat bronchoalveolar lining fluid following oral administration of the prodrug GS4104. *Antimicrob. Agents Chemother.* 41, 1949–1952. doi: 10.1128/AAC.41.9.1949

Gamblin, S. J., Haire, L. F., Russell, R. J., Stevens, D. J., Xiao, B., Ha, Y., et al. (2004). The structure and receptor binding properties of the 1918 influenza hemagglutinin. *Science* 303, 1838–1842. doi: 10.1126/science.1093155

Ge, H., Wang, Y. F., Xu, J., Gu, Q., Liu, H. B., Xiao, P. G., et al. (2010). Anti-influenza agents from traditional chinese medicine. *Nat. Prod. Rep.* 27, 1758–1780. doi: 10.1039/c0np00005a

Giannetti, A. M. (2011). From eperimental design to validated hits: a comprehensive walk-through of fragment lead identification using surface plasmon resonance. *Methods Enzymol.* 493, 169–218. doi: 10.1016/B978-0-12-381274-2.00008-X

Gong, K. K., Li, P. L., Qiao, D., Zhang, X. W., Chu, M. J., Qin, G. F., et al. (2017). Cytotoxic and antiviral triterpenoids from the mangrove plant sonneratia paracaseolaris. *Molecules* 22:E1319. doi: 10.3390/molecules22081319

Hay, A. J., Wolstenholme, A. J., Skehel, J. J., and Smith, M. H. (1985). the molecular basis of the specific anti-influenza action of amantadine. *EMBO J.* 4, 3021–3024. doi: 10.1002/j.1460-2075.1985.tb04038.x

Hayden, F. G. (2006). Antiviral resistance in influenza viruses-implications for management and pandemic response. *N. Engl. J. Med.* 354, 785–788. doi: 10.1056/NEJMp068030

Huang, J. C., Chen, F. L., Chen, H. M., Zeng, Y. E., and Xu, H. H. (2012). Chemical constituents in roots of *Ilex asprella*. *Chin. Tradit. Herb. Drugs* 43, 1475–1478.

Huang, W., Cheng, Y., Li, X., Tan, M., Wei, H., Zhao, X., et al. (2018). Neuraminidase inhibitor susceptibility profile of human influenza viruses during the 2016-2017 influenza season in Mainland China. *J. Infect. Chemother.* 24, 729–733. doi: 10.1016/j.jiac.2018.05.003

Inouye, S., and Kono, R. (1972). Hemagglutination-inhibiting (HI) antibody response against rubella virus in non-pregnant and pregnant rabbits and transmission of antibody to young. *J. Immunol.* 108, 370–376.

International Committee on Taxonomy of Viruses (2012). "Virus taxonomy: classification and nomenclature of viruses," in *Ninth Report of the International Committee on Taxonomy of Viruses*, eds F. A. Murphy, C. M. Fauquet, D. H. L. Bishop, S. A. Ghabrial, A. Jarvis, G. P. Martelli, et al. (Vienna: Springer), doi: 10.1016/B978-0-12-384684-6.00057-4

Król, E., Rychłowska, M., and Szewczyk, B. (2014). Antivirals - current trends in fighting influenza. *Acta Biochim. Pol.* 61, 495–504.

Lei, Y., Shi, S. P., Song, Y. L., Bi, D., and Tu, P. F. (2014). Triterpene saponins from the roots of *Ilex asprella*. *Chem Biodivers.* 11, 767–775. doi: 10.1002/cbdv.201300155

Lerman, S. (1987). Chemical and physical properties of the normal and aging lens: spectroscopic (Uv, fluorescence, phosphorescence, and Nmr) analyses. *Am. J. Optom. Physiol. Opt.* 64, 11–22. doi: 10.1097/00006324-198701000-00003

Li, Y., Jiang, R., Ooi, L. S., But, P. P., and Ooi, V. E. (2007). Antiviral triterpenoids from the medicinal plant schefflera heptaphylla. *Phytother. Res.* 21, 466–470. doi: 10.1002/ptr.1962

Li, Y., Wo, J. M., Liu, Q., Li, X., and Martin, R. C. (2009). Chemoprotective effects of curcuma aromatica on esophageal carcinogenesis. *Ann. Surg. Oncol.* 6, 515–523. doi: 10.1245/s10434-008-0228-0

Makau, J. N., Watanabe, K., Ishikawa, T., Mizuta, S., Hamada, T., Kobayashi, N., et al. (2017). Identification of small molecule inhibitors for influenza a virus using in silico and *in vitro* approaches. *PLoS One* 12:e0173582. doi: 10.1371/journal.pone.0173582

Morris, G. M., Huey, R., Lindstrom, W., Sanner, M. F., Belew, R. K., Goodsell, D. S., et al. (2009). AutoDock4 and AutoDockTools4: automated docking with selective receptor flexibility. *J. Comput. Chem.* 30, 2785–2791. doi: 10.1002/jcc.21256

Nogales, A., Baker, S. F., Ortiz-Riaño, E., Dewhurst, S., Topham, D. J., and Martínez-Sobrido, L. (2014). Influenza a virus attenuation by codon deoptimization of the ns gene for vaccine development. *J. Virol.* 88, 10525–10540. doi: 10.1128/JVI.01565-14

Peng, M. H., Dai, W. P., Liu, S. J., Yu, L. W., Wu, Y. N., Liu, R., et al. (2016). Bioactive glycosides from the roots of *Ilex asprella*. *Pharm. Biol.* 54, 2127–2134. doi: 10.3109/13880209.2016.1146779

Porath, J., and Flodin, P. (1959). Gel filtration: a method for desalting and group separation. *Nature* 183, 1657–1659. doi: 10.1038/1831657a0

Russell, R. J., Kerry, P. S., Stevens, D. J., Steinhauer, D. A., Martin, S. R., Gamblin, S. J., et al. (2008). Structure of influenza hemagglutinin in complex with an inhibitor of membrane fusion. *Proc. Natl. Acad. Sci. U.S.A.* 105, 17736–17741. doi: 10.1073/pnas.0807142105

Shinoda, T., Nagao, T., Nakayama, M., Serizawa, H., Koshioka, M., Okabe, H., et al. (2002). Identification of a triterpenoid saponin from a crucifer, barbarea vulgaris, as a feeding deterrent to the diamondback moth, plutella xylostella. *J. Chem. Ecol.* 28, 587–599. doi: 10.1023/A:1014500330510

Sidwell, R. W., and Smee, D. F. (2000). *In vitro* and *in vivo* assay systems for study of influenza virus inhibitors. *Antiviral Res.* 48, 1–16. doi: 10.1016/S0166-3542(00)00125-X

Song, G., Shen, X., Li, S., Li, Y., Si, H., Fan, J., et al. (2016). Structure-activity relationships of 3-O-β-chacotriosyl oleanane-type triterp-enoids as potential H5N1 entry inhibitors. *Eur. J. Med. Chem.* 119, 109–121. doi: 10.1016/j.ejmech.2016.04.061

Tahara, H., Matsuda, S., Yamamoto, Y., Yoshizawa, H., Fujita, M., Katsuoka, Y., et al. (2017). High-content image analysis (HCIA) assay has the highest correlation with direct counting cell suspension compared to the ATP, WST-8 and alamar blue assays for measurement of cytotoxicity. *J. Pharmacol. Toxicol. Methods* 88(Pt 1), 92–99. doi: 10.1016/j.vascn.2017.08.003

Waksmundzka-Hajnos, M., Joseph, S., and Teresa, K. (2008). Thin layer chromatography in phytochemistry. *Chromatogr. Sci. Seri.* 99:874. doi: 10.1201/9781420046786

Wang, H., Xu, R., Shi, Y., Si, L., Jiao, P., Fan, Z., et al. (2016). Design, synthesis and biological evaluation of novel l-ascorbic acid-conjugated pentacyclic triterpene derivatives as potential influenza virus entry inhibitors. *Eur. J. Med. Chem.* 110, 376–388. doi: 10.1016/j.ejmech.2016.01.005

Wang, X., Jia, W., Zhao, A., and Wang, X. (2006). Anti-influenza agents from plants and traditional Chinese medicine. *Phytother. Res.* 20, 335–341. doi: 10.1002/ptr.1892

Wang, Y., Ge, H., Li, Y., Xie, Y., He, Y., Xu, M., et al. (2015). Predicting dual-targeting anti-influenza agents using multi-models. *Mol. Diver.* 19, 123–134. doi: 10.1007/s11030-014-9552-4

Wintermeyer, S. M., and Nahata, M. C. (1995). Rimantadine: a clinical perspective. *Ann. Pharmacother.* 29, 299–310. doi: 10.1177/106002809502900312

Woods, J. M., Bethell, R. C., Coates, J. A., Healy, N., Hiscox, S. A., Pearson, B. A., et al. (1993). 4-guanidino-2,4-dideoxy-2,3-dehydro-N-acetylneuraminic Acid is a highly effective inhibitor both of the sialidase (Neuraminidase) and of growth of a wide range of influenza A and B viruses *in vitro*. *Antimicrob. Agents Chemother.* 37, 1473–1479. doi: 10.1128/AAC.37.7.1473

Yamashita, M., Takanori, T., Masayo, K., Akane, T., Hatsumi, N., and Shuku, K. (2009). CS-8958, a prodrug of the new neuraminidase inhibitor R-125489, shows long-acting anti-influenza virus activity. *Antimicrob. Agents Chemother.* 53, 186–192. doi: 10.1128/AAC.00333-08

Yao, Z., Li, J., Zhou, S., Zhang, Y., and Tu, P. (2009). Triterpenoids from leaves of *Ilex cornuta*. *Zhongguo Zhong Yao Za Zhi* 34, 999–1001.

Zhou, S. X., Yao, Z. R., Li, J., and Tu, P. F. (2012). Chemical constituents from leaves of *Ilex cornuta*. *Chin. Tradit. Herb. Drugs* 43, 444–447.

Zhou, Y. B., Wang, J. H., Li, X. M., Fu, X. C., Yan, Z., Zeng, Y. M., et al. (2008). Studies on the chemical constituents of *Ilex pubescens*. *J. Asian Nat. Prod. Res.* 10, 827–831. doi: 10.1080/10286020802102410

10

Laboratory Diagnosis of Respiratory Tract Infections in Children – The State of the Art

Shubhagata Das[1], Sherry Dunbar[1] and Yi-Wei Tang[2,3]*

[1] Global Scientific Affairs, Luminex Corporation, Austin, TX, United States, [2] Department of Laboratory Medicine, Memorial Sloan Kettering Cancer Center, Weill Medical College of Cornell University, New York, NY, United States, [3] Department of Pathology and Laboratory Medicine, Memorial Sloan Kettering Cancer Center, Weill Medical College of Cornell University, New York, NY, United States

***Correspondence:**
Yi-Wei Tang
tangy@mskcc.org

In the pediatric population, respiratory infections are the most common cause of physician visits. Although many respiratory illnesses are self-limiting viral infections that resolve with time and supportive care, it can be critical to identify the causative pathogen at an early stage of the disease in order to implement effective antimicrobial therapy and infection control. Over the last few years, diagnostics for respiratory infections have evolved substantially, with the development of novel assays and the availability of updated tests for newer strains of pathogens. Newer laboratory methods are rapid, highly sensitive and specific, and are gradually replacing the conventional gold standards, although the clinical utility of these assays is still under evaluation. This article reviews the current laboratory methods available for testing for respiratory pathogens and discusses the advantages and disadvantages of each approach.

Keywords: respiratory tract infection, respiratory virus, pediatric population, respiratory infection diagnosis, molecular diagnostics

INTRODUCTION

Acute respiratory tract infections are one of the leading causes of childhood morbidity and mortality worldwide, and it has been estimated that globally, respiratory infections are responsible for about 2 million deaths in children between 0 and 5 years of age (Bryce et al., 2005; Kallander et al., 2008). Approximately 80% of these respiratory infection cases are caused by viral pathogens such as influenza A and B, respiratory syncytial virus (RSV) A and B, parainfluenza virus types 1–3, adenovirus, rhinovirus, human metapneumovirus (hMPV), and others (Mahony, 2008). The non-specific clinical presentation of respiratory infections poses a considerable challenge to the differential diagnosis of these pathogens. Early and accurate diagnosis of the causative pathogens in respiratory infections is essential to administer appropriate antiviral or antibacterial therapy, initiate effective infection control measures, and reduce the length of hospital stay (Barenfanger et al., 2000; Byington et al., 2002; Akers et al., 2017). In the last decade, there has been a remarkable improvement in the diagnosis of respiratory pathogens with the availability of molecular and point-of-care (POC) testing. Although an increasing number of laboratories are adopting rapid molecular assays, conventional testing methods, such as culture and immunodiagnostics are still used. This review focuses on current laboratory methods for testing for respiratory pathogens, and discusses the advantages and disadvantages of each approach.

NON-MOLECULAR METHODS FOR DETECTION AND IDENTIFICATION OF RESPIRATORY PATHOGENS

Electron Microscopy

Electron microscopy (EM) is one of the oldest direct examination methods that has been implemented for both clinical viral diagnosis and study of viral ultrastructure and pathogenesis in developed countries (Roingeard, 2008). Historically, EM has played an instrumental role in identifying novel viral strains in several outbreak situations, such as the coronavirus associated with the severe acute respiratory syndrome (SARS) outbreak (Falsey and Walsh, 2003; Ksiazek et al., 2003). However, despite several advantages, the use of EM has been limited in respiratory viral diagnosis as it is expensive, laborious, time-consuming, and has a greater turnaround time (approximately 3–16 h including specimen preparation), and is often insensitive when compared to other diagnostic methods (Goldsmith and Miller, 2009; Zhang et al., 2013). Additionally, EM requires strict control of experimental conditions, a high concentration of viral particles ($> 10^5\ L^{-1}$), and considerable technical skill and expertise for accurate analysis.

Culture

Detection of viruses by observing the cytopathic effect and hemadsorption in cell culture has been considered the "gold standard" for diagnosis of respiratory viral pathogens for decades. Viruses such as adenovirus, influenza A/B, RSV, and human parainfluenza viruses are the most common respiratory viruses that are isolated and detected by cell culture (Olsen et al., 1993; Winn and Koneman, 2006). The traditional tube culture method is advantageous for growing a wide variety of viruses, including novel or unknown viruses, but takes days and often weeks to provide results. Over the years, modified cell culture methods such as the centrifugation enhanced shell-vial method has reduced the turnaround time from 5 to 10 days to 24 h (Dilnessa and Zeleke, 2017). Shell-vial culture using combination cell lines allows simultaneous detection of multiple respiratory viruses and, as compared to conventional culture, has similar sensitivity for parainfluenza 1-3 (87% vs. 83%) and influenza A/B (78% vs. 75%), and significantly higher sensitivity for RSV (73% vs. 42%) (LaSala et al., 2007). Despite these advantages, many clinically relevant viruses are difficult to grow in culture (such as rhinovirus and coronavirus) and may produce variable results (Ieven and Goossens, 1997; Hodinka, 2013). Additionally, multiple freezing and thawing of the samples prior to testing can reduce the viral titer, thus effecting the growth in culture. Therefore, as compared to molecular tests, both traditional tube and shell-vial culture methods are laborious, exhibit higher false negative rates, and have longer turnaround times, making viral culture less clinically relevant (Leland and Ginocchio, 2007; Ginocchio, 2007; Hematian et al., 2016).

Culture is also the gold standard for detection of atypical (bacterial) respiratory pathogens, which is followed by identification and antimicrobial susceptibility testing by various manual or automated methods (Tenover, 2011). Bacterial culture can also often be insensitive, especially when specimen adequacy is not determined by Gram stain or if specimens were collected after antibiotic exposure (ATS and IDSA, 2005; Woodhead et al., 2005; Harris et al., 2017). Bacterial culture is also labor intensive, requires substantial technical expertise, and has a typical turnaround time of 48 – 96 h if antibiotic susceptibility testing is performed, and can therefore be considered inadequate for optimal patient care and guiding effective antimicrobial therapy (Tenover, 2011).

Antigen Detection Assays

Rapid Immunoassays

Rapid immunoassays (RIAs) can deliver test results in less than 30 min and are usually performed in the POC setting, thus allowing the test results to be incorporated into the clinical decision-making algorithm (Weinberg and Walker, 2005). Among the four primary RIA formats (latex agglutination, horizontal flow devices, lateral flow devices, and optical immunoassays), the lateral-flow immunoassay (LFIA) is the most versatile and popular immunochromatographic method. RIAs are relatively inexpensive, easy to perform, and most of them have waived status in the United States according to the Clinical Laboratory Improvement Act (CLIA) guidelines, thereby making them invaluable in outpatient clinics, primary care, emergency, and low resource settings (Ginocchio, 2007). Currently, commercially available RIAs are mostly limited to the detection of influenza A virus, influenza B virus, and RSV. Numerous studies have revealed that RIAs demonstrate overall poor sensitivity for influenza and RSV (44–95%); however, they have a higher median specificity (90 to 95%) as compared to cell culture (WHO, 2005; Leland and Ginocchio, 2007; Ginocchio, 2007).

In the pediatric population, commercially available immunoassays have demonstrated high sensitivity (93%) for detection of RSV, and a systematic review of published studies has further revealed that the sensitivity of RSV RIAs is relatively higher for children (81%) than adults (29%) (Slinger et al., 2004; Chartrand et al., 2015). The higher sensitivity can be attributed to the fact that pediatric patients often shed higher titers of respiratory viruses and for a longer time as compared to adults (Englund et al., 1996; Kawai et al., 2007). Despite the overall lower sensitivity, RIAs have been deemed a valuable diagnostic tool in the emergency department as they can significantly decrease the length of stay, additional ancillary testing, and antibiotic prescriptions for those children who do test positive for influenza (Abanses et al., 2006; Blaschke et al., 2014).

Direct Fluorescent Antibody Tests

Direct fluorescent antibody (DFA) testing of nasopharyngeal wash specimens is considered a rapid and reliable method for detecting respiratory viral infections. Commercial DFA kits have demonstrated high sensitivity and specificity for multiple respiratory viruses such as hMPV (95 and 100%), adenovirus (62 and 100%), RSV (94 and 96%), and parainfluenza viruses (88 and 99.7%), although the results can be subjective and require technical expertise for accurate interpretation (Landry and Ferguson, 2000; Ohm-Smith et al., 2004; Rocholl et al., 2004;

Aslanzadeh et al., 2008; Vinh et al., 2008). The high specificity (99–100%) of DFA indicates that the test can be used as a reliable detection method, especially during the initial days of the illness, as was shown by Shafik et al. (2011) for RSV in children.

Serological Tests

Pathogen-specific antibodies typically appear about 2 weeks after the initial infection and can be detected by serological tests. Serological tests can successfully identify antibodies to most respiratory pathogens such as RSV, adenovirus, influenza A and B, parainfluenza 1-3 virus, etc., and can detect mixed infections from hospitalized children suffering from acute respiratory infections, with the exception of infants for whom an antibody response is usually undetected (Hall et al., 1991; Chkhaidze et al., 2006). However, it has been reported that serological assays are significantly less sensitive for the detection of parainfluenza virus and adenovirus when compared to molecular methods, such as RT-PCR (Kuypers et al., 2006). Kuypers et al. (2006) found that RT-PCR detected 40% more specimens from pediatric patients that were positive for at least one respiratory virus than were detected by fluorescent antibody assay (FA). FA testing, in addition to RT-PCR, is useful for epidemiological studies as it increases the probability of identifying acute viral infections and has been used for accurate assessment of respiratory viruses other than influenza in children (Sawatwong et al., 2012; Feikin et al., 2013; Zhang et al., 2017).

For bacteria, serological testing is particularly challenging, especially for identifying atypical bacterial agents such as *Mycoplasma pneumoniae*. With varied sensitivity (14% - 77%) and specificity (49% - 97%) as compared to PCR, serological testing has limited usefulness clinically (Beersma et al., 2005; Wellinghausen et al., 2006). The clinical utility of serologic tests is further limited because they require both acute and convalescent sera to monitor seroconversion or to identify a four–fold increase in antibody titer (Loeffelholz and Chonmaitree, 2010). Additionally, serological tests are not relevant for identifying frequently recurring viral infections as the serum IgM levels are lower due to repeated exposure to vaccines or circulating viruses. For optimal virus specific IgM testing, an acute-phase serum specimen should be obtained early in the course of illness (Dunn, 2015).

NUCLEIC ACID AMPLIFICATION TESTS FOR DETECTION AND IDENTIFICATION OF RESPIRATORY PATHOGENS

A wide variety of newer, nucleic acid amplification tests (NAATs) for the detection of respiratory pathogens are commercially available. These tests are listed in **Table 1** and described below according to complexity and pathogen coverage. The accuracy of respiratory virus detection by molecular tests is not only dependent on their specific assay chemistry, but is also critically affected by the type, quantity, and quality of specimens collected (Dunn, 2015). Several types of specimens can be used for detection of respiratory viruses, including: bronchoalveolar lavage (BAL), throat swab, nasopharyngeal (NP) washes, NP aspirates, lung aspirates, and NP swabs, although the appropriate specimen type depends on the specific patient population. For example, in pediatric patients, obtaining nasal washes and nasal aspirates is more technically challenging when compared to NP swabs, especially in severely ill children and in poor resource settings (Hammitt et al., 2012). It has been observed that for optimal test results, specimens should be collected within 3–5 days after onset of symptoms to ensure that the sample has a high concentration of virus particles, viral antigen or viral nucleic acids, should be transported to the testing laboratory in refrigerated condition (2–8°C) in appropriate transport media, and testing should be performed within 48 h (Grys and Smith, 2009).

High Complexity Multiplex Panel Assays

Detection of respiratory pathogens by NAATs such as PCR, nucleic acid sequence-based amplification (NASBA), transcription mediated amplification (TMA), strand displacement amplification (SDA), loop-mediated isothermal amplification (LAMP), rolling circle amplification (RCA), etc., have gained immense popularity over the past decade. Large syndromic panels that can detect multiple pathogens simultaneously are beneficial for infection control, timely treatment decisions, and are substantially less expensive than detecting individual pathogens by monoplex real-time RT-PCR (Reijans et al., 2008; Schreckenberger and McAdam, 2015). These multiplex respiratory panels vary in terms of their complexity (high, moderate, or waived), throughput, pathogens detected, ability to subtype, instrumentation (batched or random access), workflow (stepwise or integrated sample-to-answer), ease of use, and time to result (several hours to minutes) (Caliendo, 2011; Krunic et al., 2011; Mahony et al., 2011). Studies have reported increased diagnostic yield (60% vs. 35%) and considerably higher sensitivity (80–100%) and specificity (82–100%) for these assays when compared to conventional diagnostic methods such as DFA, viral isolation, and immunoassays (Reijans et al., 2008; Gharabaghi et al., 2011).

In comparison to other NAAT-based molecular methods, high-plex syndromic panels demonstrate comparable performance, although sensitivity and specificity might vary for individual targets (Sails et al., 2017). For example, greater than 99% specificity was observed for all targets except enterovirus/rhinovirus (94%), and the overall sensitivity ranged between (83–100%) when the NxTAG RPP and the Anyplex II RV16 assays were evaluated for detection of respiratory pathogens in hospitalized children (Brotons et al., 2016). Syndromic panels can also detect bacterial infections and viral-bacterial coinfections, which is vital for developing effective treatment plans and prevention strategies (Brealey et al., 2015; Brotons et al., 2016). However, for novel pathogen strains, such as Flu A(H1N1pdm2009), panel tests often fail to identify the subtype and require confirmation by other tests (Bryce et al., 2012).

TABLE 1 | Commercially available nucleic acid amplification assays for respiratory pathogens[a].

Test	Manufacturer	Technology	Targets	Sample type[b]	Turnaround time	Complexity classification
NxTAG® respiratory pathogen panel	Luminex Corporation	Real-time RT-PCR	Multiplex Panel (20 targets)	NPS	~4 h	High
eSensor® respiratory viral panel (RVP)	GenMark Diagnostics	Multiplex microarray, competitive DNA hybridization	Multiplex Panel (14 targets)	NPS	~8 h	High
Verigene® RP flex	Luminex Corporation	RT-PCR & and microarray hybridization	Multiplex Panel (16 targets)	NPS	~2 h	Moderate
ePlex® respiratory pathogen (RP) panel	GenMark Diagnostics	RT-PCR	Multiplex Panel (17 targets)	NPS	~2 h	Moderate
FilmArray® respiratory panel (RP)	BioFire Diagnostics, Inc.,	Nested multiplex RT-PCR	Multiplex Panel (20 targets)	NPS	~1 h	Moderate
FilmArray® respiratory panel 2 (RP2)	BioFire Diagnostics, Inc.,	Nested multiplex RT-PCR	Multiplex Panel (21 targets)	NPS	~45 min	Moderate
FilmArray® respiratory panel® (RP) EZ	BioFire Diagnostics, Inc.,	Nested multiplex RT -PCR	Multiplex Panel (14 targets)	NPS	~1 h	Waived
Lyra® parainfluenza virus assay	Quidel Corporation	Real-time RT-PCR	Parainfluenza virus types 1, 2, and 3	NS, NPS	~4 h	High
Lyra® RSV + hMPV assay	Quidel Corporation	Real-time RT-PCR	RSV, hMPV	NS, NPS	~4 h	High
Simplexa™ flu A/B & RSV Kit	Focus Diagnostics, Inc.,	Real-time RT-PCR	Flu A, Flu B, and RSV	TS	<4 h	High
Panther fusion flu A/B/RSV	Hologic, Inc.,	Real-time RT-PCR	Flu A, Flu B, and RSV	NPS	~2.5 h	High
Panther fusion paraflu assay	Hologic, Inc.,	Real-time RT-PCR	Parainfluenza 1, 2, and 3	NPS	~2.5 h	High
Panther fusion AdV/hMPV/RV assay	Hologic, Inc.,	Real-time RT-PCR	Adenovirus, hMPV, and Rhinovirus	NPS	~2.5 h	High
ARIES® flu A/B & RSV assay	Luminex Corporation	Real-time PCR	Flu A, Flu B, and RSV	NPS	<2 h	Moderate
ARIES® bordetella assay	Luminex Corporation	Real-time PCR	*B. pertussis, B. parapertussis*	NPS	<2 h	Moderate
Simplexa™ flu A/B & RSV direct	Focus Diagnostics, Inc.,	Real-time RT-PCR	Flu A, Flu B, and RSV	NPS	<2 h	Moderate
Xpert® flu/RSV XC	Cepheid	Real-time RT-PCR	Flu A, Flu B, and RSV	NPS, NA, and NW	<1 h	Moderate
Solana RSV + hMPV assay	Quidel Corporation	Isothermal RT-helicase-dependent amplification (HDA)	RSV, hMPV	NS, NPS	~45 min	Moderate
Illumigene® mycoplasma direct DNA amplification assay	Meridian Bioscience, Inc.,	Loop-mediated isothermal DNA amplification (LAMP)	*Mycoplasma pneumoniae*	NPS, TS	<1 h	Moderate
Illumigene pertussis DNA amplification assay	Meridian Bioscience, Inc.,	Loop-mediated isothermal DNA amplification (LAMP)	*Bordetella pertussis*	NPS	<1 h	Moderate
Xpert® xpress Flu/RSV	Cepheid	Real-time RT-PCR	Flu A, Flu B, and RSV	NPS, NA, and NW	~30 min	Waived
Xpert® xpress flu	Cepheid	Real-time RT-PCR	Flu A, Flu B	NPS, NA, and NW	~30 min	Waived
cobas® Liat influenza A/B & RSV assay	Roche Molecular Diagnostics	Real-time RT-PCR	Flu A, Flu B, and RSV	NPS	~20 min	Waived
cobas® Liat influenza A/B assay	Roche Molecular Diagnostics	Real-time RT-PCR	Flu A, Flu B	NPS	~20 min	Waived
Alere i influenza A & B 2 test	Abbott Laboratories	Isothermal nucleic acid amplification	Flu A, Flu B	NPS, NS	<15 min	Waived
Alere i RSV	Abbott Laboratories	Isothermal nucleic acid amplification	RSV	NPS, NPS in VTM	<15 min	Waived

[a]FDA 510(k) Premarket Notification (FDA, 2018a). Retrieved from https://www.accessdata.fda.gov/scripts/cdrh/cfdocs/cfpmn/pmn.cfm; [b]NPS, nasopharyngeal swab; NS, nasal swab; NA, nasal aspirate; NW, nasal wash; TS, throat swab. [c]Waived for direct NS, NPS, and NA/NW specimens; Moderate for NS and NA/NW specimens eluted in transport media.

Syndromic respiratory panels with high sample throughput can usually run 1–96 specimens and are mostly classified as high complexity assays according to CLIA guidelines, which indicates that running these panel requires considerable knowledge, training, and experience (FDA, 2018b). It has been noted that these high throughput panels are ideal for batch testing, especially during outbreak situations and respiratory viral seasons when sample volumes are unusually high (Ginocchio et al., 2009; Crawford et al., 2010; Tang et al., 2016). Despite the advantages, implementation of high throughput panels can be challenging because of demanding sample preparation, processing, and result interpretation procedures, and the turnaround time varies from approximately 5–16 h (Beckmann and Hirsch, 2016).

Moderate Complexity Multiplex Integrated Systems

Moderate complexity sample-to-answer molecular test systems have gained immense popularity over the last few years because of their ease of use, faster turnaround time, and efficient workflow. Currently, the United States. FDA-cleared sample-to-answer test systems include both low-plex, targeted assays and high-plex panels that can detect multiple pathogens and pathogen classes. These tests usually have low to moderate sample throughput (e.g., 1–12 samples/run), but have faster turnaround times when compared to batched, high throughput, multiplex panels (Popowitch et al., 2013). The high-plex, sample-to-answer panels can detect up to 12–20 pathogens based on the panel size. Most of these qualitative assays allow random access that ensures that tests can be performed on demand, and the reactions occur in closed cassettes or cartridges, thereby minimizing the risk of contamination (Poritz et al., 2011; Popowitch and Miller, 2015).

Comparative studies evaluating the performance of these assays has reported more than 95% agreement between different commercial platforms, and greater than 85% sensitivity and 99% specificity in most cases (Babady et al., 2018). However, some high-plex sample-to-answer tests have demonstrated lower sensitivity for certain pathogens such as adenovirus (57%), influenza A(H1N1pdm09) (73%), and influenza B virus (77%) (Popowitch et al., 2013). Cross-reactivity between adenovirus subtypes has also been reported for some assays, but the differentiation of these groups is not deemed clinically important for routine diagnosis (Lin et al., 2004; Gray et al., 2007).

Despite a short turnaround time of 1–2 h, the clinical utility of these assays has been questioned since no statistically significant reduction in antibiotic prescription rates or mortality has been observed between patients who tested positive for a non-influenza virus and those who tested negative (48% vs. 49% respectively) (Green et al., 2016). In some cases, a reduction in length of hospital stay (7 days vs. 9 days) and duration of isolation (75 h vs. 82 h) was observed (Rogers et al., 2015; Akers et al., 2017). The primary concerns for the high-plex sample-to-answer assays are high cost per test, and the inability to order customized, targeted panels (Ramanan et al., 2018). Multiplex assays such as the Verigene RP *Flex* panel (Luminex) offer flexible testing and payment options by allowing users to order any combination of targets for an individual sample.

Low-Plex Integrated Test Systems

Low-plex integrated respiratory test systems typically target 1–4 pathogens per assay. Comparative studies evaluating the performance of these assays has reported more than 90% concordance between different commercial platforms, and greater than 95% sensitivity and specificity in most cases (Dugas et al., 2014; Selvaraju et al., 2014; McMullen et al., 2017). The total turnaround time per sample for these assays varies between ~1–2 h, and the number of samples that can be tested in a standard 8-h work shift depends on the number of instruments available in the testing laboratory (Ling et al., 2018). Smaller panels targeting a few pathogens that can be run independently (random access) or simultaneously (random batch) could be a viable option for controlling laboratory costs. Therefore, when considering among various testing options, it is recommended that in addition to clinical performance, other assay characteristics such as ease of use, panel composition, total turnaround time, hands-on time, and cost be considered before implementing an assay in various clinical settings (Juretschko et al., 2017).

Waived Molecular Point-of-Care Tests

Nucleic acid amplification based POC testing is relatively new in the realm of respiratory viral diagnosis and has generated contradicting opinions regarding their implementation and clinical utility. Molecular POC assays have extremely short turnaround times (<30 min), minimal hands-on time (1–2 min), and can be easily operated by non-laboratory staff members, thereby making them suitable for near patient implementation and testing (Brendish et al., 2015; Peters et al., 2017; Ling et al., 2018). Currently most of the United States. FDA-cleared commercial POC assays are limited to the detection of influenza A/B and RSV viruses, with the exception of the FilmArray® RP EZ (BioFire) which detects 14 targets (FDA, 2018c). Most of the studies evaluating the clinical performance of these assays have reported high sensitivity (87–100%) and specificity (>98%) for detecting influenza A/B and RSV in pediatric and adult patients (Bell et al., 2014; Nie et al., 2014; Popowitch and Miller, 2015; Gibson et al., 2017; Ling et al., 2018). However, these studies have also shown that the clinical performance varies and sensitivity is significantly low for influenza B (45.2–54.5%); therefore, the results should be interpreted with caution and additional confirmatory testing should be considered, depending on the clinical circumstances (Jokela et al., 2015; Busson et al., 2017; Davis et al., 2017). Molecular POC tests can be costly and more prone to incorrect results and contamination, as the assays are usually performed by non-laboratory personnel and poor training, failure to follow manufacturer's instructions, and failure to perform adequate quality control might affect the accuracy of results (Azar and Landry, 2018). Currently, more evidence-based studies are required to understand the overall clinical utility of molecular POC testing, since no correlation has been observed between implementation of these tests and reduction of antibiotic usage or hospital length of stay (Andrews et al., 2017; Brendish et al., 2017).

CONCLUDING REMARKS

Molecular testing has considerably improved the diagnosis of respiratory pathogens and is being considered as the new "gold standard". Although these tests have gained immense popularity, factors such as the patient population (adult, pediatric, and immunocompromised), the size of the laboratory, the purpose of testing (routine or urgent care), and cost/benefit ratio should be considered before implementing a particular assay. For example, during the 2012–2013 influenza outbreak, two nosocomial cases were identified at Memorial Sloan Kettering Cancer Center on January 1, 2013. Despite implementing appropriate infection control measures, five more cases were identified few days later on January 7, 2013. A delay in reporting the positive influenza result was observed as the laboratory was following the routine diagnostic algorithm, and this might have resulted in the subsequent cases of nosocomial infection. Following the 2012–2013 outbreak, the laboratory implemented the FilmArray® RP for routine diagnosis and the Xpert® Xpress Flu/RSV, a rapid molecular POC system, for seasonal use during epidemics and pandemics because the needs for routine testing and urgent care are completely different in these situations. Molecular tests are highly sensitive and specific and result in higher pathogen detection, and therefore physicians and attending clinicians should evaluate test results before initiating a particular course of treatment. Rapid molecular tests are best suited for routine diagnosis and outbreak situations; whereas, conventional methods, such as cell culture or EM could be considered for identifying novel strains of the pathogens.

With the introduction of new technologies, newer assays will be developed for respiratory and other pathogens. For example, using NP swab specimens from children, Graf et al. (2016) demonstrated that untargeted next-generation sequencing-based metagenomics (mNGS) testing had excellent agreement (93%) with multiplex molecular panels and detected more viruses that were either not targeted by the panel or missed due to highly divergent genome sequences. They concluded that mNGS can be used for accurate and unbiased detection of expected or unexpected pathogens. Implementing mNGS downstream of rapid molecular panel testing has been proven useful for characterizing the nature of hospital-associated transmission events and directing the control strategies in pediatric populations during outbreak situations (Greninger et al., 2017). However, diagnostic implementation of NGS is currently limited by incomplete understanding of analytical performance, high cost of the system and complexity of sequence data analysis. Future research will be necessary to focus on demonstrating the clinical utility of these new and upcoming assays in various patient populations and in resource limited settings.

AUTHOR CONTRIBUTIONS

All authors listed have made a substantial, direct and intellectual contribution to the work, and approved it for publication.

REFERENCES

Abanses, J. C., Dowd, M. D., Simon, S. D., and Sharma, V. (2006). Impact of rapid influenza testing at triage on management of febrile infants and young children. *Pediatr. Emerg. Care* 22, 145–149. doi: 10.1097/01.pec.0000202454.19237.b0

Akers, I. E., Weber, R., Sax, H., Boni, J., Trkola, A., and Kuster, S. P. (2017). Influence of time to diagnosis of severe influenza on antibiotic use, length of stay, isolation precautions, and mortality: a retrospective study. *Influenza Other Respir. Viruses* 11, 337–344. doi: 10.1111/irv.12454

Andrews, D., Chetty, Y., Cooper, B. S., Virk, M., Glass, S. K., Letters, A., et al. (2017). Multiplex PCR point of care testing versus routine, laboratory-based testing in the treatment of adults with respiratory tract infections: a quasi-randomised study assessing impact on length of stay and antimicrobial use. *BMC Infect. Dis.* 17:671. doi: 10.1186/s12879-017-2784-z

Aslanzadeh, J., Zheng, X., Li, H., Tetreault, J., Ratkiewicz, I., Meng, S., et al. (2008). Prospective evaluation of rapid antigen tests for diagnosis of respiratory syncytial virus and human metapneumovirus infections. *J. Clin. Microbiol.* 46, 1682–1685. doi: 10.1128/jcm.00008-08

ATS and IDSA (2005). Guidelines for the management of adults with hospital-acquired, ventilator-associated, and healthcare-associated pneumonia. *Am. J. Respir. Crit. Care Med.* 171, 388–416. doi: 10.1164/rccm.200405-644ST

Azar, M. M., and Landry, M. L. (2018). Detection of influenza A and B viruses and respiratory syncytial virus using CLIA-waived point-of-care assays: a paradigm shift to molecular tests. *J. Clin. Microbiol.* 56:e00367-18. doi: 10.1128/jcm.00367-18

Babady, N. E., England, M. R., Jurcic Smith, K. L., He, T., Wijetunge, D. S., Tang, Y. W., et al. (2018). Multicenter evaluation of the ePlex respiratory pathogen panel for the detection of viral and bacterial respiratory tract pathogens in nasopharyngeal swabs. *J. Clin. Microbiol.* 56, e01658-17. doi: 10.1128/jcm.01658-17

Barenfanger, J., Drake, C., Leon, N., Mueller, T., and Troutt, T. (2000). Clinical and financial benefits of rapid detection of respiratory viruses: an outcomes study. *J. Clin. Microbiol.* 38, 2824–2828.

Beckmann, C., and Hirsch, H. H. (2016). Comparing luminex NxTAG-respiratory pathogen panel and RespiFinder-22 for multiplex detection of respiratory pathogens. *J. Med. Virol.* 88, 1319–1324. doi: 10.1002/jmv.24492

Beersma, M. F., Dirven, K., van Dam, A. P., Templeton, K. E., Claas, E. C., and Goossens, H. (2005). Evaluation of 12 commercial tests and the complement fixation test for *Mycoplasma pneumoniae*-specific immunoglobulin G (IgG) and IgM antibodies, with PCR used as the "gold standard". *J. Clin. Microbiol.* 43, 2277–2285. doi: 10.1128/jcm.43.5.2277-2285.2005

Bell, J., Bonner, A., Cohen, D. M., Birkhahn, R., Yogev, R., Triner, W., et al. (2014). Multicenter clinical evaluation of the novel Alere™ I Influenza A&B isothermal nucleic acid amplification test. *J. Clin. Virol.* 61, 81–86. doi: 10.1016/j.jcv.2014.06.001

Blaschke, A. J., Shapiro, D. J., Pavia, A. T., Byington, C. L., Ampofo, K., Stockmann, C., et al. (2014). A national study of the impact of rapid influenza testing on clinical care in the emergency department. *J. Pediatr. Infect Dis. Soc.* 3, 112–118. doi: 10.1093/jpids/pit071

Brealey, J. C., Sly, P. D., Young, P. R., and Chappell, K. J. (2015). Viral bacterial co-infection of the respiratory tract during early childhood. *FEMS Microbiol. Lett.* 362:fnv062. doi: 10.1093/femsle/fnv062

Brendish, N. J., Malachira, A. K., Armstrong, L., Houghton, R., Aitken, S., Nyimbili, E., et al. (2017). Routine molecular point-of-care testing for respiratory viruses in adults presenting to hospital with acute respiratory illness (ResPOC): a pragmatic, open-label, randomised controlled trial. *Lancet Respir. Med.* 5, 401–411. doi: 10.1016/S2213-2600(17)30120-0

Brendish, N. J., Schiff, H. F., and Clark, T. W. (2015). Point-of-care testing for respiratory viruses in adults: the current landscape and future potential. *J. Infect.* 71, 501–510. doi: 10.1016/j.jinf.2015.07.008

Brotons, P., Henares, D., Latorre, I., Cepillo, A., Launes, C., and Munoz-Almagro, C. (2016). Comparison of NxTAG respiratory pathogen panel and anyplex II RV16 tests for multiplex detection of respiratory pathogens in hospitalized children. *J. Clin. Microbiol.* 54, 2900–2904. doi: 10.1128/jcm.01243-16

Bryce, J., Boschi-Pinto, C., Shibuya, K., and Black, R. E. (2005). WHO estimates of the causes of death in children. *Lancet* 365, 1147–1152. doi: 10.1016/s0140-6736(05)71877-8

Bryce, L., Koenig, M., and Jerke, K. H. (2012). A large-scale study of respiratory virus infection over 2 years using the Luminex xTAGRVP assay. *Mil. Med.* 177, 1533–1538. doi: 10.7205/MILMED-D-12-00277

Busson, L., Mahadeb, B., De Foor, M., Vandenberg, O., and Hallin, M. (2017). Contribution of a rapid influenza diagnostic test to manage hospitalized patients with suspected influenza. *Diagn. Microbiol. Infect. Dis.* 87, 238–242. doi: 10.1016/j.diagmicrobio.2016.11.015

Byington, C. L., Castillo, H., Gerber, K., Daly, J. A., Brimley, L. A., Adams, S., et al. (2002). The effect of rapid respiratory viral diagnostic testing on antibiotic use in a children's hospital. *Arch. Pediatr. Adolesc. Med.* 156, 1230–1234. doi: 10.1001/archpedi.156.12.1230

Caliendo, A. M. (2011). Multiplex PCR and emerging technologies for the detection of respiratory pathogens. *Clin. Infect. Dis.* 52(Suppl. 4), S326–S330. doi: 10.1093/cid/cir047

Chartrand, C., Tremblay, N., Renaud, C., and Papenburg, J. (2015). Diagnostic accuracy of rapid antigen detection tests for respiratory syncytial virus infection: systematic review and meta-analysis. *J. Clin. Microbiol.* 53, 3738–3749. doi: 10.1128/jcm.01816-15

Chkhaidze, I., Manjavidze, N., and Nemsadze, K. (2006). Serodiagnosis of acute respiratory infections in children in Georgia. *Indian J. Pediatr.* 73, 569–572. doi: 10.1007/BF02759919

Crawford, J. M., Stallone, R., Zhang, F., Gerolimatos, M., Korologos, D. D., Sweetapple, C., et al. (2010). Laboratory surge response to pandemic (H1N1) 2009 outbreak, New York City metropolitan area, USA. *Emerg. Infect. Dis.* 16, 8–13. doi: 10.3201/eid1601.091167

Davis, S., Allen, A. J., O'Leary, R., Power, M., Price, D. A., Simpson, A. J., et al. (2017). Diagnostic accuracy and cost analysis of the Alere™ I Influenza A&B near-patient test using throat swabs. *J. Hosp. Infect.* 97, 301–309. doi: 10.1016/j.jhin.2017.05.017

Dilnessa, T., and Zeleke, H. (2017). Cell culture, cytopathic effect and immunofluorescence diagnosis of viral infection. *J. Microbiol. Mod. Tech.* 2, 102–110.

Dugas, A. F., Valsamakis, A., Gaydos, C. A., Forman, M., Hardick, J., Kidambi, P., et al. (2014). Evaluation of the Xpert Flu rapid PCR assay in high-risk emergency department patients. *J. Clin. Microbiol.* 52, 4353–4355. doi: 10.1128/jcm.02343-14

Dunn, J. J. (2015). "Specimen collection, transport, and processing: virology," in *Manual of Clinical Microbiology*, 11th Edn, eds J. H. Jorgensen, M. A. Pfaller, K. C. Carroll, G. Funke, S. S. Richter, M. L. Landry, et al. (Washington, DC: American Society of Microbiology), 1405–1421.

Englund, J. A., Piedra, P. A., Jewell, A., Patel, K., Baxter, B. B., and Whimbey, E. (1996). Rapid diagnosis of respiratory syncytial virus infections in immunocompromised adults. *J. Clin. Microbiol.* 34, 1649–1653.

Falsey, A. R., and Walsh, E. E. (2003). Novel coronavirus and severe acute respiratory syndrome. *Lancet* 361, 1312–1313. doi: 10.1016/s0140-6736(03)13084-x

FDA (2018a). *510(k) Premarket Notification [Online]*. Available at: https://www.accessdata.fda.gov/scripts/cdrh/cfdocs/cfpmn/pmn.cfm [accessed June 24, 2018].

FDA (2018b). *CLIA Categorizations [Online]*. Available at: https://www.fda.gov/MedicalDevices/DeviceRegulationandGuidance/IVDRegulatoryAssistance/ucm393229.htm [accessed June 24, 2018].

FDA (2018c). *Nucleic Acid Based Tests [Online]*. Available at: https://www.fda.gov/MedicalDevices/ProductsandMedicalProcedures/InVitroDiagnostics/ucm330711.htm [accessed June 24, 2018].

Feikin, D. R., Njenga, M. K., Bigogo, G., Aura, B., Gikunju, S., Balish, A., et al. (2013). Additional diagnostic yield of adding serology to PCR in diagnosing viral acute respiratory infections in Kenyan patients 5 years of age and older. *Clin. Vaccine Immunol.* 20, 113–114. doi: 10.1128/cvi.00325-12

Gharabaghi, F., Hawan, A., Drews, S. J., and Richardson, S. E. (2011). Evaluation of multiple commercial molecular and conventional diagnostic assays for the detection of respiratory viruses in children. *Clin. Microbiol. Infect.* 17, 1900–1906. doi: 10.1111/j.1469-0691.2011.03529.x

Gibson, J., Schechter-Perkins, E. M., Mitchell, P., Mace, S., Tian, Y., Williams, K., et al. (2017). Multi-center evaluation of the cobas® Liat® Influenza A/B & RSV assay for rapid point of care diagnosis. *J. Clin. Virol.* 95, 5–9. doi: 10.1016/j.jcv.2017.08.004

Ginocchio, C. C. (2007). Detection of respiratory viruses using non-molecular based methods. *J. Clin. Virol.* 40(Suppl. 1), S11–S14. doi: 10.1016/s1386-6532(07)70004-5

Ginocchio, C. C., Zhang, F., Manji, R., Arora, S., Bornfreund, M., Falk, L., et al. (2009). Evaluation of multiple test methods for the detection of the novel 2009 influenza A (H1N1) during the New York City outbreak. *J. Clin. Virol.* 45, 191–195. doi: 10.1016/j.jcv.2009.06.005

Goldsmith, C. S., and Miller, S. E. (2009). Modern uses of electron microscopy for detection of viruses. *Clin. Microbiol. Rev.* 22, 552–563. doi: 10.1128/cmr.00027-09

Graf, E. H., Simmon, K. E., Tardif, K. D., Hymas, W., Flygare, S., Eilbeck, K., et al. (2016). Unbiased detection of respiratory viruses using RNA-seq-based metagenomics: a systematic comparison to a commercial PCR panel. *J. Clin. Microbiol.* 54, 1000–1007. doi: 10.1128/JCM.03060-15

Gray, G. C., McCarthy, T., Lebeck, M. G., Schnurr, D. P., Russell, K. L., Kajon, A. E., et al. (2007). Genotype prevalence and risk factors for severe clinical adenovirus infection, United States 2004-2006. *Clin. Infect. Dis.* 45, 1120–1131. doi: 10.1086/522188

Green, D. A., Hitoaliaj, L., Kotansky, B., Campbell, S. M., and Peaper, D. R. (2016). Clinical utility of on-demand multiplex respiratory pathogen testing among adult outpatients. *J. Clin. Microbiol.* 54, 2950–2955. doi: 10.1128/jcm.01579-16

Greninger, A. L., Waghmare, A., Adler, A., Qin, X., Crowley, J. L., Englund, J. A., et al. (2017). Rule-out outbreak: 24-hour metagenomic next-generation sequencing for characterizing respiratory virus source for infection prevention. *J. Pediatr. Infect. Dis. Soc.* 6, 168–172. doi: 10.1093/jpids/pix019

Grys, T. E., and Smith, T. F. (2009). "Specimen requirements: selection, collection, transport, and processing," in *Clinical Virology Manual*, 4th Edn, eds M. J. Loeffelholz, R. L. Hodinka, S. A. Young, and B. A. Pinsky (Washington, DC: American Society of Microbiology), 18–35.

Hall, C. B., Walsh, E. E., Long, C. E., and Schnabel, K. C. (1991). Immunity to and frequency of reinfection with respiratory syncytial virus. *J. Infect. Dis.* 163, 693–698. doi: 10.1093/infdis/163.4.693

Hammitt, L. L., Murdoch, D. R., Scott, J. A. G., Driscoll, A., Karron, R. A., Levine, O. S., et al. (2012). Specimen collection for the diagnosis of pediatric pneumonia. *Clin. Infect. Dis.* 54(Suppl. 2), S132–S139. doi: 10.1093/cid/cir1068

Harris, A. M., Bramley, A. M., Jain, S., Arnold, S. R., Ampofo, K., Self, W. H., et al. (2017). Influence of antibiotics on the detection of bacteria by culture-based and culture-independent diagnostic tests in patients hospitalized with community-acquired pneumonia. *Open Forum Infect. Dis.* 4:ofx014. doi: 10.1093/ofid/ofx014

Hematian, A., Sadeghifard, N., Mohebi, R., Taherikalani, M., Nasrolahi, A., Amraei, M., et al. (2016). Traditional and modern cell culture in virus diagnosis. *Osong Public Health Res. Perspect.* 7, 77–82. doi: 10.1016/j.phrp.2015.11.011

Hodinka, R. L. (2013). Point: is the era of viral culture over in the clinical microbiology laboratory? *J. Clin. Microbiol.* 51, 2–4. doi: 10.1128/jcm.02593-12

Ieven, M., and Goossens, H. (1997). Relevance of nucleic acid amplification techniques for diagnosis of respiratory tract infections in the clinical laboratory. *Clin. Microbiol. Rev.* 10, 242–256.

Jokela, P., Vuorinen, T., Waris, M., and Manninen, R. (2015). Performance of the Alere I influenza A&B assay and mariPOC test for the rapid detection of influenza A and B viruses. *J. Clin. Virol.* 70, 72–76. doi: 10.1016/j.jcv.2015.07.294

Juretschko, S., Mahony, J., Buller, R. S., Manji, R., Dunbar, S., Walker, K., et al. (2017). Multicenter clinical evaluation of the luminex Aries Flu A/B & RSV assay for pediatric and adult respiratory tract specimens. *J. Clin. Microbiol.* 55, 2431–2438. doi: 10.1128/jcm.00318-17

Kallander, K., Hildenwall, H., Waiswa, P., Galiwango, E., Peterson, S., and Pariyo, G. (2008). Delayed care seeking for fatal pneumonia in children aged under five years in Uganda: a case-series study. *Bull. World Health Organ.* 86, 332–338. doi: 10.2471/BLT.07.049353

Kawai, N., Ikematsu, H., Iwaki, N., Kawashima, T., Maeda, T., Mitsuoka, S., et al. (2007). Longer virus shedding in influenza B than in influenza A among outpatients treated with oseltamivir. *J. Infect.* 55, 267–272. doi: 10.1016/j.jinf.2007.05.176

Krunic, N., Merante, F., Yaghoubian, S., Himsworth, D., and Janeczko, R. (2011). Advances in the diagnosis of respiratory tract infections: role of the Luminex xTAG respiratory viral panel. *Ann. N. Y. Acad. Sci.* 1222, 6–13. doi: 10.1111/j.1749-6632.2011.05964.x

Ksiazek, T. G., Erdman, D., Goldsmith, C. S., Zaki, S. R., Peret, T., Emery, S., et al. (2003). A novel coronavirus associated with severe acute respiratory syndrome. *N. Engl. J. Med.* 348, 1953–1966. doi: 10.1056/NEJMoa030781

Kuypers, J., Wright, N., Ferrenberg, J., Huang, M. L., Cent, A., Corey, L., et al. (2006). Comparison of real-time PCR assays with fluorescent-antibody assays for diagnosis of respiratory virus infections in children. *J. Clin. Microbiol.* 44, 2382–2388. doi: 10.1128/jcm.00216-06

Landry, M. L., and Ferguson, D. (2000). SimulFluor respiratory screen for rapid detection of multiple respiratory viruses in clinical specimens by immunofluorescence staining. *J. Clin. Microbiol.* 38, 708–711.

LaSala, P. R., Bufton, K. K., Ismail, N., and Smith, M. B. (2007). Prospective comparison of R-mix^{TM} shell vial system with direct antigen tests and conventional cell culture for respiratory virus detection. *J. Clin. Virol.* 38, 210–216. doi: 10.1016/j.jcv.2006.12.015

Leland, D. S., and Ginocchio, C. C. (2007). Role of cell culture for virus detection in the age of technology. *Clin. Microbiol. Rev.* 20, 49–78. doi: 10.1128/cmr.00002-06

Lin, B., Vora, G. J., Thach, D., Walter, E., Metzgar, D., Tibbetts, C., et al. (2004). Use of oligonucleotide microarrays for rapid detection and serotyping of acute respiratory disease-associated adenoviruses. *J. Clin. Microbiol.* 42, 3232–3239. doi: 10.1128/jcm.42.7.3232-3239.2004

Ling, L., Kaplan, S. E., Lopez, J. C., Stiles, J., Lu, X., and Tang, Y. W. (2018). Parallel validation of three molecular devices for simultaneous detection and identification of influenza A and B and respiratory syncytial viruses. *J. Clin. Microbiol.* 56:e01691-17. doi: 10.1128/jcm.01691-17

Loeffelholz, M., and Chonmaitree, T. (2010). Advances in diagnosis of respiratory virus infections. *Int. J. Microbiol.* 2010:126049. doi: 10.1155/2010/126049

Mahony, J. B. (2008). Detection of respiratory viruses by molecular methods. *Clin. Microbiol. Rev.* 21, 716–747. doi: 10.1128/cmr.00037-07

Mahony, J. B., Petrich, A., and Smieja, M. (2011). Molecular diagnosis of respiratory virus infections. *Crit. Rev. Clin. Lab. Sci.* 48, 217–249. doi: 10.3109/10408363.2011.640976

McMullen, P., Boonlayangoor, S., Charnot-Katsikas, A., Beavis, K. G., and Tesic, V. (2017). The performance of Luminex ARIES® Flu A/B & RSV and Cepheid Xpert® Flu/RSV XC for the detection of influenza A, influenza B, and respiratory syncytial virus in prospective patient samples. *J. Clin. Virol.* 95, 84–85. doi: 10.1016/j.jcv.2017.08.018

Nie, S., Roth, R. B., Stiles, J., Mikhlina, A., Lu, X., Tang, Y. W., et al. (2014). Evaluation of Alere I influenza A&B for rapid detection of influenza viruses A and B. *J. Clin. Microbiol.* 52, 3339–3344. doi: 10.1128/jcm.01132-14

Ohm-Smith, M. J., Nassos, P. S., and Haller, B. L. (2004). Evaluation of the Binax NOW, BD Directigen, and BD Directigen EZ assays for detection of respiratory syncytial virus. *J. Clin. Microbiol.* 42, 2996–2999. doi: 10.1128/jcm.42.7.2996-2999.2004

Olsen, M. A., Shuck, K. M., Sambol, A. R., Flor, S. M., O'Brien, J., and Cabrera, B. J. (1993). Isolation of seven respiratory viruses in shell vials: a practical and highly sensitive method. *J. Clin. Microbiol.* 31, 422–425.

Peters, R. M., Schnee, S. V., Tabatabai, J., Schnitzler, P., and Pfeil, J. (2017). Evaluation of Alere I RSV for rapid detection of respiratory syncytial virus in children hospitalized with acute respiratory tract infection. *J. Clin. Microbiol.* 55, 1032–1036. doi: 10.1128/jcm.02433-16

Popowitch, E. B., and Miller, M. B. (2015). Performance characteristics of Xpert Flu/RSV XC assay. *J. Clin. Microbiol.* 53, 2720–2721. doi: 10.1128/jcm.00972-15

Popowitch, E. B., O'Neill, S. S., and Miller, M. B. (2013). Comparison of the Biofire FilmArray RP, Genmark eSensor RVP, Luminex xTAG RVPv1, and Luminex xTAG RVP fast multiplex assays for detection of respiratory viruses. *J. Clin. Microbiol.* 51, 1528–1533. doi: 10.1128/jcm.03368-12

Poritz, M. A., Blaschke, A. J., Byington, C. L., Meyers, L., Nilsson, K., Jones, D. E., et al. (2011). FilmArray, an automated nested multiplex PCR system for multi-pathogen detection: development and application to respiratory tract infection. *PLoS One* 6:e26047. doi: 10.1371/journal.pone.0026047

Ramanan, P., Bryson, A. L., Binnicker, M. J., Pritt, B. S., and Patel, R. (2018). Syndromic panel-based testing in clinical microbiology. *Clin. Microbiol. Rev.* 31:e00024-17. doi: 10.1128/cmr.00024-17

Reijans, M., Dingemans, G., Klaassen, C. H., Meis, J. F., Keijdener, J., Mulders, B., et al. (2008). RespiFinder: a new multiparameter test to differentially identify fifteen respiratory viruses. *J. Clin. Microbiol.* 46, 1232–1240. doi: 10.1128/jcm.02294-07

Rocholl, C., Gerber, K., Daly, J., Pavia, A. T., and Byington, C. L. (2004). Adenoviral infections in children: the impact of rapid diagnosis. *Pediatrics* 113(1 Pt 1), e51–e56.

Rogers, B. B., Shankar, P., Jerris, R. C., Kotzbauer, D., Anderson, E. J., Watson, J. R., et al. (2015). Impact of a rapid respiratory panel test on patient outcomes. *Arch. Pathol. Lab. Med.* 139, 636–641. doi: 10.5858/arpa.2014-0257-OA

Roingeard, P. (2008). Viral detection by electron microscopy: past, present and future. *Biol. Cell* 100, 491–501. doi: 10.1042/bc20070173

Sails, A. D., Eltringham, G., Valappil, M., Waugh, S., and Saunders, D. (2017). Comparison of the Luminex NxTAG respiratory pathogen panel and a multiplex in-house real-time PCR panel for the detection of respiratory viruses in symptomatic patients. *J. Med. Microbiol.* doi: 10.1099/jmm.0.000562 [Epub ahead of print].

Sawatwong, P., Chittaganpitch, M., Hall, H., Peruski, L. F., Xu, X., Baggett, H. C., et al. (2012). Serology as an adjunct to polymerase chain reaction assays for surveillance of acute respiratory virus infections. *Clin. Infect. Dis.* 54, 445–446. doi: 10.1093/cid/cir710

Schreckenberger, P. C., and McAdam, A. J. (2015). Point-counterpoint: large multiplex PCR panels should be first-line tests for detection of respiratory and intestinal pathogens. *J. Clin. Microbiol.* 53, 3110–3115. doi: 10.1128/jcm.00382-15

Selvaraju, S. B., Bambach, A. V., Leber, A. L., Patru, M.-M., Patel, A., and Menegus, M. A. (2014). Comparison of the Simplexa^{TM} Flu A/B & RSV kit (nucleic acid extraction–dependent assay) and the Prodesse ProFlu + ^{TM} assay for detecting influenza and respiratory syncytial viruses. *Diagn. Microbiol. Infect. Dis.* 80, 50–52. doi: 10.1016/j.diagmicrobio.2013.11.015

Shafik, C. F., Mohareb, E. W., and Youssef, F. G. (2011). Comparison of direct fluorescence assay and real-time rt-PCR as diagnostics for respiratory syncytial virus in young children. *J. Trop. Med.* 2011:781919. doi: 10.1155/2011/781919

Slinger, R., Milk, R., Gaboury, I., and Diaz-Mitoma, F. (2004). Evaluation of the QuickLab RSV test, a new rapid lateral-flow immunoassay for detection of respiratory syncytial virus antigen. *J. Clin. Microbiol.* 42, 3731–3733. doi: 10.1128/jcm.42.8.3731-3733.2004

Tang, Y. W., Gonsalves, S., Sun, J. Y., Stiles, J., Gilhuley, K. A., Mikhlina, A., et al. (2016). Clinical evaluation of the Luminex NxTAG respiratory pathogen panel. *J. Clin. Microbiol.* 54, 1912–1914. doi: 10.1128/jcm.00482-16

Tenover, F. C. (2011). Developing molecular amplification methods for rapid diagnosis of respiratory tract infections caused by bacterial pathogens. *Clin. Infect. Dis.* 52(Suppl. 4), S338–S345. doi: 10.1093/cid/cir049

Vinh, D. C., Newby, D., Charest, H., and McDonald, J. (2008). Evaluation of a commercial direct fluorescent-antibody assay for human metapneumovirus in respiratory specimens. *J. Clin. Microbiol.* 46, 1840–1841. doi: 10.1128/jcm.01554-07

Weinberg, A., and Walker, M. L. (2005). Evaluation of three immunoassay kits for rapid detection of influenza virus A and B. *Clin. Diagn. Lab. Immunol.* 12, 367–370. doi: 10.1128/cdli.12.3.367-370.2005

Wellinghausen, N., Straube, E., Freidank, H., von Baum, H., Marre, R., and Essig, A. (2006). Low prevalence of Chlamydia pneumoniae in adults with community-acquired pneumonia. *Int. J. Med. Microbiol.* 296, 485–491. doi: 10.1016/j.ijmm.2006.05.003

WHO (2005). *WHO Recommendations on the use of Rapid Testing for Influenza Diagnosis [Online].* Available at: http://www.who.int/influenza/resources/documents/RapidTestInfluenza_WebVersion.pdf [accessed June 24, 2018].

Winn, W. C., and Koneman, E. W. (2006). *Koneman's Color Atlas and Textbook of Diagnostic Microbiology.* Philadelphia, PA: Lippincott Williams & Wilkins.

Woodhead, M., Blasi, F., Ewig, S., Huchon, G., Ieven, M., Ortqvist, A., et al. (2005). Guidelines for the management of adult lower respiratory tract infections. *Eur. Respir. J.* 26, 1138–1180. doi: 10.1183/09031936.05.00055705

Zhang, Y., Hung, T., Song, J., and He, J. (2013). Electron microscopy: essentials for viral structure, morphogenesis and rapid diagnosis. *Sci. China Life Sci.* 56, 421–430. doi: 10.1007/s11427-013-4476-2

Zhang, Y., Sakthivel, S. K., Bramley, A., Jain, S., Haynes, A., Chappell, J. D., et al. (2017). Serology enhances molecular diagnosis of respiratory virus infections other than influenza in children and adults hospitalized with community-acquired pneumonia. *J. Clin. Microbiol.* 55, 79–89. doi: 10.1128/jcm.01701-16

11

The Antihistamine Drugs Carbinoxamine Maleate and Chlorpheniramine Maleate Exhibit Potent Antiviral Activity Against a Broad Spectrum of Influenza Viruses

Wei Xu[1], Shuai Xia[1], Jing Pu[1], Qian Wang[1], Peiyu Li[1], Lu Lu[1] and Shibo Jiang[1,2]**

[1] Shanghai Public Health Clinical Center and School of Basic Medical Sciences, Key Laboratory of Medical Molecular Virology of MOE/MOH, Fudan University, Shanghai, China, [2] Lindsley F. Kimball Research Institute, New York Blood Center, New York, NY, United States

***Correspondence:**
Lu Lu
lul@fudan.edu.cn
Shibo Jiang
shibojiang@fudan.edu.cn

Influenza A viruses (IAV) comprise some of the most common infectious pathogens in humans, and they cause significant mortality and morbidity in immunocompromised people as well as children and the elderly. After screening an FDA-approved drug library containing 1280 compounds by cytopathic effect (CPE) reduction assay using the Cell Counting Kit-8, we found two antihistamines, carbinoxamine maleate (CAM) and S-(+)-chlorpheniramine maleate (SCM) with potent antiviral activity against A/Shanghai/4664T/2013(H7N9) infection with IC_{50} (half-maximal inhibitory concentration) of 3.56 and 11.84 μM, respectively. Further studies showed that CAM and SCM could also inhibit infection by other influenza A viruses, including A/Shanghai/37T/2009(H1N1), A/Puerto Rico/8/1934(H1N1), A/Guizhou/54/1989(H3N2), and one influenza B virus, B/Shanghai/2017(BY). Mice were challenged intranasally with A/H7N9/4664T/2013 (H7N9) virus and intraperitoneally injected with CAM (10 mg/kg per day) or SCM (1 mg/kg per day) for 5 days. CAM or SCM (10 mg/kg per day) were fully protected against challenge with A/Shanghai/4664T/2013(H7N9). The results from mechanistic studies indicate that both could inhibit influenza virus infection by blocking viral entry into the target cell, the early stage of virus life cycle. However, CAM and SCM neither blocked virus attachment, characteristic of HA activity, nor virus release, characteristic of NA activity. Such data suggest that these two compounds may interfere with the endocytosis process. Thus, we have identified two FDA-approved antihistamine drugs, CAM and SCM, which can be repurposed for inhibiting infection by divergent influenza A strains and one influenza B strain with potential to be used for treatment and prevention of influenza virus infection.

Keywords: antihistamine, carbinoxamine, chlorpheniramine, influenza virus, viral entry

INTRODUCTION

Influenza is an acute respiratory illness caused by influenza virus infection, resulting in more than 5 million severe cases and 650,000 deaths worldwide every year[1]. Although most influenza virus infections are self-limiting, they can sometimes be associated with severe, even fatal, disease outcomes, such as pneumonia and congestive heart failure (Rockman et al., 2017). Influenza viruses are classified into types A, B, and C. Influenza A viruses (IAVs) have undergone frequent changes through mutation or reassortment, resulting in the appearance of new strains that can cause an epidemic or pandemic[2]. For example, an outbreak of novel avian IAV influenza A virus (H7N9) infection was reported in China in April of 2013. This has caused at least 1,564 deaths during the 5 major epidemic waves that followed (Qiu et al., 2013; Zhu et al., 2016). In the past few years, several highly pathogenic avian influenza (HPAI) viruses, including H5N8, H5N6 and H10N8, were identified, raising global public health concerns (Chen et al., 2014; Xu et al., 2017; Zhang et al., 2017). This calls for rapid identification of antiviral agents to prevent and treat divergent influenza virus infection.

Currently, two major classes of antiviral drugs are available for the treatment of influenza, including M2 ion channel protein inhibitors (e.g., amantadine and rimantadine) and influenza neuraminidase inhibitors (NAIs, e.g., oseltamivir, zanamivir, and peramivir) (Ong and Hayden, 2007). M2 ion channel protein inhibitors are only active against IAVs, yet 95% of IAV strains are resistant to amantadine (Yen et al., 2005; Salter et al., 2011). Although NAIs like oseltamivir are effective against both influenza A and B viruses (Baranovich et al., 2014), a large variety of influenza virus strains have become resistant to oseltamivir because of its extensive clinical application (Matsuzaki et al., 2010; Pizzorno et al., 2014; Marjuki et al., 2015). Lack of effective treatments for influenza and the continuous emergence of drug resistance highlight the urgency of developing new drugs for treatment of influenza virus infection.

Drug discovery is extremely expensive and time-consuming. It generally takes 10–15 years and billions of dollars to reach clinical trials (DiMasi et al., 2003). Thus, for rapidly spreading and emerging infectious diseases, an alternative approach to identify new antiviral agents lies in the repurposing of existing drugs used in clinics since these FDA-approved drugs have already been proven safe in many previous clinical trials (Chong and Sullivan, 2007).

Using this strategy, some FDA-approved drugs for non-infectious diseases have shown efficacy against infection caused by such emerging viruses as Ebola virus and Zika viruses (Xu et al., 2016). Following the logic of this investigative path, we screened an FDA-approved drug library containing 1,280 compounds and found two antihistamines, carbinoxamine maleate (CAM) and S-(+)-chlorpheniramine maleate (SCM), with potent antiviral activity against A/Shanghai/4664T/2013(H7N9) infection with IC_{50} (half-maximal inhibitory concentration) at low μM level.

CAM (brand names: Palgic, Histex PD, Karbinal ER, Carboxine, Ryvent) and SCM (brand names: Chlor-Trimeton, Allergy Relief, Chlorphen) are H1-receptor blocking agent-based antihistamine drugs approved by the U.S. FDA in 1950s and 1982 for treatment of hay fever, rhinitis, urticaria, and asthma (Halpern et al., 1965; Falagas and Kasiakou, 2005; Bergen et al., 2006; Li et al., 2006; Nation et al., 2016). At present, CAM- and SCM-containing formulations are approved only for adults or children ages 2 or older. In this study, we evaluated their antiviral activity against divergent influenza A and B viruses in vitro and in vivo, specifically IAV H7N9 infection in mice, and investigated their potential mechanism of action.

[1]http://www.who.int/csr/don/26-october-2017-ah7n9-china/en/

[2]http://www.who.int/mediacentre/factsheets/fs211/en/

MATERIALS AND METHODS

Chemical Library and Compounds

The FDA-approved drug library containing 1,280 compounds was obtained from MicroSource Discovery Systems, Inc. (Gaylordsville, CT, United States). Compounds were solubilized in dimethyl sulfoxide (DMSO) at 10 mM and stored in 96-well PCR Tubes at −80°C. Carbinoxamine maleate salt (CAM) and S-(+)-Chlorpheniramine maleate salt (SCM) were purchased from Sigma-Aldrich (St. Louis, MO, United States). Favipiravir (T-705) and Oseltamivir phosphate were purchased from TargetMol Company (Boston, MA, United States).

Cells, Viruses and Plasmids

Madin-Darby canine kidney (MDCK) cells, 293T cells, U87 cells and Huh-7 cells were obtained from ATCC (Manassas, VA, United States). Cells were cultured in DMEM (Thermo Fisher Scientific, Waltham, MA, United States) containing 10% FBS (Biowest, France), penicillin 100 U/ml, and streptomycin 10 μg/ml. Influenza virus strains A/Shanghai/37T/2009(H1N1), A/Puerto Rico/8/1934(H1N1), A/Guizhou/54/1989(H3N2), A/Shanghai/4664T/2013(H7N9), and B/Shanghai/2017(BY) were obtained from the Shanghai Public Health Clinical Center (Shanghai, China). The experiments on H7N9 IAV were conducted in the BSL-3 Laboratory of Fudan University. Live viruses were propagated in MDCK cells. Virus titers were determined by a $TCID_{50}$ endpoint dilution assay. Plasmid pNL4-3.Luc.R-E- was obtained from the NIH AIDS Reagent Program (Germantown, MD, United States).

CCK-8 Assay for Measuring Cytotoxicity of the Compounds Tested

The cytotoxicity of a test compound was determined, as previously described (Furuta et al., 2002; Han et al., 2011) by measuring cell viability in the presence of various compound concentrations. Briefly, 100 μl MDCK cells (0.5×10^5 cells/ml) were dispensed into wells of a 96-well plate and incubated at 37°C/5% CO_2 for 24 h. The test compound at the serial dilution in 100 μL of DMEM without serum was added to the cells. After culture for 72 h, cell viability was measured using the Cell Counting Kit-8 (CCK-8), which was purchased from Dojindo Laboratory (Kumamoto, Japan), and using a spectrophotometer (Ultra 384, Tecan, NC, United States). The percent cytotoxicity (=100% − % cell viability) was calculated, and CC_{50} (half-maximal cytotoxic concentration) of the test compound was determined using the Calcusyn software program (Biosoft, Ferguson, MO, United States) (Chou and Talalay, 1984).

Cytopathic Effect (CPE) Reduction Assay for Measuring Inhibitory Activity of a Compound on Cell Death Caused by Influenza Virus Infection

The inhibitory activity of a test compound against influenza virus infection-induced death of MDCK cells was measured by CPE reduction assay using CCK-8 as previously described (Choi et al., 2016; Wang et al., 2017; Jin et al., 2018; Liu et al., 2018). PBS containing no inhibitor and the anti-influenza virus agent, Favipiravir (T-705), were included as the negative and positive controls, respectively. Briefly, MDCK cells were plated in wells of a 96-well plate at a density of 10^4 cells/well. After incubation at 37°C for 12 h, a mixture of a test compound (50 μL) at graded concentration in serum-free DMEM containing 2 μg/mL tosyl phenylalanyl chloromethyl ketone (TPCK)-Trypsin and 50 μL of a influenza virus (100 $TCID_{50}$) was added to the monolayer cells, followed by an incubation at 37°C for 8 h. The supernatants were replaced with DMEM medium containing 2 μg/mL TPCK-Trypsin. After culture at 37°C for 72 h, the inhibitory activity of the compound on cytopathic effect induced by viral infection was measured using CCK-8 as described above. The IC_{50} values were calculated with the Calcusyn Program (Biosoft).

A time-of-addition assay was performed as previously described (Maddry et al., 2011). Briefly, the A/Shanghai/37T/2009(H1N1) at an MOI of 0.1 was added to the monolayer MDCK cells, followed by addition of a test compound at indicated concentration of 0, 0.5, 1, 2, 4, and 12 h post-infection (p.i.). The inhibitory activity of the compound on H1N1 IAV infection was detected by CPE reduction assay using CCK-8 as described above.

Quantitative Reverse Transcription PCR (RT-qPCR) Assay for Measuring the Inhibitory Activity of a Test Compound on Expression of mRNA of Influenza a HA Gene

MDCK cells were seeded onto 12-well plates (2 × 10^5/well) and cultured overnight. The cells were infected with approximately 100 pfu/ml of the influenza A/PR/8/34 (H1N1) virus for 1h in the absence or presence of CAM and SCM at the indicated concentration and then the medium was replaced with fresh DMEM containing 1.5 μg/ml TPCK-Trypsin. After incubation at 37°C for 12 h, total RNA was isolated from cells using Trizol Reagent (TransGen, China). The First-stranded cDNA was reverse by TransScript First-Strand cDNA Synthesis SuperMix (TransGen, China) according to the instructions. The qPCR assay was performed by using the TransStart Top Green qPCR SuperMix. The primer sequences used for the influenza A HA genes are 5′-TTCCCAAGATCCATCCGGCAA-3′ (forward) and 5′-CCTGCTCGAAGACAGCCACAACG-3′ (reverse); NP genes are 5′-GACCAGGAGTGGAGGAAACA-3′ (forward) and 5′-CGGCCATAATGGTCACTCTT-3′ (reverse); and the sequences for the GAPDH gene are 5′-AGGGCAATGCCAGC CCCAGCG-3′ (forward) and; 5′-AGGCGTCGGAGGG CCCCCTC-3′ (reverse).

Indirect Immunofluorescence Assay for Measuring the Inhibitory Activity of a Test Compound on Expression of Influenza Virus Nucleoprotein (NP) in Virus-Infected Cells

MDCK cells (1 × 10^4 cells/well) were seeded onto 96-well plates at 37°C under 5% CO_2 for 8 h. The cells were washed twice with phosphate-buffered saline (PBS) and infected with 100 $TCID_{50}$ of the influenza A/PR/8/34 (H1N1) virus in the presence or absence of CAM and SCM at the indicated concentration for 1 h. The supernatant was aspirated and covered with culture medium containing 1.5 μg/ml TPCK-Trypsin. After incubation at 37°C for 12 h, the cells were fixed with 4% paraformaldehyde for 10 min, then permeabilized with 0.1% Triton™ X-100 for 10 min, blocked with 1% BSA for 1 h and labeled with a primary antibody against influenza virus A nucleoprotein (NP) (1:250 dilution, Santa Cruz, CA, United States) for 3 h. Goat anti-Mouse IgG (H + L) Highly Cross-Adsorbed Secondary Antibody Alexa Fluor® 488 conjugate (diluted 1:250) was added at 37°C for 1 h. After further washing, the nuclei were stained with DAPI for 10 min. The cells were observed and photographed by using a fluorescence microscope.

Plaque Reduction Assay for Measuring the Inhibitory Activity of a Test Compound on Plaque Formation Induced by Influenza Virus Infection

Briefly, MDCK cells were plated onto 12-well culture plates (1 × 10^6 cells/well) and cultured overnight. MDCK cells were washed twice with PBS and incubated with approximately 100 pfu/ml of the influenza A/PR/8/34 (H1N1) virus in the presence or absence of CAM and SCM at the indicated concentration for 1 h. After incubation at 37°C for 1 h, the supernatant was aspirated. The cells were washed once with PBS and were covered with DMEM containing 1% low melting agarose and 1.5 μg/ml TPCK-trypsin. After 2–3 days post-infection, the cell monolayer was fixed with 4% formalin and stained with

1% crystal violet for 1 h and the plaque forming units were counted.

Luminescence Assay for Detecting Inhibitory Activity of a Test Compound on Entry of the Pseudotyped H7N9 IAV, Nipah Virus and VSV Into Their Target Cells

Pseudotyped H7N9 IAV, Nipah virus, and vesicular stomatitis virus (VSV) were constructed, and their infectivity was evaluated as previously described (Qiu et al., 2013). For the pseudotyped H7N9 influenza virus 293T cells (5×10^5 cells/well) were seeded to six-well plate the day before transfection, and co-transfected with 2.5 μg of pcDNA3.1-HA and NA of A/Shanghai/4664T/2013(H7N9), respectively, and 10 μg of lentivirus vector pNL4-3-Luc R-E- by using VigoFect reagents (Vigorous Biotechnology, Beijing, China). For the pseudotyped Nipah virus or VSV, 293T cells were co-transfected with Nipah G protein or VSV G protein, respectively, and plasmid encoding Env-defective, lentivirus vector pNL4-3-Luc R-E- by using VigoFect reagents. After incubation at 37°C for 6 h, cells were washed with PBS 3 times and cultured in DMEM containing 10% FBS. After culture at 37°C/5% CO_2 for 2 days, supernatants containing the pseudoviruses were collected and filtered to remove cells and cell debris. The pseudoviruses were concentrated by ultracentrifugation at 25,000 rpm at 4°C for 3 h, and then their titers were determined using the Luciferase Assay System (Promega, Madison, WI, United States), following the manufacturer's instructions. Aliquots of the pseudoviruses were stored at −80°C.

The inhibitory activity of a test compound on entry of H7N9, Nipah or VSV pseudovirus into their target cells was determined as described previously (Xia et al., 2018). Briefly, MDCK cells for H7N9 pseudovirus entry, Huh-7 cells for Nipah pseudovirus entry, and U87 cells for VSV pseudovirus entry were plated in wells of a 96-well plate at a density of 10^4 cells each well, respectively. After incubation at 37°C for 12 h, a mixture of a test compound (50 μL) at a serial twofold dilution in serum-free DMEM and 50 μL of the corresponding pseudovirus was added to the corresponding cells. MDCK, Huh7 and U87 cells were infected by these control viruses, as described above, followed by incubation at 37°C for 12 h. The culture supernatants were replaced with free DMEM containing 2% FBS. After culture at 37°C for 48 h, the luciferase activity was measured using the Luciferase Assay System (Promega) with a microplate luminometer (Ultra 384, Tecan, NC, USA). The inhibitory activity of a test compound on entry of HIV-1 IIIB infection were determined as described previously (Su et al., 2017a,b). Series dilution of CAM and SCM were incubated with 50 μL 100 $TCID_{50}$ of the HIV-1 at 37°C for 1 h and then 10^4 MT-2 cells per well were added into the 96 well plate. After 12 h culture, the medium was replaced with fresh RPMI 1640 medium containing 10% FBS. After culture at 37°C for 4 days, the supernatant was mixed with 50 μL of 5% Triton X-100. The p24 antigen was detected by ELISA. The IC_{50} values were calculated with the Calcusyn Program (Biosoft).

Neuraminidase (NA) Inhibition Assay

Neuraminidase inhibition assay was performed to investigate the influence of a test compound on the release of newly produced viral particles, as described previously (Shen et al., 2018). Briefly, 15 μL of A/Puerto Rico/8/1934(H1N1) virus solution were mixed with 5 μL of a test compound at graded concentrations in wells of a 96-well black plate, followed by incubation at 37°C for 30 min. Then, 30 μL of 20 μM MU-NANA 2′-(4-Methylumbelliferyl)-alpha-D-*N*-acetylneuraminic acid sodium salt hydrate (Sigma-Aldrich, United States), as the substrate dissolved in the MES (2-(*N*-Morpholino) ethanesulfonic acid buffer (32.5 mM MES and 4 mM $CaCl_2$, pH 6.5), were added to each well, followed by incubation at 37°C for 1 h in the dark. Subsequently, 50 μL of 14 mM NaOH were added to terminate the enzymatic reaction. The fluorescence intensity of the product 4-methylumbelliferone was recorded using a microplate reader with excitation and emission wavelengths of 340 and 440 nm, respectively. The IC_{50} values were calculated with the Calcusyn Program (Biosoft).

Haemagglutination Inhibition (HI) Assay

The HI assay was performed to measure the inhibitory activity of a test compound on attachment of an influenza virus to red blood cells (RBC) through the interaction between HA on virus and receptor on RBC, as described previously (Shen et al., 2018). A/Shanghai/37T 2009(H1N1) virus or H7N9 pseudovirus at the

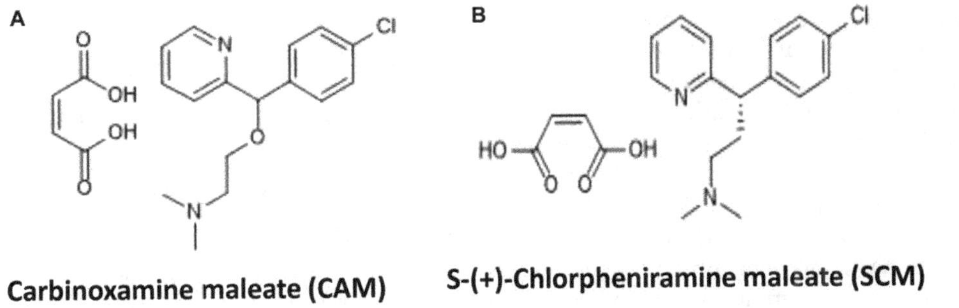

FIGURE 1 | (A,B) Chemical structures of carbinoxamine and S-(+)-Chlorpheniramine maleate. The chemical structure of compounds were download from ChemACX.Com and edited by ChemDraw Professional 16.0 software.

TABLE 1 | Anti-influenza virus activity of CAM and SCM.

		Compound	
		CAM	SCM
	CC50 (μM)	297.30 ± 11.11	285.30 ± 10.89
Influenza A [A/Puerto Rico/8/1934(H1N1)]	IC50 (μM)	4.53 ± 1.51	8.41 ± 2.18
	SI	65.73	33.92
Influenza A [A/Guizhou/54/1989(H3N2)]	IC50 (μM)	8.83 ± 2.94	13.70 ± 1.74
	SI	33.67	20.82
Influenza A [A/Shanghai/37T/2009(H1N1)]	IC50 (μM)	4.24 ± 0.39	24.74 ± 2.57
	SI	70.11	11.53
Influenza B [B/Shanghai/2017(BY)]	IC50 (μM)	15.54 ± 6.40	18.33 ± 2.33
	SI	19.13	15.56
Influenza A [A/H7N9/4664T/2013 (H7N9)]	IC50 (μM)	3.56 ± 1.09	11.84 ± 2.64
	SI	83.51	24.09

CC_{50}, half-maximal cytotoxic concentration; IC_{50}, half-maximal inhibitory concentration; SI, selectivity index (=CC_{50}/IC_{50}).

concentration of 4 HA units were prepared. Compounds with twofold serial dilution with PBS were mixed with equal volume of influenza virus solution (4 HAU per 25 μL). After incubation at room temperature for 1 h, 50 μL of 1% chicken RBC in PBS were added to the mixture. HI was observed and recorded after 1h at room temperature.

Animal Experiment for Evaluating the *in vivo* Inhibitory Activity of a Test Compound on Influenza Virus in Mice

The animal experimental procedure was carried out according to ethical guidelines and approval by Shanghai Public Health Clinical Center Animal Welfare and Ethics Committee (2017-A046-01). The animal studies with infectious H7N9 IAV were conducted in a Biosafety Level 3 facility of Fudan University with Institutional Biosafety Committee approval.

Female C57BL/6 mice (4–8 weeks old, specific-pathogen-free) purchased from Shanghai Lingchang BioTech co., Ltd. (Shanghai, China) and randomly divided into 7 groups ($n = 12$): mock-infection group, PBS group, CAM high dose group (10 mg/kg/day), CAM low dose group (1 mg/kg/day), SCM high dose group (10 mg/kg/day), SCM low dose group (1 mg/kg/day) and OSE group (1 mg/kg/day). Except for mice in the mock-infection control group that received 20 μL DMEM and 20 μL PBS, mice in the treatment groups were anesthetized by intraperitoneal injection of pelltobarbitalum natricum (He et al., 2016; Yamayoshi et al., 2017) and challenged intranasally with A/H7N9/4664T/2013 (H7N9) (3.1×10^7 $TCID_{50}$ in 20 μL DMEM), following by i.p. application of 20 μL PBS (for PBS control group) or a compound in 20 μL PBS (for each compound-treatment group). On the 6th day post infection, 3 mice in each group were euthanized with CO_2 inhalation and their left lungs were removed. The lungs were then immersed in TRIzol™ reagent and frozen at −80°C. Total RNA was isolated from lung homogenates. The levels of viral RNA were determined by two-step RT-qPCR kit (TransGen, China). The right lungs were placed in 4% paraformaldehyde at 4°C for hematoxylin-eosin (H&E) staining and histological analysis. The body weight of the mice was monitored daily for 14 days after infection. Survival curves were generated according to the Kaplan–Meier method and the differences was calculated by Log-rank (Mantel-Cox) Test (GraphPad Prism 6.0).

Histopathological Analysis

The formalin-fixed paraffin-embedded tissues were cut into 4 μm sections and stained with hematoxylin and eosin (H&E). Observation and description were made after scanning in the panoramic scanner (3D HISTECH Pannoramic MIDI, Hungary). Blinded sections were examined by two independent pathologists and scored for the following indicative parameters: (A) alveolar congestion, (B) hemorrhage, (C) Neutrophilic infiltration, (D) hyaline membrane formation, (E) thickness of the alveolar wall (0 = non-observed damage, 1 = mild damage, 2 = moderate damage, 3 = severe damage, and 4 = maximal damage). Ten non-overlapping microscopic images were obtained from each tissue sample with 40x objective for observation.

Immunohistochemical Assay

Immunohistochemical staining of viral NP was performed. The right lung of each mouse was fixed in 10% buffered formalin solution for 7 days and embedded in paraffin. The embedded tissue was cut into 4 μm sections and stained with a primary mouse polyclonal antibody against NP of influenza A virus (Santa Cruz Biotechnology, Santa Cruz, CA, United States) at 1:1000 and a secondary HRP-labeled goat anti-mouse IgG antibody (Thermo Fisher Scientific) at 1:200. The integrated optical density (IOD) value was measured by Image-Pro Plus 6.0 software (Media Cybernetics, Inc., Rockville, MD, United States). The images were captured under an optical microscope (×200). The same brown and yellow color was selected as the unified standard to judge the positivity of all images. The IOD values in three randomly selected views were determined. The mean IOD value was considered as the relative expression levels of viral NP.

RESULTS

CAM and SCM Exhibited Potent and Broad Antiviral Activity Against Influenza Virus Infection in MDCK Cells, as well as Low Cytotoxicity

To identify chemical compounds with broad antiviral activity against divergent influenza viruses, we previously screened a FDA-approved drug library that includes 1280 FDA-approved drugs (Gaylordsville, CT, United States) against H7N9 influenza virus infection by CPE reduction assay using CCK-8 for

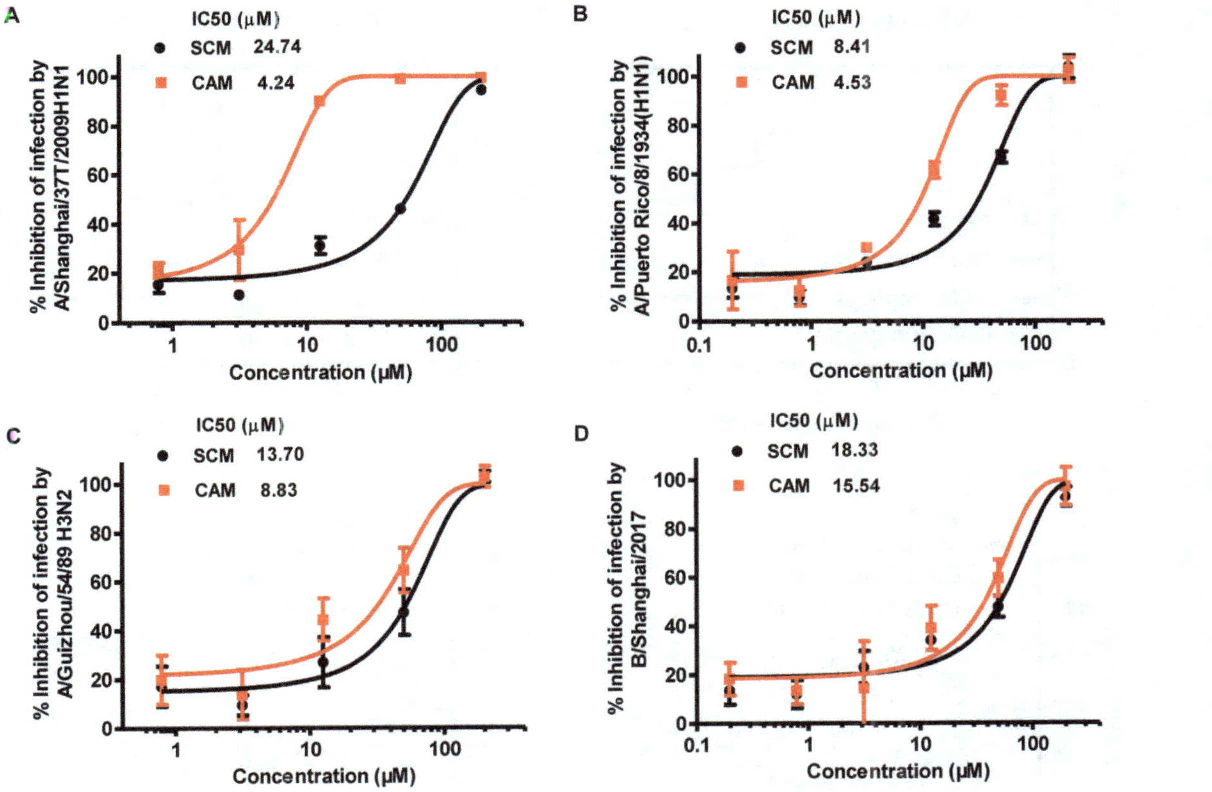

FIGURE 2 | Inhibition of CAM and SCM on influenza virus infection in vitro. The IC_{50} values of CAM and SCM were measured for their inhibition of infection by: **(A)** A/Shanghai/37T/2009(H1N1); **(B)** A/Puerto Rico/8/1934(H1N1); **(C)**: A/Guizhou/54/1989(H3N2); **(D)** B/Shanghai/2017(BY) in MDCK cells at 100 $TCID_{50}$ in the presence of increasing concentrations of the compounds. The inhibitory activity of CAM and SCM on cytopathic effect (CPE) caused by influenza virus infection was determined at 72 h post infection by CPE reduction assay using CCK-8. Data are expressed as mean ± standard error (SE) of triplicate assays, and the experiment was repeated at least twice.

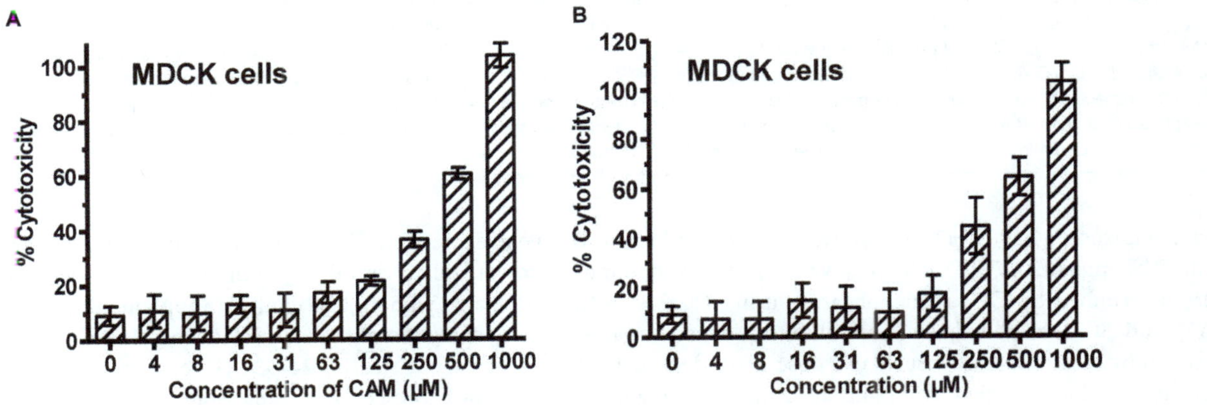

FIGURE 3 | Cytotoxicity of CAM **(A)** and SCM **(B)** to MDCK cells. MDCK cells were incubated with the test compounds at graded concentration for 72 h before the cell viability was measured by CCK-8 assay. The samples were tested in triplicate. CC_{50} was calculated as described in the "Materials and Methods." Data are expressed as mean ± standard error (SE) of triplicate assays, and the experiment was repeated at least twice.

identifying compounds with inhibitory activity against influenza virus infection-induced cell death at the concentrations of the compounds below their CC_{50}. We found two antihistamines, carbinoxamine maleate (CAM) and S-(+)-chlorpheniramine maleate (SCM) (**Figure 1**), with potent antiviral activity against infection of A/Shanghai/4664T/2013(H7N9) with IC_{50} of 3.56 and 11.84 μM, respectively (**Table 1**). We then further evaluated their inhibitory activity against three different influenza A virus subtypes isolated from humans, including A/Shanghai/37T/2009(H1N1), A/Puerto Rico/8/1934(H1N1),

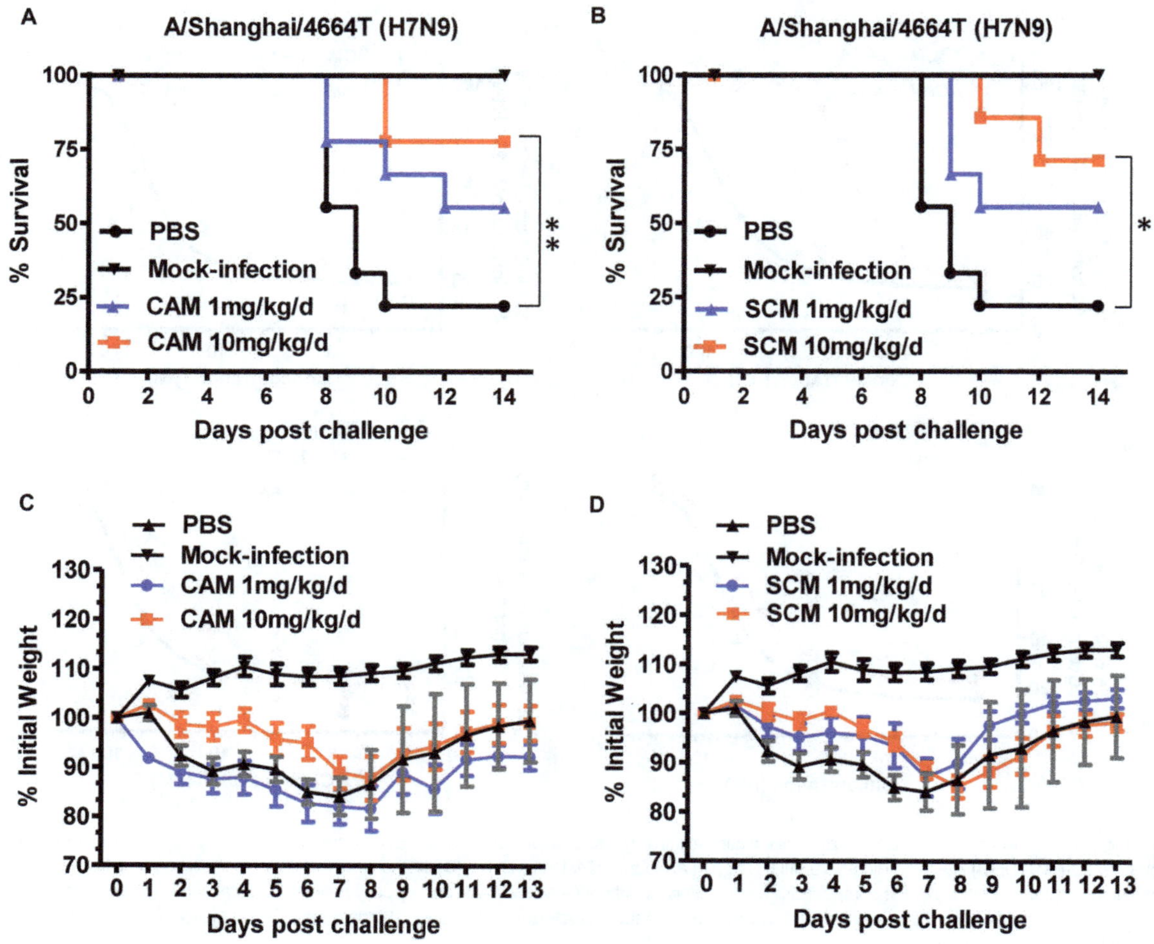

FIGURE 4 | Evaluation of CAM and SCM for efficacy against a highly pathogenic influenza A/4664T/2013 (H7N9) virus infection in C57BL/6 mice. **(A)** Survival of H7N9 infected mice treated with CAM (1 mg/kg/day or 10 mg/kg/day); **(B)** Survival of H7N9 infected mice treated with SCM (1 mg/kg/day or 10 mg/kg/day); Changes in body weight of virus-infected mice treated with CAM **(C)** or SCM **(D)**. C57BL/6 mice anesthetized with pelltobarbitalum natricum (10 mg/ml) were infected with 3.1×10^7 $TCID_{50}$ of the influenza A virus strain (A/4664T/2013 H7N9). CAM and SCM (1 mg/kg/day or 10 mg/kg/day) was intraperitoneally administered to C57BL/6 mice 1 h post infection once daily for 5 days. PBS and oseltamivir phosphate (OSE, 1 mg/kg/day) were used as a negative and positive controls, respectively. Survival curves were generated according to the Kaplan–Meier method and the differences were analyzed by Log-rank (Mantel-Cox) Test (GraphPad Prism 6.0). The data were obtained from a single experiment. *Indicates a statistically significant difference ($P < 0.05$) and **represents significant difference at $P < 0.01$ in survival rate between treated group and the PBS group.

and A/Guizhou/54/1989(H3N2), as well as one influenza B virus, B/Shanghai/2017(BY). The IC_{50} values of the compounds were determined by CPE reduction assay using CCK-8. Both CAM and SCM exhibited effective inhibitory activity against infection by these influenza viruses in a dose-dependent manner with IC_{50} values ranging from 4.2 to 24.7 μM (**Figure 2** and **Table 1**). Favipiravir (T-705) exhibited potent antiviral activity against A/Guizhou/54/89(H3N2) infection with IC_{50} of 0.746 μM (**Supplementary Figure S4**). We then performed a plaque reduction assay and found that CAM and SCM were effective in reducing plaque formation caused by A/Shanghai/37T/2009(H1N1) and A/Guizhou/54/1989(H3N2) infection with IC_{50} in a range of 2.7–14.5 μM (**Supplementary Table S4**).

The *in vitro* antiviral efficacy of CAM and SCM was also evaluated by using RT-qPCR assay for assessing the levels of viral gene expression. The results showed that CAM and SCM could downregulate viral RNA synthesis in a dose-dependent manner, compared with the PBS control (**Supplementary Figures S1A,B**). The expression of the viral NP in the MDCK cells infected with the influenza A/PR/8/341934 (H1N1) was analyzed by indirect immunofluorescence staining assay. As shown in **Supplementary Figure S1C**, addition of CAM and SCM at 10 μM resulted in marked reduction in the number of fluorescent-staining cells, compared to the PBS control. All these results indicate that CAM and SCM possess relatively broad-spectrum antiviral activities against divergent influenza A strains and one influenza B strain.

We then determined the cytotoxicity of these compounds to MDCK cells using CCK-8 assay and found that both CAM and SCM exhibited low cytotoxicity to MDCK cells with CC_{50} values of 297 ± 11 and 285 ± 11 μM, respectively

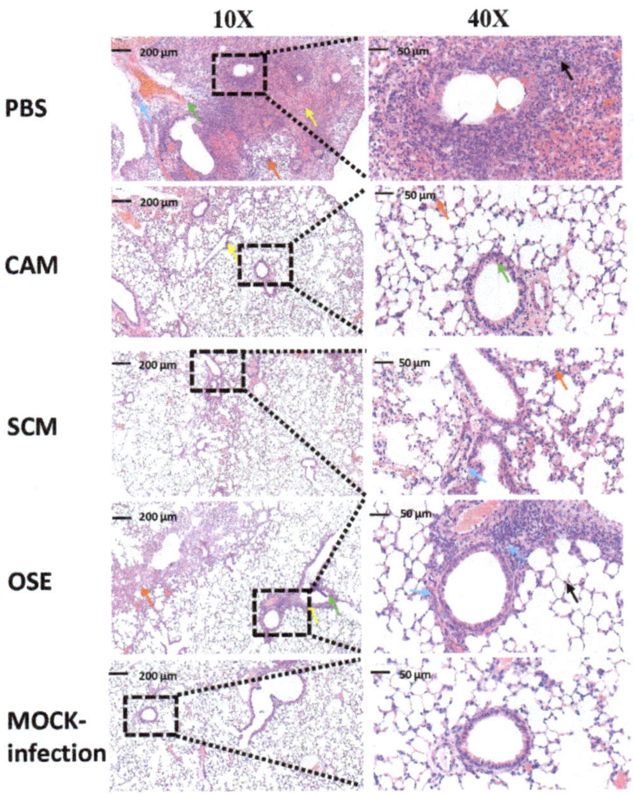

FIGURE 5 | CAM and SCM effectively attenuated the lung pathology of A/4664T/2013 (H7N9) influenza virus-infected mice. The representative histopathologic changes of the lung tissues showed that less inflammatory infiltrate was observed in CAM- and SCM-treated groups compared with the PBS group. Lungs were fixed in 10% neutral-buffered formalin for 7 days and were cut into 4-µm-thick sections and stained with hem-atoxylin-eosin (H&E) staining. The digital images of whole-lung sections were captured by using a panoramic scanner slide scanner (3D HISTECH Pannoramic MIDI, Hungary). All micrographs were taken at ×10 or ×40 magnification. The inflammatory situations are symbolized by the arrow color. Black arrows represented neutrophils. Red arrows showed inflammatory cell infiltration and blue arrow showed more inflammatory cell infiltration. Thickening of alveolar wall (yellow arrow) and epithelial cell shedding (green arrow) were observed in the PBS group.

(**Figure 3** and **Table 1**). Accordingly, the selectivity index ($SI = CC_{50}/IC_{50}$) of CAM and SCM were in the range of 12 – 84 (**Table 1**). These data suggest that both CAM and SCM have effective *in vitro* anti-influenza virus activity with low cytotoxicity.

CAM and SCM Protect Against H7N9 Influenza Virus Infection in Mice

To evaluate the *in vivo* efficacy of CAM and SCM for protection against H7N9 IAV infection, C57BL/6 mice were inoculated with 3.1×10^7 $TCID_{50}$ A/Shanghai/4664T/2013(H7N9) and intraperitoneally injected with CAM and SCM at both high dose (10 mg/kg/day) and low dose (1 mg/kg/day), respectively, daily for 5 days beginning 1 h after infection. Mice in the positive and negative control groups were treated with OSE, a neuraminidase inhibitor (Tamiflu, 1 mg/kg/day), or PBS, respectively. As shown in **Figure 4**, the mice intraperitoneally injected with CAM and SCM were protected from challenge with H7N9 IAV in a dose-dependent manner. The survival rates of the mice treated with CAM or SCM at high dose (10 mg/kg/day) for 5 days were 77.7 and 71.4%, respectively, while those of mice treated with OSE or PBS were 66.6 and 22.2%, respectively.

We then examined the lung tissues of H7N9- or mock-infected mice treated or untreated with CAM or SCM for the virus gene (mRNA for HA) expression by using a two-step RT-qPCR kit. The results showed that both CAM and SCM could significantly downregulate the expression of viral gene in the mouse lung tissues (**Supplementary Figure S2**). The viral NP mRNA levels in the H7N9-infected mice treated with OSE, high dose of CAM, high and low doses of SCM, and the mock-infected mice were significantly lower than that in the H7N9-infected mice without treatment (PBS control) (**Supplementary Figure S2**). These results suggest that like OSE, both CAM and SCM are highly effective in inhibiting H7N9 replication in the mouse lung tissues.

Subsequently, we examined the lung tissues of H7N9- or mock-infected mice treated or untreated with CAM or SCM for the histopathological changes. As shown in **Figure 5**, no signs of pathological changes were observed in the mock-infected (i.e., normal) mice. In the PBS treatment group, the structure of focal alveoli was destroyed, and alveolar walls were blurred. A large number of inflammatory cell infiltrates, including neutrophils (black arrows) and macrophages (red arrows), were seen. Meanwhile, exudation of protein-rich edema fluid (yellow arrows) was found in some alveolar spaces and bronchial lumens, and severe inflammatory cell infiltration (green arrow) was observed around the blood vessels. In the CAM treatment group, some inflammatory cell infiltrates (red arrows) were seen in the alveolar wall and around the blood vessels (yellow arrows). Bronchial epithelial cells were tightly arranged with clear boundaries. Thus, CAM treatment could effectively attenuate histopathological appearance and mitigate inflammatory responses. The histopathological changes of the lung tissues in mice treated with OSE were very similar to those in mice treated with CAM and SCM, in which only a few inflammatory cell infiltrates (blue arrows) were visible around the bronchi and blood vessels, and some loose cytoplasmic ribosomes in local bronchial epithelial cells were seen (yellow arrows). A qualitative histological assessment of the lung tissues was performed by two independent pathologists in a blinded manner. The mean cumulative histological scores in the CAM-, SCM-, OSE-treatment groups and the mock-infection group were significantly lower than that in PBS control group (**Supplementary Table S1**). The ratio of the alveolar/parenchymal area in the CAM-, SCM-, OSE-treatment groups and the mock-infection group were also remarkably lower than that in PBS control group (**Supplementary Table S2**). We also performed an immunohistochemical staining assay to quantitatively evaluate the expression of the viral NP in the lung tissues of mice infected with H7N9 influenza virus.

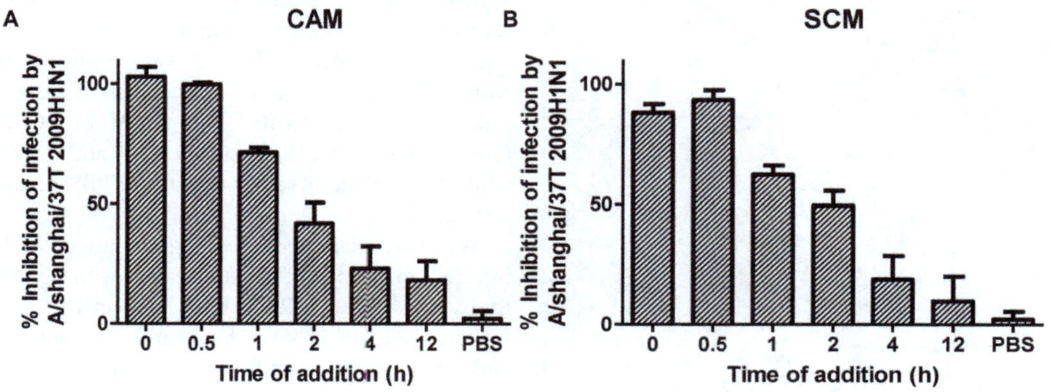

FIGURE 6 | (A,B) Time of addition assay for analysis of mechanism of CAM and SCM against influenza A/shanghai/37T (2009H1N1) infection. MDCK cells cultured in DMEM supplemented with 10% FBS (Biowest, France), penicillin (100 U/ml), and streptomycin (10 μg/ml) at 37°C/5% CO_2 were infected with influenza A/shanghai/37T (2009H1N1) at 0.1 MOI in DMEM containing 2 μg/mL TPCK-Trypsin. CAM and SCM diluted in DMEM to give a final concentration of 20 μM were added to mixture of virus and cells at 0, 0.5, 1, 2, 4, and 12 h post infection. Inhibition activity of CAM and SCM was measured by CPE reduction assay using CCK-8, according to the manufacturer's instruction. The data were presented as means ± SE of triplicate assays and the experiment was repeated at least twice.

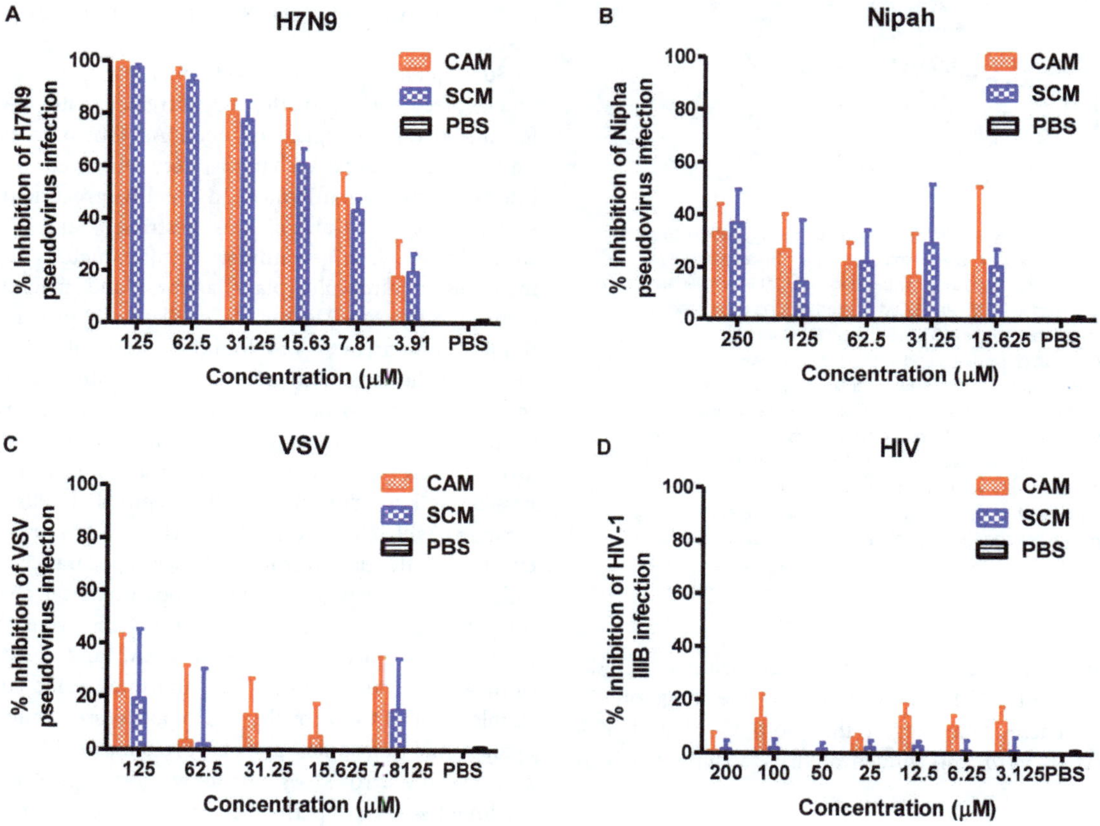

FIGURE 7 | CAM and SCM inhibited the entry of H7N9 pseudovirus into MDCK cells. **(A)** CAM and SCM inhibited the entry of A/Shanghai/4664T/2013(H7N9) pseudovirus into MDCK cells. **(B)** CAM and SCM did not inhibit entry of Nipha pseudovirus into Huh7 cells. **(C)** CAM and SCM exhibited no inhibitory activity on VSV pseudovirus entry into U87 cells. **(D)** CAM and SCM did not inhibit HIV-1 IIIB infection in MT-2 cells. The data were presented as means ± SE of triplicate assays and the experiment was repeated at least twice.

We found that the integrated optical density (IOD) in the CAM-, SCM-, and OSE-treatment groups was significantly lower than that in PBS control group (**Supplementary Figure S3** and **Supplementary Table S3**). All these results suggest that like OSE, CAM and SCM can effectively inhibit the influenza A H7N9 virus infection *in vivo* and attenuated the histopathological changes in the lungs of virus-infected mice.

CAM and SCM Inhibited Influenza Virus Infection at an Early Step of Infection

The influenza replication cycle consists of several steps. To elucidate the mechanism of action of CAM and SCM, a time-of-addition experiment was performed, as described previously (Droebner et al., 2017). CAM and SCM were added to MDCK cells at 0, 0.5, 1, 2, 4, and 12 h, respectively, after infection with A/Shanghai/37T/2009(H1N1) at MOI of 0.1. As shown in **Figure 6**, CAM and SCM exerted 99 and 93% inhibition on A/Shanghai/37T/2009(H1N1) infection, respectively, when added to cells at 0.5 h p.i., while their inhibitory activity was reduced to 23 and 19%, respectively, when they were added to cells at 4 h p.i. These results indicate that CAM and SCM inhibit influenza virus infection at an early step, possibly the viral entry stage.

CAM and SCM Inhibited the Entry of H7N9 Pseudovirus Into MDCK Cells

To determine whether CAM and SCM could block the entry of the influenza virus into the target cells, we used the plasmid Env-H7N9-pNL4-3.luc.R-E- to construct pseudotyped H7N9 influenza virus particles, which express the two envelope proteins of the influenza A virus, HA and NA. The effect of CAM and SCM on the entry of this pseudotyped H7N9 IAV was detected by single-cycle pseudovirus infection assay. Pseudovirus expressing VSV G protein or Nipha virus (NiV) G protein was included as control. The result showed that CAM and SCM could effectively inhibit H7N9 pseudovirus infection in a dose-dependent manner with IC_{50} of 8.98 ± 3.93 and 10.85 ± 1.19 μM, respectively (**Figure 7A**), while CAM and SCM had no effect on infection by Nipha pseudovirus (**Figure 7B**) or VSV-G pseudovirus (**Figure 7C**), suggesting that antiviral ability might be related to HA or NA. Since these pseudoviruses contain the HIV-1 NL4-3 internal genes, we further investigated if these two compounds would have any effect on live HIV-1 IIIB infection. We found that neither CAM nor SCM had inhibitory effect on HIV-1 IIIB infection (**Figure 7D**). Collectively, these results indicate that both CAM and SCM are able to block the entry of influenza virus into the target cell, which represents the early step of virus replication.

CAM and SCM Had No Effect on Virus Attachment to Host Cells or on Viral NA Activity

HA is a major membrane glycoprotein responsible for virus-cell receptor interaction and virus attachment to the target cell, the first step of viral entry (Fan et al., 2015), while NA is

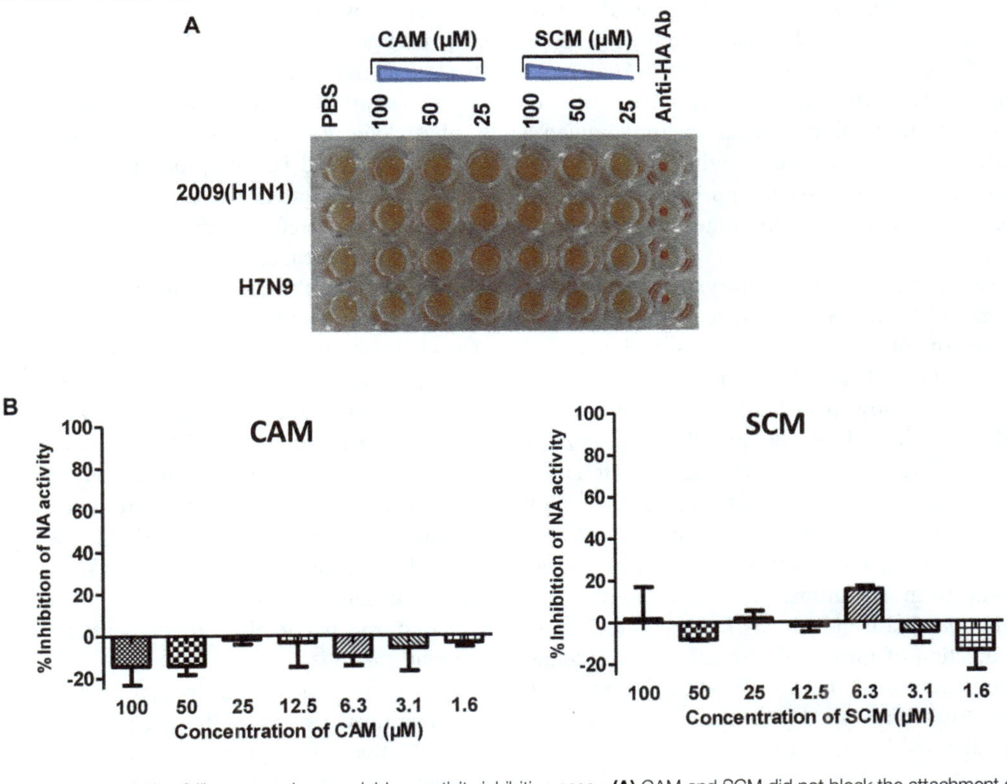

FIGURE 8 | Haemagglutination inhibition (HI) assay and neuraminidase activity inhibition assay. **(A)** CAM and SCM did not block the attachment of influenza virus to chicken RBCs. Twenty-five μL of A/shanghai/37T/2009H1N1 and pseudoviruses of H7N9 (~4 hemagglutination units) were mixed with an equal volume of CAM and SCM at 100, 50, and 25 μM, respectively, or anti-H1N1 antibody (10 μg/ml) as the positive control. After incubated at room temperature for 1 h, 50 μL of 1% (v/v) chicken RBCs were added, followed by an incubation at room temperature for 1 h. Haemagglutination was observed and record. **(B)** The inhibition of CAM and SCM on NA activity. The data were presented as means ± SE of triplicate assays and the experiment was repeated at least twice.

another membrane glycoprotein responsible for the release of the newly produced viral particles (NA activity). We performed a haemagglutination inhibition (HI) assay using chicken red blood cells (RBCs) to determine whether CAM or SCM could bind to HA on the virus surface to effectively inhibit the HI activity of HA. As shown in **Figure 8**, CAM and SCM at the concentration as high as 100 μM could not inhibit HA-mediated RBC agglutination (**Figure 8A**), nor could it inhibit NA activity (**Figure 8B**). These results suggest that CAM and SCM may not interfere with HA-mediated virus attachment and NA-mediated virus release, but other steps of viral entry.

DISCUSSION

In recent years, a number of avian influenza viruses, such as H7N9, H5N6, H10N8 and H9N2, have gained the ability to cross the species barrier to infect humans, posing a significant threat to public health worldwide (Chen et al., 2014; Bi et al., 2016; Zhu et al., 2016; Yao et al., 2018). Five major epidemic waves of H7N9 IAV infection have occurred since it first emerged in March 2013[2]. People infected with the H7N9 virus suffer from severe pneumonia and its complications, which can be fatal (Zhu et al., 2016). Although the NA inhibitor oseltamivir has been widely used to treat influenza virus infection, long-term oseltamivir treatment often leads to the emergence of drug-resistant viruses (Khodadad et al., 2015; Kiso et al., 2017). It has been reported that almost all seasonal influenza H1N1 viruses circulating in the United States in 2008–2009 were oseltamivir-resistant isolates (Kao et al., 2010). This calls for the development of new antiviral therapeutics against influenza viruses with resistance to the current antiviral drugs. Small-molecule compounds with broad-spectrum antiviral activity could offer a second line of defense when influenza epidemics or pandemics occur.

By screening an FDA-approved drug library, we identified two antihistamine drugs, CAM and SCM, which have had clinical application in the treatment of hay fever, rhinitis, urticaria, and asthma, with potent antiviral activity against avian influenza virus H7N9 with IC_{50} at low μM level. More importantly, both drugs could also inhibit infection by other influenza A viruses, such as 2009(H1N1), 1934(H1N1), and 1989(H3N2) strains, as well as an influenza B virus, B/Shanghai/2017(BY), suggesting that both CAM and SCM have broad antiviral activity against divergent influenza A strains and one influenza B strain. The result from an animal study showed that i.p. injection of CAM or SCM at 10 mg/kg/day for 5 days resulted in full protection of mice against challenge with lethal dose of avian influenza virus H7N9, indicating that these two antihistamine drugs have good potential for clinical use in the treatment, or, possibly, prevention of influenza virus infection.

The life cycle of the influenza virus can be divided into seven stages, as follows: (1) Attachment - HA, which can be cleaved into HA1 and HA2 subunits (Skehel, 2009), binds to sialic acid receptors on the host cell surface, facilitating viral entry into the cell (Yang et al., 2013). (2) Endocytosis - When virions are transported into the endocytic vesicle, the low pH environment (5.0–5.5) triggers the conformation of HA to mediate fusion of the viral and endosomal membranes (Xu and Wilson, 2011). These events are followed by (3) transcription, Translation, Replication, (4) packaging and (5) release of the newly produced viral particles out of the cell (Das et al., 2010; Lai et al., 2016). To determine which stage was targeted by CAM and SCM, we conducted time-of-addition and pseudovirus entry experiments. We found that both CAM and SCM target at the early stage of influenza virus life cycle by blocking entry of the influenza virus into the host cell. As described above, the entry stage consists of the early step of viral attachment to cells and late stage of viral endocytosis. Our study has shown that neither CAM nor SCM can block the attachment of 2009 H1N1 virus to chicken RBCs, suggesting that these two antihistamine drugs do not affect viral attachment to host cells, but may target the other steps of viral entry. More recently, Kouznetsova et al. (2014) and He et al. (2015) have reported that chlorcyclizine HCl (CCZ), an over-the-counter antihistamine drug for allergy symptoms, exhibits potent inhibitory activity against HCV infection by targeting viral entry into host cells, although the exact mechanism of action has not been clarified. Kouznetsova et al. (2014) and He et al. (2015) identified 53 compounds that block Ebola virus-like particle entry, three of which are antihistamine drugs, Clemastine, Maprotiline, and Benztropine. Similarly, however, they have not determined which stage of viral entry is targeted by these antihistamine drugs. Therefore, further studies on the mechanism(s) of action of these antihistamine drugs against viral infection are warranted. Histamine is a physiologically active substance that binds and activates histamine H1 and H2 receptors in the respiratory tract, brain, skin vasculature, and heart. Antihistamine drugs block the action of histamine, therefore reducing such symptoms as sneezing, rhinitis, rhinorrhea, erythema, pruritus, and urticaria. The first generation of antihistamines, for instance, CAM or SCM, have the ability to cross the blood-brain barrier and penetrate human central nervous cells to bind histamine receptors because of their anti-cholesterol properties. In the present study, we found that both CAM and SCM also possess the ability to inhibit influenza virus infection. Therefore, application of CAM or SCM for treatment of influenza may have complementary effect, i.e., inhibiting influenza virus infection and attenuating the inflammatory responses and allergic syndromes caused by viral infection. Furthermore, CAM or SCM may be use prophylactically in healthy individuals during an influenza epidemic or pandemic for prevention of influenza virus infection.

In summary, based on an FDA-approved drug library, we have identified two FDA-approved antihistamine drugs, CAM and SCM, that exhibit potent inhibitory activity against divergent influenza A strains and one influenza B strain and that protect mice from fatal challenge of avian H7N9 influenza virus. These antihistamine drugs inhibit influenza virus infection by targeting the early stage of virus life cycle, viral entry into the host cells. These results suggest that both CAM and SCM have potential for clinical use in the treatment and prevention of influenza virus infection.

AUTHOR CONTRIBUTIONS

SJ and LL conceived and designed the experiments. WX, SX, JP, PL, and QW performed the experiments. WX, LL, and SJ analyzed the data and wrote the manuscript.

ACKNOWLEDGMENTS

We would like to thank Zhiping Sun for his guidance and help in the BSL-3 Laboratory.

REFERENCES

Baranovich, T., Burnham, A. J., Marathe, B. M., Armstrong, J., Guan, Y., Shu, Y. L., et al. (2014). The neuraminidase inhibitor oseltamivir is effective against A/Anhui/1/2013 (H7N9) influenza virus in a mouse model of acute respiratory distress syndrome. *J. Infect. Dis.* 209, 1343–1353. doi: 10.1093/infdis/jit554

Bergen, P. J., Li, J., Rayner, C. R., and Nation, R. L. (2006). Colistin methanesulfonate is an inactive prodrug of colistin against *pseudomonas aeruginosa*. *Antimicrob. Agents. Chemother.* 50, 1953–1958. doi: 10.1128/Aac.00035-06

Bi, Y. H., Chen, J. J., Zhang, Z. J., Li, M. X., Cai, T. L., Sharshov, K., et al. (2016). Highly pathogenic avian influenza H5N1 Clade 2.3.2.1c virus in migratory birds, 2014-2015. *Virol. Sin.* 31, 300–305. doi: 10.1007/s12250-016-3750-4

Chen, H., Yuan, H., Gao, R., Zhang, J., Wang, D., Xiong, Y., et al. (2014). Clinical and epidemiological characteristics of a fatal case of avian influenza A H10N8 virus infection: a descriptive study. *Lancet* 383, 714–721. doi: 10.1016/S0140-6736(14)60111-2

Choi, J. G., Jin, Y. H., Kim, J. H., Oh, T. W., Yim, N. H., Cho, W. K., et al. (2016). In vitro anti-viral activity of psoraleae semen water extract against influenza A viruses. *Front. Pharmacol.* 7:460. doi: 10.3389/fphar.2016.00460

Chong, C. R., and Sullivan, D. J. (2007). New uses for old drugs. *Nature* 448, 645–646. doi: 10.1038/448645a

Chou, T. C., and Talalay, P. (1984). Quantitative analysis of dose-effect relationships: the combined effects of multiple drugs or enzyme inhibitors. *Adv. Enzyme. Regul.* 22, 27–55. doi: 10.1016/0065-2571(84)90007-4

Das, K., Aramini, J. M., Ma, L. C., Krug, R. M., and Arnold, E. (2010). Structures of influenza A proteins and insights into antiviral drug targets. *Nat. Struct. Mol. Biol.* 17, 530–538. doi: 10.1038/nsmb.1779

DiMasi, J. A., Hansen, R. W., and Grabowski, H. G. (2003). The price of innovation: new estimates of drug development costs. *J. Health. Econ.* 22, 151–185. doi: 10.1016/S0167-6296(02)00126-1

Droebner, K., Haasbach, E., Dudek, S. E., Scheuch, G., Nocker, K., Canisius, S., et al. (2017). Pharmacodynamics, pharmacokinetics, and antiviral activity of BAY 81-8781, a novel NF-kappaB inhibiting anti-influenza drug. *Front. Microbiol.* 8:2130. doi: 10.3389/fmicb.2017.02130

Falagas, M. E., and Kasiakou, S. K. (2005). Colistin: the revival of polymyxins for the management of multidrug-resistant gram-negative bacterial infections. *Clin. Infect. Dis.* 40, 1333–1341. doi: 10.1086/429323

Fan, X., Hashem, A. M., Chen, Z., Li, C., Doyle, T., Zhang, Y., et al. (2015). Targeting the HA2 subunit of influenza A virus hemagglutinin via CD40L provides universal protection against diverse subtypes. *Mucosal Immunol.* 8, 211–220. doi: 10.1038/mi.2014.59

Furuta, Y., Takahashi, K., Fukuda, Y., Kuno, M., Kamiyama, T., Kozaki, K., et al. (2002). In vitro and in vivo activities of anti-influenza virus compound T-705. *Antimicrob. Agents Chemother.* 46, 977–981. doi: 10.1128/Aac.46.4.977-981.2002

Halpern, B. N., Hazard, J., Klotz, A., and Ky, N. T. (1965). Advantage of adding an injectable solution of dexchlorpheniramine maleate to allergen extracts in specific desensitization. *Rev. Fr. Allergol.* 5, 241–243.

Han, S. B., Shin, Y. J., Hyon, J. Y., and Wee, W. R. (2011). Cytotoxicity of voriconazole on cultured human corneal endothelial cells. *Antimicrob. Agents Chemother.* 55, 4519–4523. doi: 10.1128/AAC.00569-11

He, B., Fu, Y., Xia, S., Yu, F., Wang, Q., Lu, L., et al. (2016). Intranasal application of polyethyleneimine suppresses influenza virus infection in mice. *Emerg. Microbes. Infect.* 5:e41. doi: 10.1038/emi.2016.64

He, S., Lin, B., Chu, V., Hu, Z., Hu, X., Xiao, J., et al. (2015). Repurposing of the antihistamine chlorcyclizine and related compounds for treatment of hepatitis C virus infection. *Sci. Transl. Med.* 7:282ra49. doi: 10.1126/scitranslmed.3010286

Jin, J., Chen, S., Wang, D., Chen, Y., Wang, Y., Guo, M., et al. (2018). Oroxylin a suppresses influenza A virus replication correlating with neuraminidase inhibition and induction of IFNs. *Biomed. Pharmacother.* 97, 385–394. doi: 10.1016/j.biopha.2017.10.140

Kao, R. Y., Yang, D., Lau, L. S., Tsui, W. H. W., Hu, L. H., Dai, J., et al. (2010). Identification of influenza a nucleoprotein as an antiviral target. *Nat. Biotechnol.* 28, 600–605. doi: 10.1038/nbt.1638

Khodadad, N., Moattari, A., Abadi, M. S. S., Kadivar, M. R., Sarvari, J., Tavakoli, F., et al. (2015). Prevalence of influenza A(H1N1)pdm09 virus resistant to oseltamivir in Shiraz, Iran, during 2012-2013. *Jundishapur J. Microb.* 8:e23690. doi: 10.5812/jjm.23690

Kiso, M., Iwatsuki-Horimoto, K., Yamayoshi, S., Uraki, R., Ito, M., Nakajima, N., et al. (2017). Emergence of oseltamivir-resistant h7N9 influenza viruses in immunosuppressed cynomolgus macaques. *J. Infect. Dis.* 216, 582–593. doi: 10.1093/infdis/jix296

Kouznetsova, J., Sun, W., Martinez-Romero, C., Tawa, G., Shinn, P., Chen, C. Z., et al. (2014). Identification of 53 compounds that block Ebola virus-like particle entry via a repurposing screen of approved drugs. *Emerg. Microbes. Infect.* 3:e84. doi: 10.1038/emi.2014.88

Lai, K. K., Cheung, N. N., Yang, F., Dai, J., Liu, L., Chen, Z. W., et al. (2016). Identification of novel fusion inhibitors of influenza A virus by chemical genetics. *J. Virol.* 90, 2690–2701. doi: 10.1128/Jvi.02326-15

Li, J., Nation, R. L., Turnidge, J. D., Milne, R. W., Coulthard, K., Rayner, C. R., et al. (2006). Colistin: the re-emerging antibiotic for multidrug-resistant gram-negative bacterial infections. *Lancet Infect. Dis.* 6, 589–601. doi: 10.1016/S1473-3099(06)70580-1

Liu, C., Jiang, L., Liu, L., Sun, L., Zhao, W., Chen, Y., et al. (2018). Induction of avian beta-defensin 2 is possibly mediated by the p38 MAPK signal pathway in chicken embryo fibroblasts after newcastle disease virus infection. *Front. Microbiol.* 9:751. doi: 10.3389/fmicb.2018.00751

Maddry, J. A., Chen, X., Jonsson, C. B., Ananthan, S., Hobrath, J., Smee, D. F., et al. (2011). Discovery of novel benzoquinazolinones and thiazoloimidazoles, inhibitors of influenza H5N1 and H1N1 Viruses, from a cell-based high-throughput screen. *J. Biomol. Screen.* 16, 73–81. doi: 10.1177/1087057110384613

Marjuki, H., Mishin, V. P., Chesnokov, A. P., Jones, J., De La Cruz, J. A., Sleeman, K., et al. (2015). Characterization of drug-resistant influenza A(H7N9) variants isolated from an oseltamivir-treated patient in Taiwan. *J. Infect. Dis.* 211, 249–257. doi: 10.1093/infdis/jiu447

Matsuzaki, Y., Mizuta, K., Aoki, Y., Suto, A., Abiko, C., Sanjoh, K., et al. (2010). A two-year survey of the oseltamivir-resistant influenza A(H1N1) virus in Yamagata, Japan and the clinical effectiveness of oseltamivir and zanamivir. *Virol. J.* 7:53. doi: 10.1186/1743-422X-7-53

Nation, R. L., Garonzik, S. M., Li, J., Thamlikitkul, V., Giamarellos-Bourboulis, E. J., Paterson, D. L., et al. (2016). Updated US and European dose recommendations for intravenous colistin: how do they perform? *Clin. Infect. Dis.* 62, 552–558. doi: 10.1093/cid/civ964

Ong, A. K., and Hayden, F. G. (2007). John F Enders lecture 2006: antivirals for influenza. *J. Infect. Dis.* 196, 181–190. doi: 10.1086/518939

Pizzorno, A., Abed, Y., Plante, P. L., Carbonneau, J., Baz, M., Hamelin, M. E., et al. (2014). Evolution of oseltamivir resistance mutations in influenza A(H1N1) and

A(H3N2) viruses during selection in experimentally infected mice. *Antimicrob. Agents. Chemother.* 58, 6398–6405. doi: 10.1128/Aac.02956-14

Qiu, C., Huang, Y., Zhang, A., Tian, D., Wan, Y., Zhang, X., et al. (2013). Safe pseudovirus-based assay for neutralization antibodies against influenza A(H7N9) virus. *Emerg. Infect. Dis.* 19, 1685–1687. doi: 10.3201/eid1910.130728

Rockman, S., Lowther, S., Camuglia, S., Vandenberg, K., Taylor, S., Fabri, L., et al. (2017). Intravenous immunoglobulin protects against severe pandemic influenza infection. *eBioMedicine* 19, 119–127. doi: 10.1016/j.ebiom.2017.04.010

Salter, A., Laoi, B. N., and Crowley, B. (2011). Emergence and phylogenetic analysis of amantadine-resistant influenza a subtype H3N2 viruses in Dublin, Ireland, over six seasons from 2003/2004 to 2008/2009. *Intervirology* 54, 305–315. doi: 10.1159/000321358

Shen, X. T., Zhu, Z. B., Ding, Y., Wu, W. J., Yang, J., and Liu, S. W. (2018). An oligothiophene compound neutralized influenza A viruses by interfering with hemagglutinin. *Biochim. Biophys. Acta Biomembr.* 1860, 784–791. doi: 10.1016/j.bbamem.2017.12.006

Skehel, J. (2009). An overview of influenza haemagglutinin and neuraminidase. *Biologicals* 37, 177–178. doi: 10.1016/j.biologicals.2009.02.012

Su, S., Ma, Z., Hua, C., Li, W., Lu, L., and Jiang, S. (2017a). Adding an artificial tail-anchor to a peptide-based HIV-1 fusion inhibitor for improvement of its potency and resistance profile. *Molecules* 22:E1996. doi: 10.3390/molecules22111996

Su, S., Wang, Q., Xu, W., Yu, F., Hua, C., Zhu, Y., et al. (2017b). A novel HIV-1 gp41 tripartite model for rational design of HIV-1 fusion inhibitors with improved antiviral activity. *AIDS* 31, 885–894. doi: 10.1097/QAD.0000000000001415

Wang, J., Yan, Y. T., Fu, S. Z., Peng, B., Bao, L. L., Zhang, Y. L., et al. (2017). Anti-influenza virus (H5N1) activity screening on the phloroglucinols from rhizomes of dryopteris crassirhizoma. *Molecules* 22:E431. doi: 10.3390/molecules22030431

Xia, S., Xu, W., Wang, Q., Wang, C., Hua, C., Li, W., et al. (2018). Peptide-based membrane fusion inhibitors targeting HCoV-229E spike protein HR1 and HR2 domains. *Int. J. Mol. Sci.* 19:E487. doi: 10.3390/ijms19020487

Xu, M., Lee, E. M., Wen, Z., Cheng, Y., Huang, W. K., Qian, X., et al. (2016). Identification of small-molecule inhibitors of Zika virus infection and induced neural cell death via a drug repurposing screen. *Nat. Med.* 22, 1101–1107. doi: 10.1038/nm.4184

Xu, R., and Wilson, I. A. (2011). Structural characterization of an early fusion intermediate of influenza virus hemagglutinin. *J. Virol.* 85, 5172–5182. doi: 10.1128/JVI.02430-10

Xu, W., Dai, Y., Hua, C., Wang, Q., Zou, P., Deng, Q., et al. (2017). Genomic signature analysis of the recently emerged highly pathogenic A(H5N8) avian influenza virus: implying an evolutionary trend for bird-to-human transmission. *Microbes Infect.* 19, 597–604. doi: 10.1016/j.micinf.2017.08.006

Yamayoshi, S., Uraki, R., Ito, M., Kiso, M., Nakatsu, S., Yasuhara, A., et al. (2017). A broadly reactive human anti-hemagglutinin stem monoclonal antibody that inhibits influenza A virus particle release. *eBioMedicine* 17, 182–191. doi: 10.1016/j.ebiom.2017.03.007

Yang, J., Li, M., Shen, X., and Liu, S. (2013). Influenza A virus entry inhibitors targeting the hemagglutinin. *Viruses* 5, 352–373. doi: 10.3390/v5010352

Yao, Y. F., Zhang, T., Yang, W. H., Shao, Z. Y., He, B., Chen, X. B., et al. (2018). Avian influenza A (H7N9) virus in a wild land bird in central china, late 2015. *Virol. Sin.* 33, 96–99. doi: 10.1007/s12250-018-0001-x

Yen, H. L., Monto, A. S., Webster, R. G., and Govorkova, E. A. (2005). Virulence may determine the necessary duration and dosage of oseltamivir treatment for highly pathogenic A/Vietnam/1203/04 influenza virus in mice. *J. Infect. Dis.* 192, 665–672. doi: 10.1086/432008

Zhang, Y., Chen, M., Huang, Y., Zhu, W., Yang, L., Gao, L., et al. (2017). Human infections with novel reassortant H5N6 avian influenza viruses in China. *Emerg. Microbes. Infect.* 6:e50. doi: 10.1038/emi.2017.38

Zhu, H., Lam, T. T., Smith, D. K., and Guan, Y. (2016). Emergence and development of H7N9 influenza viruses in China. *Curr. Opin. Virol.* 16, 106–113. doi: 10.1016/j.coviro.2016.01.020

12

Genotypic Diversity and Epidemiology of Human Rhinovirus among Children with Severe Acute Respiratory Tract Infection in Shanghai, 2013–2015

Yanjie Zhao[1,2†], *Jun Shen*[3†], *Bingjie Wu*[1], *Gaoshan Liu*[1], *Roujian Lu*[1,2*] *and Wenjie Tan*[1,2*]

[1] *Key Laboratory of Laboratory Medicine, Ministry of Education, Institute of Medical Virology, Wenzhou Medical University, Wenzhou, China,* [2] *National Institute for Viral Disease Control and Prevention, Chinese Center for Disease Control and Prevention, Beijing, China,* [3] *Infectious Disease Department, Children's Hospital of Fudan University, Shanghai, China*

***Correspondence:**
Roujian Lu
xiaolu017@sina.com
Wenjie Tan
tanwj28@163.com

† *These authors have contributed equally to this work.*

Human rhinovirus (HRV), and particularly HRV-C, is increasingly recognized as a cause of severe acute respiratory infections (SARIs). However, little is known about the genotypic diversity and epidemiology of HRV among children with SARI. Thus, we investigated the genotypic diversity and epidemiology of HRV in children with SARI in China over a 2-year period. In total 1,003, nasopharyngeal aspirates were collected from children hospitalized with SARI in Shanghai from 2013 to 2015. HRV was screened for by a PCR method targeting the viral 5′ UTR and was genotyped by sequencing of the VP4–VP2 region of the HRV genome. We also screened for 15 other common respiratory viruses to assess the prevalence of co-infection with HRV. The patient demographic and clinical data were reviewed. HRV was detected in 280 (27.9%) of the 1,003 specimens: HRV-A in 140 (14.0%), HRV-B in 21 (2.1%), HRV-C in 56 (5.6%), and HRV-untyped in 63 (6.3%). A phylogenetic analysis identified 77 genotypes (43 HRV-A, 10 HRV-B, and 24 HRV-C), among which A78, A12, A89, B70, C2, C6, and C24 predominated. HRV-A was detected mainly in winter 2013 and autumn 2014, while HRV-C detection peaked in autumn 2013 and 2014. The detection frequency of HRV-A was highest in patients <5 years old. Most HRV co-infections involved adenovirus, human bocavirus, and/or human respiratory syncytial virus. In conclusion, HRV-A and -C predominate in children with SARI in Shanghai. Among the 77 genotypes detected, A78, A12, A89, B70, C2, C6, and C24 were the most frequent. The HRV species responsible for SARIs differs according to season and age.

Keywords: human rhinovirus, genotype, severe acute respiratory infections, children, epidemiology

INTRODUCTION

Human rhinovirus (HRV), a single-stranded positive-sense RNA virus, belongs to the genus Enterovirus and family Picornaviridae, and is classified as HRV-A, -B, or -C. HRV-A and HRV-B were discovered in the 1950s (Price, 1956), while HRV-C was identified using molecular techniques in 2006 (Lamson et al., 2006; Lau et al., 2007). According to the 2017 International Committee on the Taxonomy of Viruses (ICTV) release[1], a total of 168 HRV genotypes (80 HRV-A, 32 HRV-B, and 56 HRV-C) are recognized (Kuroda et al., 2015).

Human rhinovirus genomic RNA is approximately 7.2 kb that consisting of a single open reading frame (ORF) encodes 11 proteins, with 5′ and 3′ untranslated regions (UTR) at both end, respectively. The ORF encodes a poly-protein which is cleaved by viral proteases to produce 11 proteins including four structural viral proteins (VP) 1 to 4. Compared to the rest of the HRV genome, the capsid proteins exhibit a high degree of heterogeneity resulting in a wide range of antigenic diversity. RT-PCR assays targeted the 5′-UTR are usually used for HRV clinical detection. HRV species and types are classified almost exclusively now based on VP1 or VP4/VP2 sequence alignments (Wisdom et al., 2009).

Human rhinovirus is a frequently detected respiratory virus in children with mild acute respiratory infection (ARI), but may also lead to more-severe respiratory tract symptoms, such as pneumonia, bronchiolitis, and asthma. HRV is, after respiratory syncytial virus (RSV), the second most frequent viral cause of community-acquired pneumonia and other severe acute respiratory infections (SARIs) (Honkinen et al., 2012; Esposito et al., 2013). HRV-C is more frequently associated with wheezing episodes, asthma exacerbations, and lower respiratory tract infections compared with HRV-A and -B (Linsuwanon et al., 2009; Gern, 2010; Bizzintino et al., 2011). However, there is reportedly no relationship between disease severity and HRV species (Lee et al., 2012; Chen et al., 2015; van der Linden et al., 2016).

Data on the genotypic diversity and epidemiology of HRVs in children with SARI are sparse. Thus, we evaluated the predominant HRV species and genotypes, and their associations with the clinical characteristics, of 1,003 children hospitalized with SARI from 2013 to 2015 in Shanghai, China.

MATERIALS AND METHODS

Ethics Issues

All aspects of the study were performed in accordance with the national ethics regulations and approved by the Ethics Committee of the Children's Hospital of Fudan University (Jun Shen; CHFU2013016) as well as the Ethics Committee of National Institute for Viral Disease Control and Prevention (RL; IVDC2013022). Participants were received "Written Informed Consent" on the study's purpose and of their right to keep information confidential. Written consent was obtained from all participants or their guardians.

Patients and Sample Collection

From June 2013 to August 2015, 1,003 nasopharyngeal aspirates (NPAs) were collected from children hospitalized with SARI in the Children's Hospital of Fudan University, Shanghai, China. The revised World Health Organization SARI case definition (World Health Organization [WHO], 2011) was adopted and cases with clinical suspicion of SARI for children was enrolled (Zhang et al., 2013; Wang et al., 2016). Eligibility and classification of the clinical syndromes of SARI were determined from individual's original record of medical history and examination. The criteria of hospitalized patient inclusion were: sudden onset of fever >38°C and cough or sore throat and difficulty breathing (dyspnea, oxygen saturation < 90%). Additional criteria were a normal or low leukocyte count, or lower chest wall indrawing. Demographic data and clinical findings at the time of diagnosis were recorded on a standard form. All NPA samples were stored at −80°C until use.

HRV Detection and Genotyping

Viral nucleic acid was extracted from 200 μL of sample using QIAamp MinElute Virus Spin Kits (Qiagen, Germany). cDNA was synthesized using an AMV reverse transcriptase and random hexamer primers (Promega, United States), as described previously (Lu et al., 2012). Nested RT-PCR targeting of the 5′-UTR was employed for HRV screening, and of the VP4–VP2 regions for genotyping. All (totally nine, except HEV IS only) of HRV or HRV/HEV primers from 5-UTR to VP4–VP2 were used to detect HRV, as described previously (Wisdom et al., 2009). Specimens from which amplification of the VP4–VP2 regions failed were defined as untyped. PCR products were confirmed by sequencing. Phylogenetic analysis was conducted using Molecular Evolutionary Genetics Analysis (MEGA) software (ver. 7).

Detection of Common Respiratory Viruses

Human rhinovirus-positive specimens were screened for influenza virus types A and B, parainfluenza virus types 1 to 3, RSV, picornaviruses (enteroviruses and rhinoviruses), and adenovirus (AdV) using three multiple-nested-PCR assays; and for human metapneumovirus (hMPV), human bocavirus (HBoV), and human coronavirus 229E/OC43/NL63/HKU1 using nested-PCR assays. The multiple-nested and nested PCRs were performed as described previously (da Silva Filho et al., 2012; Lu et al., 2012). All PCR products of 15 common respiratory viruses were confirmed by sequencing.

Statistical Analysis

Data analysis was performed using PASW (ver. 18; SPSS Inc., United States) and GraphPad Prism software (ver. 5.0; GraphPad Software, Inc., United States). Age, maximum body temperature, laboratory parameters, clinical features, and HRV prevalence were compared by χ^2-test or Fisher's exact test for categorical variables, and by two-tailed paired Student's *t*-test for continuous variables. A value of $P < 0.05$ was considered indicative of statistical significance.

RESULTS

Epidemiology of HRV

In total, 1,003 NPAs were collected. The male: female ratio was 609:394 (1.55:1) and the median age was 1 year (range:

[1]http://ictvonline.org/virusTaxonomy.asp

10 days to 15 years). HRV was detected in 280 (27.9%) of the 1,003 specimens: HRV-A in 140 (14.0%), HRV-B in 21 (2.1%), HRV-C in 56 (5.6%), and HRV-untyped in 63 (6.3%). The HRV detection rates are shown in **Table 1**. The detection rates of HRV-A and -B differed significantly ($P < 0.001$). In general, the 5′-UTR region highly conserved between HRV and enterovirus, causing cross-reactivity in RT-PCR assay for the two viruses. In the current study, 42 enterovirus positive samples also were detected by nested RT-PCR targeting of the HRV 5′-UTR.

Human rhinovirus infected significantly more males than females (65.7% vs. 34.3%, $P = 0.044$), and HRV was detected in patients of all ages, although HRV-B was not detected in those aged 3–4 years (**Table 1**). The detection frequency of HRV-A was significantly lower in patients aged 5–9 years ($P = 0.008$), but the frequencies of detection of HRV-B, -C, and -untyped did not differ according to age.

The seasonal distribution of HRV is shown in **Figure 1**. HRV-A was detected most frequently and peaked in winter 2013 and autumn 2015. HRV-C detection peaked in autumn (17.1% in 2013 and 20.7% in 2014). HRV-B was detected year-round at similar frequencies in all seasons. Detection of HRV-untyped peaked in summer and spring 2014 and was at a low level thereafter.

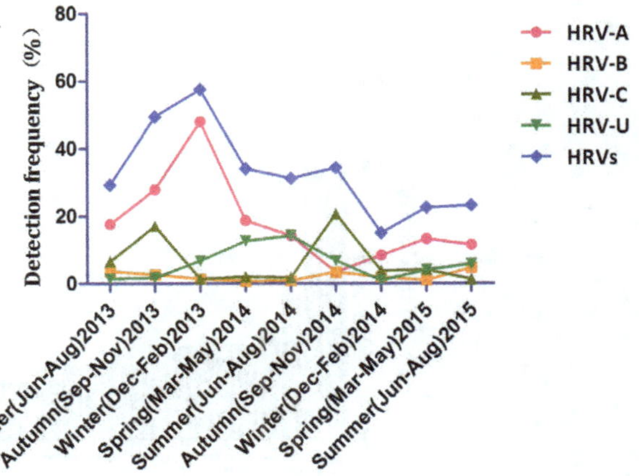

FIGURE 1 | Temporal distribution of the HRV species between June 2013 and August 2015 inclusive.

Genotypic Diversity of HRV

Sequence analysis based on 420 bp of the VP4–VP2 region of 217 of 280 the HRV strains yielded 77 genotypes: 43 HRV-A (most frequently detected: −A78 [17/140, 12.1%], followed by −A12 [15/140, 10.7%], −A89 [8/140, 5.7%], −A61 [*N* = 6], and −A1, −A22, −A56, and A-58 [*N* = 5 each]), 10 HRV-B (most frequently detected: −B70 [5/21, 23.8%], followed by −B86 and −B97 [3/21, 14.3%]) and 24 HRV-C (most frequently detected: −C2, −C6, and −C24, [6/56, 10.7%], followed by −C16 [5/56, 8.9%] and −C4 and −C53 [4/56, 7.1%]) (**Figure 2**).

Clinical Characteristics

The clinical characteristics of the patients with HRV infections are listed in **Table 2**. All HRV-positive patients presented with SARI. Fever, cough, gasping, cyanosis, and diarrhea were the most common symptoms at presentation. There was no significant difference in clinical symptoms according to HRV species, except that cough and cyanosis were less frequent in patients infected with HRV-A and HRV-C, respectively ($P = 0.048$ and 0.005).

Co-infection With Other Respiratory Viruses

Of the 280 HRV-positive patients, 131 (46.8%) were co-infected—102 with one other virus, 21 with two other viruses, and 8 with three other viruses (**Table 3**). Most such co-infections involved AdV, HBoV, and RSV (39.7, 38.2, and 17.6%, respectively). The patients with co-infections did not have more serious disease (data not shown).

DISCUSSION

We evaluated the HRV genotype distribution in children with SARI in the Children's Hospital of Fudan University, Shanghai,

TABLE 1 | Population demographic of HRV-positive specimens.

Variable	HRV-A (*N* = 140)	HRV-B (*N* = 21)	HRV-C (*N* = 56)	Untyped (*N* = 63)	Total (*N* = 280)
Gender					
Male	91 (65%)	14 (66.7%)	34 (60.7%)	44 (69.8%)	184 (65.7%)
Female	49 (35%)	7 (33.3%)	22 (39.3%)	19 (30.2%)	96 (34.3%)
P-value	0.263	0.573	1.000	0.126	0.044*
Age group (years)					
<1 Year	78 (55.7%)	7 (33.3%)	24 (42.9%)	32 (50.8%)	141 (50.3%)
1–2 Years	33 (23.6%)	7 (33.3%)	14 (25%)	13 (20.6%)	67 (23.9%)
3–4 Years	17 (12.1%)	0	11 (19.6%)	8 (12.7%)	36 (12.9%)
5–9 Years	9 (6.4%)	6 (28.6%)	5 (8.9%)	9 (14.3%)	29 (10.3%)
10–14 Years	3 (2.1%)	1 (4.8%)	2 (3.6%)	1 (1.6%)	7 (2.5%)
P-value	0.008*	0.124	0.235	0.810	0.055

*$P < 0.05$.

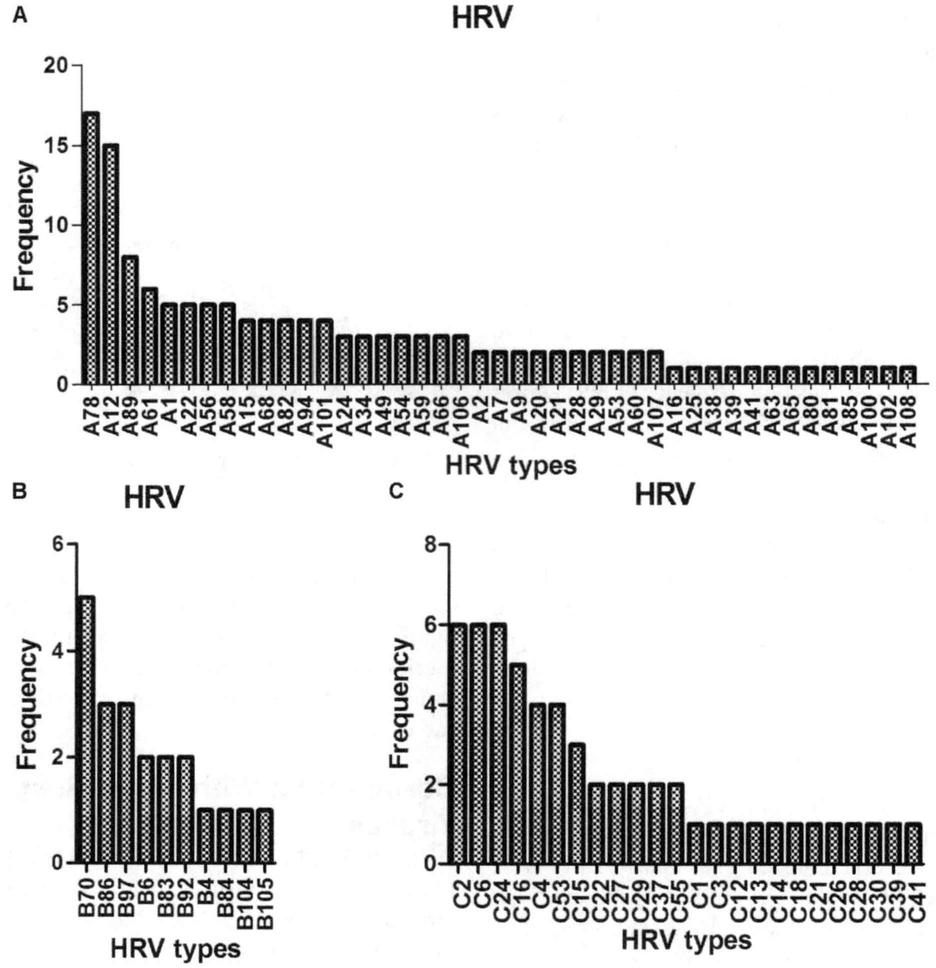

FIGURE 2 | Detection of HRV genotypes in the study **(A–C)**.

TABLE 2 | Clinical characteristics of patients with HRV infections in the study.

Characteristics	HRV-A (*N* = 140)	HRV-B (*N* = 21)	HRV-C (*N* = 56)	HRV-Untyped (*N* = 63)	*P*-value
Fever (mean/median)	39.0/39.0	39.2/39.0	39.1/39.0	38.7/39.0	
Cough	119 (85%)	21 (100%)	52 (92.8%)	56 (88.9%)	0.048*
Gasping	53 (37.9%)	8 (38.1%)	23 (41.1%)	22 (34.9%)	0.924
Cyanosis	17 (12.1%)	3 (14.3%)	0	7 (11.1%)	0.005*
Diarrhea	17 (12.1%)	1 (4.8%)	4 (7.1%)	11 (17.5%)	0.228
Bronchitis	9 (6.4%)	1 (5%)	9 (16.1%)	5 (7.9%)	0.206
Bronchial asthma	2 (1.4%)	0	1 (1.8%)	2 (3.2%)	0.699
Pneumonia	95 (67.9%)	16 (76.2%)	37 (66.1%)	41 (65.1%)	0.804
Severe pneumonia	15 (11.0%)	4 (19.0%)	4 (7.1%)	9 (14.3%)	0.435
Respiratory failure	11 (7.1%)	1 (4.8%)	6 (10.7%)	7 (11.1%)	0.732
Death	0	0	0	2 (3.2%)	0.111

*$P < 0.05$.

China from June 2013 to August 2015. Of the 1,003 samples, 280 (27.9%) were positive for HRV (HRV-A, 50.0%; HRV-B, 7.5%; HRV-C, 20%; and HRV-untyped, 22.5%). This HRV detection rate is consistent with prior studies (11.0–40.6%) worldwide, as are the proportions of the three HRV species (HRV-A, 44.4–56%; HRV-B, 2–12%; and HRV-C, 25–45.3%) (Xiang et al., 2010; Henquell et al., 2012; Rahamat-Langendoen et al., 2013; Marcone et al., 2014; Tsatsral et al., 2015; Xiao et al., 2015; Milanoi et al., 2016; van der Linden et al., 2016; Blaschke et al., 2018). This prevalence of HRV-untyped is higher than in a

TABLE 3 | Co-detections of HRV and other respiratory virus in the study.

2 Virus (*N* = 102)		**3 Viruses (*N* = 21)**		**4 Viruses (*N* = 8)**	
HRV+ADV	36	HRV+ADV+HBoV	7	HRV+ADV+HBoV+HCoV	2
HRV+HBoV	32	HRV+HBoV+hRSV	3	HRV+PIV+HBoV+ENV	1
HRV+hRSV	16	HRV+ADV+hRSV	2	HRV+PIV+ADV+ENV	1
HRV+PIV	7	HRV+ADV+PIV	1	HRV+PIV+HBoV+ADV	1
HRV+HCoV	7	HRV+ADV+ENV	1	HRV+hRSV+HBoV+ADV	1
HRV+FluA	2	HRV+ADV +HCoV	1	HRV+FluA+ADV+hRSV	1
HRV+ENV	2	HRV+HBoV+PIV	1	HRV+HMPV+HBoV+ ENV	1
HRV+HMPV	1	HRV+HBoV+HCoV	1		
		HRV+hRSV+HCoV	1		
		HRV+FluA+HMPV	1		
		HRV+FluA+HBoV	1		
		HRV+ENV +HCoV	1		

HRV, human rhinovirus; ADV, adenovirus; HBoV, human bocavirus; hRSV, human respiratory syncytial virus; PIV, parainfluenza virus; HCoV, human coronavirus; FluA, influenza type A; ENV, enterovirus; HMPV, human metapneumovirus.

recent study in Chongqing (13%) (Xiao et al., 2015), perhaps because our study involved patients with SARI. We achieved identical results using another nested-PCR detection primer also targeting the VP4–VP2 region (data not shown). Further research on whether these HRV-untyped contain new genotypes is warranted.

We detected 77 HRV genotypes in Shanghai from 2013 to 2015 (43 HRV-A, 10 HRV-B, and 24 HRV-C). The predominant HRV-A genotypes were A-78, A-12, A-89, and A-61; those of HRV-B were B-70, B-86, and B-97; and the predominant HRV-C genotypes were C-2, C-6, C-24, and C-16. Variation in the prevalent HRV genotype has been reported by others. In Amsterdam, 129 HRV genotypes were detected in inpatients and outpatients: A-12, A-78, and C-2 predominated (van der Linden et al., 2016). In Buenos Aires, 30 HRV genotypes were detected in children with acute respiratory infections: A-101, A-49, and C-10 predominated (Marcone et al., 2014). In Asia, 59, 36, and 28 HRV genotypes were detected in Mongolia, Beijing, and Cambodia, respectively: A-46, A-12, A-78, B-79, B-86, C-2, and C-36; A-12 and B42; and A-89, A-78, B-79, and C-6, respectively, predominated (Xiang et al., 2010; Naughtin et al., 2015; Tsatsral et al., 2015). Therefore, a large number of HRV genotypes circulate simultaneously, and some genotypes (such as A-12, A-78, and C-2) are the more prevalent types across worldwide although various predominant genotype patterns were reported geographically.

Human rhinovirus circulated throughout this 2-year study with peaks in winter 2013 and autumn 2014; HRV-C predominated in autumn. This seasonal pattern is similar to those reported previously (Xiang et al., 2010; Marcone et al., 2014; van der Linden et al., 2016). Also, HRV-A was detected most frequently in those <5 years old, while the frequency of detection of HRV-B and -C did not differ by age. In contrast, in Mongolia, HRV-A and -C are detected more frequently in younger children, and -B more frequently in older children (Tsatsral et al., 2015).

Human rhinovirus-A and HRV-C are reportedly associated with more severe illness (Miller et al., 2011; Fawkner-Corbett et al., 2016); however, others have reported no link between species and disease severity (Xiang et al., 2010; Henquell et al., 2012; Rahamat-Langendoen et al., 2013; Marcone et al., 2014). In this study, there were no significant differences in clinical symptoms among the three HRV species, except that cough and cyanosis were less frequent in patients with HRV-A and HRV-C, respectively. HRV-C infection in boys under 5 years old with acute asthma significantly increases the risk of moderate/severe exacerbations (Lambert et al., 2017). Moreover, of 570 HRV-positive hospitalized patients with community-acquired pneumonia, 57 (10%) had viremia; the vast majority (98.2%) of viremic patients were infected with HRV-C. The frequency of HRV viremia was higher in patients 1–2 years of age, and patients with viremia were more likely to have severe clinical symptoms, such as chest retraction, wheezing, and asthma (Lu et al., 2017). Therefore, particular HRV species may be associated with disease severity at specific situations which further research is warranted.

Almost half (46.8%) of the HRV-positive patients were co-infected with other respiratory viruses, most frequently ADV, HBoV, and hRSV. This may reflect the viruses in circulation at the time, consistent with previous reports (Xiang et al., 2010; van der Linden et al., 2016; Blaschke et al., 2018). Additionally, for those patients infected with 2–4 respiratory viruses, further research is necessary to demonstrate the dominant virus by qPCR positive with CT value and impact on disease severity.

In summary, we report for in detail the first time the variety of HRV genotypes in circulation and their distribution according to season and age group, as well as their clinical symptoms, in children hospitalized with SARI in China during a 2-year period. Our data shown that HRV was detected in 280 (27.9%) of the 1,003 NPAs from children with SARI in Shanghai, in which HRV-A and -C were predominate. Among the 77 HRV genotypes detected, A78, A12, A89, B70, C2, C6, and C24 were the most frequent. The HRV species responsible for SARIs differs according to season and age.

AUTHOR CONTRIBUTIONS

RL, JS, and WT conceived and designed the experiments. YZ, RL, JS, BW, and GL performed the experiments. RL, JS, and WT analyzed the data. RL and WT wrote the manuscript.

FUNDING

This work was supported by the Control and Prevention of Major Infectious Disease of China (2017ZX10104001-002-003 and 2014ZX10004001-002), and the National Key Research and Development Program of China (2016YFD0500301 and 2016YFC1200200). The funders had no role in the study design, data collection and analysis, decision to publish, or preparation of the manuscript.

ACKNOWLEDGMENTS

The authors would like to thank the staffs of the Children Hospital of Fudan University, Shanghai, China for providing samples.

REFERENCES

Bizzintino, J., Lee, W. M., Laing, I. A., Vang, F., Pappas, T., Zhang, G., et al. (2011). Association between human rhinovirus C and severity of asthma in children. *Eur. Respir. J.* 37, 1037–1042. doi: 10.1183/09031936.00092410

Blaschke, A. J., Korgenski, E. K., Wilkes, J., Presson, A. P., Thorell, E. A., Pavia, A. T., et al. (2018). Rhinovirus in febrile infants and risk of bacterial infection. *Pediatrics* 141:e20172384. doi: 10.1542/peds.2017-2384

Chen, W. J., Arnold, J. C., Fairchok, M. P., Danaher, P. J., McDonough, E. A., Blair, P. J., et al. (2015). Epidemiologic, clinical, and virologic characteristics of human rhinovirus infection among otherwise healthy children and adults: rhinovirus among adults and children. *J. Clin. Virol.* 64, 74–82. doi: 10.1016/j.jcv.2015.01.007

da Silva Filho, L. V., Zerbinati, R. M., Tateno, A. F., Boas, L. V., de Almeida, M. B., Levi, J. E., et al. (2012). The differential clinical impact of human coronavirus species in children with cystic fibrosis. *J. Infect. Dis.* 206, 384–388. doi: 10.1093/infdis/jis274

Esposito, S., Daleno, C., Prunotto, G., Scala, A., Tagliabue, C., Borzani, I., et al. (2013). Impact of viral infections in children with community-acquired pneumoniae: results of a study of 17 respiratory viruses. *Influenza Other Respir. Viruses* 7, 18–26 doi: 10.1111/j.1750-2659.2012.00340.x

Fawkner-Corbett, D. W., Khoo, S. K., Duarte, C. M., Bezerra, P. G., Bochkov, Y. A., Gern, J. E., et al. (2016). Rhinovirus-C detection in children presenting with acute respiratory infection to hospital in Brazil. *J. Med. Virol.* 88, 58–63 doi: 10.1002/jmv.24300

Gern, J. E. (2010). The ABCs of rhinoviruses, wheezing, and asthma. *J. Virol.* 84, 7418–7426. doi: 10.1128/JVI.02290-09

Henquell, C., Mirand, A., Deusebis, A. L., Regagnon, C., Archimbaud, C., Chambon, M., et al. (2012). Prospective genotyping of human rhinoviruses in children and adults during the winter of 2009-2010. *J. Clin. Virol.* 53, 280–284 doi: 10.1016/j.jcv.2011.10.009

Honkinen, M., Lahti, F., Osterback, R., Ruuskanen, O., and Waris, M. (2012). Viruses and bacteria in sputum samples of children with community-acquired pneumonia. *Clin. Microbiol. Infect.* 18, 300–307 doi: 10.1111/j.1469-0691.2011.03603.x

Kuroda, M., Niwa, S., Sekizuka, T., Tsukagoshi, H., Yokoyama, M., Ryo, A., et al. (2015). Molecular evolution of the VP1, VP2, and VP3 genes in human rhinovirus species C. *Sci. Rep.* 5:8185. doi: 10.1038/srep08185

Lambert, K. A., Prendergast, L. A., Dharmage, S. C., Tang, M., O'Sullivan, M., Tran, T., et al. (2017). The role of human rhinovirus (HRV) species on asthma exacerbation severity in children and adolescents. *J. Asthma* 55, 596–602. doi: 10.1080/02770903.2017.1362425

Lamson, D., Renwick, N., Kapoor, V., Liu, Z., Palacios, G., Ju, J., et al. (2006). MassTag polymerase-chain-reaction detection of respiratory pathogens, including a new rhinovirus genotype, that caused influenza-like illness in New York State during 2004-2005. *J. Infect. Dis.* 194, 1398–1402. doi: 10.1086/508551

Lau, S. K. P., Yip, C. C. Y., Tsoi, H. W., Lee, R. A., So, L. Y., Lau, Y. L., et al. (2007). Clinical features and complete genome characterization of a distinct human rhinovirus (HRV) genetic cluster, probably representing a previously undetected HRV species HRV-C, associated with acute respiratory illness in children. *J. Clin. Microbiol.* 45, 3655–3664 doi: 10.1128/JCM.01254-07

Lee, W. M., Lemanske, R. F. Jr., Evans, M. D., Vang, F., Pappas, T., Gangnon, R., et al. (2012). Human rhinovirus species and season of infection determine illness severity. *Am. J. Respir. Crit. Care Med.* 186, 886–891. doi: 10.1164/rccm.201202-0330OC

Linsuwanon, P., Payungporn, S., Samransamruajkit, R., Posuwan, N., Makkoch, J., Theanboonlers, A., et al. (2009). High prevalence of human rhinovirus C infection in Thai children with acute lower respiratory tract disease. *J. Infect.* 59, 115–121. doi: 10.1016/j.jinf.2009.05.009

Lu, R., Yu, X., Wang, W., Duan, X., Zhang, L., Zhou, W., et al. (2012). Characterization of human coronavirus etiology in Chinese adults with acute upper respiratory tract infection by real-time RT-PCR assays. *PLoS ONE* 7:e38638. doi: 10.1371/journal.pone.0038638

Lu, X., Schneider, E., Jain, S., Bramley, A. M., Hymas, W., Stockmann, C., et al. (2017). Rhinovirus viremia in patients hospitalized with community-acquired pneumonia. *J. Infect. Dis.* 216, 1104–1111. doi: 10.1093/infdis/jix455

Marcone, D. N., Culasso, A., Carballal, G., Campos, R., and Echavarría, M. (2014). Genetic diversity and clinical impact of human rhinoviruses in hospitalized and outpatient children with acute respiratory infection, Argentina. *J. Clin. Virol.* 61, 558–564. doi: 10.1016/j.jcv.2014.10.006

Milanoi, S., Ongus, J. R., Gachara, G., Coldren, R., and Bulimo, W. (2016). Serotype and genetic diversity of human rhinovirus strains that circulated in Kenya in 2008. *Influenza Other Respir. Viruses* 10, 185–191. doi: 10.1111/irv.12373

Miller, E. K., Williams, J. V., Gebretsadik, T., Carroll, K. N., Dupont, W. D., Mohamed, Y. A., et al. (2011). Host and viral factors associated with severity of human rhinovirus-associated infant respiratory tract illness. *J. Allergy Clin. Immunol.* 127, 883–891. doi: 10.1016/j.jaci.2010.11.041

Naughtin, M., Sareth, R., Sentilhes, A. C., Vong, S., Joffret, M. L., Cornillot, E., et al. (2015). Genetic diversity of human rhinoviruses in Cambodia during a three-year period reveals novel genetic types. *Infect. Genet. Evol.* 35, 42–49. doi: 10.1016/j.meegid.2015.07.030

Price, W. H. (1956). The isolation of a new virus associated with respiratory clinical disease in humans. *Proc. Natl. Acad. Sci. U.S.A.* 42, 892–896 doi: 10.1073/pnas.42.12.892

Rahamat-Langendoen, J. C., Riezebos-Brilman, A., Hak, E., Schölvinck, E. H., and Niesters, H. G. (2013). The significance of rhinovirus detection in hospitalized children: clinical, epidemiological and virological features. *Clin. Microbiol. Infect.* 19, 435–442. doi: 10.1111/1469-0691.12242

Tsatsral, S., Xiang, Z., Fuji, N., Maitsetseg, C., Khulan, J., Oshitani, H., et al. (2015). Molecular Epidemiology of the Human Rhinovirus Infection in Mongolia during 2008-2013. *Jpn. J. Infect. Dis.* 68, 280–287. doi: 10.7883/yoken.JJID.2014.090

van der Linden, L., Bruning, A. H., Thomas, X. V., Minnaar, R. P., Rebers, S. P., Schinkel, J., et al. (2016). A molecular epidemiological perspective of rhinovirus types circulating in Amsterdam from 2007 to 2012. *Clin. Microbiol. Infect.* 22, 1002–1002. doi: 10.1016/j.cmi.2016.08.007

Wang, Y., Zhu, N., Li, Y., Lu, R., Wang, H., Liu, G., et al. (2016). Metagenomic analysis of viral genetic diversity in respiratory samples from children with severe acute respiratory infection in China. *Clin. Microbiol. Infect.* 22, 458–459. doi: 10.1016/j.cmi.2016.01.006

Wisdom, A., Leitch, E. C., Gaunt, E., Harvala, H., and Simmonds, P. (2009). Screening respiratory samples for detection of human rhinoviruses (HRVs) and enteroviruses: comprehensive VP4-VP2 typing reveals high incidence and genetic diversity of HRV species C. *J. Clin. Microbiol.* 47, 3958–3967. doi: 10.1128/JCM.00993-09

World Health Organization [WHO] (2011). *Global Technical Consultation: Global Standards and Tools for Influenza Surveillance*. Geneva: World Health Organization, 2011.

Xiang, Z., Gonzalez, R., Xie, Z., Xiao, Y., Liu, J., Chen, L., et al. (2010). Human rhinovirus C infections mirror those of human rhinovirus A in children with community-acquired pneumonia. *J. Clin. Virol.* 49, 94–99. doi: 10.1016/j.jcv.2010.07.013

Xiao, Q., Zheng, S., Zhou, L., Ren, L., Xie, X., Deng, Y., et al. (2015). Impact of Human Rhinovirus Types and Viral Load on the Severity of Illness in Hospitalized Children With Lower Respiratory Tract Infections. *Pediatr. Infect. Dis. J.* 34, 1187–1192. doi: 10.1097/INF.0000000000000879

Zhang, C., Zhu, N., Xie, Z., Lu, R., He, B., Liu, C., et al. (2013). Viral etiology and clinical profiles of children with severe acute respiratory infections in China. *PLoS ONE* 8:e72606. doi: 10.1371/journal.pone.0072606

13

Enterovirus D68 – The New Polio?

*Hayley Cassidy, Randy Poelman, Marjolein Knoester, Coretta C. Van Leer-Buter and Hubert G. M. Niesters**

Department of Medical Microbiology and Infection Prevention, Division of Clinical Virology, University of Groningen, University Medical Center Groningen, Groningen, Netherlands

***Correspondence:**
Hubert G. M. Niesters
h.g.m.niesters@umcg.nl

Enterovirus D68 (EV-D68) has emerged over the recent years, with large outbreaks worldwide. Increased occurrence has coincided with improved clinical awareness and surveillance of non-polio enteroviruses. Studies showing its neurotropic nature and the change in pathogenicity have established EV-D68 as a probable cause of Acute Flaccid Myelitis (AFM). The EV-D68 storyline shows many similarities with poliovirus a century ago, stimulating discussion whether EV-D68 could be ascertaining itself as the "new polio." Increasing awareness amongst clinicians, incorporating proper diagnostics and integrating EV-D68 into accessible surveillance systems in a way that promotes data sharing, will be essential to reveal the burden of disease. This will be a necessary step in preventing EV-D68 from becoming a threat to public health.

Keywords: Enterovirus D68, emerging, pathogenicity, surveillance, outbreak response

INTRODUCTION

Enterovirus D68: The Virus

Enterovirus D68 is a single-stranded positive-sense RNA virus of the *Picornaviridae* family, belonging to the species enterovirus D. EV-D68 was first isolated from respiratory samples in 1962 in California, United States from four pediatric patients presenting with acute respiratory symptoms. The four isolates obtained from the patients were referred to as the Fermon, Franklin, Robinson,and Rhyne strains, each presenting with similar antigenic properties. As a representative strain of the new serotype, the Fermon strain was selected (Imamura and Oshitani, 2015). Since its first description, EV-D68 has been classified into three genetic clades, A, B and C. Subclades A1, A2, B1, and B2 have evolved and can be further identified depending on enterovirus typing, targeting either VP1 or VP4-2 capsid protein (Nix et al., 2006; Esposito et al., 2015). EV-D68 was also previously known as rhinovirus 87 until it was re-classified in 2002 (Blomqvist et al., 2002). EV-D68 is unusual in that it has shared characteristics from two key members of the *Picornaviridae* family; enterovirus and rhinovirus. Firstly, it has a lower optimal growth temperature of 33°C (the temperature of the nose), allowing better replication in the nasal cavity than other EV, and secondly it is acid

Abbreviations: AFM, acute flaccid myelitis; AFP, acute flaccid paralysis; CDC, Centers for Disease Control and Prevention; CNS, central nerve system; CSF, cerebral spinal fluid; EC50, lower effective concentration; ECDC, European Centre for Disease Prevention and Control; ENPEN, European Non-Polio Enterovirus Network; ESCV, European Society of Clinical Virology; EV, enteroviruses; EV-A71, enterovirus A71; EV-D68, enterovirus D68; FDA, Food and Drug Administration; GBS, Guillain-Barré syndrome; GPEI, Global Polio Eradication Initiative; hIVIG, human intravenous immunoglobulin; ICAM-5, neuron-expressed intercellular adhesion molecule 5; IP, intraperitoneally; MRI, magnetic resonance imaging; NCIRD, The National Center for Immunization and Respiratory Diseases; NGS, next generation sequencing; NNDSS, National Notifiable Diseases Surveillance System; PAHO, Pan American Health Organization; RNA, ribonucleic acid; RT-PCR, reverse transcriptase PCR; USA, United States; UTR, untranslated region; VP1, viral protein 1; VP4-2, Complete viral protein 4 and partial viral protein 2; WHO, World Health Organization; WNV, West Nile virus.

sensitive, meaning it is unable to adequately survive during passage in the stomach (Foster et al., 2015). Phylogeny however, shows that EV-D68 is genetically more closely related to EV than to rhinoviruses. Studies into the cellular receptors of EV-D68 have shown that it targets the α2-6-linked sialic acid, which is present on cells in the upper respiratory tract, indicating tropism toward this area (Imamura et al., 2014). This critical difference in tropism is significant when comparing EV-D68 to poliovirus, which predominantly reproduces in the gastrointestinal tract. It is likely that most EV-D68 infections are asymptomatic or present with a mild respiratory illness however, it is difficult to know it's true circulation and burden on the community. Nevertheless, studies have indicated that circulation of EV-D68 increases over the summer-autumn season like with other EV (Tokarz et al., 2012).

The Beginning of Enterovirus Awareness – The Polio Era

Enteroviruses are thought to have existed and coevolved with humanity for thousands of years. One of the oldest records of enterovirus is an Egyptian carving thought to illustrate a priest with a small, weakened limb, which is considered a typical feature of a past polio infection. The causative agent of poliomyelitis (poliovirus), was not discovered until 1908 (Paul, 1971). It was not only the first enterovirus to be discovered, but also caused the most devastating and widespread morbidity and mortality of all the enterovirus genotypes. Poliovirus infection can result in a variety of symptoms, of which AFP that can cause lifelong disability and may result in death, is the most typical clinical entity. Awareness of polio increased during the 20th century. This is largely attributed to President Franklin Roosevelt, himself paralyzed from polio, who was instrumental in founding the National Foundation for Infantile Paralysis which started mass worldwide vaccination campaigns (Noor and Krilov, 2016). The first poliovirus vaccine was an inactivated injectable vaccine, developed by Jonas Salk in 1955. The second vaccine administered orally, was a vaccine developed by Albert Sabin in 1961 (Noor and Krilov, 2016). These primary awareness programs, together with the vaccination campaign, initiated in the fifties, paved the way for the GPEI created in 1988, which aimed to eradicate the virus. Over the subsequent years, following the initial discovery of poliovirus, over 100 enterovirus serotypes have now been discovered with nearly 70 species infecting humans (Craighead, 2000). Non-polio EV can cause a variety of clinical syndromes, ranging from hand-foot and mouth disease to aseptic meningitis.

sThe introduction of the poliovirus vaccine dramatically reduced the incidence of infections globally, with only small clusters sporadically occurring. According to the GPEI, only two countries, Afghanistan and Pakistan still report endemic wild-type poliovirus in circulation in 2018 (The Global Poliovirus Eradication Initiative [GPEI], 2018). Recently, the GPEI also reported a few new cases of vaccine-derived poliovirus in the Democratic Republic of the Congo, Nigeria, Somalia and Papua New Guinea (The Global Poliovirus Eradication Initiative [GPEI], 2018). Therefore, cases of AFP outside these countries have decreased to very low numbers. Remaining cases of AFP are also linked to GBS and neurological infections caused by other viruses such as WNV and more recently, non-polio EV.

The Rise in Awareness of EV-D68

In the majority of patients, EV-D68 only causes mild respiratory illness. However, the co-occurrence of EV-D68 and a predominantly severe respiratory disease on one side and neurological complications of "polio-like" paralysis on the other side has established EV-D68 as an emerging pathogen (Holm-Hansen et al., 2016). While EV-D68 has been known as a respiratory pathogen since its first description in 1962, the apparent change in pathogenicity into a virus capable of causing AFP over a relatively short period of time, has led to increased interest and awareness of the virus in recent years. This is reflected in the number of published papers. **Figure 1** reveals the result of a PubMed search for Enterovirus-D68. With the disappearance of poliovirus as a major threat to public health, enterovirus networks such as the ENPEN, have been set up along with established networks such as the ESCV to focus on non-polio EV which may become new challenges (Harvala et al., 2018). EV-D68 has become a compelling topic for research over the recent years, due to a mix of increased prevalence, pathology and awareness. This review will explore the EV-D68 story further.

Epidemiology: From Sporadic Respiratory Virus to Emerging Neuropathogenic Threat

Enterovirus D68 had only been reported sporadically worldwide since 2010. Indeed before 2014, only sporadic outbreaks were reported in the US, the Philippines, Japan and the Netherlands (Rahamat-Langendoen et al., 2011; Gong et al., 2016). Significantly, there were only 26 cases reported in the United States between 1970 and 2005 and only 699 cases described in Europe, Southeast Asia and Africa between 1970 and 2013 (Holm-Hansen et al., 2016; Wang et al., 2017). However, it must be noted that specific testing for EV-D68 or routine

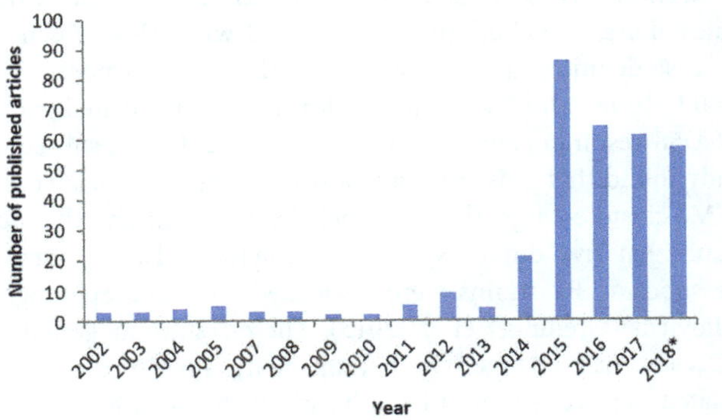

FIGURE 1 | The number of published articles on PubMed describing Enterovirus-D68 from January 2002 to October2018. The number of published articles for each year is in accordance with EV-D68 interest from the previous year. *Until October.

typing for EV was and is not standard practice in the majority of laboratories and assuredly not for testing respiratory samples. Therefore the true burden of disease is not known and trends have been likely to be missed. A study published in 2012 reports the analysis of trends in EV-D68 circulation across the United States and in Africa over two decades (Tokarz et al., 2012). This was a direct result of increasing sporadic reports of respiratory disease associated with EV-D68 across North America, Europe and Asia. The study found the genome had undergone a rearrangement from the initial Fermon strain in the spacer region of the 5′UTR, which is known to affect the translational efficiency and thought to increase the virulence. Further rearrangement led to a separation into clades A, B and C, with additional deletions within each clade. Interestingly, another study (Kaida et al., 2017) reported clade B had specific substitutions in the BC-loop, which is found on the surface canyon of the VP1 protein, known to have a role in antigenicity. This evolution may have had significant implications in the run up to the 2014 outbreak, but remains unclear so far.

The 2014 Outbreak

In August 2014, the United States and Canada experienced the first few cases of what resulted in the largest known EV-D68 outbreak in history. An unprecedented number of cases, particularly in young children, of severe-respiratory illness was linked to EV-D68 infections. Unexpectedly, this outbreak of severe respiratory infections coincided with an upsurge in AFP. Many of the affected children were also shown to have concurrent EV-D68 infections. The Polio and Picornavirus Laboratory Branch of the CDC tested 56 respiratory samples and found EV-D68 to be the most commonly detected pathogen, with an overall rate of 20% (11/56) in samples tested. Furthermore the detection increased to 47% (8/17) in samples collected near onset of respiratory illness (≤7 days) (Sejvar et al., 2016). Fifty-five CSF specimens were also tested and found to have one positive EV-D68 sample (also positive for Epstein-Barr virus) (Sejvar et al., 2016). The paralysis seen in patients infected with EV-D68 was clinically defined as AFM which was essentially, an acute onset of AFP with MRI scans showing motor neuron damage in the myelum. This will be discussed more in detail later in see section "EV-D68 Case Definition." In 2014, in the United States alone, 120 children were reported with AFM which met the case definition (Messacar et al., 2016). Furthermore, over a 1000 hospital admissions and 12 deaths were associated with an EV-D68 respiratory infection (Levy et al., 2015). A subsequent study found that most EV-D68 positive samples associated with AFM, clustered into the B1 subclade. Interestingly, the study found that five out of six coding polymorphisms present in the subclade B1 strains were associated with neuropathogenic poliovirus (Greninger et al., 2015). These results suggested that the virus had changed in pathogenicity since the originally isolated Fermon strain, a hypothesis which was also supported by results of studies in mice models (Hixon et al., 2017b), which will be discussed later.

At that time, severe respiratory outbreaks of EV-68 were reported from several countries across Europe in 2014. During these outbreaks, cases of AFM were identified, including one in France and in the United Kingdom and two in Norway (Lang et al., 2014; Pfeiffer et al., 2015; Varghese et al., 2015; Holm-Hansen et al., 2016). It is still unclear how frequently EV-D68 causes AFM compared to the number of respiratory infections caused by this virus. Estimating this frequency is currently impossible, firstly as the background circulation of this relatively emerging virus is unknown and secondly, only children with severe respiratory illness were tested in the 2014 outbreak in the United States and in Canada, therefore there is no information on the frequency at which EV-D68 causes mild symptoms. One study investigated EV-D68 detection by country, mostly in Northern and Western Europe, during the United States outbreak (Poelman et al., 2015b). Out of 17,248 respiratory (majority) specimens tested, 4273 had confirmed picornavirus detection with 389 samples positive for EV-D68. In Southern and Eastern Europe, too few samples were tested to draw any conclusions. Hence, crucial information about how large the threat of EV-D68 could be, is still missing.

Regarding poliomyelitis, studies have shown that 1 in 200 poliovirus infections led to irreversible paralysis, with 5–10% of paralysis cases resulting in death due to breathing difficulties (World Health Organization [WHO], 2018). As AFP is not a reportable disease in many countries, as long as it is not caused by poliovirus, it is impossible to say how many potential cases of EV-D68 associated AFM have occurred during upsurges of EV-D68 in the past few years. As the link between EV-D68 and AFM had not been established at that time, many children who presented with sudden paralysis were not adequately sampled to detect EV-D68. Subsequent data from the EV-D68 outbreak in the United States and Canada in 2014 indicates that neurological complications could occur in 1 out of 100 symptomatic cases with a total of 1153 confirmed EV-D68 respiratory infections, and 12 EV-D68 positive AFM cases during this period (Sejvar et al., 2016). Similarly, in Europe, out of 389 confirmed positive samples in 2014, four AFM cases and one death were associated with EV-D68 (Poelman et al., 2015b; Varghese et al., 2015). Limited EV-D68 detection was seen both in the United States and in Europe in 2015 (Wang et al., 2017).

The 2016 Outbreak

In 2016, a new upsurge in the number of EV-D68 cases was first reported from the Netherlands. The majority of patients presented with severe respiratory illness, but one case of AFM was seen in a 4-year-old boy (Knoester et al., 2017). Phylogenetic analysis of the samples revealed a different clustering to the 2014 outbreak strains. Simultaneously, similar upsurges were described by groups in Norway, Denmark, Germany, France, Spain, Portugal, Sweden, Wales (United Kingdom), Scotland (United Kingdom) and in the United States (Dyrdak et al., 2016; ECDC, 2016; Wang et al., 2017). In addition, cases of EV-D68 were also linked with AFM in Wales (2 cases), Scotland (5 cases), England (1 case), Sweden (3 cases), Italy (2 cases), Spain (3 cases), France (at least 1) and Argentina (15 cases) with strains clustering with a divergent B3 lineage (Antona et al., 2016; Dyrdak et al., 2016, ECDC, 2016; PAHO/WHO, 2016; Williams et al., 2016; Cabrerizo et al., 2017; Esposito et al., 2017; Giombini et al., 2017; Kirolos et al., 2017; Stacpoole et al., 2017). A subsequent surveillance study (Knoester et al., 2018) presented the results of a survey which found a total of 29 cases reported of EV-D68 infections associated with AFM in Europe in 2016. Interestingly, a higher number of EV-D68-associated AFM cases were reported in Europe in 2016 compared to 2014; 29 versus four cases in 2014. This could suggest the "new" circulating B3 subclade is more neuropathogenic or perhaps more transmissible than the B1 clade, which was most frequently reported in 2014. However, this most likely is due to increased surveillance and awareness established in 2014. In the United States, 149 AFM cases were reported in 2016, yet the exact number of AFM cases associated with EV-D68 is not known. Although there were fewer reported EV-D68 infections in 2016 in the United States overall, some AFM cases associated with EV-D68 were reported by Wang et al., 2017.

Diagnosing an Enterovirus D68 Infection

Sample Collection

Depending on the clinical picture, several diagnostic samples can and should be collected to detect EV, such as CSF, feces, respiratory material and serum/plasma (Harvala et al., 2018). As most EV are transmitted via the fecal-oral route and replicate in the intestine, high viral loads are usually present in feces, therefore an effective material for detection and genotyping. Genotyping or serotyping are necessary and mandatory in cases of AFP to exclude poliovirus, and stool samples are essential to achieve this. However, EV-D68 is not readily detected in fecal samples, in addition it has a rhinovirus-like replication cycle in the nasal cavity. Indeed, the recently published PAHO/WHO report now recommends including a respiratory sample if AFP is suspected (PAHO/WHO report, 2017). Animal models have shown that EV-D68 can also disseminate to the CNS by retrograde axonal transport (Morrey et al., 2018). Multiple material types should therefore be collected if a patient presents with CNS symptoms: stool, CSF, blood and respiratory samples (Harvala et al., 2018).

Molecular Testing for Pan-Enterovirus Detection

Molecular testing is recognized as the gold standard for diagnosing an enterovirus infection. RT-PCR targeting the 5′UTR region has been established as a routine molecular test in many laboratories throughout Europe and other parts of the world (Harvala et al., 2018). It is used as a broad spectrum assay to detect the presence of EV, without regard to specific subtypes. The majority of assays are laboratory developed tests and can be used to screen a panel of suspected pathogens or to detect a specific target. Rapid and self-contained specimen-to-result tests such as the FilmArray system (BioFire/bioMerieux, Salt Lake City, United States) have also been used to screen and identify enterovirus /rhinovirus simultaneously by combining a nested multiplex PCR with melting curve analysis (Poritz et al., 2011). However, further tests would be needed as the FilmArray cannot distinguish enterovirus from rhinovirus. Additional FDA approved tests for enterovirus detection are the Cepheid GeneXpert and SmartCycler (Cepheid, Sunnyvale, California, United States). Finally, cell cultures can be used, however, they are not suitable for all enterovirus strains and further identification is required, using serotyping methods or real-time RT PCR.

A specific RT-PCR was developed to detect EV-D68 during a European surveillance project in 2014 (Poelman et al., 2015b). During an EV-D68 season (Summer-Autumn) or during an upsurge of the virus, a specific RT-PCR could be used for rapid diagnostics and patient management, and is particularly useful in the work-up of severe respiratory infections and AFM. During the 2014 outbreak, a study was carried out where the FilmArray system was used to detect positive enterovirus samples through its enterovirus/rhinovirus signals in a respiratory panel (Shibib et al., 2016). It was consequently found that a positive detection in the Rhinovirus 1 and 4 targets led to a high association (13.1× more likely) of EV-D68 found in subsequent samples sent to the CDC for confirmation. Further point of care tests were also evaluated during the outbreak. Similarly, the GenMark eSensor respiratory viral panel (Carlsbad, California, United States) was found to pick up low-positive rhinoviruses which were later found to be EV-D68 in 67% of samples, with a 94% sensitivity and 88% specificity rate (McAllister et al., 2015). This was subsequently noted due to cross-reactivity with rhinoviruses (McAllister et al., 2015; Diaz-Decaro et al., 2018).

Molecular Testing for Genotyping

Sanger sequencing of the VP1, and occasionally VP4-2 structural proteins, following detection of a positive EV sample is considered the gold standard for the determination of specific EV genotypes, according to World Health Organization (WHO) guidelines and Nix et al., 2006. Type specific RT-PCR and Sanger sequencing techniques have been used increasingly during outbreaks of EV-A71 in Asia and EV-D68 in the United States and Europe (Poelman et al., 2015a; Duong et al., 2016). Sequencing has transformed diagnostics, increasing the amount of knowledge on pathogens, their circulation and phylogeny. Phylogenetic analysis can be used more efficiently to look for genetic relationships within the EV subtype. However, typing enterovirus remains difficult due to vast variations in the genome (Midgley et al., 2015).

The development of these molecular tests has also allowed for the rapid detection and reporting of results in real time. A steady flow of epidemiological data should be available from health agencies or regional centers and fed back to the performing labs, and vice versa. This is not always optimal, and improvements could be achieved through for example the Antimicrobial, Infection and Prevention and Diagnostic stewardship model (Dik et al., 2016).

Next Generation Sequencing

Next generation sequencing, in comparison to the Sanger targeted approach, allows for the sequencing of multiple reads at once by reading optical signals after each base addition (Escalona et al., 2016). Useful information about changes in tropism or pathogenicity has been obtained by NGS. A retrospective study into the diversity of EV-D68 during the United States outbreak in 2014 using NGS technologies (metagenomic shotgun sequencing) revealed specific polymorphisms C3277A and A4020G, which triggered functional mutations at cleavage sites

$2A^{pro}$ and $3C^{pro}$ respectively (Huang et al., 2015). These amino acid substitutions are suspected to alter protease activity and increase replication and transmission rates. The group also found similar mutations in a 2013 strain (US/CO/13-60), thought to be an ancestor of the 2014 outbreak strains. Indeed these coding polymorphisms were found to be present in poliovirus, as mentioned previously (Huang et al., 2015).

EV-D68 ASSOCIATION WITH ACUTE FLACCID MYELITIS (AFM)

The Strength of EV-D68 Association With AFM

The upsurge in infection and awareness has led to the expansion of current scientific knowledge, with several groups now investigating the depth of the association of EV-D68 with AFM. Many begin by describing the paralleling of numbers from the CDC for EV-D68 infections and the cases of AFM for 2014–2018 (**Figure 2**; Dyda et al., 2018; Messacar et al., 2018). From looking at the literature, during and after the United States 2014 outbreak, similar upsurges of severe respiratory and neurological symptoms were found worldwide, most notably in Northern Europe. The association was further strengthened by a group (Aliabadi et al., 2016) which found infection with EV-D68 resulted in a higher odds ratio than two control groups (10× and 4.5× respectfully) for AFM presentation. Furthermore, the respiratory prodromal phase prior to paralysis in 65% of patients (Martin et al., 2016), along with a high involvement of the cranial and spinal cord, appear to be more specifically associated with an EV-D68 infection (Messacar et al., 2018). Additionally, AFM mainly affects children, similarly to EV-D68, which indicates a specific target population (Dyda et al., 2018).

One of the challenges of the association is that EV-D68 is not always detected in clinical samples from AFM patients. One group (Greninger et al., 2015) found EV-D68 in respiratory samples in approximately 48% of AFM patients (25 cases), where no other pathogen including EV-D68, could be detected in CSF samples. Indeed, as discussed previously, detection of EV-D68 in CSF is uncommon. This has only been reported in a handful of cases (Kreuter et al., 2011; Esposito et al., 2016; Giombini et al., 2017; Ruggieri et al., 2017). A recent paper (Morrey et al., 2018) investigated this link through mouse models, deficient in interferon responses. Mice were challenged IP with EV-D68 of a known viral load. These researchers detected EV-D68 in the spinal cord just at early onset of paralysis, compared with the muscle injection site, which persisted for 6 weeks. The fact that the virus does not reside in the spinal cord for long could reflect the challenges in EV-D68 detection in CSF samples. Other viruses causing neurological disease including poliovirus, EV-A71, WNV and Rabies are similarly absent from CSF (Huang and Shih, 2015). Awareness of research in this area is particularly important for clinicians, as once an association is proven, they may be more inclined to take a respiratory sample and request for EV-D68 testing as well, during suspected AFM cases.

Experiments Revealing the Neurotropic Nature of EV-D68

The unprecedented upsurge in AFM associated with EV-D68 has led to many questions into why this emerging virus has become

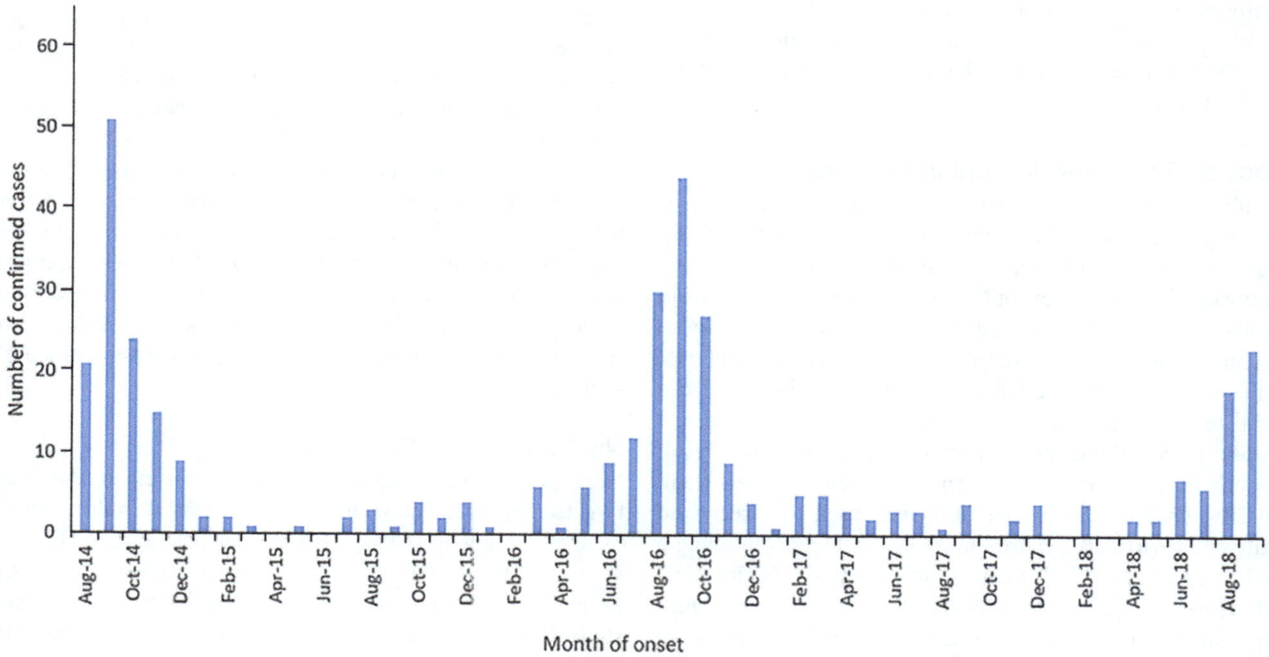

FIGURE 2 | The number of confirmed United States AFM cases, published on the CDC by month of onset from August 2014-October 2018. The high number of confirmed AFM cases coincided with the 2014, 2016 and 2018 EV-D68 outbreaks. Figure taken from the NCIRD, AFM in the United States 2018.

so pathogenic, leading to the polio-like paralysis observed. At present the exact mechanism which EV-D68 uses to instigate infection remains largely unknown. Studies have shown that poliovirus can gain access to the CNS through axonal transport and neuromuscular junctions (Ohka et al., 1998; Huang and Shih, 2015), and it could be possible that EV-D68 follows a similar mechanism. A recent study in an EV-D68 mouse model, links paralysis to infections with EV-D68 through intramuscular injection by using various strains of the virus, including the 2014 outbreak strains. These injections resulted in the loss of motor neurons in the anterior horn of the corresponding spinal cord segments, leading to paralyzed limbs. The study goes on to suggest that replication of the virus in the motor neurons causes the damage, paralleling the development of neurological symptoms (Hixon et al., 2017b). Significantly, the study fulfills Koch's postulates by activating paralysis in naïve mice from EV-D68 isolated from the spinal cord of a paralyzed mouse.

Much is still unknown about the exact mechanism EV-D68 uses to gain entry and replicate. Recently, a group investigating the life cycle of EV-D68 has started to answer some of the questions (Baggen et al., 2018). It was found that EV-D68 binds to synthetic glycoproteins through a terminally linked sialic acid. This binding induces a conformational change in the viral capsid, which commences the uncoating process, to inject the RNA and initiate the replication (Baggen et al., 2018). Sialic acid has been understood to be a binding site for other EV, such as Coxsackievirus A24, which was associated with acute haemorrhagic conjunctivitis (Baggen et al., 2018).

Wei et al. (2016) identified ICAM-5 as a possible entry receptor for EV-D68. EV-D68 was believed to bind to the ICAM-5-Fc receptor, where sialic acid was thought to induce a conformation change. Crucially, the telencephalon region of the brain was found to have enhanced ICAM-5 expression, this receptor could help explain the neurotropism of this virus (Wei et al., 2016; Messacar et al., 2018). Herpes Simplex Virus-1, another well-known neurotropic virus, also interacts with ICAM-5 to mediate cytokine secretion during infection (Tse et al., 2009). Although these studies shed a light on how EV-D68 may achieve its neuro-invasive capability, many more questions remain concerning the factors which determine the variability in disease severity which is seen in clinical cases. It is possible that changes in the genome, through mutational or selection pressure, led to an altered pathogenicity. Evidence in favor of this hypothesis has been shown by other authors, describing genogroup replacement between 2006 and 2014 (Xiang et al., 2016), and specific mutations in the puff region (key neutralization site) of VP2 in EV-D68 strains, which were isolated from patients with severe respiratory infections. Xiang et al. (2016) goes on to describe a mutational difference between the sequences obtained from the United States and China strains. In the United States strains there was a mutation in the pseudoknot structure in 3′-UTR, resulting in an altered phenotype comparatively to the Chinese strains. This could account for the differences in outbreaks between the United States and China in 2014.

EV-D68 Case Definition

Although EV-D68 has shown similar neurological presentation to poliovirus, as well as similar MRI features, it has its own specific case definition. In response to the increased number of severe respiratory infections and number of acute paralysis cases during the 2014 outbreak the CDC proposed the case definition; "*onset of acute limb weakness on or after August 1, 2014, and a magnetic resonance image (MRI) showing a spinal cord lesion largely restricted to gray matter in a patient age ≤ 21 years*" (Washington State Department of Health, 2016). AFP patients who presented with pleocytosis (white blood cells $>5\ mm^3$) in their CSF who had a negative or no MRI result were recommended as a probable case. The terms AFM and AFP are used interchangeably in articles and reports from 2014. Adding to the confusion is the restriction of the AFM case definition to individuals younger than 21 years of age, as it is currently understood that AFM does occur in adults as well. Although mostly children with a chronic illness were affected, children and adults without any known underlying condition were also reported (Williams et al., 2016; Stacpoole et al., 2017). Additionally, it must be updated in accordance with increased data gained from reports.

The establishment of a case definition for AFM was particularly important as other diseases such as GBS, may also present with AFP. Although, paralysis tends to be more symmetrical in GBS (Jasti et al., 2016). Cases of EV-D68 associated AFM could be diagnosed as "atypical-GBS," unless an MRI scan is made or electromyography examinations are carried out. Typically, EV-D68 associated AFM develops following acute febrile respiratory syndrome, up to 2 weeks prior to onset of weakness (Tyler, 2015). Prodromal symptoms compatible with respiratory infections including shortness of breath (82%), cough (82%), and rhinorrhoea or nasal congestion (71%) (Martin et al., 2016) could be incorporated into the case definition.

Clinical Characteristics and Diagnosis of EV-D68 AFM

Patients presenting with a suspected EV-D68 associated AFM should undergo a series of examinations to confirm this diagnosis. One of the most valuable examinations, MRI, was used extensively during the 2014 outbreak to facilitate the establishment of a case definition. Patients can present with a variety of symptoms varying from cough, runny nose and diarrhea to muscles aches, fever and in some cases respiratory distress, particularly in children younger than five (National Center for Immunization and Respiratory Diseases [NCIRD], Division of Viral Diseases, 2017; Knoester et al., 2018). AFM symptoms are typically described as asymmetric motor weakness mostly affecting the upper limbs in the majority of current known cases. The weakness is flaccid, with deep-tendon reflexes reduced or absent (CDC and NCIRD, 2015). The cranial nerves are commonly affected with symptoms such as facial weakness, dysarthria and dysphagia being described (Tyler, 2015). Most patients did undergo a spinal tap on presentation, which showed cerebrospinal fluid pleocytosis in the majority of cases (Tyler, 2015). An MRI scan is essential for the diagnosis, as it shows lesions in the anterior horn of the gray matter along the spinal cord and sometimes in the brainstem (Tyler, 2015). As shown in the MRI images (**Figures 3,4**), these distinctive lesions point at the involvement of the spinal cord motor neurons. It must be noted that the lesions seen on the MRI scans during cases of EV-D68 associated AFM are identical to lesions in the spinal cord which are found in poliomyelitis. Diagnosing a case of AFM requires input from radiologists, clinical virologists, pediatricians and neurologists and highlights the need for communication between specialists to ensure a case is recognized, with the appropriate samples and tests requested, including PCR and MRI scans.

Treatment Options

Increasing reports of enhanced pathogenicity and the severity of the paralysis in the affected individuals have led to urgency in finding an effective treatment for EV-D68. At present, there is no vaccine or therapy which exists against EV-D68. A study carried out by Rhoden et al. (2015) evaluated several anti-viral candidates for EV-D68, with some promising results; V-7404, a protease inhibitor currently in development to treat poliovirus in immunodeficient patients; DAS181, similarly in development however to treat Influenza and Parainfluenza virus infections, and finally Rupintrivir, another protease inhibitor, not currently being developed further. Both V-7404 and Rupintrivir were able to inhibit all four tested EV-D68 strains (one Fermon and three 2014 outbreak strains). DAS181, which works as a sialidase was comparable in effectiveness, with a slightly EC50. However, these results were only obtained from *in vitro* testing, and clinical studies with these agents will not be available in the intermediate future.

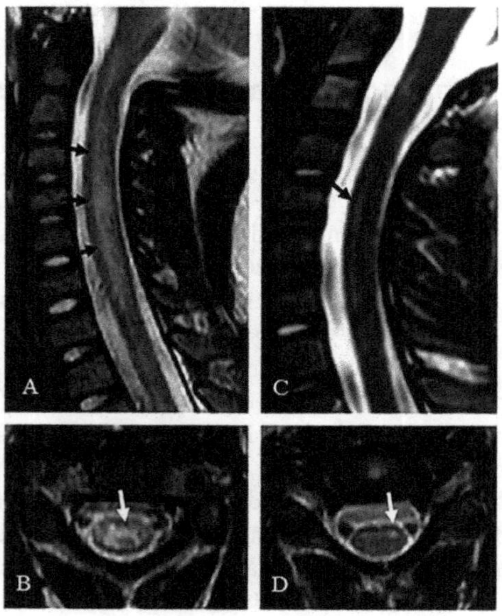

FIGURE 3 | MRI of a suspected EV-D68 AFM patient. The MRI presents sagittal **(A,C)** and axial images **(B,D)** of the central nerves system. **(A)** Presents a case where the whole central gray matter was involved, producing a characteristic "H" pattern on axial image **(B)**. **(C)** Presents a case where T2 hyperintensity was confined to the left anterior horn cells, which is demonstrated on the axial image **(D)**. Taken from Maloney et al., 2015.

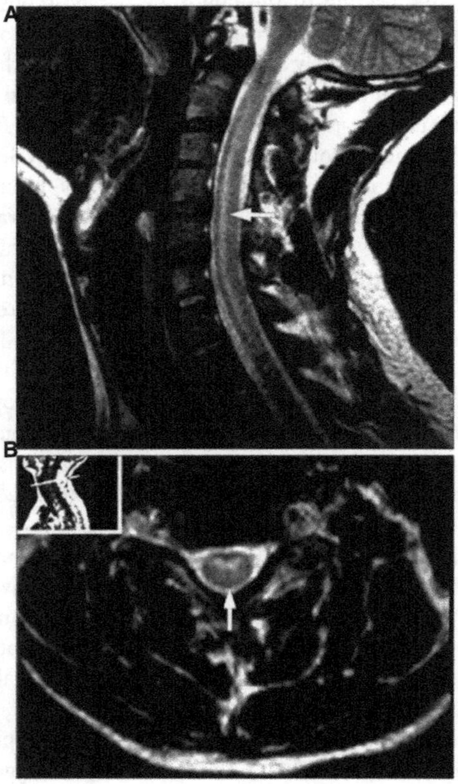

FIGURE 4 | MRI of a poliovirus AFM patient. The MRI presents a sagittal **(A)** and an axial image **(B)** of the central nerves system. **(A)** presents a case showing hyperintensities involving the anterior horn cells from C3 to C7. **(B)** demonstrates the same case as an axial image. Taken from Haq and Wasay (2006).

A further study (Tyler, 2015) investigated the use of an already FDA approved drug, Fluoxetine, a serotonin inhibitor normally used as an antidepressant. The study found Fluoxetine inhibited the replication of EV-D68 in HeLa cells by a direct interaction with the 2C protein, which is thought to have a function in assembly. It is unknown if the tested strain was from the 2014 outbreak. However, Fluoxetine administration was noted to result in low maximal plasma levels, which could lead to problems in *in vivo* investigations (Rhoden et al., 2015).

As EV-D68 is a relatively emerging pathogen in terms of increased pathogenicity in recent years, treatment options are still far off. Exploring existing treatments for viruses, other than EV-D68, which present with similar symptoms, is therefore an attractive strategy (CDC and NCIRD, 2014). Recently, investigations were carried out (Hixon et al., 2017a) into three different empiric therapies that could decrease the severity of paralysis in a mouse model. The mice were intramuscularly injected with one of the 2014 outbreak strains. Positive results were obtained with hIVIG, which reduced paralysis and spinal cord viral loads. Fluoxetine was shown to have a neutral effect, contrasting to Tyler, 2015 and dexamethasone worsened outcomes for the mice, causing increased mortality, possibly due to reducing the immune response and increasing viral replication. Disadvantageous results of corticosteroid treatment were also seen when these agents were used in an outbreak of neuro-invasive EV-A71 in Cambodia (World Health Organization [WHO], 2012). So far this research presents promising results for hIVIG therapy (pre and early post-infection) by providing potential protection against one of the most severe manifestations of an EV-D68 infection. Indeed, hIVIG therapy has been used previously and has arguably been successful in a least one suspected AFM case associated with WNV (Walid and Mahmoud, 2009). However, a further study (Chong et al., 2018) found hIVIG given to patients initially after onset of neurological symptoms, led to a poor prognosis.

As permanent functional impairment appears to be common in EV-D68 associated AFM (Messacar et al., 2016), solutions are also being sought to improve the outcome of patients after the paralysis has become irreversible. A potentially promising technique is nerve and muscle transfer, which was historically used for poliomyelitis associated paralysis (Messacar et al., 2016). As such, one study (Saltzman et al., 2016) describes the results of a trial involving nerve transfers in several patients following AFM associated EV-D68. In most of the cases proximal nerves were transferred, with one case undergoing bilateral nerve transfers. The study showed promising results with some muscle strength regained over a 6-month follow-up.

Non-polio Enterovirus Awareness and Its Subsequent Increased Surveillance

In the United States, published results from various surveillance studies are presented through the CDC. However, EV-D68 is only voluntarily reported in most states in the United States and is not a national notifiable disease (CDC and NNDSS, 2018). Similarly, the ECDC does not have an active surveillance system in place and relies on member states to provide updates on circulation of various EV. Therefore non-polio enterovirus surveillance in Europe can also depend on local interests of specific laboratories and national health institutes. As it is not mandatory to report EV-D68 in Europe (except Norway), and just in a few states in the United States, little real-time information is known on the exact numbers. This is a current challenge for EV-D68 data. However this may change now that the PAHO/WHO has introduced the recommendation of including respiratory samples in suspected EV-D68 cases (PAHO/WHO report, 2017).

Several surveillance systems are in place throughout Europe. One example is the enhanced non-polio EV surveillance system implemented in Denmark in which respiratory samples were included, along with clinical description and genetic characterisation of the viruses (Barnadas et al., 2017). Similarly, in collaboration with the Dutch National Institute of Health, the TYPENED initiative [Typing network Netherlands] is involved in sequencing and collection of data (Niesters et al., 2013). In France, two EV National Reference Laboratories (in Clermont-Ferrand and Lyon) report the number of enterovirus infections and type of samples analyzed on a regular basis.[1] (Schuffenecker et al., 2016). Additionally, networks such as ENPEN exist to increase knowledge and communicate both epidemiological and clinical data during outbreaks, and to chart emerging infections. Such networks have been instrumental in raising awareness of EV-D68 and other non-polio EV through an email alert system and conferences (Harvala et al., 2018).

DISCUSSION

Burden of Disease and the Problems of Underdiagnosing

Enterovirus D68 made headlines worldwide in 2014 as a mysterious, relatively unknown virus was capable of causing severe illness. The CDC currently monitors and provides monthly updates on the incidence of AFM, which subsequently revealed another upsurge in 2016. Since no recent data has been published on the number of confirmed EV-D68 infections or the number of AFM cases in Europe, more testing and communication is required to understand both the EV-D68 infection patterns and the frequency at which this virus causes AFM. Specific EV-D68 assays have been developed to rapidly diagnose infections. Despite the existing evidence for the association between EV-D68 and AFM (Hixon et al., 2017b; Messacar et al., 2018), EV-D68 is overlooked due to insufficient knowledge, sampling, laboratory testing and communication between healthcare professionals and little surveillance from public health authorities.

Future Perspective and Directions

The current surveillance systems for poliovirus such as GPEI, environmental and AFP surveillance have been instrumental in nearly eradicating polio. Integrating EV-D68 into these established surveillance systems, would be highly effective in understanding the true burden of disease and prepare hospitals and laboratories for upcoming outbreaks. NGS has the potential to be a powerful tool in investigating emerging and untypeable pathogens. It could also be used to understand the host-pathogen relationship during an infection and to understand the evolution of these viruses. However, there are still both technical and financial obstacles left to overcome before its used in routine practice (Rutvisuttinunt et al., 2017).

Further outbreaks of EV-D68 can be expected and could subsequently lead to an increase in EV-D68 associated AFM cases. EV-D68 numbers and AFM cases have increased in autumn of 2018. This has been communicated by the EV-D68 network made up of virologists and clinicians who collaborated during the 2014 and 2016 outbreaks. This has included two recent AFM cases from the Netherlands. Preliminary typing results obtained from the University Medical Center Groningen, the Netherlands, have indicated that recent EV-D68 samples have clustered into the B3 and A2 subclades. It is imperative to have effective and streamlined diagnostic procedures along with stewardship models to deal with the potential increase in cases. As a result, awareness needs to be created targeting clinicians and hospital wards in order to make clinical staff are aware of the virus. Continued interdisciplinary communication is important to ensure EV-D68 is translated across each medical field appropriately.

[1] http://cnr.chu-clermontferrand.fr/CNR/

As effective treatment of EV-D68 infections and AFM are thus far unsubstantial, the focus may need to be placed on the development of a vaccine. Currently efficient vaccines are available for a few members of the enterovirus genus i.e., poliovirus and EV-A71 (Klein and Chong, 2015). These viruses however, have shown high incidences therefore it could be questioned whether a vaccine should be developed for EV-D68 at this time for economic reasons. Yet these vaccines have transformed the fight against these fatal EV. Using current knowledge and approaches, development of a vaccine against EV-D68 is technically achievable. A group recently published the results of a trial involving insect cell-expressed EV-D68 virus-like particle as a promising candidate for an EV-D68 vaccine (Dai et al., 2018). At present, the number of infections and life-threating cases do not reflect those of poliovirus, possibly due to lack of reporting with the current voluntary reporting systems. Only increased surveillance and diagnosis will make it possible to expose the extent of the EV-D68 threat.

AUTHOR CONTRIBUTIONS

HC drafted the manuscript. RP, MK, CVL-B, and HN revised the work critically and gave final approval before publication.

REFERENCES

Aliabadi, N., Messacar, K., Pastula, D., Robinson, C., Leshem, E., Sejvar, J., et al. (2016). Enterovirus D68 infection in children with acute flaccid Myelitis, Colorado, USA, 2014. *Emerg. Infect. Dis.* 22, 1387–1394. doi: 10.3201/eid2208.151949

Antona, D., Kossorotoff, M., Schuffenecker, I., Mirand, A., Leruez-Ville, M., Bassi, C., et al. (2016). Severe paediatric conditions linked with EV-A71 and EV-D68, France, May to October 2016. *Euro Surveill.* 21:30402. doi: 10.2807/1560-7917.ES.2016.21.46.30402

Baggen, J., Thibaut, H., Strating, J., and Van Kuppeveld, F. (2018). The life cycle of non-polio enteroviruses and how to target it. *Nat. Rev. Microbiol.* 16, 368–381. doi: 10.1038/s41579-018-0005-4

Barnadas, C., Midgley, S., Skov, M., Jensen, L., Poulsen, M., and Fischer, T. (2017). An enhanced *Enterovirus* surveillance system allows identification and characterization of rare and emerging respiratory enteroviruses in Denmark, 2015–16. *J. Clin. Virol.* 93, 40–44. doi: 10.1016/j.jcv.2017.05.017

Blomqvist, S., Savolainen, C., Råman, L., Roivainen, M., and Hovi, T. (2002). Human rhinovirus 87 and enterovirus 68 represent a unique serotype with rhinovirus and enterovirus features. *J. Clin. Microbiol.* 40, 4218–4223. doi: 10.1128/JCM.40.11.4218-4223.2002

Cabrerizo, M., García-Iñiguez, J. P., Munell, F., Madurga-Revilla, P., Rodrigo, C., Martínez-Sapiña, A., et al. (2017). First cases of severe flaccid paralysis associated with enterovirus D68 infection in Spain, 2015–2016. *Pediatr. Infect. Dis. J.* 36, 1214–1216. doi: 10.1097/INF.0000000000001668

CDC and NCIRD (2018). *Acute Flaccid Myelitis Investigation.* Available at: https://www.cdc.gov/acute-flaccid-myelitis/afm-surveillance.html [accessed July 03, 2018]

CDC and NCIRD (2014). *Acute Flaccid Myelitis: Interim Considerations for Clinical Management.* Available at: https://www.cdc.gov/acute-flaccid-myelitis/hcp/clinical-management.html [accessed July 03, 2018]

CDC and NCIRD (2015). *For Clinicians: Diagnosing Acute Flaccid Myelitis (AFM) in the United States.* Available at: https://www.cdc.gov/acute-flaccid-myelitis/downloads/afm-presentation.pdf [accessed July 03, 2018]

CDC and NNDSS (2018). *National Notifiable Conditions.* Available at: https://wwwn.cdc.gov/nndss/conditions/notifiable/2018/ [accessed April 16, 2018].

Chong, P., Kira, R., Mori, H., Okumura, A., Torisu, H., Yasumoto, S., et al. (2018). Clinical features of acute flaccid myelitis temporally associated with an enterovirus D68 outbreak: results of a nationwide survey of acute flaccid paralysis in Japan, August-December 2015. *Clin. Infect. Dis.* 66, 653–664. doi: 10.1093/cid/cix860

Craighead, J. (ed.) (2000). "Enteroviruses," in *Pathology and Pathogenesis of Human Viral Disease*, (Amsterdam: Elsevier), 1–28. doi: 10.1016/B978-012195160-3/50002-9

Dai, W., Zhang, C., Zhang, X., Xiong, P., Liu, Q., Gong, S., et al. (2018). A virus-like particle vaccine confers protection against enterovirus D68 lethal challenge in mice. *Vaccine* 36, 653–659. doi: 10.1016/j.vaccine.2017.12.057

Diaz-Decaro, J., Green, N., and Godwin, H. (2018). Critical evaluation of FDA-approved respiratory multiplex assays for public health surveillance. *Expert Rev. Mol. Diagn.* 18, 631–643. doi: 10.1080/14737159.2018.1487294

Dik, J.-W., Poelman, R., Friedrich, A., Panday, P., Lo-Ten-Foe, J., Van Assen, S., et al. (2016). An integrated stewardship model: antimicrobial, infection prevention and diagnostic (AID). *Future Microbiol.* 11, 93–102. doi: 10.2217/fmb.15.99

Duong, V., Mey, C., Eloit, M., Zhu, H., Danet, L., Huang, Z., et al. (2016). Molecular epidemiology of human enterovirus 71 at the origin of an epidemic of fatal hand, foot and mouth disease cases in Cambodia. *Emerg. Microbes. Infect.* 5:e104. doi: 10.1038/emi.2016.101

Dyda, A., Stelzer-Braid, S., Adam, D., Chughtai, A., Raina MacIntyre, C., Amalie, D., et al. (2018). The association between acute flaccid myelitis (AFM) and *Enterovirus* D68 (EV-D68) – what is the evidence for causation? *Euro Surveill.* 23:17-00310. doi: 10.2807/1560-7917.ES.2018.23.3.17-00310

Dyrdak, R., Grabbe, M., Hammas, B., Ekwall, J., Hansson, K. E., Luthander, J., et al. (2016). Outbreak of enterovirus D68 of the new B3 lineage in Stockholm, Sweden, August to September 2016. *Euro Surveill.* 21:30403. doi: 10.2807/1560-7917.ES.2016.21.46.30403

ECDC. (2016). *Rapid Risk Assessment – Enterovirus Detections Associated with Severe Neurological Symptoms in Children and Adults in European Countries.* Solna Municipality: ECDC.

Escalona, M., Rocha, S., and Posada, D. (2016). A comparison of tools for the simulation of genomic next-generation sequencing data. *Nat. Rev. Genet.* 17, 459–469. doi: 10.1038/nrg.2016.57

Esposito, S., Bosis, S., Niesters, H., and Principi, N. (2015). Enterovirus D68 infection. *Viruses* 7, 6043–6050. doi: 10.3390/v7112925

Esposito, S., Chidini, G., Cinnante, C., Napolitano, L., Giannini, A., Terranova, L., et al. (2017). Acute flaccid myelitis associated with enterovirus-D68 infection in an otherwise healthy child. *Virol. J.* 14:4. doi: 10.1186/s12985-016-0678-0

Esposito, S., Lunghi, G., Zampiero, A., Tagliabue, C., Orlandi, A., Torresani, E., et al. (2016). Enterovirus-D68 in the cerebrospinal fluid of two children with aseptic meningitis. *Pediatr. Infect. Dis. J.* 35, 589–591. doi: 10.1097/INF.0000000000001085

Foster, C. B., Friedman, N., Carl, J., and Piedimonte, G. (2015). Enterovirus D68: a clinically important respiratory enterovirus. *Cleve. Clin. J. Med.* 82, 26–31. doi: 10.3949/ccjm.82a.14166

Giombini, E., Rueca, M., Barberi, W., Iori, A. P., Castilletti, C., Scognamiglio, P., et al. (2017). Enterovirus D68–associated acute flaccid myeltis in immunocompromised women in Italy. *Emerg. Infect. Dis.* 23, 1690–1693. doi: 10.3201/eid2310.170792

Gong, Y.-N., Yang, S.-L., Shih, S.-R., Huang, Y.-C., Chang, P.-Y., Huang, C.-G., et al. (2016). Molecular evolution and the global reemergence of enterovirus D68 by genome-wide analysis. *Medicine* 95:e4416. doi: 10.1097/MD.0000000000004416

Greninger, A., Naccache, S., Messacar, K., Clayton, A., Yu, G., Somasekar, S., et al. (2015). A novel outbreak enterovirus D68 strain associated with acute flaccid myelitis cases in the USA (2012-14): a retrospective cohort study. *Lancet Infect. Dis.* 15, 671–682. doi: 10.1016/S1473-3099(15)70093-9

Haq, A., and Wasay, M. (2006). Magnetic resonance imaging in poliomyelitis. *JAMA Neurol.* 63:778. doi: 10.1001/archneur.63.5.778

Harvala, H., Broberg, E., Benschop, K., Berginc, N., Ladhani, S., Susi, P., et al. (2018). Recommendations for enterovirus diagnostics and characterisation within and beyond Europe. *J. Clin. Virol.* 101, 11–17. doi: 10.1016/j.jcv.2018.01.008

Hixon, A., Clarke, P., and Tyler, K. (2017a). Evaluating treatment efficacy in a mouse model of enterovirus D68-associated paralytic myelitis. *J. Infect. Dis.* 216, 1245–1253. doi: 10.1093/infdis/jix468

Hixon, A., Yu, G., Leser, J., Yagi, S., Clarke, P., Chiu, C., et al. (2017b). A mouse model of paralytic myelitis caused by enterovirus D68. *PLoS Pathogens* 13:e1006199. doi: 10.1371/journal.ppat.1006199

Holm-Hansen, C., Midgley, S., and Fischer, T. (2016). Global emergence of enterovirus D68: a systematic review. *Lancet Infect. Dis.* 16, e64–e75. doi: 10.1016/S1473-3099(15)00543-5

Huang, H., and Shih, S. (2015). Neurotropic enterovirus infections in the central nervous system. *Viruses* 7, 6051–6066.doi:10.3390/v7112920

Huang, W., Wang, G., Zhuge, J., Nolan, S., Dimitrova, N., and Fallon, J. (2015). Whole-Genome sequence analysis reveals the enterovirus D68 isolates during the United States 2014 outbreak mainly belong to a novel clade. *Sci. Rep.* 5:15223. doi: 10.1038/srep15223

Imamura, T., Okamoto, M., Nakakita, S.-I., Suzuki, A., Saito, M., Tamaki, R., et al. (2014). Antigenic and receptor binding properties of enterovirus. *J. Virol.* 88, 2374–2384. doi: 10.1128/JVI.03070-13

Imamura, T., and Oshitani, H. (2015). Global reemergence of enterovirus D68 as an important pathogen for acute respiratory infections. *Rev. Med. Virol.* 25, 102–114. doi: 10.1002/rmv.1820

Jasti, A., Selmi, C., Sarmiento-Monroy, J., Vega, D., Anaya, J., and Gershwin, M. (2016). Guillain-Barré syndrome: causes, immunopathogenic mechanisms and treatment. *Expert Rev. Clin. Immunol.* 12, 1175–1189. doi: 10.1080/1744666X.2016.1193006

Kaida, A., Iritani, N., Yamamoto, S., Kanbayashi, D., Hirai, Y., Togawa, M., et al. (2017). Distinct genetic clades of enterovirus D68 detected in 2010, 2013, and 2015 in Osaka City, Japan. *PLoS One* 12:e0184335. doi: 10.1371/journal.pone.0184335

Kirolos, A., Mark, K., Waugh, C., Shetty, J., McCallum, A., Templeton, K., et al. (2017). Cluster of acute flaccid paralysis in children following enterovirus D68 infection in Scotland. *Eur. J. Public Health.* 27:ckx187.697. doi: 10.1093/eurpub/ckx187.697

Klein, M., and Chong, P. (2015). Is a multivalent hand, foot, and mouth disease vaccine feasible? *Hum. Vaccin. Immunother.* 11, 2688–2704. doi: 10.1080/21645515.2015.1049780

Knoester, M., Helfferich, J., Poelman, R., Van Leer-Buter, C., Brouwer, O., and Niesters, H. (2018). Twenty-Nine cases of enterovirus-D68 associated acute flaccid myelitis in Europe 2016; A case series and epidemiologic overview. *Pediatr. Infect. Dis. J.* doi: 10.1097/INF.0000000000002188 [Epub ahead of print].

Knoester, M., Schölvinck, E., Poelman, R., Smit, S., Vermont, C., Niesters, H., et al. (2017). Upsurge of enterovirus D68, the Netherlands, 2016. *Emerg. Infect. Dis.* 23, 140–143. doi: 10.3201/eid2301.161313

Kreuter, J. D., Barnes, A., McCarthy, J. E., Schwartzman, J. D., Oberste, M. S., Rhodes, C. H., et al. (2011). A fatal central nervous system enterovirus 68 infection. *Arch. Pathol. Lab. Med.* 135, 793–796. doi: 10.1043/2010-0174-CR.1

Lang, M., Mirand, A., Savy, N., Henquell, C., Maricet, S., Perignon, R., et al. (2014). Acute flaccid paralysis following enterovirus D68 associated pneumonia, France, 2014. *Euro Surveill.* 19:20952. doi: 10.2807/1560-7917.ES2014.19.44.20952

Levy, A., Roberts, J., Lang, J., Tempone, S., Kesson, A., Dofai, A., et al. (2015). Enterovirus D68 disease and molecular epidemiology in Australia. *J. Clin. Virol.* 69, 117–121. doi: 10.1016/j.jcv.2015.06.079

Maloney, J., Mirsky, D., Messacar, K., Dominguez, S., Schreiner, T., and Stence, N. (2015). MRI findings in children with acute flaccid paralysis and cranial nerve dysfunction occurring during the 2014 enterovirus D68 outbreak. *Am. J. Neuroradiol.* 36, 245–250. doi: 10.3174/ajnr.A4188

Martin, G., Li, R., Cook, V., Carwana, M., Tilley, P., Sauve, L., et al. (2016). Respiratory presentation of pediatric patients in the 2014 enterovirus D68 outbreak. *Can. Respir. J.* 2016:8302179. doi: 10.1155/2016/8302179

McAllister, S., Schleiss, M., Arbefeville, S., Steiner, M., Hanson, R., Pollock, C., et al. (2015). Epidemic 2014 enterovirus D68 cross-reacts with human rhinovirus on a respiratory molecular diagnostic platform. *PLoS One* 10:e0118529. doi: 10.1371/journal.pone.0118529

Messacar, K., Asturias, E., Hixon, A., Van Leer-Buter, C. M., Niesters, H., Tyler, K., et al. (2018). Personal view enterovirus D68 and acute flaccid myelitis—evaluating the evidence for causality. *Lancet Infect. Dis.* 18, e239–e247. doi: 10.1016/S1473-3099(18)30094-X

Messacar, K., Schreiner, T., Van Haren, K., Yang, M., Glaser, C., Tyler, K., et al. (2016). Acute flaccid myelitis: a clinical review of US cases 2012–2015. *Ann. Neurol.* 80, 326–338. doi: 10.1002/ana.24730

Midgley, C., Watson, J., Nix, W., Curns, A., Rogers, S., Brown, B., et al. (2015). Severe respiratory illness associated with a nationwide outbreak of enterovirus D68 in the USA (2014): a descriptive epidemiological investigation. *Lancet Respir. Med.* 3, 879–887. doi: 10.1016/S2213-2600(15)00335-5

Morrey, J., Wang, H., Hurst, B., Zukor, K., Siddharthan, V., Van Wettere, A., et al. (2018). Causation of acute flaccid paralysis by myelitis and myositis in enterovirus-D68 infected mice deficient in interferon αβ/γ receptor deficient mice. *Viruses* 10:E33. doi: 10.3390/v10010033

National Center for Immunization and Respiratory Diseases [Ncird], Division of Viral Diseases (2017). *Enterovirus D68*. Available at: https://www.cdc.gov/non-polio-enterovirus/about/ev-d68.html [accessed April 11, 2018]

Niesters, H., Rossen, J., van der Avoort, H., Baas, D., Benschop, K., Claas, E., et al. (2013). Laboratory-based surveillance in the molecular era: the TYPENED model, a joint data-sharing platform for clinical and public health laboratories. *Euro Surveill.* 18:20387. doi: 10.2807/ese.18.04.20387-en

Nix, A. W., Oberste, M., and Pallansch, M. (2006). Sensitive, seminested PCR amplification of VP1 sequences for direct identification of all enterovirus serotypes from original clinical specimens. *J. Clin. Microbiol.* 44, 2698–2704. doi: 10.1128/JCM.00542-06

Noor, A., and Krilov, L. (2016). Enterovirus infections. *Pediatr. Rev.* 37, 505–515. doi: 10.1542/pir.2016-0103

Ohka, S., Yang, W.-X., Terada, E., Iwasaki, K., and Nomoto, A. (1998). Retrograde transport of intact poliovirus through the axon via the fast transport system. *Virology* 250, 67–75. doi: 10.1006/viro.1998.9360

PAHO/WHO. (2016). *Report From: The Argentina International Health Regulations National Focal Point.* Washington, DC: PAHO.

PAHO/WHO report. (2017). *Epidemiological Alert Acute Flaccid Myelitis Associated with Enterovirus D68 in the Context of Acute Flaccid Paralysis Surveillance.* Washington, DC: PAHO.

Paul, J. (1971). *A History of Poliomyelitis*. New Haven, CT: Yale University Press.

Pfeiffer, H., Bragstad, K., Skram, M., Dahl, H., Knudsen, P., Chawla, M., et al. (2015). Two cases of acute severe flaccid myelitis associated with enterovirus D68 infection in children, Norway, autumn 2014. *Euro Surveill.* 20:21062. doi: 10.2807/1560-7917.ES2015.20.10.21062

Poelman, R., Schölvinck, E., Borger, R., Niesters, H., and Van Leer-Buter, C. (2015a). The emergence of enterovirus D68 in a Dutch University Medical Center and the necessity for routinely screening for respiratory viruses. *J. Clin. Virol.* 62, 1–5. doi: 10.1016/j.jcv.2014.11.011

Poelman, R., Schuffenecker, I., Van Leer-Buter, C., Josset, L., Niesters, H., Lina, B., et al. (2015b). European surveillance for enterovirus D68 during the emerging North-American outbreak in 2014. *J. Clin. Virol.* 71, 1–9. doi: 10.1016/j.jcv.2015.07.296

Poritz, M., Blaschke, A., Byington, C., Meyers, L., Nilsson, K., Jones, D., et al. (2011). Filmarray, an automated nested multiplex PCR system for multi-pathogen detection: development and application to respiratory tract infection. *PLoS One* 6:e26047. doi: 10.1371/journal.pone.0026047

Rahamat-Langendoen, J., Riezebos-Brilman, A., Borger, R., van der Heide, R., Brandenburg, A., Schölvinck, E., et al. (2011). Upsurge of human enterovirus 68 infections in patients with severe respiratory tract infections. *J. Clin. Virol.* 52, 103–106. doi: 10.1016/j.jcv.2011.06.019

Rhoden, E., Zhang, M., Nix, W., and Oberste, M. (2015). In vitro efficacy of antiviral compounds against enterovirus D68. *Antimicrob. Agents Chemother.* 59, 7779–7781. doi: 10.1128/AAC.00766-15

Ruggieri, V., Paz, M. I., Peretti, M. G., Rugilo, C., Bologna, R., Freire, C., et al. (2017). Enterovirus D68 infection in a cluster of children with acute flaccid myelitis, Buenos Aires, Argentina, 2016. *Eur. J. Paediatr. Neurol.* 21, 884–890. doi: 10.1016/j.ejpn.2017.07.008

Rutvisuttinunt, W., Klungthong, C., Thaisomboonsuk, B., Chinnawirotpisan, P., Ajariyakhajorn, C., Manasatienkij, W., et al. (2017). Retrospective use of next-generation sequencing reveals the presence of Enteroviruses in acute influenza-like illness respiratory samples collected in South/South-East Asia during 2010–2013. *J. Clin. Virol.* 94, 91–99. doi: 10.1016/j.jcv.2017.07.004

Saltzman, E., Vu, A., Schwenker, A., Raney, S., Sneag, D., Yakuboff, K., et al. (2016). Nerve transfers for enterovirus D68-induced acute flaccid myelitis. *HAND* 11:97S. doi: 10.1016/j.pediatrneurol.2018.07.018

Schuffenecker, I., Mirand, A., Josset, L., Henquell, C., Hecquet, D., Pilorgé, L., et al. (2016). Epidemiological and clinical characteristics of patients infected with enterovirus D68, France, July to December 2014. *Euro Surveill.* 21:30226. doi: 10.2807/1560-7917.ES.2016.21.19.30226

Sejvar, J., Lopez, A., Cortese, M., Leshem, E., Pastula, D., Miller, L., et al. (2016). Acute flaccid myelitis in the United States, August-December 2014: results of nationwide surveillance. *Clin. Infect. Dis.* 63, 737–745. doi: 10.1093/cid/ciw372

Shibib, D., Matushek, S., Beavis, K., Gawel, S., and Charnot-Katsikas, A. (2016). BioFire film array respiratory panel for detection of enterovirus D68. *J. Clin. Microbiol.* 54, 457–459. doi: 10.1128/JCM.02339-15

Stacpoole, S., Molyneux, A., and Bäumer, D. (2017). Acute segmental poliomyelitis-like flaccid paralysis in an adult in the UK, associated with enterovirus D68. *Pract. Neurol.* 17, 297–301. doi: 10.1136/practneurol-2017-001609

The Global Poliovirus Eradication Initiative [GPEI] (2018). *Global Polio Eradication Initiative.* Available at http://polioeradication.org/where-we-work/polio-endemic-countries/ [accessed June 03, 2018] doi: 10.1136/practneurol-2017-001609

Tokarz, R., Firth, C., Madhi, S., Howie, S., Wu, W., Sall, A., et al. (2012). Worldwide emergence of multiple clades of enterovirus 68. *J. Gen. Virol.* 93(Pt 9), 1952–1958. doi: 10.1099/vir.0.043935-0

Tse, M., Lane, C., Mott, K., Onlamoon, N., Hsiao, H., and Perng, G. (2009). ICAM-5 modulates cytokine/chemokine production in the CNS during the course of herpes simplex virus type 1 infection. *J. Neuroimmunol.* 213, 12–19. doi: 10.1016/j.jneuroim.2009.06.007

Tyler, K. (2015). Rationale for the evaluation of fluoxetine in the treatment of enterovirus d68-associated acute flaccid myelitis. *JAMA Neurol.* 72, 493–494. doi: 10.1001/jamaneurol.2014.4625

Varghese, R., Iyer, A., Hunter, K., Cargill, J., and Cooke, R. (2015). Sampling the upper respiratory tract for enteroviral infection is important in the investigation of an acute neurological illness in children. *Eur. J. Paediatr. Neurol.* 19, 494–495. doi: 10.1016/j.ejpn.2015.03.009

Walid, M., and Mahmoud, A. (2009). Successful treatment with intravenous immunoglobulin of acute flaccid paralysis caused by West Nile Virus. *Perm. J.* 13, 43–46. doi: 10.7812/TPP/09-028

Wang, G., Zhuge, J., Huang, W., Nolan, S., Gilrane, V., Yin, C., et al. (2017). Enterovirus D68 subclade B3 strain circulating and causing an outbreak in the United States in 2016. *Sci. Rep.* 7:1242. doi: 10.1038/s41598-017-01349-4

Washington State Department of Health (2016). *Communicable Disease Epidemiology. Acute Flaccid Myelitis and Poliomyelitis Reporting and Investigation Guideline.* Chesterfield: DCHS.

Wei, W., Guo, H., Chang, J., Yu, Y., Liu, G., Zhang, N., et al. (2016). ICAM-5 Telencephalin is a functional entry. *Cell Host Microbe* 20, 631–641. doi: 10.1016/j.chom.2016.09.013

Williams, C., Thomas, R., Pickersgill, T., Lyons, M., Lowe, G., Stiff, R., et al. (2016). Cluster of atypical adult Guillain-Barré syndrome temporally associated with neurological illness due to EV-D68 in children, South Wales, United Kingdom, October 2015 to January 2016. *Euro Surveill.* 21:30119. doi: 10.2807/1560-7917.ES.2016.21.4.30119

World Health Organization [WHO] (2018). *Poliomyelitis.* Available at: http://www.who.int/mediacentre/factsheets/fs114/en/ [accessed April 11, 2018]

World Health Organization [WHO] (2012). *(Emergencies Preparedness, Response) Severe Complications of Hand, Foot and Mouth Disease (HFMD) Caused by EV-71 in Cambodia – Conclusion of the Joint Investigation.* Available at: http://www.who.int/csr/don/2012_07_13/en/. [accessed April 11, 2018]

Xiang, Z., Xie, Z., Liu, L., Ren, L., Xiao, Y., Paranhos-Baccalà, G., et al. (2016). Genetic divergence of enterovirus D68 in China and the United States. *Sci. Rep.* 6:27800. doi: 10.1038/srep27800

14

Diagnostic Parameters of Adenoviremia in Pediatric Stem Cell Transplant Recipients

*Karin Kosulin[1], Herbert Pichler[2], Anita Lawitschka[2], René Geyeregger[1] and Thomas Lion[1,3]**

[1] *Molecular Microbiology, Children's Cancer Research Institute, Vienna, Austria,* [2] *Stem Cell Transplant Unit, St. Anna Children's Hospital, Vienna, Austria,* [3] *Department of Pediatrics, Medical University of Vienna, Vienna, Austria*

Correspondence:
Thomas Lion
thomas.lion@ccri.at

Despite recent progress in the diagnostic risk assessment of human adenovirus (HAdV) infections in immunocompromised patients, clinical complications mediated by these viruses continue contributing to significant morbidity and mortality, particularly in the pediatric hematopoietic allogeneic stem cell transplant (HSCT) setting. Current data highlight the importance of monitoring stool samples to assess the risk of invasive HAdV infections in children undergoing HSCT. The advent of novel, more effective antiviral treatment options might permit successful virus control even at the stage of systemic infection, thus increasing the interest in optimized HAdV monitoring in peripheral blood (PB). We have screened over 300 pediatric HCST recipients by serial monitoring of stool and PB specimens, and identified 31 cases of invasive HAdV infection by quantitative pan-adenovirus RQ-PCR analysis of consecutive PB specimens. The diagnostic parameters assessed included HAdV peak levels (PL) and the time-averaged area under the curve (AAUC) of virus copy numbers. The predictive value for patient outcome reflected by non-relapse and HAdV-related mortality was determined. The patients were assigned to quartiles based on their PL and AAUC, and the readouts were highly correlated ($p < 0.0001$). Non-relapse mortality in patients by AAUC quartile (lowest to highest) was 26, 50, 75, and 86%, respectively, and AAUC was strongly correlated with non-relapse mortality ($p < 0.0001$), while the association between PL and non-relapse mortality was less pronounced ($p = 0.013$). HAdV-related mortality was absent or very low in patients within the two lower quartiles of both PL and AAUC, and increased to $\geq$70% in the upper two quartiles. Despite the significant correlation of PL and AAUC with patient outcome, it is necessary to consider that the risk of non-relapse mortality even within the lowest quartile was still relatively high, and it might be difficult therefore to translate the results into differential treatment approaches. By contrast, the correlation with HAdV-related mortality might permit the identification of a low-risk patient subset. Nevertheless, the well-established correlation of HAdV shedding into the stool and intestinal expansion of the virus with the risk of invasive infection will expectedly remain an essential diagnostic parameter in the pediatric HSCT setting.

Keywords: human adenovirus, pediatric stem cell transplant recipients, viremia, area under the curve, non-relapse mortality

INTRODUCTION

The incidence and severity of invasive HAdV infections in allogeneic HSCT recipients correlate with different factors including the level of immune system impairment, mediated in part by the conditioning regimen and the employment of strongly T-cell depleting strategies (Saif et al., 2015; Rustia et al., 2016). Preemptive treatment with cidofovir has been regarded as a standard of care in HSCT recipients displaying viremia (Matthes-Martin et al., 2012), but the response rates were suboptimal. The ability to control the infection by current therapeutic modalities, including also adoptive transfer of HAdV-specific T-cells, has been suggested to depend on timely onset of treatment (Lion et al., 2003; Feuchtinger et al., 2006; Geyeregger et al., 2014; Lion, 2014; Feucht et al., 2015). This notion has sparked the search for diagnostic parameters permitting early risk assessment of impending invasive infection and disseminated disease. In the pediatric HSCT setting, monitoring of serial stool specimens during the post-transplant period was shown to facilitate early HAdV detection, and expansion of viral loads in stool with peak levels exceeding 10E6 virus copies/g was demonstrated to confer a very high risk for systemic infection (Lion et al., 2010; Jeulin et al., 2011). In children undergoing HSCT, HAdV expansion in stool was reported to almost invariably precede invasive infection defined by the detection of viremia (Lion et al., 2010; Lion, 2014). The absolute level of virus copy numbers in stool identified as critical may vary depending on the specific techniques of quantitative analysis used by different laboratories (Lion et al., 2010; Jeulin et al., 2011; Legoff et al., 2017; Hum et al., 2018). In this regard, documentation of rapidly rising HAdV copy numbers in serial stool specimens may be a more universal parameter for risk assessment of imminent invasive infection (Lion, 2014). Recent data indicate that a proportion of children carry persistent HAdV in the gastrointestinal (GI) tract, with most prominent occurrence in the ileum (Kosulin et al., 2016c). The observed rates of HAdV persistence in the GI tract and reactivation of the virus post-transplant were similar, suggesting that intestinal virus persistence could be a key risk factor for ensuing HAdV-related complications after HSCT (Kosulin et al., 2016c). More recent findings revealed that intestinal HAdV shedding prior to transplantation confers a highly significant risk for early and rapid post-transplant expansion of the virus, leading to an elevated incidence of invasive infections associated with pronounced morbidity and mortality (Kosulin et al., 2018). The important role of stool monitoring is well-documented in the pediatric setting, but may be of lesser relevance in adult HSCT recipients in whom intestinal HAdV persistence and reactivation have not been documented to date. However, individual reports on transplant-related mortality in patients with adenoviremia suggest that these infections can also be severe and potentially life-threatening outside the pediatric setting (Ganzenmueller et al., 2011; Sive et al., 2012; Taniguchi et al., 2012; Lee et al., 2016; Ramsay et al., 2017). Due to the fact that the number of HAdV types has been steadily increasing as a result of homologous recombination events (Ismail et al., 2018), the current spectrum has expanded by almost forty newly recognized virus types over the last decade (http://hadvwg.gmu.edu/), reflecting the generation of recombinant viruses with potentially altered tissue tropism and pathogenicity. This implies that the methods used for diagnostic screening must be regularly controlled and adapted, if necessary, in order to ensure reliable detection of all known HAdV types (Kosulin et al., 2016a). Although many pediatric transplant centers have already adopted serial HAdV monitoring in stool samples as part of the routine diagnostic program, the decision to initiate antiviral treatment is still mostly based on detection of the virus in peripheral blood, with attempts to define thresholds of viral copy numbers deemed adequate for the onset of therapy (Teramura et al., 2004; Lindemans et al., 2010; Lee et al., 2013). Based on the observations that delayed treatment initiation by the available therapeutic modalities at the stage of invasive infection carries a considerable risk of failure, it has been suggested that, at least in the pediatric setting, it might be beneficial to start therapy guided by regular monitoring of stool specimens, before the HAdV infection becomes invasive (Lion, 2014; Hiwarkar et al., 2018). However, employment of the novel antiviral agent brincidofovir was shown in clinical studies to permit efficient HAdV elimination even in patients displaying viremia, and the efficacy of this drug was independent from immune reconstitution, in contrast to treatment with cidofovir (Florescu et al., 2012; Grimley et al., 2017; Hiwarkar et al., 2017). These clinical observations highlighted the need to establish improved diagnostic parameters based on the screening of peripheral blood samples. Serial monitoring of HAdV plasma levels has been commonly used to assess the response to therapy, but the possible role of the duration of adenoviremia reflecting the overall systemic exposure to the virus has not been investigated. A holistic measure that combines both parameters could permit improved monitoring of responses to different therapeutic interventions. To address this notion, we have evaluated the impact of peak HAdV levels and the area under the curve indicating virus plasma levels over time as diagnostic and prognostic parameters in pediatric HSCT recipients.

PATIENTS AND METHODS

Patients

Serial samples including stool and peripheral blood specimens derived from 304 patients who were treated by allogeneic stem cell transplantation at the St. Anna Children's Hospital, Vienna, Austria, between the years 2000 and 2015, were investigated. Patient and transplant characteristics were published previously (Kosulin et al., 2018), and the most important parameters are displayed in **Table 1**. The samples were acquired within the routine HAdV screening program starting prior to conditioning, and thereafter at weekly intervals for a minimum of 100 days post-transplant. The present study was restricted to the analysis of test results derived from routine diagnostic analyses, with available written informed consents provided by individual patients and/or their parents. In line with previously published definitions (Lion et al., 2010), disseminated HAdV disease was diagnosed by the detection of multiple organ involvement (e.g., hepatitis, encephalitis, retinitis) in the presence of two or more HAdV-positive PCR assays in peripheral blood and other sites tested (e.g., cerebrospinal

TABLE 1 | Patient characteristics.

Pat.	Age	Underlying disease	Donor type	Conditioning	Engraftment (day post HSCT)				GvHD grade
					Leuko>200/μl	Leuko>1,000/μl	Gran>500/μl	T cells>300μl	
1	1.3	Immunodeficiency	UD	RIC	22	47	99	68	0
2	12.2	Acute leukemia	UD	MA	23	26	24	268	0
3	1.7	Acute leukemia	UD	MA	16	20	21	75	1
4	8.2	Metabolic disease	UD	RIC	10	13	14	74	1
5	3.6	Immunodeficiency	UD	RIC	1	17	18	96	3
6	13.4	Lymphoma	UD	MA	12	14	24	n.a.	0
7	7.4	SAA	UD	RIC	17	20	21	64	4
8	5.1	DA	UD	RIC	13	16	15	n.a.	4
9	3.2	Immunodeficiency	MSD	RIC	21	35	41	115	0
10	16.6	Solid tumor	MMFD	RIC	11	13	13	n.a.	0
11	14.1	Acute leukemia	UD	MA	28	40	40	97	0
12	9.2	Acute leukemia	UD	MA	15	19	18	51	0
13	3.7	Solid tumor	MMFD	RIC	9	12	12	162	0
14	2.2	Solid tumor	MMFD	RIC	17	19	19	n.a.	0
15	10.5	Acute leukemia	UD	MA	16	19	19	n.a.	0
16	7.4	Chronic leukemia	UD	MA	17	32	32	n.a.	4
17	13.6	Lymphoma	UD	MA	28	32	34	111	1
18	9.4	Acute leukemia	MSD	MA	9	11	14	23	4
19	20.1	Acute leukemia	UD	RIC	24	30	29	n.a.	3
20	8.6	Acute leukemia	MMFD	MA	12	13	13	n.a.	0
21	15.7	Acute leukemia	UD	MA	22	24	24	53	3
22	0.6	Immunodeficiency	MMFD	RIC	15	20	20	357	0
23	17.5	Thalassemia	UD	RIC	13	16	15	92	0
24	7.2	Immunodeficiency	UD	RIC	n.a.	n.a.	n.a.	n.a.	0
25	5.6	Lymphoma	UD	MA	14	20	23	n.a.	0
26	8.8	Acute leukemia	UD	MA	17	19	19	n.a.	4
27	0.5	Immunodeficiency	UD	RIC	9	10	10	n.a.	0
28	18.4	Immunodeficiency	UD	RIC	13	n.a.	n.a.	n.a.	0
29	2.1	Acute leukemia	MMFD	MA	13	18	19	n.a.	4
30	17.5	Acute leukemia	UD	RIC	12	n.a.	21	n.a.	0
31	10.0	Acute leukemia	UD	MA	11	12	12	n.a.	0

SAA, severe aplastic anemia; DA, dyserythropoietic anemia; UD, unrelated donor; MSD, matched sibling donor; MMFD, mismatched family donor; RIC, reduced intensity conditioning; MA, myeloablative conditioning; Leuko, leukocytes; Gran, granulocytes; GvHD, Graft vs. host disease; n.a., not achieved or patient died.

fluid, BAL, respiratory secretions, urine), in absence of other identifiable causes. All patients with fever, unexplained symptoms, or laboratory test abnormalities were carefully tested for infections and for GvHD. HAdV-associated death was defined as multiple organ failure in the presence of increasing or persisting adenoviral load in peripheral blood, in association with HAdV detection from multiple other sites, if pertinent.

Antiviral prophylaxis in the HSCT recipients included acyclovir 30 mg/kg per day intravenously from day −7 until day +28 for HSV-IgG positive patients and ganciclovir 10 mg/kg for CMV-IgG positive patients with CMV-IgG negative donors. Patients with a positive PCR test in peripheral blood for CMV or HAdV were regarded as eligible for preemptive antiviral treatment, regardless of the viral load. Treatment was initiated upon availability of PCR results, generally within 48–72 h after sampling. Patients with CMV-DNAemia received primary preemptive therapy with ganciclovir and, in case of persistent DNAemia, secondary preemptive treatment with cidofovir, until two consecutive negative results were obtained. Patients with adenovirus-DNAemia received preemptive treatment with cidofovir, sometimes in combination with ribavirin, if HAdV species C was present, until resolution of DNAemia. In cases of failed response to antivirals and absence of HAdV-specific T-cells, adoptive T-cell transfer with donor-derived HAdV-specific T cells was offered (Lion et al., 2010; Geyeregger et al., 2014).

Isolation of Viral DNA

The QIAamp DNA Mini Kit (Qiagen) was used for extraction of DNA from peripheral blood (PB) specimens, and isolation of DNA from stool samples was done by employing the QIAamp DNA Stool Mini Kit (Qiagen), in line with recommendations provided by the manufacturer.

RQ-PCR Analysis

For HAdV-screening, a pan-adenovirus real-time quantitative (RQ)-PCR assay was used involving the ABI 7500 Sequence Detectors (Thermo Fisher Scientific, Waltham, MA, USA), as specified in earlier reports (Ebner et al., 2005; Kosulin et al., 2016a,b). Samples revealing HAdV-positive test results by the screening assay indicated above were subjected to HAdV species identification by specific PCR tests (Lion et al., 2003). The limit of detection provided by the RQ-PCR tests employed was ten virus DNA copies per PCR reaction, and samples revealing ≥500 DNA copies/ml plasma were deemed HAdV-positive. Accordingly, the presence of adenoviremia was defined as the detectability of HAdV in peripheral blood at or above the indicated level. The HAdV virus burden over time was assessed by calculating the time-averaged area under the curve (AAUC) over 16 weeks from the onset of viremia with ≥1,000 copies/ml. For AAUC calculation, positive values below the lower limit of quantification and negative values within the 16-weeks observation time were also considered, and were assigned arbitrary values of 499 and 99, respectively.

Statistics

The correlation between HAdV peak plasma levels and AAUC quartiles was assessed using the Pearson correlation supplemented by analysis of variance (ANOVA). Fine-Gray models were used to examine the association between AAUC ($\log_{10}$ copies/ml) and time to non-relapse mortality within 1 year of transplant, where relapse was considered as a competing risk and AAUC was included as a continuous covariate. HAdV-related mortality was analyzed similarly, with both relapse and non-HAdV associated deaths handled as competing risks. Hazard ratios (HR) and associated 95% confidence intervals (CI) were determined, to assess the relative risk for mortality in relation to a 1 $\log_{10}$ increase in AAUC ($\log_{10}$ copies/ml). Patients were divided into quartiles based on the PL and AAUC levels, and the median values for each quartile were determined. The quartiles of PL were approximated by logical grouping according to the thresholds indicated below, resulting in seven patients assigned to each of the first three quartiles and ten patients to the highest quartile. HRs and 95% CI were determined by comparing the median value of the lowest quartile vs. median values of the other three quartiles. All analyses were repeated to additionally examine the association of peak HAdV viremia and mortality. Pearson correlation and ANOVA were conducted using the GraphPad Prism 5 software, and Fine-Gray models were run using SAS version 9.4.

RESULTS

Occurrence of Adenoviremia and Outcome

Within the cohort of 304 pediatric patients who underwent allogeneic HSCT at our center, screening by a universal RQ-PCR assay covering the entire spectrum of known HAdV species and types, 31 (10.2%) developed viremia, with HAdV detection of more than 10E3 virus copies/ml at a minimum of two subsequent time points. In nearly all patients who experienced invasive infection, the virus was detectable in stool at levels above the critical threshold of 10E6 copies/g prior to or at the onset of viremia. The only exceptions observed included a few patients in whom no stool data were available for several weeks prior to the onset of viremia (**Table 2**). The distribution of HAdV species detected in PB, displaying predominance of species C and A, corresponded to that detected in children with intestinal persistence of the virus (Kosulin et al., 2016c) (**Table 2**). Concurrent infections with other DNA viruses were frequent 28/31 (90%), most commonly with CMV, EBV and BKV (**Table 2**). During the observation time of 100 days post-transplant, first onset of viremia was detected between days 1 and 93, with a median on day 34 (**Table 2**). The overall mortality in patients with adenoviremia was 68% (21/31), and lethal outcome affected also six of nine patients who had received adoptive transfer of HAdV-specific T-cells in addition to standard treatment with cidofovir ± ribavirin (**Table 2**). The cause of death was attributable to HAdV-related disease in 39% (12/31), while the remaining patients succumbed to relapse of the underlying disease or other infectious or non-infectious complications (**Table 2**).

Temporal Correlation Between Intestinal Adenovirus Reactivation and Onset of Viremia

Nearly all transplant recipients were screened for the presence of HAdV in serial stool specimens already prior to conditioning, and the virus copy numbers were assessed at weekly intervals at least until day 100 post-transplant. In line with our earlier observations (Lion et al., 2010), the onset of HAdV viremia was almost invariably preceded by detection of the virus in stool (**Table 2**). The presence of virus loads exceeding 10E6 copies per gram of stool, a threshold previously demonstrated to confer a very high risk of invasive infection, predated the onset of viremia by a median of 11 days (range 0–79; **Table 2**), corroborating the paramount importance of stool surveillance as a basis for timely risk assessment of impending HAdV viremia in the pediatric allogeneic HSCT setting.

Peak Adenovirus Levels and Viral Burden Over Time (AAUC) in Peripheral Blood

All patients with viremia had HAdV peak levels (PL) of at least 10E3 virus copies/ml PB, and the highest virus copy number observed in the cohort presented was 10E9/ml. The approximate assignment of patients to quartiles based on their peak HAdV copy numbers/ml PB revealed the following distribution: quartile 1, <10E4 (median 1 × 10E3); quartile 2, <10E5 (median 1 × 10E4); quartile 3, <10E6 (median 2 × 10E5); quartile 4, ≥10E6 (median 8.5 × 10E6). In order to determine the overall exposure of patients to the viral burden over time, the AAUC ($\log_{10}$ copies/ml) was calculated for each patient with viremia, as exemplified in **Figure 1**, yielding values between 2.05 and 5.76. The division of patients into quartiles according to their respective AAUC resulted in the following distribution: quartile 1: <2.50 (median 2.09); quartile 2: <3.25 (median 2.75); quartile 3: <4.0 (median 3.47); quartile 4: ≥4.0 (median

TABLE 2 | Virus detection and outcome.

Pat.	1st HAdV pos. in stool (day post HSCT)	>10E6 HAdV copies/g stool (day post HSCT)	1st HAdV pos. in PB (day post HSCT)	HAdV species	HAdV-specific T cell transfer	Cause of death	Co-infections
1	−5	5	19	A		Encephalomyelitis	CMV
2	21	21	27	A		–	BKV, EBV, HSV-1
3	−14	−14	1	C		–	–
4	−9	4	26	A		Relapse	HHV-6
5	5	13	13	C		–	BKV, EBV, A. spp.
6	10	48	85	C		Relapse	BKV, HSV-1
7	−14	28	49	A	YES	–	BKV, PVB19, CMV, HSV-1, HHV-6,-7
8	17	17	19	A	YES	HAdV, CMV	CMV, *C. albicans*
9	−14	6	13	C		–	EBV, HSV1, HHV-6, NV
10	6	11	35	A	YES	SIRS	CMV, EBV
11	13	27	34	C		CNS-LPD, CMV	BKV, CMV, EBV
12	−14	61	72	C	YES	–	BKV, EBV, HHV-6
13	6	14	93	A	YES	–	CMV
14	14	14	21	A		–	EBV, HSV-1, HHV-7
15	n.a.	n.a.	40	C		SIRS	EBV
16	39	54	60	A		VOD	BKV, *C. albicans*
17	7	36	48	C		HAdV	BKV
18	34	34	48	A, C		HAdV	BKV, EBV, HHV-6
19	80	87	94	C		HAdV	CMV, *C. albicans*
20	−14	n.a.*	11	n.d.		HAdV	HHV-6, C.
21	53	67	67	C		HAdV	BKV, CMV, EBV, HHV-7, PVB19, *C. albicans*
22	−14	−14	1	E, F		–	BKV, InfA
23	5	12	50	C		–	CMV
24	−9	n.a.	1	C		HAdV	*A. fumigatus, C. albicans*
25	−7	65	85	C	YES	Relapse	EBV
26	61	68	75	C		Bacterial sepsis	BKV, CMV
27	−14	−14	1	A		HAdV	EBV
28	−2	5	12	C		HAdV	CMV, *C. albicans, C. glabrata*
29	−10	34	34	C	YES	HAdV	–
30	9	10	31	B, E	YES	HAdV	BKV, CMV, A. spp., *C. krusei*
31	17	20	28	C	YES	HAdV	BKV, CMV

*CNS-LPD, central nervous system lymphoproliferative disorder; SIRS, Systemic Inflammatory Response Syndrome; VOD, veno-occlusive disease; BKV, BK virus; CMV, Cytomegalovirus; EBV, Epstein-Barr virus; HHV-6, human herpesvirus 6; HHV-7, human herpesvirus 7; HSV-1, herpes simplex virus 1; InfA, Influenza A virus; NV, Norovirus; PVB19, Parvovirus B19; C., Candida; A., Aspergillus; spp., species; n.a., no available analysis prior to viremia; *No quantitative detection of virus copies available; n.d., not determined.*

4.92). ANOVA showed a significant association of HAdV PL values with individual AAUC quartiles ($p = 0.0001$; **Figure 2A**), and direct comparison between PL and AAUC values in each patient revealed a significant correlation ($p < 0.0001$; R-squared 0.81; **Figure 2B**).

Correlation of Peak Adenovirus Levels and Viral Burden Over Time (AAUC) With Patient Outcome

The HAdV peak viral load and AAUC were both correlated with non-relapse and HAdV-related mortality. An increasing rate of non-relapse mortality was observed with rising AAUC, revealing 25% in quartile 1, 50% in quartile 2, 75% in quartile 3, and 86% in quartile 4. The correlation was less clear for the quartiles of PL, with 43% in quartile 1, 57% in quartile 2, 43% in quartile 3, and 80% in quartile 4. HAdV AAUC was strongly associated with non-relapse mortality ($p < 0.0001$, HR 1.7, 95% CI 1.3–2.2) and HAdV-related mortality ($p < 0.0001$, HR 2.2, 95% CI 1.7–2.9). Hazard ratios relating HAdV AAUC quartiles are summarized in **Table 3**. Similarly, the PL of HAdV viremia was also associated with non-relapse mortality, albeit with less pronounced significance ($p = 0.013$, HR 1.3, 95% CI 1.1–1.6), and revealed a highly significant correlation with HAdV-related mortality ($p = 0.0001$, HR 1.7, 95% CI 1.3–2.2). The corresponding hazard ratios are summarized in **Table 4**.

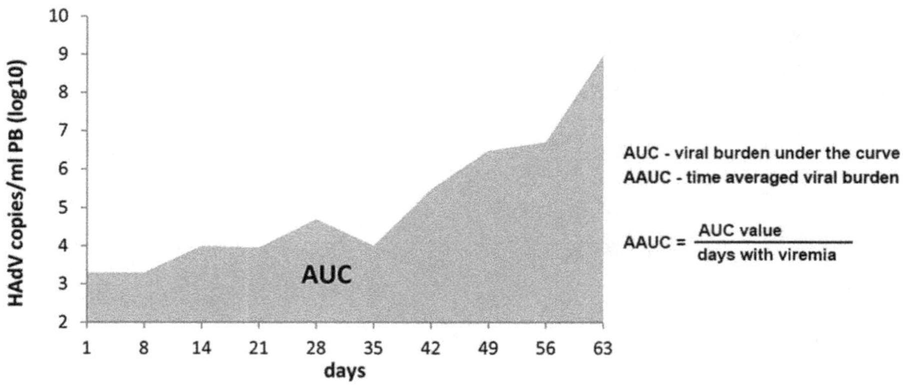

FIGURE 1 | Area under the curve (AUC) and average time-dependent AUC (AAUC). An exemplary AUC of a patient who died from HAdV disease on day 63 after HSCT is shown. The formula underlying the calculation of AAUC is indicated. The denominator for AAUC is not just days with viremia; days alive and without viremia would contribute to averaging viral burden over time (i.e., through 16 weeks, if the patient is alive and available for follow-up at that time).

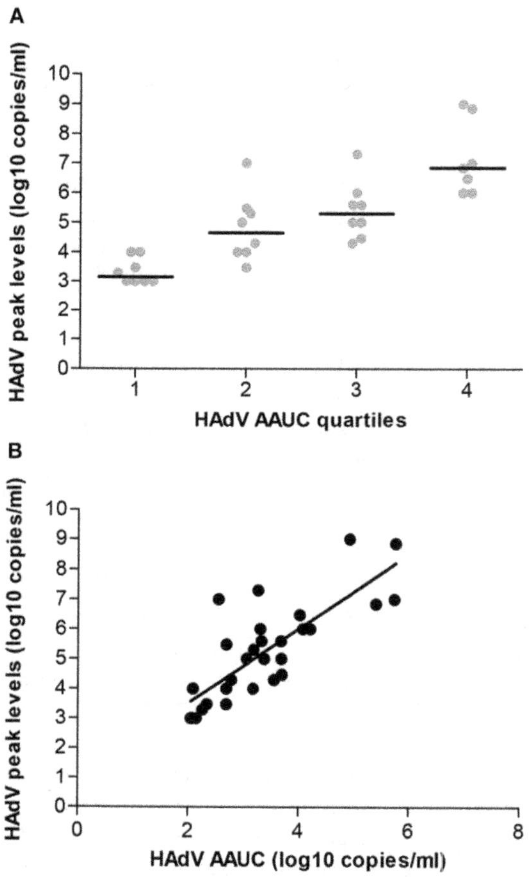

FIGURE 2 | Correlation of HAdV peak levels in peripheral blood with viral burden over time. **(A)** The individual HAdV copy numbers assigned to AAUC quartiles are given (ANOVA variance analysis $p < 0.0001$). **(B)** The Pearson correlation shows a highly significant correlation between the AAUC values and the HAdV copy number peak values ($p < 0.0001$; $r = 0.7977$).

All patients with viremia received antiviral treatment with cidofovir (±ribavirin), and HAdV-specific T-cells derived from the original HSCT donor were provided to nine refractory patients (see **Table 2**). This immunotherapeutic intervention displayed good efficacy in three patients who cleared the infection upon T-cell therapy. However, four patients, including those who had received delayed adoptive transfer of HAdV-specific T-cells, had prolonged viremia with high HAdV burden, and ultimately succumbed to disseminated viral disease, while the remaining two T-cell recipients died from reasons unrelated to HAdV infection. Overall, non-relapse mortality was high in all patients who developed viremia (21/31; 68%), and could be attributed to probable HAdV disease in several instances (12/21; 57%) (**Table 2**).

TABLE 3 | Adenovirus AAUC (log_{10} copies/mL) vs. mortality.

Quartile (Range)	Non-relapse mortality HR (95% CI)	HAdV-related mortality HR (95% CI)
4th (4.0–5.8)	4.4 (2.1–9.2)	9.2 (4.3–19.9)
3rd (3.3–3.7)	2.1 (1.5–3.0)	3.0 (2.0–4.3)
2nd (2.6–3.2)	1.4 (1.2–1.7)	1.7 (1.4–2.0)
1st (2.1–2.3)	Reference	Reference

TABLE 4 | Peak adenovirus levels (log_{10} copies/mL) vs. mortality.

Range	Non-relapse mortality HR (95% CI)	HAdV-related mortality HR (95% CI)
≥6.0	2.8 (1.2–6.2)	7.3 (2.6–20.4)
5.0–<6.0	1.8 (1.1–2.9)	3.2 (1.8–5.9)
4.0–<5.0	1.3 (1.1–1.6)	1.7 (1.3–2.2)
<4.0	Reference	Reference

DISCUSSION

In the present study, we have addressed the potential prognostic relevance of peak HAdV levels in peripheral blood as well as the viral burden over time as diagnostic parameters in pediatric HSCT recipients. These parameters appeared highly correlated ($p < 0.0001$), although some patients with high PL had lower

HAdV AAUC due to the relatively short duration of viremia. However, the number of patients with discrepant assignment to PL vs. AAUC quartiles was too small to determine an impact on outcome. This partial discordance might conceivably be attributable to the effect of antiviral therapy including cidofovir (±ribavirin) and HAdV-specific T-cells.

The correlation of high HAdV load in PB with lethal outcome of the infection in the allogeneic HSCT setting, and consequently, the importance of quantitative monitoring of HAdV DNaemia, have been discussed previously (Ganzenmueller et al., 2011; Lion, 2014; Hiwarkar et al., 2017). Novel treatment options including particularly the antiviral agent brincidofovir, which has documented efficacy in patients with invasive HAdV infection (Florescu et al., 2012; Grimley et al., 2017; Hiwarkar et al., 2017; Ramsay et al., 2017; Lopez et al., 2018), highlight the need for additional PB-based diagnostic parameters permitting the assessment of viral response to treatment and prediction of outcome. The total adenoviral burden over a fixed time period, calculated as HAdV AAUC, captures both peak and duration of viremia. Moreover, the variability in follow-up time inferred by early mortality is controlled by the AAUC. This parameter is an established virological endpoint for quantifying the course and severity of disease in acute lytic viral infections, and has been used previously as a primary endpoint in clinical studies of investigational antivirals (Pulido et al., 2004; Lamarca et al., 2006; DeVincenzo et al., 2014; Vegvari et al., 2016). The employment of AAUC in the present study revealed a clear correlation with patient outcome based on non-relapse mortality, which displayed a continuous increase along the quartiles (**Figure 2A**). The risk of non-relapse mortality was ≥50% in patients assigned to AAUC quartiles 2–4, but it is necessary to consider that the proportion of lethal outcomes within quartile 1 was still as high as 25%. The same principal consideration applies to the peak HAdV levels in PB, where non-relapse mortality was above 40%, regardless of the PL quartile. Despite the more or less pronounced differences between individual AAUC and PL quartiles, these observations indicate that non-relapse mortality was high in all patients who had developed viremia. The number of viremic patients included in the present study is certainly limited, and interpretation of the data must therefore be performed with great caution. Nevertheless, the findings suggest that the onset of viremia at any level may represent a high-risk situation requiring improved clinical management to decrease the mortality rate. In fact, based on the observations presented, differential treatment approaches based on the assignment to different PL or AAUC quartiles would not seem pertinent, but measures that can reduce peak viral load and AAUC are likely to improve outcomes. The recently reported superior efficacy of brincidofovir in comparison to cidofovir in pediatric HSCT recipients with HAdV viremia (Hiwarkar et al., 2017) might, at least in part, be attributable to the fact that oral brincidofovir delivers the antiviral effect directly to the GI tract, which appears to be the primary site of viral replication in this setting.

Invasive HAdV infections represented by viremia occur primarily by representatives of the species A, B, and C, and, in line with published data, the latter species was also most prevalent in viremic patients in the present study. This observation is supported by the predominance of HAdV species C in children with persistence of the virus in the gastrointestinal tract, which is the main site of reactivation and expansion in the pediatric allogeneic HSCT setting, as demonstrated previously (Kosulin et al., 2016c). Other HAdV species (D-G) are far less frequently detected in peripheral blood, and mostly occur in combination with one of the common species (Lion, 2014). There is no evidence, however, that the presence of any particular HAdV species or type in peripheral blood, either alone or in combination, has any relevant impact on the response to antiviral treatment. Neither cidofovir nor brincidofovir reveal any differences in their efficacy against various HAdV species. Only ribavirin, which has occasionally been used in addition to cidofovir, may only be effective, if at all in the clinical setting, against HAdV species C (Lion, 2014). Although HAdV-specific T-cells might conceivably display differential efficacy depending on the species present, there are currently no data supporting the notion that the HAdV species present could affect outcome of the disease.

Current data support the notion that the prevention of invasive HAdV infection should be the paramount aim in order to reduce transplant-related mortality in HSCT recipients. In the pediatric transplant setting, the role of HAdV reactivation and expansion in the intestinal tract has been clearly established as a pre-eminent risk factor for ensuing invasive infection (Lion et al., 2010; Jeulin et al., 2011; Legoff et al., 2017; Hum et al., 2018; Kosulin et al., 2018), and the expected clinical availability of effective antiviral treatment options displaying relatively low toxicity might greatly facilitate stool-guided preemptive therapy (Hiwarkar et al., 2018). The observation that serial HAdV monitoring of stool specimens in children undergoing allogeneic HSCT permits reliable assessment of the risk for invasive HAdV infection is well-documented (Lion et al., 2010; Lion, 2014; Hiwarkar et al., 2018). It was shown that the median time span between the documentation of HAdV copy numbers in stool exceeding the critical threshold of 10E6/g and the onset of viremia was 11 days (Lion et al., 2010; Lion, 2014), thereby providing a rational window of opportunity for early initiation of treatment, in an attempt to prevent systemic infection and disseminated disease. The proposed algorithm for HAdV monitoring and treatment in the pediatric HSCT setting based on serial monitoring of stool samples (Lion, 2014) may remain relevant even if more effective treatment options permitting control of the disease at the stage of viremia become readily available, because early containment of the infection at the pre-invasive stage could be perceived as a preferable strategy with regard to the expected outcome. Besides the considerations pertaining to the importance of preventing invasive infection, the parameters investigated in the present study indicated an intriguing correlation with HAdV-related mortality, which was very low in the AAUC quartiles 1 and 2, and in the PL quartile 1, respectively, including a single patient who has died from probable HAdV infection. Hence, these findings would indicate that virus levels in PB below 10E4 copies/ml and AAUC levels below 3.2 confer a low probability of succumbing to the viral infection, thereby providing diagnostic markers of potential prognostic relevance.

It is necessary to bear in mind, however, that the commonly used definitions of probable or proven HAdV disease may not be universally employed (Lion et al., 2010; Matthes-Martin et al., 2012), and unequivocal attribution of the cause of death to HAdV may be difficult to establish without autopsy and proof of (multiple) organ involvement. Since in severely immunocompromised transplant recipients, co-infections with multiple (viral and other) pathogens are not uncommon, as indicated in **Table 2**, the assignment of the cause of death is supported, in part, by the clinical findings compatible with specific infections and, in part, by the diagnostic monitoring of individual pathogens in the presence of concomitant infections. In case of HAdV-related mortality, which is often associated with multi-organ failure, lethal outcome is generally preceded by high or steadily increasing copy numbers of the virus in serial peripheral blood specimens (Lion et al., 2003; Lion, 2014). If other concomitant infections (including particularly CMV, which can cause similar clinical symptoms), are detectable at low or declining copy numbers during HAdV predominance, the latter virus may be regarded as the main culprit. Nevertheless, the partially discrepant observations between non-relapse and HAdV-related mortality in the present study may indicate that the former term, which also encompasses graft-vs.-host disease, treatment-related toxicity and other infections, may overestimate the actual contribution of HAdV to lethal outcome. In this regard, it would be of interest to employ more extensive diagnostics to facilitate reliable assessment of the actual pathogenetic role of HAdV in organ damage and mortality. Despite the recent insights and the progress in the molecular monitoring of invasive HAdV infections in the HSCT setting, optimal diagnostic surveillance remains a challenging task.

AUTHOR CONTRIBUTIONS

KK analyzed and interpreted the data, designed the study. HP and AL provided patient samples and were involved in data collection. RG was involved in data analysis and interpretation. TL designed the study, was involved in data interpretation and manuscript preparation.

REFERENCES

DeVincenzo, J. P., Whitley, R. J., Mackman, R. L., Scaglioni-Weinlich, C., Harrison, L., Farrell, E., et al. (2014). Oral GS-5806 activity in a respiratory syncytial virus challenge study. *N. Engl. J. Med.* 371, 711–722. doi: 10.1056/NEJMoa1401184

Ebner, K., Suda, M., Watzinger, F., and Lion, T. (2005). Molecular detection of the entire spectrum of human adenoviruses by a two-reaction RQ-PCR assay. *J. Clin. Microbiol.* 43, 3049–3053. doi: 10.1128/JCM.43.7.3049-3053.2005

Feucht, J., Opherk, K., Lang, P., Kayser, S., Hartl, L., Bethge, W., et al. (2015). Adoptive T-cell therapy with hexon-specific Th1 cells as a treatment of refractory adenovirus infection after HSCT. *Blood* 125, 1986–1994. doi: 10.1182/blood-2014-06-573725

Feuchtinger, T., Matthes-Martin, S., Richard, C., Lion, T., Fuhrer, M., Hamprecht, K., et al. (2006). Safe adoptive transfer of virus-specific T-cell immunity for the treatment of systemic adenovirus infection after allogeneic stem cell transplantation. *Br. J. Haematol.* 134, 64–76. doi: 10.1111/j.1365-2141.2006.06108.x

Florescu, D. F., Pergam, S. A., Neely, M. N., Qiu, F., Johnston, C., Way, S., et al. (2012). Safety and efficacy of CMX001 as salvage therapy for severe adenovirus infections in immunocompromised patients. *Biol. Blood Marrow Transplant.* 18, 731–738. doi: 10.1016/j.bbmt.2011.09.007

Ganzenmueller, T., Buchholz, S., Harste, G., Dammann, E., Trenschel, R., and Heim, A. (2011). High lethality of human adenovirus disease in adult allogeneic stem cell transplant recipients with high adenoviral blood load. *J. Clin. Virol.* 52, 55–59. doi: 10.1016/j.jcv.2011.06.005

Geyeregger, R., Freimuller, C., Stemberger, J., Artwohl, M., Witt, V., Lion, T., et al. (2014). First-in-man clinical results with good manufacturing practice (GMP)-compliant polypeptide-expanded adenovirus-specific T cells after haploidentical hematopoietic stem cell transplantation. *J. Immunother.* 37, 245–249. doi: 10.1097/CJI.0000000000000034

Grimley, M. S., Chemaly, R. F., Englund, J. A., Kurtzberg, J., Chittick, G., Brundage, T. M., et al. (2017). Brincidofovir for asymptomatic adenovirus viremia in pediatric and adult allogeneic hematopoietic cell transplant recipients: a randomized placebo-controlled phase II trial. *Biol. Blood Marrow Transplant.* 23, 512–521. doi: 10.1016/j.bbmt.2016.12.621

Hiwarkar, P., Amrolia, P., Sivaprakasam, P., Lum, S. H., Doss, H., O'Rafferty, C., et al. (2017). Brincidofovir is highly efficacious in controlling adenoviremia in pediatric recipients of hematopoietic cell transplant. *Blood* 129, 2033–2037. doi: 10.1182/blood-2016-11-749721

Hiwarkar, P., Kosulin, K., Cesaro, S., Mikulska, M., Styczynski, J., Wynn, R., et al. (2018). Management of adenovirus infection in patients after haematopoietic stem cell transplantation: state-of-the-art and real-life current approach: a position statement on behalf of the Infectious Diseases Working Party of the European Society of Blood and Marrow Transplantation. *Rev. Med. Virol.* 28:e1980. doi: 10.1002/rmv.1980

Hum, R. M., Deambrosis, D., Lum, S. H., Davies, E., Bonney, D., Guiver, M., et al. (2018). Molecular monitoring of adenovirus reactivation in faeces after haematopoietic stem-cell transplantation to predict systemic infection: a retrospective cohort study. *Lancet Haematol.* 5, e422–e429. doi: 10.1016/S2352-3026(18)30130-3

Ismail, A. M., Cui, T., Dommaraju, K., Singh, G., Dehghan, S., Seto, J., et al. (2018). Genomic analysis of a large set of currently-and historically-important human adenovirus pathogens. *Emerg. Microbes Infect.* 7:10. doi: 10.1038/s41426-017-0004-y

Jeulin, H., Salmon, A., Bordigoni, P., and Venard, V. (2011). Diagnostic value of quantitative PCR for adenovirus detection in stool samples as compared with antigen detection and cell culture in haematopoietic stem cell transplant recipients. *Clin. Microbiol. Infect.* 17, 1674–1680. doi: 10.1111/j.1469-0691.2011.03488.x

Kosulin, K., Berkowitsch, B., and Lion, T. (2016a). Modified pan-adenovirus real-time PCR assay based on genome analysis of seventy HAdV types. *J. Clin. Virol.* 80, 60–61. doi: 10.1016/j.jcv.2016.05.001

Kosulin, K., Berkowitsch, B., Matthes, S., Pichler, H., Lawitschka, A., Potschger, U., et al. (2018). Intestinal adenovirus shedding before allogeneic stem cell transplantation is a risk factor for invasive infection post-transplant. *EBioMedicine* 28, 114–119. doi: 10.1016/j.ebiom.2017.12.030

Kosulin, K., Dworzak, S., Lawitschka, A., Matthes-Leodolter, S., and Lion, T. (2016b). Comparison of different approaches to quantitative adenovirus detection in stool specimens of hematopoietic stem cell transplant recipients. *J. Clin. Virol.* 85, 31–36. doi: 10.1016/j.jcv.2016.10.021

Kosulin, K., Geiger, E., Vecsei, A., Huber, W. D., Rauch, M., Brenner, E., et al. (2016c). Persistence and reactivation of human adenoviruses in the gastrointestinal tract. *Clin. Microbiol. Infect.* *22*, 381 e381–381 e388. doi: 10.1016/j.cmi.2015.12.013

Lamarca, A., Clumeck, N., Plettenberg, A., Domingo, P., Fu, K., Craig, C., et al. (2006). Efficacy and safety of a once-daily fixed-dose combination of abacavir/lamivudine compared with abacavir twice daily and lamivudine once daily as separate entities in antiretroviral-experienced HIV-1-infected patients (CAL30001 Study). *J. Acquir. Immune Defic. Syndr.* 41, 598–606. doi: 10.1097/01.qai.0000214821.33905.5c

Lee, Y. J., Chung, D., Xiao, K., Papadopoulos, E. B., Barker, J. N., Small, T. N., et al. (2013). Adenovirus viremia and disease: comparison of T cell-depleted and conventional hematopoietic stem cell transplantation recipients from a single institution. *Biol. Blood Marrow Transplant.* 19, 387–392. doi: 10.1016/j.bbmt.2012.10.014

Lee, Y. J., Huang, Y. T., Kim, S. J., Maloy, M., Tamari, R., Giralt, S. A., et al. (2016). Adenovirus viremia in adult CD34(+) selected hematopoietic cell transplant recipients: low incidence and high clinical impact. *Biol. Blood Marrow Transplant.* 22, 174–178. doi: 10.1016/j.bbmt.2015.08.019

Legoff, J., Resche-Rigon, M., Bouquet, J., Robin, M., Naccache, S. N., Mercier-Delarue, S., et al. (2017). The eukaryotic gut virome in hematopoietic stem cell transplantation: new clues in enteric graft-versus-host disease. *Nat. Med.* 23, 1080–1085. doi: 10.1038/nm.4380

Lindemans, C. A., Leen, A. M., and Boelens, J. J. (2010). How I treat adenovirus in hematopoietic stem cell transplant recipients. *Blood* 116, 5476–5485. doi: 10.1182/blood-2010-04-259291

Lion, T. (2014). Adenovirus infections in immunocompetent and immunocompromised patients. *Clin. Microbiol. Rev.* 27, 441–462. doi: 10.1128/CMR.00116-13

Lion, T., Baumgartinger, R., Watzinger, F., Matthes-Martin, S., Suda, M., Preuner, S., et al. (2003). Molecular monitoring of adenovirus in peripheral blood after allogeneic bone marrow transplantation permits early diagnosis of disseminated disease. *Blood* 102, 1114–1120. doi: 10.1182/blood-2002-07-2152

Lion, T., Kosulin, K., Landlinger, C., Rauch, M., Preuner, S., Jugovic, D., et al. (2010). Monitoring of adenovirus load in stool by real-time PCR permits early detection of impending invasive infection in patients after allogeneic stem cell transplantation. *Leukemia* 24, 706–714. doi: 10.1038/leu.2010.4

Lopez, S. M. C., Michaels, M. G., and Green, M. (2018). Adenovirus infection in pediatric transplant recipients: are effective antiviral agents coming our way? *Curr. Opin. Organ Transplant.* 23, 395–399. doi: 10.1097/MOT.0000000000000542

Matthes-Martin, S., Feuchtinger, T., Shaw, P. J., Engelhard, D., Hirsch, H. H., Cordonnier, C., et al. (2012). European guidelines for diagnosis and treatment of adenovirus infection in leukemia and stem cell transplantation: summary of ECIL-4 (2011). *Transpl. Infect. Dis.* 14, 555–563. doi: 10.1111/tid.12022

Pulido, F., Katlama, C., Marquez, M., Thomas, R., Clumeck, N., Pedro Rde, J., et al. (2004). A randomized study investigating the efficacy and safety of amprenavir in combination with low-dose ritonavir in protease inhibitor-experienced HIV-infected adults. *HIV Med.* 5, 296–302. doi: 10.1111/j.1468-1293.2004.00224.x

Ramsay, I. D., Attwood, C., Irish, D., Griffiths, P. D., Kyriakou, C., and Lowe, D. M. (2017). Disseminated adenovirus infection after allogeneic stem cell transplant and the potential role of brincidofovir–case series and 10 year experience of management in an adult transplant cohort. *J. Clin. Virol.* 96, 73–79. doi: 10.1016/j.jcv.2017.09.013

Rustia, E., Violago, L., Jin, Z., Foca, M. D., Kahn, J. M., Arnold, S., et al. (2016). Risk factors and utility of a risk-based algorithm for monitoring cytomegalovirus, Epstein-Barr virus, and adenovirus infections in pediatric recipients after allogeneic hematopoietic cell transplantation. *Biol. Blood Marrow Transplant.* 22, 1646–1653. doi: 10.1016/j.bbmt.2016.05.014

Saif, M. A., Borrill, R., Bigger, B. W., Lee, H., Logan, A., Poulton, K., et al. (2015). *In vivo* T-cell depletion using alemtuzumab in family and unrelated donor transplantation for pediatric non-malignant disease achieves engraftment with low incidence of graft vs. host disease. *Pediatr. Transplant.* 19, 211–218. doi: 10.1111/petr.12416

Sive, J. I., Thomson, K. J., Morris, E. C., Ward, K. N., and Peggs, K. S. (2012). Adenoviremia has limited clinical impact in the majority of patients following alemtuzumab-based allogeneic stem cell transplantation in adults. *Clin. Infect. Dis.* 55, 1362–1370. doi: 10.1093/cid/cis689

Taniguchi, K., Yoshihara, S., Tamaki, H., Fujimoto, T., Ikegame, K., Kaida, K., et al. (2012). Incidence and treatment strategy for disseminated adenovirus disease after haploidentical stem cell transplantation. *Ann. Hematol.* 91, 1305–1312. doi: 10.1007/s00277-012-1440-3

Teramura, T., Naya, M., Yoshihara, T., Kanoh, G., Morimoto, A., and Imashuku, S. (2004). Adenoviral infection in hematopoietic stem cell transplantation: early diagnosis with quantitative detection of the viral genome in serum and urine. *Bone Marrow Transplant.* 33, 87–92. doi: 10.1038/sj.bmt.1704320

Vegvari, C., Hadjichrysanthou, C., Cauet, E., Lawrence, E., Cori, A., de Wolf, F., et al. (2016). How can viral dynamics models inform endpoint measures in clinical trials of therapies for acute viral infections? *PLoS ONE* 11:e0158237. doi: 10.1371/journal.pone.0158237

15

Viral Respiratory Infections in the Neonatal Intensive Care Unit

Karin Pichler[1]*, *Ojan Assadian*[2] *and Angelika Berger*[1]

[1] Division of Neonatology, Intensive Care and Neuropediatrics, Department of Pediatrics and Adolescent Medicine, Medical University of Vienna, Vienna, Austria, [2] Department for Hospital Epidemiology and Infection Control, Medical University of Vienna, Vienna, Austria

Correspondence:
Karin Pichler
karin.a.pichler@meduniwien.ac.at

Although infrequent, respiratory viral infections (RVIs) during birth hospitalization have a significant impact on short- and long-term morbidity in term and preterm neonates. RVI have been associated with increased length of hospital stay, severe disease course, unnecessary antimicrobial exposure and nosocomial outbreaks in the neonatal intensive care unit (NICU). Virus transmission has been described to occur via health care professionals, parents and other visitors. Most at risk are infants born prematurely, due to their immature immune system and the fact that they stay in the NICU for a considerable length of time. A prevalence of RVIs in the NICU in symptomatic infants of 6–30% has been described, although RVIs are most probably underdiagnosed, since testing for viral pathogens is not performed routinely in symptomatic patients in many NICUs. Additional challenges are the wide range of clinical presentation of RVIs, their similarity to bacterial infections and the unreliable detection methods prior to the era of molecular biology based technologies. In this review, current knowledge of early-life RVI in the NICU is discussed. Reviewed viral pathogens include human rhinovirus, respiratory syncytial virus and influenza virus, and discussed literature is restricted to reports based on modern molecular biology techniques. The review highlights therapeutic approaches and possible preventive strategies. Furthermore, short- and long-term consequences of RVIs in infants hospitalized in the NICU are discussed.

Keywords: viral respiratory tract infections, neonatal intensive care unit, preterm infant, human rhinovirus, respiratory syncytial virus, human metapneumovirus, influenza virus

INTRODUCTION

Respiratory viral infections (RVIs) are increasingly recognized to be more prevalent in the neonatal intensive care unit (NICU) than previously considered (Ronchi et al., 2014). So far, RVIs have frequently been undiagnosed or have been identified only late in the course of an infectious episode because of their subtle clinical presentation (Ronchi et al., 2014). If infants presented with clinical deterioration the standard approach in many NICUs usually is to evaluate for bacterial sepsis, but the possibility that a viral pathogen may be the causative agent still is not being considered routinely. The currently established work-up strategy is supported by abundantly available diagnostic methods with a focus on bacterial agents and a still limited diagnostic accuracy with low sensitivity in increasingly available viral point-of care tests based on antigen detection (Casiano-Colón et al., 2003).

Only the emergence of new diagnostic methods such as the multiplex reverse transcription-polymerase chain reaction enzyme-linked immunosorbent assay (multiplex RT-PCR ELISA) facilitated the identification of virus or virus genome in pediatric patients (Woo et al., 1997; Meerhoff et al., 2010; Krause et al., 2014). PCR based technologies provide results with high sensitivity and specificity and allow screening for a large number of different viruses from a single specimen. Early virus detection is particularly important in the vulnerable infant hospitalized in a NICU. Immediate implementation of effective isolation and infection prevention measures are necessary to prevent further viral transmission, especially in modern, family centered NICUs. These units bear increased risks of virus transmission as they provide kangaroo care, 24-h visiting policies, and are not only open to parents and siblings, but do also encourage their involvement. Early virus detection also facilitates the withholding or discontinuation of avoidable antimicrobial therapy, contributing to NICU specific stewardship initiatives (Cantey and Patel, 2014). In this review, current knowledge of and literature on early-life RVI in the NICU is discussed on the basis of human rhinovirus, respiratory syncytial virus, and influenza virus. Only original research articles based on modern molecular biology techniques and published in English as well as reporting hospital-acquired RVIs were included.

Anectodal reports have also been published on other than the mentioned viruses such as parainfluenza virus type 3. However, in all of these reports viruses were detected using immunofluorescence techniques (Singh-Naz et al., 1990; Simmonds et al., 2009; Dunn et al., 2017; Maeda et al., 2017). Since this review focuses on reports using PCR-based diagnostics, reports on parainfluenza virus were not included.

Occurrence and Impact of Viral Respiratory Tract Infections

Although molecular biology based detection methods have already been established 20 years ago, data on the occurrence of RVIs in the NICU is still limited (Ronchi et al., 2014). In infants hospitalized in the NICU and evaluated for late-onset sepsis, the incidence of RVIs was reported to be 6.6–8% (Ronchi et al., 2014; Cerone et al., 2017; Kidszun et al., 2017). An observational study from the Netherlands found an overall incidence of RVIs in the NICU of around 1% (Verboon-Maciolek et al., 2005).

Lately, concern of increased nosocomial respiratory virus infection rates arose, because of family centered care and liberalization of visiting policies in NICUs, especially for siblings. Data in this regard are controversial. Some studies noted an increase in symptomatic RVI due to sibling visits (Schwab et al., 1983; Solheim and Spellacy, 1988; Moore et al., 2003; Peluso et al., 2015; Horikoshi et al., 2018). Peluso et al. hypothesized that findings might differ in open-ward NICUs vs. NICUs with single-patient rooms (Peluso et al., 2015), whereas others did not note such an increase. Details on the studies investigating the occurrence of RVIs in the NICU including detected viruses are given in **Table 1**.

Although the reported incidences seem to be relatively low, relevant short and long-term consequences of early-life RVIs shall be considered (Bennett et al., 2012; Ronchi et al., 2014; Kidszun et al., 2017). Early-life RVIs have been reported to be associated with increased length of hospital stay, severe disease, otherwise avoidable antimicrobial exposure, and nosocomial outbreaks in the NICU (Gelber and Ratner, 2002; Kidszun et al., 2014). A study from the UK reported that 51% of preterm infants with a RVI needed escalation of respiratory support during the episode with more respiratory pressure support and twice as many required home oxygen. Furthermore, the frequency of broncho-pulmonary dysplasia (BPD) was significantly higher among these infants (Bennett et al., 2012). The majority of patients hospitalized in a NICU, have an immature and inexperienced innate and adaptive immune system (van den Berg et al., 2010). Their innate cytokine response against viruses can be inadequate or, conversely, overwhelming and thus associated with increased disease severity (Perez et al., 2015).

The long-term impact of early-life RVIs is lesser explopored. One study showed an association with lung function abnormalities in susceptible infants, particularly recurrent wheeze and asthma at follow-up at school age (Jackson, 2014). Bennett et al. (2012) reported complications such as longer length of stay and prolonged ventilatory support as well as more than twice the rate of BPD in infants without overt symptoms of RVI but positive virus detection during birth hospitalization. However, it is debatable whether the detection of a virus in nasopharyngeal aspirates truly proves an active respiratory viral infection (Pavia, 2011). Especially viruses like rhinovirus, adenovirus, and enterovirus have frequently been identified in asymptomatic infants (van Benten et al., 2003; Rhedin et al., 2014). Also, during routine surveillance monitoring, respiratory viruses are found in up to 52% of infants in the NICU (Smit et al., 2013). Thus, it remains unresolved how these findings should be applied to preterm infants during birth hospitalization.

Several studies (Jefferson et al., 2011; Bennett et al., 2012; Kujari et al., 2014; French et al., 2016) reported strategies that aimed to reduce nosocomial RVI in the NICU. The most effective infection prevention practices proved to be cohorting of infected patients, staff protective equipment such as gowns and gloves, hand hygiene policies and restriction of visitors during periods of high community RVI prevalence. However, the majority of these infection prevention measures have been implemented during outbreak situations, and the effect of single measures was never explored systematically in prospective controlled studies. It must, however, be acknowledged that designing prospective studies investigating the preventive efficacy of one single intervention in the clinical practice of a NICU comes with practical and ethical limitations.

Influenza

Influenza virus infections have long been thought to be uncommon in neonates due to the presence of maternal antibodies (Puck et al., 1980) and the fact that neonates generally have reduced contact with adults or children infected with influenza virus (Wilkinson et al., 2006). However, there is an increasing number of reports on influenza infections in neonates and descriptions of influenza spread within neonatal units. Importantly, cases of severe influenza and mortality in

TABLE 1 | Studies investigating the occurrence of RVIs in the NICU (LOS, late onset sepsis; RSV, respiratory syncytial virus; HRV, human rhinovirus; LOS, late-onset sepsis; NICU, neonatal intensive care unit; RTVI, respiratory tract viral infection; PMA, post menstrual age).

Study	Study group	Duration of the study	Prevalence (virus-positive/examined individuals)	Detected viruses
Cerone et al., 2017, USA	All infants evaluated for LOS	26 month	29/357 (8%), 3 infants were co-infected with more than one virus	RSV (n = 14), HRV (n = 11), others (n = 7)
Kidszun et al., 2017, Germany	All infants evaluated for LOS	43 month	6/137 (6.8%)	Picornavirus (n = 4), RSV (n = 2)
Caserta et al., 2017, USA	All infants in the NICU <36 weeks PMA	2 month	4/618 (0.6%), 50% asymptomatic	RSV (n = 1), HRV (n = 1), coronavirus 4 (n = 1), Influenza B (n = 1)
Zinna et al., 2016, UK	Retrospective case-control study of infants with PCR positive RVI	6 years	95/275	HRV (n = 65), parainfluenza virus type 3 (n = 6), RSV (n = 5), others (n = 19)
Kidszun et al., 2014, Germany	All infants evaluated for LOS	19 month	6/60 (10%)	Picornavirus (n =5), RSV (n = 1)
Ronchi et al., 2014, USA	All infants evaluated for LOS	12 month	8/100 (8%)	Entero-/rhinoviruses (n = 2), HRV (n = 2), coroncavirus (n = 2), parainfluenza viruses (n = 2)
Bennett et al., 2012, USA	All infants in the NICU <33 weeks PMA	12 month	26/50 (52%), 30% asymptomatic	Parainfluenza viruses (n = 20), RSV (n = 15), metapneumovirus (n = 9), others (n = 11)
Diniz et al., 2005, Portugal	Infants with acute respiratory failure and need of mechanical ventilation <37 weeks PMA	2 years	23/78 (29.5%)	RSV (n = 11), influenza A (n = 8), co-infection with 2 viruses (n = 4)

the newborn and especially the preterm infant have also been reported (Wilkinson et al., 2006; Sert et al., 2010).

Influenza is an RNA virus of the *Orthomyxoviridae* family, classified into types A, B, and C. Influenza type A is responsible for most clinical infection in humans, whereas type B accounts only for 11% of human infections and type C causes only mild illness (Woods and Abramson, 2005). Transmission occurs mainly by aerosol. Transmission by large droplets and self-inoculation of the nasal mucosa by contaminated hands has also been described several times (Tellier, 2009). The incubation period of influenza ranges from 1 to 5 days. Viral shedding occurs 1 day before clinical symptoms appear through the duration of the symptomatic period (Gelber and Ratner, 2002). Protection and treatment are limited in neonates and especially preterm infants (Whitley and Monto, 2006) as current influenza vaccines are not effective in infants under 6 month of age (Principi and Esposito, 2004). An important prevention method is annual vaccination against influenza of parents, other caregivers and health care workers. However, low compliance, particularly in health care workers, has been repeatedly reported (Kassianos et al., 2018) also among health care workers in the NICU (Milupi et al., 2012; Tsagris et al., 2012). Thus, infected NICU staff may be the source of nosocomial outbreaks, particularly during the early onset phase of the infection and when pressure to present at work is high during critically staffed periods. Despite the obviously possible vicious circle of low immunization rate among healthcare workers—increased likelihood of influenza infection—decreased staffing—increased pressure to present at work even when prodromal symptoms start, we did not identify epidemiological work focusing on the effect of these interconnections.

In the era of PCR-based detection methods 5 outbreaks of influenza have been reported in NICUs (**Table 2**) (Rocha et al., 2010; Pannaraj et al., 2011; Vij et al., 2011; Milupi et al., 2012; Tsagris et al., 2012). All these outbreaks occurred during the 2009–2010 H1N1 pandemic and reported influenza A/H1N1/2009 as causing virus. The affected infants presented mainly with respiratory symptoms including desaturation, tachypnea, increased secretions, apnea and need for mechanical ventilation. Additionally bradycardia, pyrexia, and rales were observed. Such clinical features may be difficult to distinguish from bacterial sepsis. One infant was reported to develop clinical seizures during infection with influenza A/H1N1/2009 (Vij et al., 2011). This infant was born at 29 weeks postmenstrual age (PMA) and was 21 days old at the onset of influenza infection. Because of the seizures a cerebrospinal fluid analysis was performed with normal results. However, it was not sent for influenza A/H1N1/2009 PCR. Also, a cranial MRI did not reveal any abnormalities and the patient fully recovered from the influenza infection. Seizures have been described in association with influenza infections in older children along with neurologic manifestations including encephalopathy (Ekstrand et al., 2010; Kedia et al., 2011).

Next to these outbreak descriptions there are a few case reports on influenza infections in infants hospitalized in the NICU. A publication from Israel reports on a preterm infant of 32 weeks PMA, who developed respiratory failure on day of life 50 due to Influenza A/H1N1. The infant received the neuraminidase inhibitor oseltamivir in therapeutic dosage and was discharged in good health at day of life 60 (Barak et al., 2010). In contrast, Jajoo et al. from India published a case of a preterm infant of 32 weeks PMA who presented with respiratory failure on day

TABLE 2 | Influenza outbreaks in the NICU detected by RT-PCR including details on affected infants, clinical symptoms, and infection control measures taken.

Study	Date	NICU	Pathogen	Affected infants	Symptoms	Median age at symptoms onset (range)	Infection control measures	Source of the outbreak	Health care workers vaccination rate
Milupi et al., 2012, UK	4-day period in Jan 2011	Level II	Influenza A/H1N1/2009	3 preterm infants born at 28, 30, and 31 weeks PMA	Bradycardia, desaturation, tachypnea, apnea	21 (13–28)	Oseltamivir treatment of affected infants, cohorting, admission stop for 3 days, enhanced surveillance for 2 weeks	Unknown	40%
Tsagris et al., 2012, Greece	February 2011	Level III	Influenza A/H1N1/2009	3 preterm infants born at 24, 28, and 35 weeks PMA	Apnoea, pyrexia, rhinits	67 (47–84)	Oseltamivir treatment of affected infants, oseltamivir prophylaxis in all other infants in the NICU, RT-PCR before discontinuation of therapy, cohortation and care in isolated incubators, admission stop	Non-vaccinated staff members	15%
Pannaraj et al., 2011, USA	June and July 2009	Level III	Influenza A/H1N1/2009	11 infants born at 26–40 weeks PMA	Influenza like illness	72 (5–192)	Oseltamivir treatment of affected infants, oseltamivir prophylaxis in all other infants in the NICU, isolation and cohortating, visitor restriction, monitoring for symptoms in health care personnel, admission stop	One ill family member	Not specified
Vij et al., 2011, USA	October-November 2009	Level II and III	Influenza A/H1N1/2009	3 infants born at 25, 28, and 29 weeks PMA	Increased secretions, increased oxygen requirements, apnea, rales, need for mechanical ventilation, seizures, increased abdominal girth	29 (16–51)	Cohortating and isolation of affected infants	Unknown	Not specified
Rocha et al., 2010, Portugal	November 2009	Level III	Influenza A/H1N1	12 infants born at 28–40 weeks PMA	Respiratory deterioration including need for mechanical ventilation	18 (3–38)	Oseltamivir treatment of affected infants, oseltamivir prophylaxis in all other infants in the NICU, cohorting	Index case identified	Not specified

of life 6. The infant was diagnosed with influenza A/H1N1 on day of life 10 and oseltamivir was started in therapeutic dosage. Nevertheless, the infants' pneumonia continued to worsen and the infant died on day of life 16 due to refractory shock and multiorgan dysfunction (Jajoo and Gupta, 2010). To the best of our knowledge this is the only infant reported to have died in the NICU due to influenza A infection, whereas all other reported infants recovered fully from the infection. This is in contrast to reports in other healthcare settings and older patients, where epidemic and pandemic influenza was associated with significant mortality in infants (Bhat et al., 2005). The reason for the relatively low mortality of infants affected from influenza in the NICU is unclear. An important fact might be increased awareness of NICU staff especially in times of pandemics and consecutively early diagnosis and prompt initiation of supportive therapy.

In most of the reported outbreaks and also in the case reports of influenza infection in the NICU, the affected infants were treated with the neuraminidase inhibitor oseltamivir (Bhat et al., 2005; Jajoo and Gupta, 2010; Rocha et al., 2010; Pannaraj et al., 2011; Milupi et al., 2012; Tsagris et al., 2012). Exposed infants commonly received oseltamivir prophylaxis (Rocha et al., 2010; Pannaraj et al., 2011; Milupi et al., 2012; Tsagris et al., 2012). In one NICU outbreak scenario infants diagnosed with influenza were only cohorted and isolated without any drug treatment. Also these infants had a favorable outcome (Vij et al., 2011).

Oseltamivir is a neuraminidase inhibitor effective against both influenza A and B. It is converted to its active metabolite, oseltamivir carboxylate by hepatic esterases and then renally eliminated through both glomerular filtration and tubular secretion processes. These processes are diminished in neonates and young adults and do not reach adult capacity until 6–12 months of age (Abdel-Rahman et al., 2011). Oseltamivir has been shown to reduce the duration of illness in previously healthy children by 26% (36 h; Matheson et al., 2007). Furthermore, it significantly reduced complications of influenza, particularly otitis media. Safety concerns about the use of neuraminidase inhibitors in infants have been raised after an animal trial conducted by the US Food and Drug Administration (Wooltorton, 2004). In this trial 7-day old rats were fed with excessively high doses of oseltamivir (~250 times the dose recommended in children). Many of the rats died consecutively. Nevertheless in 2009 during the H1N1 pandemic, the U.S. Food and Drug Administration released an Emergency Use Authorization (EUA) for oseltamivir in infants <1 year of age. The recommendation for dosage was initially age-dependent and was then corrected to a weight-based dosing approach, i.e., 3 mg/kg/dose orally twice daily for children 0 to <12 month based on the CASG (collaborative Antiviral Study Group of the National Institutes of Health NIH, USA) study results. Acosta et al. subsequently conducted a study to determine the dosing in preterm infants (Acosta et al., 2010). Results from this study suggest a therapeutic oseltamivir dosage of ~1 mg/kg/dose twice daily as well as a prophylactic oseltamivir dosage of ~1 mg/kg/dose once a day in premature neonates <37 weeks PMA (Acosta et al., 2010). Both treatment and prophylaxis with oseltamivir must be started within 48 h of the onset of symptoms or of exposure to be effective (Munoz, 2003; Matheson et al., 2007). In both outbreak reports and case reports where oseltamivir was used in therapeutic and/or prophylactic dose, no serious side effects, especially no central nervous system toxicity was observed (Bhat et al., 2005; Jajoo and Gupta, 2010; Rocha et al., 2010; Pannaraj et al., 2011; Vij et al., 2011; Milupi et al., 2012; Tsagris et al., 2012). Only mild gastrointestinal symptoms like diarrhea were reported. Laboratory investigations monitoring hematology, renal, and hepatic functions were not altered due to therapy with oseltamivir. Thus, oseltamivir in the currently recommended dosage seems to be safe also in the smallest infants and can be considered as therapeutic option during outbreak situations in the NICU.

Human Rhinovirus

Human rhinovirus (HRV) is among the most frequent causes of upper and lower respiratory tract infections in infants hospitalized in the NICU (van Piggelen et al., 2010; Steiner et al., 2012). HRV is classified into 3 species, A, B and C, within the genus *Enterovirus* of the *Picornaviridae* family. More than 150 different HRV genotypes are known so far. HRV infections do not provide protective immunity against other genotypes because of a low cross-neutralization between serotypes (Jacobs et al., 2013). This might be an explanation for the frequent occurrence of HRV infections. Rhinovirus species C has been associated with more severe illness in several reports, especially in preterm infants, compared to species A or B (Reid et al., 2011; Marcone et al., 2018). Treatment of HRV infection is limited to symptomatic treatment.

Five reports on HRV outbreaks in hospitalized NICU patients have been identified (**Table 3**). HRV species C was detected as causative agent in three of these reports (Reid et al., 2011; Reese et al., 2016; Marcone et al., 2018), whereas in the other two HRV species was not elucidated due to lack of genotyping (van Piggelen et al., 2010; Steiner et al., 2012). HRV affected both term and preterm infants. Mean age at onset of symptoms was 58 days (range 5–282 days). The most frequent symptoms were nasal congestion, increased respiratory secretions and increased work of breathing. Almost all reported infants needed increased respiratory support and increased oxygen supplementation during the course of the HRV infection (van Piggelen et al., 2010; Reid et al., 2011; Steiner et al., 2012; Reese et al., 2016; Marcone et al., 2018). In the report of van Piggelen et al. from the Netherlands (van Piggelen et al., 2010), which included 11 patients of 26–41 weeks PMA, all infants needed mechanical ventilation during the infectious episode. Generally, severe respiratory failure due to HRV infection does not seem to be uncommon (Reid et al., 2011; Steiner et al., 2012; Reese et al., 2016; Marcone et al., 2018) and has been described even in an otherwise healthy term newborn (Broberg et al., 2011). In contrast, all patients requiring mechanical ventilation during HRV infection in the report of Steiner et al. had major co-morbidities besides prematurity (giant thoracic lymphangioma, neuromuscular impairment owing to severe perinatal asphyxia and to suspected metabolic disorder, respectively; Steiner et al., 2012). Furthermore, Steiner et al. reported that presence of apneas during HRV infection correlated with a more severe disease course (Steiner et al., 2012).

All infants reported in the literature recovered from HRV infection. One study (van Piggelen et al., 2010) reported that 4 infants developed recurrent respiratory tract infections in the first year of life, which, according to the authors, could not be explained solely by prematurity. No other data is available on possible long-term consequences of HRV infection in this early period of life.

Also, only limited data exists about nosocomial HRV transmission (Reid et al., 2011; Reese et al., 2016; Marcone et al., 2018). It is known that HRV can remain viable from hours to days on environmental surfaces at ambient temperature. Thus, transmission can occur both via direct contact or aerosolization (Jacobs et al., 2013). A further challenge of HRV is that virus shedding has been reported to occur up to 44 days in otherwise healthy preterm infants (Steiner et al., 2012; Marcone et al., 2018). Management of these infants with a positive PCR result but resolved clinical signs in the NICU is problematic. To date there are no studies correlating viral loads with either infectiousness or the presence of infectious viral particles.

Respiratory Syncytial Virus (RSV)

RSV is an enveloped, non-segmented, negative-sense RNA virus belonging to the *Pneumoviridae* family and is classified in the genus orthopneumovirus. It is divided into two antigenic subgroups, A and B. RSV is the leading cause of hospitalization for respiratory illness in children under 12 month of age (Iwane et al., 2004). It causes seasonal outbreaks worldwide. Symptoms of RSV infection range from afebrile cough and congestion to severe bronchiolitis or pneumonia with respiratory failure. Most at risk for severe RSV infection are infants aged <6 months, preterm infants born prior to 35 weeks PMA and infants and children with underlying lung disease or congenital heart disease (Boyce et al., 2000). Some studies reported more severe disease courses in RSV subtype A infections as compared to subytpe B (Halasa et al., 2005; Buonocore et al., 2012).

RSV spreads by close contact via direct inoculation of large-particle aerosols or self-inoculation after touching contaminated surfaces. RSV is also able to spread hemtogenously from the primary site of infection to remote extra-pulmonary tissue (Eisenhut, 2006). The virus replicates in the nasal or ocular mucosal epithelium (Goldmann, 2000). Although RSV is relatively labile, the virus can survive for 6–12 h on surfaces, providing the opportunity for environmental nosocomial transmission. Homaira et al. examined clothing of health care workers and visitors as potential source of RSV infection in the NICU and detected RSV-RNA only at a low viral load on clothing of health care workers (Homaira et al., 2016). An older study found that freshly obtained secretions from infected infants survive on clothing of health care workers for ~40 min (Hall et al., 1980). Thus, carriage on clothing may contribute to nosocomial infections in the NICU.

RSV detection rates in NICUs in the absence of outbreaks seem to be low. Studies indicated rates from 1 to 4% during winter epidemics (Berger et al., 2010; Homaira et al., 2016). However, nosocomial RSV infections have been reported to cause

TABLE 3 | HRV outbreaks in the NICU including details of affected infants, symptoms, and infection control measures.

Study	Date	NICU	Pathogen	Affected infants	Symptoms	Median age at symptoms onset (range)	Infection control measures	Source of the outbreak
Marcone et al., 2018, Argentina	Winter 2014	Level III	Four different rhinovirus genotypes (C43, C1, C6, and A63-like)	2 extremely preterm, 3 very preterm, 1 late preterm infant	Symptoms of lower respiratory tract infection, need for oxygen supplementation	42 days (8–62 days)	Contact isolation	Unknown
Reese et al., 2016, USA	Not specified	Level II-III	HRV species C	2 infants born at 25 weeks PMA and 31 weeks PMA	Symptoms of lower respiratory tract infection, need for oxygen supplementation	44 days (16–73)	Not specified	Unknown
Steiner et al., 2012, Austria	11 month in 2011	Level III	HRV, genotyping not performed	16 infants born at 24–36 weeks PMA	Nasal congestion and increased work of breathing, need for increased respiratory support and increased oxygen supplementation, apnea	79 days (38–169)	Not specified	Unknown
Reid et al., 2011, Australia	March 2010	Level III	HRV species C	7 preterm infants born at 25–29 weeks PMA	Increased respiratory secretions, unstable body temperature, apnea, increase in supplemental oxygen therapy	75 (14–282)	Cohorting, droplet and contact precautions, screening of contacts	Unknown
van Piggelen et al., 2010, The Netherlands	2003–2008	Not specified	HRV, genotyping not performed	11 infants born at 26–41 weeks PMA	Respiratory distress, apnea, rhinorrhea and hypothermia, atelectasis, increased secretions	49 (5–94)	Not specified	Unknown

more severe courses than community acquired RSV infections (Simon et al., 2008) and lead to high morbidity, significant mortality and substantial increase in health care costs (Halasa et al., 2005). There is a limited number of reports in the literature on nosocomially acquired RSV infections among both term and preterm infants in the NICU (Bont, 2009). Four NICU outbreaks of RSV were reported using RT-PCR technology for virus detection (Halasa et al., 2005; Visser et al., 2008; O'Connell et al., 2011; Hammoud et al., 2016; **Table 4**). In all these reports infants presented with signs of respiratory deterioration and need of increased respiratory support. In general, RSV infections in the NICU occurred mostly late in the clinical course, i.e., with a mean age of more than one month (**Table 4**). However, individual infections as early as on day 10 of life were reported (**Table 4**). Many infants needed mechanical ventilation in the course of the RSV infection. One case was reported to require extracorporal membrane oxygenation (ECMO; Halasa et al., 2005). Still, most infants recovered from the RSV infection. In the study of Berger et al. (2010) patients, parents and staff were screened for RSV in a NICU for a period of 8 weeks. Only 4 of 1,002 samples tested positive for RSV. The only infant, however, diagnosed with RSV infection in this study had a fatal outcome. This infant was a preterm 26 weeks PMA infant with first symptoms of RSV infection on day of life 42 after an uneventful clinical course, which emphasizes the risk of an adverse outcome of nosocomial RSV infections especially in premature infants. Also in the study of Visser et al. which reports an outbreak of RSV in a South African kangaroo mother care unit, 2 infants died due to a fatal course of RSV infection. Both patients were male and born at 28 and 32 weeks PMA, respectively. The first child suffered from a dual infection with RSV A and B while the second was infected with RSV B (Visser et al., 2008).

Because of the high mortality and morbidity reported in special patient groups, prophylactic immunization with palivizumab is recommended monthly during the RSV season (Simoes, 1999; American Academy of Pediatrics Bronchiolitis Guidelines Committee, 2014). Palivizumab is a monoclonal antibody that is usually administered prior to hospital discharge to be protective against community-acquired RSV infection (American Academy of Pediatrics Bronchiolitis Guidelines Committee, 2014). If administered correctly, palivizumab has been shown to be safe and effective in reducing the number of RSV-related hospitalization in randomized, multicenter, placebo-controlled trials (1998; Wegzyn et al., 2014). Also, in the reported outbreak scenarios the authors chose to administer palivizumab either to all infants hospitalized in the NICU (O'Connell et al., 2011; Hammoud et al., 2016) or to a subgroup of NICU patients who were considered to be at particularly increased risk of nosocomial RSV infection (Halasa et al., 2005) and reported successful termination of the outbreak. Despite these anecdotal reports, immunoprophylaxis with palivizumab is currently not recommended for the prevention of health care-associated RSV infections (American Academy of Pediatrics Bronchiolitis Guidelines Committee, 2014).

Several authors highlight that of all infection control methods, adequate hand washing/hand disinfection, rapid screening for

TABLE 4 | Outbreaks of RSV in the NICU including details on affected patients, clinical symptoms, and infection control measures.

Study	Date	NICU	Pathogen	Affected Infants	Symptoms	Median age at onset of symptoms (range)	Infection control measures	Source of the outbreak
Hammoud et al., 2016, Kuwait	February 2012	Not specified	RSV	13 infants at 26–33 weeks PMA	Respiratory symptoms requiring increased ventilatory support	38 days (10–160 days)	Palivizumab given to all NICU patients, general infection control measures	Index case identified
O'Connell et al., 2011, Ireland	February 2010	Level III	RSV A	4 infants in the NICU	Respiratory deterioration	22 days (31–59 days)	Palivizumab given to all NICU patients, respiratory and contact precautions, no transfer of infants between the rooms, admissions limited to unforeseen emergencies, increased frequency of cleaning, cohorting of affected infants	Index case identified
Visser et al., 2008, South Africa	March–May 2006	Kangaroo mother care ward	RSV A and B	23 infants 27–38 weeks PMA	Pneumonia with need for oxygen supplementation and/or intubation	Not specified	Not specifeid	Index cases identified
Halasa et al., 2005, USA	January–February 2002	Level III	RSV B	9 infants at 30–36 weeks PMA	Cough and congestion, increased oxygen requirement, apnea and respiratory failure	34 days (11–69 days)	Palivizumab given to all NICU patients not infected with RSV, cohorting of infected infants, contact precautions	Index case identified

Only reports using PCR-based diagnostic techniques were included.

infection and cohorting of infected patients are most effective to prevent RSV transmission in NICUs and pediatric wards (Groothuis et al., 2008).

CONCLUSION

RVIs are still an under-diagnosed and underestimated entity in the NICU. Although incidences of RVIs are relatively low and outbreaks are rare, RVIs can cause significant morbidity in neonates and especially preterm infants. Thus, PCR based virus detection methods should be considered in infants hospitalized in the NICU with signs of respiratory deterioration in order to allow rapid diagnosis of RVIs and to implement rapidly effective isolation and infection prevention measures to prevent both severe disease in theses infants and viral spread in the unit.

AUTHOR CONTRIBUTIONS

KP and OA performed the review of the current literature as well as data analysis. KP and AB drafted the manuscript. All authors have read and approved the final manuscript.

ACKNOWLEDGMENTS

We acknowledge Ms. Brigitte Wildner for her valuable help in literature search.

REFERENCES

(1998). Palivizumab, a humanized respiratory syncytial virus monoclonal antibody, reduces hospitalization from respiratory syncytial virus infection in high-risk infants. The impact-rsv study group. *Pediatrics* 102(3 Pt 1):531–7.

Abdel-Rahman, S. M., Newland, J. G., and Kearns, G. L. (2011). Pharmacologic considerations for oseltamivir disposition: focus on the neonate and young infant. *Paediatr Drugs* 13, 19–31. doi: 10.2165/11536950-000000000-00000

Acosta, E. P., Jester, P., Gal, P., Wimmer, J., Wade, J., Whitley, R. J., et al. (2010). Oseltamivir dosing for influenza infection in premature neonates. *J. Infect. Dis.* 202, 563–566. doi: 10.1086/654930

American Academy of Pediatrics Bronchiolitis Guidelines Committee (2014). Updated guidance for palivizumab prophylaxis among infants and young children at increased risk of hospitalization for respiratory syncytial virus infection. *Pediatrics* 134, 415–420. doi: 10.1542/peds.2014-1665

Barak, S., Kushnir, A., Chulski, E., and Miron, D. (2010). Influenza A/H1N1 virus in very low-birth-weight premature infant: case report. *Am. J. Perinatol.* 27, 513–515. doi: 10.1055/s-0030-1247606

Bennett, N. J., Tabarani, C. M., Bartholoma, N. M., Wang, D., Huang, D., Riddell, S. W., et al. (2012). Unrecognized viral respiratory tract infections in premature infants during their birth hospitalization: a prospective surveillance study in two neonatal intensive care units. *J. Pediatr.* 161, 814–818. doi: 10.1016/j.jpeds.2012.05.001

Berger, A., Obwegeser, E., Aberle, S. W., Langgartner, M., and Popow-Kraupp, T. (2010). Nosocomial transmission of respiratory syncytial virus in neonatal intensive care and intermediate care units: a prospective epidemiologic study. *Pediatr. Infect. Dis. J.* 29, 669–670. doi: 10.1097/INF.0b013e3181d76d61

Bhat, N., Wright, J. G., Broder, K. R., Murray, E. L., Greenberg, M. E., Glover, M. J., et al. (2005). Influenza-associated deaths among children in the united states, 2003-2004. *N. Engl. J. Med.* 353, 2559–2567. doi: 10.1056/NEJMoa051721

Bont, L. (2009). Nosocomial RSV infection control and outbreak management. *Paediatr. Respir. Rev.* 10(Suppl. 1):16–17. doi: 10.1016/S1526-0542(09)70008-9

Boyce, T. G., Mellen, B. G., Mitchel, E. F., Wright, P. F., and Griffin, M. R. (2000). Rates of hospitalization for respiratory syncytial virus infection among children in medicaid. *J. Pediatr.* 137, 865–870. doi: 10.1067/mpd.2000.110531

Broberg, E., Niemel,ä, J., Lahti, E., Hyypiä, T., Ruuskanen, O., and Waris, M. (2011). Human rhinovirus c–associated severe pneumonia in a neonate. *J. Clin. Virol.* 51, 79–82. doi: 10.1016/j.jcv.2011.01.018

Buonocore, G., Bracci, R., and Weindling, A. M. (2012). *Neonatology: A Practical Approach to Neonatal Diseases.* Milan: Springer.

Cantey, J. B., and Patel, S. J. (2014). Antimicrobial stewardship in the NICU. *Infect. Dis. Clin. North Am.* 28, 247–261. doi: 10.1016/j.idc.2014.01.005

Caserta, M. T., Yang, H., Gill, S. R., Holden-Wiltse, J., and Pryhuber, G. (2017). Viral respiratory infections in preterm infants during and after hospitalization. *J. Pediatr.* 182, 53.e3–58.e3. doi: 10.1016/j.jpeds.2016.11.077

Casiano-Colón, A. E., Hulbert, B. B., Mayer, T. K., Walsh, E. E., and Falsey, A. R. (2003). Lack of sensitivity of rapid antigen tests for the diagnosis of respiratory syncytial virus infection in adults. *J. Clin. Virol.* 28, 169–174. doi: 10.1016/S1386-6532(03)00002-7

Cerone, J. B., Santos, R. P., Tristram, D., Lamson, D. M., Stellrecht, K. A., St George, K., et al. (2017). Incidence of respiratory viral infection in infants with respiratory symptoms evaluated for late-onset sepsis. *J. Perinatol.* 37, 922–926. doi: 10.1038/jp.2017.69

Diniz, E. M., Vieira, R. A., Ceccon, M. E., Ishida, M. A., and Vaz, F. A. (2005). Incidence of respiratory viruses in preterm infants submitted to mechanical ventilation. *Rev. Inst. Med. Trop. Sao. Paulo* 47, 37–44. doi: 10.1590/S0036-46652005000100007

Dunn, G. L., Tapson, H., Davis, J., and Gobin, M. (2017). Outbreak of piv-3 in a neonatal intensive care unit in England. *Pediatr. Infect. Dis. J.* 36, 344–345. doi: 10.1097/INF.0000000000001443

Eisenhut, M. (2006). Extrapulmonary manifestations of severe RSV bronchiolitis. *Lancet* 9540:988. doi: 10.1016/S0140-6736(06)69409-9

Ekstrand, J. J., Herbener, A., Rawlings, J., Turney, B., Ampofo, K., Korgenski, E. K., et al. (2010). Heightened neurologic complications in children with pandemic H1N1 influenza. *Ann. Neurol.* 68, 762–766. doi: 10.1002/ana.22184

French, C. E., McKenzie, B. C., Coope, C., Rajanaidu, S., Paranthaman, K., Pebody, R., et al. (2016). Risk of nosocomial respiratory syncytial virus infection and effectiveness of control measures to prevent transmission events: a systematic review. *Influenza Other Respir. Viruses* 10, 268–290. doi: 10.1111/irv.12379

Gelber, S. E., and Ratner, A. J. (2002). Hospital-acquired viral pathogens in the neonatal intensive care unit. *Semin. Perinatol.* 26, 346–356. doi: 10.1053/sper.2002.36268

Goldmann, D. A. (2000). Transmission of viral respiratory infections in the home. *Pediatr. Infect. Dis. J.* 19(Suppl. 10), S97–S102. doi: 10.1097/00006454-200010001-00002

Groothuis, J., Bauman, J., Malinoski, F., Eggleston, M. (2008). Strategies for prevention of RSV nosocomial infection. *J. Perinatol.* 28, 319–23. doi: 10.1038/jp.2008.37

Halasa, N. B., Williams, J. V., Wilson, G. J., Walsh, W. F., Schaffner, W., and Wright, P. F. (2005). Medical and economic impact of a respiratory syncytial virus outbreak in a neonatal intensive care unit. *Pediatr. Infect. Dis. J.* 24, 1040–1044. doi: 10.1097/01.inf.0000190027.59795.ac

Hall, C. B., Douglas, R. G., and Geiman, J. M. (1980). Possible transmission by fomites of respiratory syncytial virus. *J. Infect. Dis.* 141, 98–102. doi: 10.1093/infdis/141.1.98

Hammoud, M. S., Al-Taiar, A., Raina, A., Elsori, D., Al-Qabandi, S., and Al-Essa, M. (2016). Use of palivizumab with other infection control measures to control respiratory syncytial virus outbreaks in neonatal care units. *J. Trop. Pediatr.* 62, 409–414. doi: 10.1093/tropej/fmw025

Homaira, N., Sheils, J., Stelzer-Braid, S., Lui, K., Oie, J. L., Snelling, T., et al. (2016). Respiratory syncytial virus is present in the neonatal intensive care unit. *J. Med. Virol.* 88, 196–201. doi: 10.1002/jmv.24325

Horikoshi, Y., Okazaki, K., Miyokawa, S., Kinoshita, K., Higuchi, H., Suwa, J., et al. (2018). Sibling visits and viral infection in the neonatal intensive care unit. *Pediatr. Int.* 60, 153–156. doi: 10.1111/ped.13470

Iwane, M. K., Edwards, K. M., Szilagyi, P. G., Walker, F. J., Griffin, M. R., Weinberg, G. A., et al. (2004). Population-based surveillance for hospitalizations associated with respiratory syncytial virus, influenza virus, and parainfluenza viruses among young children. *Pediatrics* 113, 1758–1764. doi: 10.1542/peds.113.6.1758

Jackson, D. J. (2014). Early-life viral infections and the development of asthma: a target for asthma prevention? *Curr. Opin. Allergy Clin. Immunol.* 14, 131–136. doi: 10.1097/ACI.0000000000000047

Jacobs, S. E., Lamson, D. M., St George, K., and Walsh, T. J. (2013). Human rhinoviruses. *Clin. Microbiol. Rev.* 26, 135–162. doi: 10.1128/CMR.00077-12

Jajoo, M., and Gupta, R. (2010). H1N1 influenza in a preterm neonate. *Indian J. Pediatr.* 77, 1045–1046. doi: 10.1007/s12098-010-0166-2

Jefferson, T., Del Mar, C. B., Dooley, L., Ferroni, E., Al-Ansary, L. A., Bawazeer, G. A., et al. (2011). Physical interventions to interrupt or reduce the spread of respiratory viruses. *Cochrane Database Syst. Rev.* 6:CD006207. doi: 10.1002/14651858.CD006207.pub4

Kassianos, G., Kuchar, E., Nitsch-Osuch, A., Kyncl, J., Galev, A., Humolli, I., et al. (2018). Motors of influenza vaccination uptake and vaccination advocacy in healthcare workers: a comparative study in six european countries. *Vaccine* 28, 6546–6552. doi: 10.1016/j.vaccine.2018.02.031

Kedia, S., Stroud, B., Parsons, J., Schreiner, T., Curtis, D. J., Bagdure, D., et al. (2011). Pediatric neurological complications of 2009 pandemic influenza A (H1N1). *Arch. Neurol.* 68, 455–462. doi: 10.1001/archneurol.2010.318

Kidszun, A., Hansmann, A., Winter, J., Gröndahl, B., Knuf, M., Weise, K., et al. (2014). Detection of respiratory viral infections in neonates treated for suspicion of nosocomial bacterial sepsis: a feasibility study. *Pediatr. Infect. Dis. J.* 33, 102–104. doi: 10.1097/INF.0000000000000008

Kidszun, A., Klein, L., Winter, J., Schmeh, I., Gröndahl, B., Gehring, S., et al. (2017). Viral infections in neonates with suspected late-onset bacterial sepsis-a prospective cohort study. *Am. J. Perinatol.* 34, 1–7. doi: 10.1055/s-0036-1584150

Krause, J. C., Panning, M., Hengel, H., and Henneke, P. (2014). The role of multiplex PCR in respiratory tract infections in children. *Dtsch. Arztebl. Int.* 111, 639–645. doi: 10.3238/arztebl.2014.0639

Kujari, A. M., Waris, M., Lehtonen, L., and Ruuskanen, O. (2014). Respiratory viral infections are not uncommon in neonatal intensive care units. *Acta Paediatr.* 103, e225–e228. doi: 10.1111/apa.12590

Maeda, H., Haneda, K., and Honda, Y. (2017). Parainfluenza virus type 3 outbreak in a neonatal intensive care unit. *Pediatr. Int.* 59, 1219–1222. doi: 10.1111/ped.13389

Marcone, D. N., Carballal, G., Irañeta, M., Rubies, Y., Vidaurreta, S. M., and Echavarría, M. (2018). Nosocomial transmission and genetic diversity of rhinovirus in a neonatal intensive care unit. *J Pediatr.* 193, 252.e1–255.e1. doi: 10.1016/j.jpeds.2017.09.013

Matheson, N. J., Harnden, A. R., Perera, R., Sheikh, A., and Symmonds-Abrahams, M. (2007). Neuraminidase inhibitors for preventing and treating influenza in children. *Cochrane Database Syst. Rev.* 24:CD002744. doi: 10.1002/14651858.CD002744.pub2

Meerhoff, T. J., Houben, M. L., Coenjaerts, F. E., Kimpen, J. L., Hofland, R. W., Schellevis, F., et al. (2010). Detection of multiple respiratory pathogens during primary respiratory infection: nasal swab versus nasopharyngeal aspirate using real-time polymerase chain reaction. *Eur. J. Clin. Microbiol. Infect. Dis.* 29, 365–371. doi: 10.1007/s10096-009-0865-7

Milupi, M., Madeo, M., Brooke, N., and Ahmad, S. J. (2012). Neonatal influenza A/H1N1/2009 outbreak in a UK district general hospital. *J. Hosp. Infect.* 81, 131–133. doi: 10.1016/j.jhin.2012.04.005

Moore, K. A., Coker, K., Du Buisson, A. B., Swett, B., and Edwards, W. H. (2003). Implementing potentially better practices for improving family-centered care in neonatal intensive care units: successes and challenges. *Pediatrics* 111(4 Pt 2), e450–e460.

Munoz, F. M. (2003). Influenza virus infection in infancy and early childhood. *Paediatr. Respir. Rev.* 4, 99–104. doi: 10.1016/S1526-0542(03)00027-7

O'Connell, K., Boo, T. W., Keady, D., Niriain, U., O'Donovan, D., Commane, M., et al. (2011). Use of palivizumab and infection control measures to control an outbreak of respiratory syncytial virus in a neonatal intensive care unit confirmed by real-time polymerase chain reaction. *J. Hosp. Infect.* 77, 338–342. doi: 10.1016/j.jhin.2010.12.012

Pannaraj, P. S., Tam, B., and Akan, D. (2011). Oseltamivir treatment and prophylaxis in a neonatal intensive care unit during a 2009 H1N1 influenza outbreak. *J. Perinatol.* 31, 487–493. doi: 10.1038/jp.2010.159

Pavia, A. T. (2011). Viral infections of the lower respiratory tract: old viruses, new viruses, and the role of diagnosis. *Clin. Infect. Dis.* 52(Suppl. 4), S284–S289. doi: 10.1093/cid/cir043

Peluso, A. M., Harnish, B. A., Miller, N. S., Cooper, E. R., and Fujii, A. M. (2015). Effect of young sibling visitation on respiratory syncytial virus activity in a NICU. *J. Perinatol.* 35, 627–630. doi: 10.1038/jp.2015.27

Perez, G. F., Pancham, K., Huseni, S., Jain, A., Rodriguez-Martinez, C. E., Preciado, D., et al. (2015). Rhinovirus-induced airway cytokines and respiratory morbidity in severely premature children. *Pediatr. Allergy Immunol.* 26, 145–152. doi: 10.1111/pai.12346

Principi, N., and Esposito, S. (2004). Are we ready for universal influenza vaccination in paediatrics? *Lancet Infect. Dis.* 4, 75–83. doi: 10.1016/S1473-3099(04)00926-0

Puck, J. M., Glezen, W. P., Frank, A. L., and Six, H. R. (1980). Protection of infants from infection with influenza A virus by transplacentally acquired antibody. *J. Infect. Dis.* 142, 844–849. doi: 10.1093/infdis/142.6.844

Reese, S. M., Thompson, M., Price, C. S., and Young, H. L. (2016). Evidence of nosocomial transmission of human rhinovirus in a neonatal intensive care unit. *Am. J. Infect. Control* 44, 355–357. doi: 10.1016/j.ajic.2015.10.018

Reid, A. B., Anderson, T. L., Cooley, L., Williamson, J., and Mcgregor, A. R. (2011). An outbreak of human rhinovirus species C infections in a neonatal intensive care unit. *Pediatr. Infect. Dis. J.* 30, 1096–1095. doi: 10.1097/INF.0b013e31822938d7

Rhedin, S., Lindstrand, A., Rotzén-Östlund, M., Tolfvenstam, T., Ohrmalm, L., Rinder, M. R., et al. (2014). Clinical utility of PCR for common viruses in acute respiratory illness. *Pediatrics* 133, e538–e545. doi: 10.1542/peds.2013-3042

Rocha, G., Pissarra, S., Silva, G., and Guimares, H. (2010). Experience with oseltamivir in term and preterm newborns. *Res. Gate* 5, 327–331. doi: 10.3233/JPI-2010-0270

Ronchi, A., Michelow, I. C., Chapin, K. C., Bliss, J. M., Pugni, L., Mosca, F. (2014). Viral respiratory tract infections in the neonatal intensive care unit: the virion-i study. *J. Pediatr.* 165, 690-6. doi: 10.1016/j.jpeds.2014.05.054

Schwab, F., Tolbert, B., Bagnato, S., and Maisels, M. J. (1983). Sibling visiting in a neonatal intensive care unit. *Pediatrics* 71, 835–838.

Sert, A., Yazar, A., Odabas, D., and Bilgin, H. (2010). An unusual cause of fever in a neonate: influenza A (H1N1) virus pneumonia. *Pediatr. Pulmonol.* 45, 734–736. doi: 10.1002/ppul.21245

Simmonds, A., Munoz, J., Montecalvo, M., Clones, B., and Lagamma, E. F. (2009). Outbreak of parainfluenza virus type 3 in a neonatal intensive care unit. *Am. J. Perinatol.* 26, 361–364. doi: 10.1055/s-0028-1110087

Simoes, E. A. (1999). Respiratory syncytial virus infection. *Lancet* 354, 847–852. doi: 10.1016/S0140-6736(99)80040-3

Simon, A., Müller, A., Khurana, K., Engelhart, S., Exner, M., Schildgen, O., et al. (2008). Nosocomial infection: a risk factor for a complicated course in children with respiratory syncytial virus infection–results from a prospective multicenter german surveillance study. *Int. J. Hyg. Environ. Health* 211, 241–250. doi: 10.1016/j.ijheh.2007.07.020

Singh-Naz, N., Willy, M., and Riggs, N. (1990) Outbreak of parainfluenza virus type 3 in a neonatal nursery. *Pediatr. Infect. Dis. J.* 9, 31–33 doi: 10.1097/00006454-199001000-00007

Smit, P. M., Pronk, S. M., Kaandorp, J. C., Weijer, O., Lauw, F. N., Smits, P. H., et al. (2013). RT-PCR detection of respiratory pathogens in newborn children admitted to a neonatal medium care unit. *Pediatr. Res.* 73, 355–361. doi: 10.1038/pr.2012.176

Solheim, K., and Spellacy, C. (1988). Siblings visitation: effects on newborn infection rates. *J. Obstet. Gynecol. Neonatal Nurs.* 17, 43–48. doi: 10.1111/j.1552-6909.1988.tb00413.x

Steiner, M., Strassl, R., Straub, J., Böhm, J., Popow-Kraupp, T., and Berger, A. (2012). Nosocomial rhinovirus infection in preterm infants. *Pediatr. Infect. Dis. J.* 31, 1302–1304. doi: 10.1097/INF.0b013e31826ff939

Tellier, R. (2009). Aerosol transmission of influenza A virus: a review of new studies. *J. R. Soc. Interface* 6(Suppl. 6):S783–S790. doi: 10.1098/rsif.2009.0302.focus

Tsagris, V., Nika, A., Kyriakou, D., Kapetanakis, I., Harahousou, E., Stripeli, F., et al. (2012). Influenza A/H1N1/2009 outbreak in a neonatal intensive care unit. *J. Hosp. Infect.* 81, 36–40. doi: 10.1016/j.jhin.2012.02.009

van Benten, I., Koopman, L., Niesters, B., Hop, W., van Middelkoop, B., de Waal, L., et al. (2003). Predominance of rhinovirus in the nose of symptomatic and asymptomatic infants. *Pediatr. Allergy Immunol.* 14, 363–370. doi: 10.1034/j.1399-3038.2003.00064.x

van den Berg, J. P., Westerbeek, E. A., Berbers, G. A., van Gageldonk, P. G., van der Klis, F. R., and van Elburg, R. M. (2010). Transplacental transport of igg antibodies specific for pertussis, diphtheria, tetanus, haemophilus influenzae type b, and neisseria meningitidis serogroup C is lower in preterm compared with term infants. *Pediatr. Infect. Dis. J.* 29, 801–805. doi: 10.1097/INF.0b013e3181dc4f77

van Piggelen, R. O., van Loon, A. M., Krediet, T. G., and Verboon-Maciolek, M. A. (2010). Human rhinovirus causes severe infection in preterm infants. *Pediatr. Infect. Dis. J.* 29, 364–365. doi: 10.1097/INF.0b013e3181c6e60f

Verboon-Maciolek, M. A., Krediet, T. G., Gerards, L. J., Fleer, A., and van Loon, T. M. (2005). Clinical and epidemiologic characteristics of viral infections in a neonatal intensive care unit during a 12-year period. *Pediatr. Infect. Dis. J.* 24, 901–904. doi: 10.1097/01.inf.0000180471.03702.7f

Vij, N. K., Stryker, C. C., Esper, F. P., Jacobs, M. R., and Gonzalez, B. E. (2011). Influenza A/H1N1/09-10 infections in a NICU during the 2009-2010 H1N1 pandemic. *Pediatrics* 128, e1297–e1301. doi: 10.1542/peds.2011-0219

Visser, A., Delport, S., and Venter, M. (2008). Molecular epidemiological analysis of a nosocomial outbreak of respiratory syncytial virus associated pneumonia in a kangaroo mother care unit in south africa. *J. Med. Virol.* 80, 724–732. doi: 10.1002/jmv.21128

Wegzyn, C., Toh, L. K., Notario, G., Biguenet, S., Unnebrink, K., Park, C., et al. (2014). Safety and effectiveness of palivizumab in children at high risk of serious disease due to respiratory syncytial virus infection: a systematic review. *Infect. Dis. Ther.* 3, 133–158. doi: 10.1007/s40121-014-0046-6

Whitley, R. J., and Monto, A. S. (2006). Prevention and treatment of influenza in high-risk groups: Children, pregnant women, immunocompromised hosts, and nursing home residents. *J. Infect. Dis.* 194(Suppl. 2):S133–S138. doi: 10.1086/507548

Wilkinson, D. J., Buttery, J. P., and Andersen, C. C. (2006). Influenza in the neonatal intensive care unit. *J. Perinatol.* 26, 772–776. doi: 10.1038/sj.jp.7211625

Woo, P. C., Chiu, S. S., Seto, W. H., and Peiris, M. (1997). Cost-effectiveness of rapid diagnosis of viral respiratory tract infections in pediatric patients. *J. Clin. Microbiol.* 35, 1579–1581.

Woods, C. R., and Abramson, J. S. (2005). The next influenza pandemic: will we be ready to care for our children? *J. Pediatr.* 147, 147–155. doi: 10.1016/j.jpeds.2005.04.066

Wooltorton, E. (2004). Oseltamivir (Tamiflu) unsafe in infants under 1 year old. *CMAJ* 170:336.

Zinna, S., Lakshmanan, A., Tan, S., McClaughry, R., Clarkson, M., Soo, S., et al. (2016). Outcomes of nosocomial viral respiratory infections in high-risk neonates. *Pediatrics* 138: e20161675. doi: 10.1542/peds.2016-1675

Prevalence of Common Respiratory Viral Infections and Identification of Adenovirus in Hospitalized Adults in Harbin, China 2014 to 2017

*Yingchen Wang[1†], Tuo Dong[1†], Guiyun Qi[2], Lixin Qu[1], Wei Liang[1], Binbin Qi[1], Zhe Zhang[1], Lei Shang[1], Hong Gao[1], Xiqiao Du[1], Bing Lu[1], Yan Guo[3], Zhenwei Liu[1], Huisong Yu[1], Qi Cui[1], Xiaocen Wang[1], Ye Li[1], Weiyuan Guo[2] and Zhangyi Qu[1,4]**

[1] Department of Microbiology, Public Health College, Harbin Medical University, Harbin, China, [2] Department of Clinical Laboratory, The Second Affiliated Hospital of Harbin Medical University, Harbin, China, [3] Department of Ear Nose Throat, The Second Affiliated Hospital of Harbin Medical University, Harbin, China, [4] Department of Natural Focus Disease Control, Institute of Environment-Associated Disease, Sino-Russia Joint Medical Research Center, Harbin Medical University, Harbin, China

***Correspondence:**
Zhangyi Qu
hmu635@126.com

† These authors have contributed equally to this work

Background: Respiratory infections pose a great challenge in global health, and the prevalence of viral infection in adult patients has been poorly understood in northeast China. Harbin is one of the major cities in northeast China, and more than half of any given year in Harbin is occupied by winter. To reveal the viral etiology and seasonality in adult patients from Harbin, a 4-year consecutive survey was conducted in Harbin, China.

Methods: From January 2014 to December 2017, specimens were obtained from adult patients admitted to the Second Affiliated Hospital of Harbin Medical University with lower respiratory tract infections. Sputum samples were examined by direct immunofluorescence assays to detect seven common respiratory viruses, including influenza virus (type A and B), parainfluenza virus (type 1 to 3), respiratory syncytial virus and adenovirus. Adenovirus positive samples were seeded onto A549 cells to isolate viral strains. Phylogenetic analysis was conducted on the highly variable region of adenoviral hexon gene.

Results: A total of 1,300 hospitalized adult patients with lower respiratory tract infections were enrolled, in which 189 patients (14.5%) were detected as having at least one viral infection. The co-infection rate in this study was 25.9% (49/189). The dominant viral pathogen from 2014 to 2017 was parainfluenza virus, with a detection rate of 7.2%, followed by influenza virus, respiratory syncytial virus and adenovirus. Based on the climate seasons determined by daily average temperature, the highest overall viral detection rate was detected in spring (22.0%, 52/236), followed by winter (13.4%, 109/813), autumn (11.4%, 13/114) and summer (10.9%, 15/137). Adenovirus type 3 strains with slight variations were isolated from positive cases, which were closely related to the GB strain from the United States, as well as the Harbin04B strain isolated locally.

Conclusion: This study demonstrated that common respiratory viruses were partially responsible for hospitalized lower respiratory tract infections in adult patients from Harbin, China, with parainfluenza virus as the dominant viral pathogen. Climate seasons could be rational indicators for the seasonality analysis of airborne viral infections. Future surveillance on viral mutations would be necessary to reveal the evolutionary history of respiratory viruses.

Keywords: human adenovirus, respiratory viral infections, lower respiratory tract infections, adult patients, epidemiology

INTRODUCTION

Lower respiratory tract infections are a persistent public health problem, causing more than two million deaths per year worldwide, with a rate of 36 deaths per 100,000 population (GBD 2016 Causes of Death Collaborators, 2017). The morbidity and mortality of respiratory infections could be even worse in developing countries, including China. Viral infections played an important role in pediatric lower respiratory tract infections, and the corresponding common viral pathogens were influenza A and B virus (IAV and IBV), parainfluenza virus (PIV, type 1 to 3), respiratory syncytial virus (RSV) and human adenovirus (ADV) (Pavia, 2011). These seven viruses were also common in respiratory infections of the adult population in Shandong province, China (Liu et al., 2015). To the best of our knowledge, there were no commercial vaccines available for most of these viruses, except for influenza A and B viruses (Lambkin-Williams et al., 2018).

The etiology of respiratory infection in the adult population has been overlooked, at least in China, although there are plenty of reports on the epidemiology of respiratory viral infection in the pediatric population (Wang et al., 2016). China is a vast country with notable variations in climate characteristics among different regions. Due to the differences in socioeconomic, geographic or climate factors, the epidemiological features of viral infection in the respiratory tract show dramatic variation among different study populations (Sloan et al., 2011; Lu et al., 2013; He et al., 2014; Rehder et al., 2015).

Harbin is one of the major metropolises in northeast China, hosting more than eight million people. The winter in Harbin lasts for more than half a year, while the summer is short, resulting in the length of four seasons being unequal. Viral respiratory infections in the pediatric population from Harbin were reported by the authors' team in 2009 (Zhang et al., 2009), in which the adult population was not included. A clear picture of the viral etiology in hospitalized adults with respiratory infections ought to be critical for both public health policy makers and clinical practitioners.

Phylogenetic history of several respiratory viruses isolated from China in recent years have been well established, including the influenza virus (Wang et al., 2018; Yang et al., 2018), the PIV (Pan et al., 2017) and the RSV (Liu et al., 2014; Zou et al., 2016). The information about adenoviral evolutionary history in China was limited to outbreak reports and novel strains identification (Lu et al., 2014; Li et al., 2018), leaving a gap for circulating stains among adult patients.

Human adenovirus is one of the common pathogens in respiratory infections and could be divided into seven species (Ismail et al., 2018). The most recent reported human adenovirus type is type 85 in species D, which was isolated from Japan (Hashimoto et al., 2018). Human adenovirus species B type 55 (HAdv B55) was reported to be responsible for adult pneumonia outbreaks in Beijing China during 2011 with the genome identity as 99.87%, comparing to the prototype strain of HAdv B55 in 2006 (Cheng et al., 2018). Adenoviral infections in children from Harbin were found to be ADV species B, as reported by the authors, while the viral type among adult patients is still poorly understood.

The adenoviral virion was composed of 252 capsomeres, containing 240 hexons and 12 pentons, while each penton was anchored by one fiber (or two fibers in several types) (Nemerow et al., 2012). The knob region in adenoviral fiber was responsible for cellular attachment through host receptors including CAR, CD46, DSG-1 and sialic acids (Baker et al., 2018; Lenman et al., 2018). The RGD loop of penton could be recognized by the host cell's integrin (Veesler et al., 2014). The hexon protein is the major neutralizing antigen of adenoviruses (Madisch et al., 2005), while the hyper variable region (HVR) in hexon protein hosts its type specific epitopes reported by the authors' team (Yuan et al., 2009). Experiments on chimeric adenoviral capsids showed that the replacement of HVRs in hexon could alter the viral serotypes (Qiu et al., 2012; Tian et al., 2018). The hexon specific $CD4^{+}$ and $CD8^{+}$ T cells have been proved to be an effective treatment for human adenoviral infections in clinical settings (Zandvliet et al., 2010; Feucht et al., 2015). Recent reports indicated that antibodies against fiber knob or penton base may also be involved in the neutralization of adenoviruses (Yu et al., 2013; Tomita et al., 2018). To the best of our knowledge, the hypervariable region of adenoviral hexon protein plays an essential role in viral type-specific immunity.

In this report, the prevalence of common viruses in the lower respiratory tract infection of hospitalized adult patients from Harbin, China was explored in hopes of revealing the clinical and pathogenic features of respiratory viruses. Adenoviral strains were isolated from positive cases to identify potential molecular variations within its hypervariable regions.

MATERIALS AND METHODS

Specimens and Clinical Data Collection

From January 2014 to December 2017, sputum samples were collected from 1,300 adult patients hospitalized for lower respiratory tract infections in the Second Affiliated Hospital of Harbin Medical University. All patients enrolled in this study lived in urban and suburban areas of Harbin without travel histories within 3 months before admission and sampling. All patients were older than 18 years and suffering from at least one complaint, including fever with body temperature $\geq$ 38°C, cough, expectoration, hemoptysis, chest tightness (chest pain), or dyspnea. The sputum samples were expectorated spontaneously into sterile containers and delivered to the laboratory within 2 h, tested immediately or stored at −80°C prior to use.

Patients' clinical data, including symptoms, history of illness, clinical diagnoses and laboratory test results were surveyed through the hospital's health information system. This study had been approved by the ethical review committees of Harbin Medical University in accordance with the Declaration of Helsinki. Both informed and written consents were obtained from each participant who provided specimens.

Detection of Respiratory Viruses

The presence of common respiratory viruses, including PIV type 1 to 3, influenza virus A and B virus (IAV and IBV), RSV, and human ADV was determined by the D^3 Ultra^{TM} DFA Respiratory Virus Screening Kit (Diagnostic Hybrids, Inc., Athens, OH, United States).

Cell Culture and Virus Isolation

Virus isolation for the ADV-positive specimens was performed using the A549 cell line (provided by the Cancer Hospital of Harbin Medical University) following the protocol described previously (Smith et al., 1986; Huang et al., 2013). In brief, Cells seeded with clinical samples were incubated at 37°C for 4 days. If there was no observed cytopathic effect, two additional blind passages of the culture were performed to avoid false negative results. The cultures with ADV-like cytopathic effects were passaged again to confirm viral presence.

Preparation of Nucleic Acids

The viral DNA of human ADV was extracted from infected cells using the AxyPrep Multisource Genomic DNA Miniprep Kit (Axygen Biosciences) according to the manufacturer's instructions and eluted in 100 μl elution buffer.

PCR Amplification and Sequence Typing

The highly variable region in the adenoviral hexon gene was amplified using the following primer pairs: forward, 5′-CAATTCACTCGCTCCTA-3′ and reverse, 5′-GTGGAAAGGCACATAACG-3′. All primers were synthesized by Comate Bioscience Co., Ltd. PCR was performed with the Platinum PCR SuperMix (Invitrogen) following the manufacturer's instructions. A total reaction volume of 50 μL contained 5 μL of 10 × PCR buffer (Takara Bio Premix Ex Taq^{TM}), 200 nM of each primer, 200 nM of each dNTPS, 2 μL of each DNA sample, 0.25 μL Taq enzyme (Takara Bio Premix Ex Taq^{TM}), and sterile water. The cycling conditions were 5 min at 95°C, followed by 35 cycles of 30 s at 95°C, 30 s at 55°C, and 30 s at 72°C, with a final 5-min extension at 72°C. DNA extracted from the A549 cell culture and sterile water were used as negative controls. The amplicons were bi-directionally sequenced using the Sanger sequencing method with an ABI PRISM 3130 genetic analyzer (Comate Bioscience Co., Ltd., Jilin, China).

Air Temperature Data and Climate Seasons

The daily average air temperature from January 1st, 2014 to December 31st, 2017 in Harbin city was kindly provided by the Harbin Meteorological Observatory. Historical temperature datasets covering 1981–2010 in Harbin were accessible from the China Meteorological Data Service Center. Climate seasons were determined based on the smoothed daily average temperature curve according to the Chinese national standard No: QX/T 152-2012 (Administration, 2012). In brief, spring starts when the daily average temperature permanently rose above 10°C, while summer comes when it rose above 22°C permanently. The autumn starts when the daily temperature drops to 22°C permanently and the winter begins at 10°C. "Permanently" means the daily temperature has remained above or below the threshold for at least five consecutive days. The details can be found in the **Supplementary Table S1**.

Statistical Analysis

Statistical analysis was conducted using the R language (version 3.4.2). The prevalence (detection percentage) of viruses was calculated by dividing the sum of positive cases by the number of cases in total. Chi-square tests or Fisher's exact tests were selected for comparing the cross tables of categorical variables. The Wilcoxon rank-sum or Kruskal–Wallis tests were chosen for continuous variable comparisons as appropriate. Datasets were visualized by an Excel spreadsheet.

Phylogenetic Analysis

The quality of sequencing data was checked manually via Chromas software version 2.4 (Technelysium Pty Ltd., South Brisbane, QLD, Australia), before contigs for each isolate were assembled using UGENE (Protsyuk et al., 2015) Software suite (version 1.9) guided by the published hexon gene sequence of human adenoviruses. Similar strains to the isolates in this report were found from the GenBank database via the BLAST search method (Boratyn et al., 2013). Fifty-eight nucleotide sequences of the hexon gene covering all seven species of human ADV were selected as the reference in this study. Before the tree building process, multiple sequences were aligned by MUSCLE (Edgar, 2004) software (version 3.6). The unrooted Neighbor-Joining tree was reconstructed using the kimura 2 parameters distance, whose robustness was tested by the bootstrap method with 1,000 replications implemented in MEGA (Kumar et al., 2018) software (version

TABLE 1 | Demographic and clinical characteristics summary of enrolled patients.

Characteristics	All patients n = 1300), no.(%)	Overall viral detection		*P*-value
		Positive, (*n* = 189), no.(%)	Negative, (*n* = 1111) no.(%)	
Male	710(54.6)	104(55.0)	606(54.5)	0.902
Age, median (IQR)	61(51 – 71)	63(54 – 69)	61(51 – 71)	0.730[a]
Age groups in years				0.104
18–49	288(22.2)	38(20.1)	250(22.5)	
50–69	652(50.2)	108(57.1)	544(49.0)	
≥70	360(27.7)	43(22.8)	317(28.5)	
Surveillance year				0.017
2014	299(23.0)	29(15.3)	270(24.3)	
2015	280(21.5)	52(27.5)	228(20.5)	
2016	327(25.2)	53(28)	274(24.7)	
2017	394(30.3)	55(29.1)	339(30.5)	
Climate season				0.003
Spring	236(18.2)	52(27.5)	184(16.6)	
Summer	137(10.5)	15(7.9)	122(11.0)	
Autumn	114(8.8)	13(6.9)	101(9.1)	
Winter	813(62.5)	109(57.7)	704(63.4)	
Calendar season[b]				0.002
Spring	481(37.0)	81(42.9)	400(36.0)	
Summer	203(15.6)	25(13.2)	178(16.0)	
Autumn	476(36.6)	52(27.5)	424(38.2)	
Winter	140(10.8)	31(16.4)	109(9.8)	
Clinical diagnosis				0.025
Pneumonia	556(42.8)	99(52.4)	457(41.1)	
Bronchitis	496(38.2)	69(36.5)	427(38.4)	
COPD	128(9.8)	11(5.8)	117(10.5)	
Asthma	20(1.5)	1(0.5)	19(1.7)	
Bronchiectasia	45(3.5)	5(2.6)	40(3.6)	
Other LRI	55(4.2)	4(2.1)	51(4.6)	
Days of hospitalization, median (IQR)	13(9 – 17)	12(9 – 19)	13(9 – 17)	0.306[a]
Chronic diseases[c]	583(44.8)	68(36.0)	515(46.4)	0.008
Clinical signs				
Fever	658(50.6)	91(48.1)	567(51.0)	0.463
Cough	628(48.3)	101(53.4)	527(47.4)	0.127
Expectoration	453(34.8)	70(37.0)	383(34.5)	0.494
Hemoptysis	49(3.8)	8(4.2)	41(3.7)	0.717
Chest tightness	606(46.6)	72(38.1)	534(48.1)	0.011
Dyspnea	343(26.4)	41(21.7)	302(27.2)	0.113

[a] *Wilcoxon test.* [b] *Calendar seasons defined by Spring (February to April), Summer (May to July), Autumn (August to October) and Winter (November to January of the next year).* [c] *Chronic diseases refers to chronic respiratory disease, cancer, diabetes mellitus, chronic cardiac diseases, cerebrovascular disease, chronic kidney disease and other chronic disease lasting for more than 1 year.*

10.0.1). The parsimony tree was also built on the same dataset.

RESULTS

Demographic and Clinical Characteristics

In total, 1,300 hospitalized adult patients with respiratory infection were enrolled from January 2014 to December 2017 in Harbin city. Among these patients, 710 were male and 590 were female, as shown in **Table 1**. The age of the population in this study varied from 18 to 97 years old, while the median age was 61 with an interquartile range (IQR) from 51 to 71. These 1,300 patients were divided into three age groups: (1) young group (18–49 years old), 288 patients; (2) middle age group (50–69 years old), 652 patients; and (3) senior citizen group (>70 years old), 360 patients.

The hospital days for these patients varied from 1 to 242 days with a median of 13 days. Of all the patients, 556 were diagnosed with pneumonia, 496 with bronchitis, 128 with COPD (Chronic obstructive pulmonary disease), 45 with bronchiectasis, 20 with asthma and 51 with other infections. Some clinical signs were more frequent among cases with certain diagnoses. In all, 370 (66.5%) pneumonia cases complained of fever, while only 185 (37.3%) cases with bronchitis had fever ($P < 0.001$). Cough was the chief complaint of the bronchial infections ($P < 0.001$), including bronchitis (56.0%), COPD (55.5%) and asthma (60.0%). Out of 1,300 enrolled patients and 583 were diagnosed with chronic diseases, including chronic respiratory disease, cancer, diabetes mellitus, chronic cardiac diseases, cerebrovascular disease, chronic kidney disease, and other chronic diseases lasting more than 1 year.

Detection Percentage of Seven Viruses

Among the 1,300 total patients, 189 (14.5%) cases were determined to be positive with at least one of seven viruses, including influenza virus (A and B), PIV (type 1, 2, and 3), RSV and ADV. One hundred and forty patients were infected with only one virus as the single infection, and 49 patients were co-infected with more than one virus. Double infections were observed in 43 cases, while triple infection was found in six cases. As shown in **Table 2**, the most frequent single infection was PIV (59 cases) and the major double infection was combined influenza and parainfluenza viruses (17 cases). The details were accessible from the **Supplementary Table S2.**

Age and Gender Distribution

The median age of the viral positive group was 63 (IQR 54–69) and the negative group was 61 (IQR 51–71). The age difference between the viral infection positive and negative group was not statistically significant ($p = 0.730$). The viral detection rate varied from 16.6% (108/652) in the middle age group to 11.9% (43/360) in the senior citizen group, but the difference was not statistically significant ($p = 0.104$). There was no significant difference in the viral infections between genders ($p = 0.902$).

Year and Seasonal Distribution

The virus detection rate among the study years varied significantly ($p = 0.017$) from 18.6% (52/280) in 2015 to 9.7% (29/299) in 2014, as shown in **Table 1**. The detection rate was not equal among calendar seasons ($p = 0.002$) or climate seasons ($p = 0.003$). Based on the climate seasons, the highest overall detection rate was in spring (22.0%, 52/236), followed by winter (13.4%, 109/813), autumn (11.4%, 13/114), and summer (10.9%, 15/137).

For individual virus positive samples, certain viruses were more frequently detected in spring than in other seasons, including influenza virus (8.9%, 21/236), PIV (9.7%, 23/236), and RSV (9.3%, 22/236), as shown in **Table 3**. ADV was more frequently detected in winter, with a detection rate of 1.8% (15/813). PIV was the dominant viral pathogen during the study period, accounting for 65.5% (19/29) of the viral infection cases in 2014, 40.3% (21/52) in 2015, 54.7% (29/53) in 2016, and 43.6% (24/55) in 2017. As shown in **Table 3**, viral co-infections were more not equally distributed among seasons, with the highest ratio in spring at 7.2% (17/236, $p = 0.022$).

TABLE 2 | Summary of detected viral infections (2014-2017).

Co-infection level	Flu	PIV	RSV	ADV	Cases
1-Single	+	−	−	−	43
	−	+	−	−	59
	−	−	+	−	32
	−	−	−	+	6
2-Double	+	+	−	−	17
	+	−	+	−	8
	+	−	−	+	3
	−	+	+	−	8
	−	+	−	+	5
	−	−	+	+	2
3-Triple	+	+	+	−	1
	+	−	+	+	2
	−	+	+	+	3
Total					189

Flu (influenza virus, including type A and B), PIV (parainfluenza virus, including type 1 to 3), RSV (respiratory syncytial virus), and ADV (adenovirus).

Daily Distribution With Air Temperature

Overall detected respiratory viral positive cases were plotted against daily average air temperature in **Figure 1**. The low temperature over days was a strong indicator for respiratory viral infections. Positive cases were rare in summer, which began late in June and ended in mid of August. One exception was found in the summer in 2017 which was related to a sudden drop of air temperature from 27.2°C on 18th July to 18.8°C on 27th July 2017.

Viral Infection and Clinical Characteristics

The overall percentage of viral infection was significantly connected with clinical diagnoses ($p = 0.025$), as shown in **Table 1**. The highest detection rate was observed in the pneumonia group (17.8%, 99/556), followed by bronchitis (13.9%, 69/496), while the lowest detection rate was found in the asthma group (5%, 1/20). Chest tightness was the only symptom that showed statistically significant difference ($p = 0.011$) between the positive (38.1%, 72/189) and negative (48.1%, 534/1111) group of viral infections. The respiratory viral infection did not prolong hospital stay statistically ($p = 0.306$), although the median days in the hospital for the positive viral infection group was 12 (IQR 9–17), which was shorter than 13 in the negative group (IQR 9–17). Overall, the viral detection rate was relatively lower in the chronic diseases group (11.7% vs. 16.9%), with statistical significance ($p = 0.008$). Detection rates varied among different chronic diseases, but the difference was not significant ($p = 0.467$). The viral co-infection ratio among different diagnosed groups was not significant ($p = 0.372$).

Isolation and Phylogenetic Analysis of Adenovirus

Two strains of human ADV were isolated from two patients diagnosed with pneumonia, respectively. The Harbin17B strain

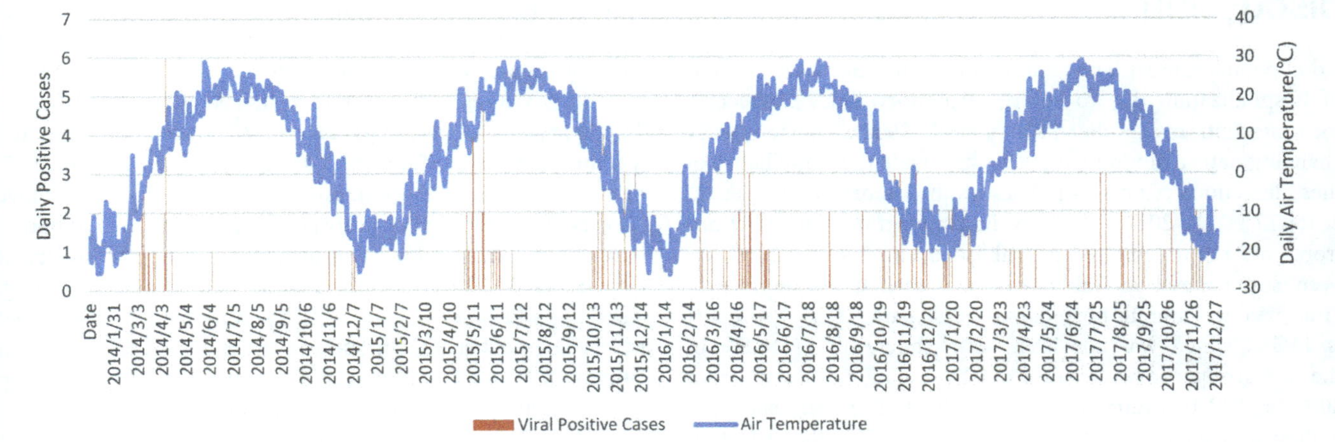

FIGURE 1 | Daily overall viral positive cases against air temperature. Notes: Date string was formatted as YYYY/MM/DD.

TABLE 3 | Respiratory virus detection percentages within clinical groups.

	Total cases (*n*)	Flu, *n*(%)	PIV, *n*(%)	RSV, *n*(%)	ADV, *n*(%)	Single infection, *n*(%)	Double infection, *n*(%)	Triple infection, *n*(%)	Positive cases, *n*(%)
Overall	1300	74(5.7)	93(7.2)	56(4.3)	21(1.6)	140(10.8)	43(3.3)	6(0.5)	189(14.5)
Age in years									
18-49	288	11(3.8)	16(5.6)	13(4.5)	7(2.4)	30(10.4)	7(2.4)	1(0.3)	38(13.2)
50-69	652	39(6.0)	56(8.6)	34(5.2)	11(1.7)	79(12.1)	26(4.0)	3(0.5)	108(16.6)
≥70	360	24(6.7)	21(5.8)	9(2.5)	3(0.8)	31(8.6)	10(2.8)	2(0.6)	43(11.9)
Surveillance year									
2014	299	12(4.0)	19(6.4)	9(3.0)	7(2.3)	14(4.7)	12(4.0)	3(1.0)	29(9.7)
2015	280	21(7.5)	21(7.5)	17(6.1)	5(1.8)	41(14.6)	10(3.6)	1(0.4)	52(18.6)
2016	327	19(5.8)	29(8.9)	12(3.7)	4(1.2)	42(12.8)	11(3.4)	0(0.0)	53(16.2)
2017	394	22(5.6)	24(6.1)	18(4.6)	5(1.3)	43(10.9)	10(2.5)	2(0.5)	55(14.0)
Climate seasons									
Spring	236	21(8.9)	23(9.7)	22(9.3)	4(1.7)	35(14.8)	16(6.8)	1(0.4)	52(22.0)
Summer	137	10(7.3)	5(3.6)	2(1.5)	1(0.7)	13(9.5)	1(0.7)	1(0.7)	15(10.9)
Autumn	114	6(5.3)	4(3.5)	5(4.4)	1(0.9)	10(8.8)	3(2.6)	0(0.0)	13(11.4)
Winter	813	37(4.6)	61(7.5)	27(3.3)	15(1.8)	82(10.1)	23(2.8)	4(0.5)	109(13.4)
Clinical diagnoses									
Pneumonia	556	35(6.3)	51(9.2)	31(5.6)	12(2.2)	73(13.1)	22(4.0)	4(0.7)	99(17.8)
Bronchitis	496	29(5.8)	30(6.0)	20(4.0)	9(1.8)	52(10.5)	15(3.0)	2(0.4)	69(13.9)
COPD	128	5(3.9)	9(7.0)	2(1.6)	0(0.0)	6(4.7)	5(3.9)	0(0.0)	11(8.6)
Asthma	20	0(0.0)	0(0.0)	1(5.0)	0(0.0)	1(5.0)	0(0.0)	0(0.0)	1(5.0)
Bronchiectasia	45	3(6.7)	2(4.4)	1(2.2)	0(0.0)	4(8.9)	1(2.2)	0(0.0)	5(11.1)
Other LRI	55	2(3.6)	1(1.8)	1(1.8)	0(0.0)	4(7.3)	0(0.0)	0(0.0)	4(7.3)

Flu (influenza virus, including type A and B), PIV (parainfluenza virus, including type 1 to 3), RSV (respiratory syncytial virus), and ADV (adenovirus).

came from a male patient aged 69 whose samples were collected in December 2017. The other strain, named Harbin17A, was isolated from a male patient aged 24 whose samples were collected in January 2017. Based on the evolutionary tree reconstruction of the hexon gene sequencing data, both strains isolated in this study were identified as human ADV species B type 3. These two strains were nearly identical, with the closest evolutionary distance to the strain GB (GenBank: AY599834; ATCC: VR-3) from the United States as well as the Harbin04B strain from a previous local epidemic, as shown in **Figure 2.** The parsimony tree was similar in topology with neighbor-joining tree (figure not shown in the article). Multiple sequence alignments indicated that, compared with the GB strain, the Harbin17A and Harbin17B strain shared a variable site in the 482nd codon (GB numbering) of the hexon gene hosting an A to C mutation, resulting in threonine (T) to proline (P) mutation of the amino acid sequences. The Harbin04B strain had a threonine on the same site in the hexon protein encoded by the codon ACU, which was identical to the Harbin17A and Harbin17B strain.

DISCUSSION

Adult populations with respiratory infections bear heavy burdens of hospitalization due to severe respiratory illness, especially for senior citizens (Muller-Pebody et al., 2006). The constantly changing nature of viral pathogens has made the surveillance of these infections critical to public health authorities (Zou et al., 2016; Li et al., 2017). The key indicators for viral infections from this report and recent published surveys in China has been summarized in **Table 4**. The overall detection rate of viral infection among hospitalized adult patients in this report is 14.5%, which was consistent with the result of 16.8% in the age group above 14 years old by a national survey from 2009 to 2013 in China (Feng et al., 2014). The dominant viral pathogen throughout this study period was PIV, with a detection rate of 7.2%, followed by influenza virus. The national survey on hospitalized patients with respiratory infection in China from 2009 to 2013 showed that influenza virus had the highest detection rate of 8.0% in adult patients. The detection rate of respiratory viruses in the over 16 years age group was 24.2% in Shandong province of China (Liu et al., 2015) and was dominated by influenza virus (8.7%) from 2011 to 2013. From 2012 to 2015, the respiratory viral detection rate in hospitalized patients above 14 years old within Beijing and Shandong China was reported to be 38.9%, in which influenza virus had the highest frequency of 8.0% (Yu et al., 2018). Compared with recent surveys in Beijing, Shandong and other regions in China, this report showed that the PIV dominated epidemic seasons from 2014 to 2017 in adult patients in Harbin, which should be important for preparing future epidemic control strategies in public health.

The viral infection rate within asthma subgroup of this report was 5%, and it was one patient with RSV among 20 asthma

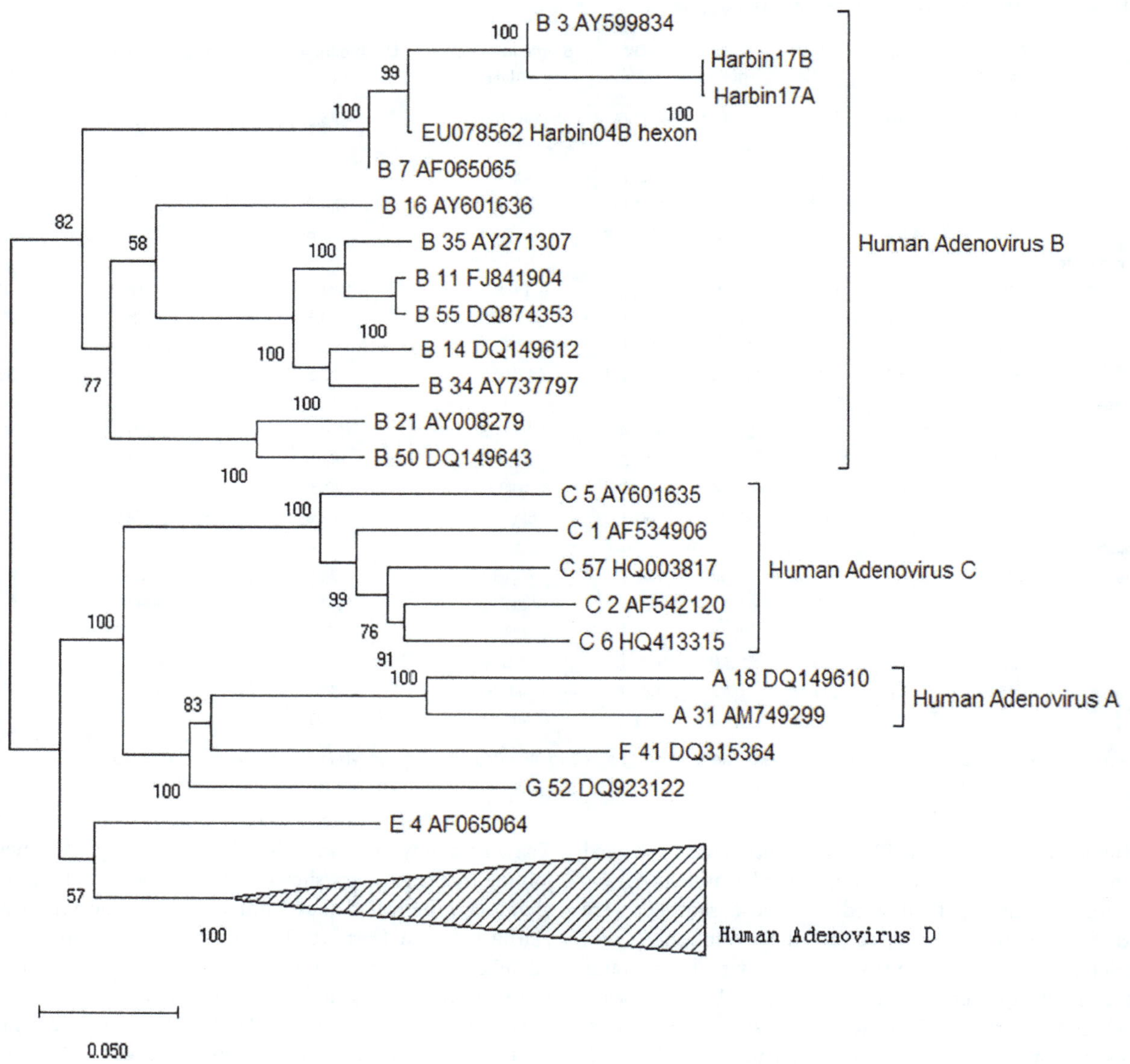

FIGURE 2 | Phylogenetic tree of human adenoviruses based on the highly variable region in the hexon gene.

TABLE 4 | Summary of detected viral infections in adult patients among this study and recent reports.

Surveillance area	Surveillance period	Age in years	Total cases	Viral positive cases	Flu A and B (%)	PIV (%)	RSV (%)	ADV (%)	hBoV (%)	HMPV (%)	HcoV (%)	HRV (%)	Co-detection (%)	Reference
Harbin	2014-2017	≥18	1300	189(14.5)	74(5.7)	93(7.2)	56(4.3)	21(1.6)	–(–)	–(–)	–(–)	–(–)	43(3.31)	This report
Shandong	2011-2013	≥16	240	58(24.2)	21(8.7)	15(6.3)	5(2.1)	6(2.5)	–(–)	1(0.4)	12(5.0)	6(2.5)	6(2.5)	Liu et al., 2015
Beijing and Shandong	2012-2015	≥14	1431	556(38.9)	114(8.0)	84(5.9)	37(2.6)	78(5.5)	28(2.0)	47(3.3)	54(3.8)	114(8.0)	–(–)	Yu et al., 2018
24 Provinces in China	2009-2013	≥15	7732	1300(16.8)	625(8.1)	133(1.7)	125(1.6)	132(1.7)	26(0.3)	64(0.8)	107(1.4)	–(–)	88(1.1)	Feng et al., 2014

Flu (influenza virus, including type A and B), PIV (parainfluenza virus, including type 1 to 3), RSV (respiratory syncytial virus), ADV (adenovirus), hBoV (Human bocavirus), HMPV (Human metapneumovirus), HCoV (Human coronavirus), HRV (Human Rhinoviruses), "-", not reported.

patients in total as shown in **Table 3**. Asthma is related to viral infection, while the detection rates varies among different pathogens. A recently published meta-analysis showed that the mean prevalence of RSV, influenza virus, PIV and ADV was 13.6%, 10%, 5.6%, and 3.8%, respectively (Zheng et al., 2018). The apparently low detection rate within asthma group in this report could be possibly caused by the sampling bias due to the limited subgroup size.

Air temperature was a major meteorological variable associated with respiratory viral infection (Chan et al., 2015). Harbin city is located at 46 degrees north latitude with an annual average temperature of 4.9 degrees Celsius. Climate seasons are not in equal length in Harbin, according to historical statistics from 1981 to 2010. The longest season in Harbin is winter, which starts on the 4th of October and lasts 201 days, followed by spring on the 23rd of April with 61 days. Starting on the 23rd of June, summers in Harbin are relatively short at 53 days, while autumn is 50 days and is the shortest season, starting on the 15th of August. In routine epidemiological analysis, 12 months in a year were usually divided into four seasons equally, which is not the case in Harbin and possibly compromises contagious disease seasonality prediction. Based on climate seasons defined by the daily average air temperature, influenza, parainfluenza and RSV detected in this report all presented significant seasonal peaks in spring, although similar phenomena were absent within the calendar seasons.

Sputum samples were acceptable both in viral culture and antigen detection in respiratory infections compared with nasopharyngeal swabs and aspirates (Covalciuc et al., 1999), although they were not frequently collected in recent surveys on lower respiratory tract infected adult patients from China. Detection of respiratory virus in sputum samples has been proven effective on a small scale, either by the immunofluorescence method (Honkinen et al., 2012) or the PCR method (Branche et al., 2014). This report provided a medium scale test on the validity or effectiveness of respiratory viral detection from sputum samples with 1,300 cases.

In this report, two nearly identical strains were isolated from pneumonia patients in Harbin, possessing high similarity with the local strain Harbin04B and the strain GB. The Harbin04B strain was isolated from a pediatric patient in Harbin (Zhang et al., 2009). ADV strain GB was named VR-3 in the ATCC database, which was isolated from an adult patient with common cold in Maryland, United States in 1953 (Huebner et al., 1954). The similarity of these strains across Asian and American continents through several decades may result from the globalization movement in modern China. It could also be explained by another hypothesis based on the evolution history of adenoviruses. On the geological scale, Homo sapiens inherit human adenoviruses from our ancestors within the Hominidae, resulting in an evolutionary rate of human ADV as low as 2.8E-8 substitution per site per year (Hoppe et al., 2015). Considering its 36 kbp genome, we would have to wait a millennium (or 992 years exactly) before a single site mutation within an adenoviral genome occurred naturally.

There were a few limitations to this study. First, the 4 years of investigation on a single city in this present report was relatively short and much more localized than other long-term or national surveillance, which may lead to a bias of the viral etiology. Second, the enrolled population in this study consisted of adult patients only, while the samples from pediatric patients were not collected simultaneously. The comparison of the viral prevalence status between adult and pediatric populations in this study was difficult. Third, the bacterial culture results of the clinical samples were not included in this report, which prevents us from drawing a comprehensive picture on the pathogens associated with lower respiratory tract infections.

CONCLUSION

In this report, 14.5% of lower respiratory tract infections in hospitalized adults from Harbin were found to be related with common respiratory viruses. The PIV dominated viral infection from 2014 to 2017 with detection rates of 7.2%. Climate seasons based on daily temperature records were found to be reliable in seasonality analysis. ADV type 3 strains with slight variations were isolated from positive cases. Further surveillance would be important to continuously monitoring the viral etiology in adult patients both local and abroad.

AUTHOR CONTRIBUTIONS

ZQ, YW, and TD designed this study and prepared the manuscript. GQ, YG, and WG collected the specimens. YW, TD, and YG conducted the epidemiological investigation. TD, LQ, WL, BQ, ZZ, LS, HG, XD, BL, ZL, HY, QC, XW, and YL performed the laboratory experiments. YW and TD analyze the data and made the figures and tables. All authors reviewed the manuscript.

FUNDING

This study was supported by the National Natural Science Foundation of China (Grant No. 31370074, 81172725, and 30771909), the Natural Science Foundation of Heilongjiang Province (Grant No. QC2016107), the Heilongjiang Academy of Medical Sciences (Grant No. 201612 and 201717), the innovative scientific research funding projects of Harbin Medical University (Grant No. 2016JCZX19), the Postdoctoral Fellowship of Heilongjiang Province of China (Grant No. LBH-Z15152) and the scientific and technological transformative project from Sino-Russia Joint Medical Research Center of Harbin Medical University.

ACKNOWLEDGMENTS

We gratefully acknowledge the Harbin Meteorological Observatory and the China Meteorological Data Service Center for providing air temperature datasets in this report.

REFERENCES

Administration, C. M. (2012). *Division of Climatic Season*. Beijing: China Meteorological Press.

Baker, A. T., Aguirre-Hernandez, C., Hallden, G., and Parker, A. L. (2018). Designer oncolytic adenovirus: coming of age. *Cancers* 10:E201. doi: 10.3390/cancers10060201

Boratyn, G. M., Camacho, C., Cooper, P. S., Coulouris, G., Fong, A., Ma, N., et al. (2013). BLAST: a more efficient report with usability improvements. *Nucleic Acids Res.* 41, W29–W33. doi: 10.1093/nar/gkt282

Branche, A. R., Walsh, E. E., Formica, M. A., and Falsey, A. R. (2014). Detection of respiratory viruses in sputum from adults by use of automated multiplex PCR. *J. Clin. Microbiol.* 52, 3590–3596. doi: 10.1128/JCM.01523-14

Chan, P. K., Tam, W. W., Lee, T. C., Hon, K. L., Lee, N., Chan, M. C., et al. (2015). Hospitalization incidence, mortality, and seasonality of common respiratory viruses over a period of 15 years in a developed subtropical city. *Medicine* 94:e2024. doi: 10.1097/MD.0000000000002024

Cheng, Z., Yan, Y., Jing, S., Li, W. G., Chen, W. W., Zhang, J., et al. (2018). Comparative genomic analysis of re-emergent human adenovirus type 55 pathogens associated with adult severe community-acquired pneumonia reveals conserved genomes and capsid proteins. *Front. Microbiol.* 9:1180. doi: 10.3389/fmicb.2018.01180

Covalciuc, K. A., Webb, K. H., and Carlson, C. A. (1999). Comparison of four clinical specimen types for detection of influenza A and B viruses by optical immunoassay (FLU OIA test) and cell culture methods. *J. Clin. Microbiol.* 37, 3971–3974.

Edgar, R. C. (2004). MUSCLE: multiple sequence alignment with high accuracy and high throughput. *Nucleic Acids Res.* 32, 1792–1797. doi: 10.1093/nar/gkh340

Feng, L., Li, Z., Zhao, S., Nair, H., Lai, S., Xu, W., et al. (2014). Viral etiologies of hospitalized acute lower respiratory infection patients in China, 2009-2013. *PLoS One* 9:e99419. doi: 10.1371/journal.pone.0099419

Feucht, J., Opherk, K., Lang, P., Kayser, S., Hartl, L., Bethge, W., et al. (2015). Adoptive T-cell therapy with hexon-specific Th1 cells as a treatment of refractory adenovirus infection after HSCT. *Blood* 125, 1986–1994. doi: 10.1182/blood-2014-06-573725

GBD 2016 Causes of Death Collaborators (2017). Global, regional, and national age-sex specific mortality for 264 causes of death, 1980-2016: a systematic analysis for the global burden of disease study 2016. *Lancet* 390, 1151–1210. doi: 10.1016/S0140-6736(17)32152-9

Hashimoto, S., Gonzalez, G., Harada, S., Oosako, H., Hanaoka, N., Hinokuma, R., et al. (2018). Recombinant type human mastadenovirus D85 associated with epidemic keratoconjunctivitis since 2015 in Japan. *J. Med. Virol.* 90, 881–889. doi: 10.1002/jmv.25041

He, Y., Lin, G. Y., Wang, Q., Cai, X. Y., Zhang, Y. H., Lin, C. X., et al. (2014). A 3-year prospective study of the epidemiology of acute respiratory viral infections in hospitalized children in Shenzhen. China. *Influenza Other Respir. Viruses* 8, 443–451. doi: 10.1111/irv.12257

Honkinen, M., Lahti, E., Osterback, R., Ruuskanen, O., and Waris, M. (2012). Viruses and bacteria in sputum samples of children with community-acquired pneumonia. *Clin. Microbiol. Infect.* 18, 300–307. doi: 10.1111/j.1469-0691.2011.03603.x

Hoppe, E., Pauly, M., Gillespie, T. R., Akoua-Koffi, C., Hohmann, G., Fruth, B., et al. (2015). Multiple cross-species transmission events of human adenoviruses (HAdV) during hominine evolution. *Mol. Biol. Evol.* 32, 2072–2084. doi: 10.1093/molbev/msv090

Huang, G., Yu, D., Zhu, Z., Zhao, H., Wang, P., Gray, G. C., et al. (2013). Outbreak of febrile respiratory illness associated with human adenovirus type 14p1 in Gansu Province, China. *Influenza Other Respir. Viruses* 7, 1048–1054. doi: 10.1111/irv.12118

Huebner, R. J., Rowe, W. P., Ward, T. G., Parrott, R. H., and Bell, J. A. (1954). Adenoidal-pharyngeal-conjunctival agents: a newly recognized group of common viruses of the respiratory system. *N. Engl. J. Med.* 251, 1077–1086. doi: 10.1056/NEJM195412302512701

Ismail, A. M., Cui, T., Dommaraju, K., Singh, G., Dehghan, S., Seto, J., et al. (2018). Genomic analysis of a large set of currently-and historically-important human adenovirus pathogens. *Emerg. Microbes Infect.* 7:10. doi: 10.1038/s41426-017-0004-y

Kumar, S., Stecher, G., Li, M., Knyaz, C., and Tamura, K. (2018). MEGA X: molecular evolutionary genetics analysis across computing platforms. *Mol. Biol. Evol.* 35, 1547–1549. doi: 10.1093/molbev/msy096

Lambkin-Williams, R., Noulin, N., Mann, A., Catchpole, A., and Gilbert, A. S. (2018). The human viral challenge model: accelerating the evaluation of respiratory antivirals, vaccines and novel diagnostics. *Respir. Res.* 19:123. doi: 10.1186/s12931-018-0784-1

Lenman, A., Liaci, A. M., Liu, Y., Frangsmyr, L., Frank, M., Blaum, B. S., et al. (2018). Polysialic acid is a cellular receptor for human adenovirus 52. *Proc. Natl. Acad. Sci. U.S.A.* 115, E4264–E4273. doi: 10.1073/pnas.1716900115

Li, J., Lu, X., Sun, Y., Lin, C., Li, F., Yang, Y., et al. (2018). A swimming pool-associated outbreak of pharyngoconjunctival fever caused by human adenovirus type 4 in Beijing, China. *Int. J. Infect. Dis.* 75, 89–91. doi: 10.1016/j.ijid.2018.08.009

Li, M., Zhao, N., Luo, J., Li, Y., Chen, L., Ma, J., et al. (2017). Genetic characterization of continually evolving highly pathogenic H5N6 influenza viruses in China, 2012-2016. *Front. Microbiol.* 8:260. doi: 10.3389/fmicb.2017.00260

Liu, J., Mu, Y., Dong, W., Yao, F., Wang, L., Yan, H., et al. (2014). Genetic variation of human respiratory syncytial virus among children with fever and respiratory symptoms in Shanghai, China, from 2009 to 2012. *Infect. Genet. Evol.* 27, 131–136. doi: 10.1016/j.meegid.2014.07.011

Liu, T., Li, Z., Zhang, S., Song, S., Julong, W., Lin, Y., et al. (2015). Viral etiology of acute respiratory tract infections in hospitalized children and adults in shandong province, China. *Virol. J.* 12, 168. doi: 10.1186/s12985-015-0388-z

Lu, Q. B., Tong, Y. G., Wo, Y., Wang, H. Y., Liu, E. M., Gray, G. C., et al. (2014). Epidemiology of human adenovirus and molecular characterization of human adenovirus 55 in China, 2009-2012. *Influenza Other Respir. Viruses* 8, 302–308. doi: 10.1111/irv.12232

Lu, Y., Wang, S., Zhang, L., Xu, C., Bian, C., Wang, Z., et al. (2013). Epidemiology of human respiratory viruses in children with acute respiratory tract infections in Jinan, China. *Clin. Dev. Immunol.* 2013:210490. doi: 10.1155/2013/210490

Madisch, I., Harste, G., Pommer, H., and Heim, A. (2005). Phylogenetic analysis of the main neutralization and hemagglutination determinants of all human adenovirus prototypes as a basis for molecular classification and taxonomy. *J. Virol.* 79, 15265–15276. doi: 10.1128/JVI.79.24.15265-15276.2005

Muller-Pebody, B., Crowcroft, N. S., Zambon, M. C., and Edmunds, W. J. (2006). Modelling hospital admissions for lower respiratory tract infections in the elderly in England. *Epidemiol. Infect.* 134, 1150–1157. doi: 10.1017/S0950268806006376

Nemerow, G. R., Stewart, P. L., and Reddy, V. S. (2012). Structure of human adenovirus. *Curr. Opin. Virol.* 2, 115–121. doi: 10.1016/j.coviro.2011.12.008

Pan, Y., Zhang, Y., Shi, W., Peng, X., Cui, S., Zhang, D., et al. (2017). Human parainfluenza virus infection in severe acute respiratory infection cases in Beijing, 2014-2016: a molecular epidemiological study. *Influenza Other Respir. Viruses* 11, 564–568. doi: 10.1111/irv.12514

Pavia, A. T. (2011). Viral infections of the lower respiratory tract: old viruses, new viruses, and the role of diagnosis. *Clin. Infect. Dis.* 52(Suppl. 4), S284–S289. doi: 10.1093/cid/cir043

Protsyuk, I. V., Grekhov, G. A., Tiunov, A. V., and Fursov, M. Y. (2015). Shared Bioinformatics Databases within the Unipro UGENE Platform. *J. Integr. Bioinform.* 12, 24–34. doi: 10.2390/biecoll-jib-2015-257

Qiu, H., Li, X., Tian, X., Zhou, Z., Xing, K., Li, H., et al. (2012). Serotype-specific neutralizing antibody epitopes of human adenovirus type 3 (HAdV-3) and HAdV-7 reside in multiple hexon hypervariable regions. *J. Virol.* 86, 7964–7975. doi: 10.1128/JVI.07076-11

Rehder, K. J., Wilson, E. A., Zimmerman, K. O., Cunningham, C. K., and Turner, D. A. (2015). Detection of multiple respiratory viruses associated with mortality and severity of illness in children. *Pediatr. Crit. Care Med.* 16, e201–e206. doi: 10.1097/PCC.0000000000000492

Sloan, C., Moore, M. L., and Hartert, T. (2011). Impact of pollution, climate, and sociodemographic factors on spatiotemporal dynamics of seasonal respiratory viruses. *Clin. Transl. Sci.* 4, 48–54. doi: 10.1111/j.1752-8062.2010.00257.x

Smith, C. D., Craft, D. W., Shiromoto, R. S., and Yan, P. O. (1986). Alternative cell line for virus isolation. *J. Clin. Microbiol.* 24, 265–268.

Tian, X., Qiu, H., Zhou, Z., Wang, S., Fan, Y., Li, X., et al. (2018). Identification of a critical and conformational neutralizing epitope in human adenovirus type 4 hexon. *J. Virol.* 92, e1643-17. doi: 10.1128/JVI.01643-17

Tomita, K., Sakurai, F., Iizuka, S., Hemmi, M., Wakabayashi, K., Machitani, M., et al. (2018). Antibodies against adenovirus fiber and penton base proteins inhibit adenovirus vector-mediated transduction in the liver following systemic administration. *Sci. Rep.* 8:12315. doi: 10.1038/s41598-018-30947-z

Veesler, D., Cupelli, K., Burger, M., Graber, P., Stehle, T., and Johnson, J. E. (2014). Single-particle EM reveals plasticity of interactions between the adenovirus penton base and integrin alphaVbeta3. *Proc. Natl. Acad. Sci. U.S.A.* 111, 8815–8819. doi: 10.1073/pnas.1404575111

Wang, H., Zheng, Y., Deng, J., Wang, W., Liu, P., Yang, F., et al. (2016). Prevalence of respiratory viruses among children hospitalized from respiratory infections in Shenzhen. *China Virol. J.* 13:39. doi: 10.1186/s12985-016-0493-7

Wang, X., Wu, P., Pei, Y., Tsang, T. K., Gu, D., Wang, W., et al. (2018). Assessment of human-to-human transmissibility of avian influenza A(H7N9) virus across five waves by analyzing clusters of case-patients in mainland China, 2013-2017. *Clin. Infect. Dis.* doi: 10.1093/cid/ciy541 [Epub ahead of print].

Yang, J., Lau, Y. C., Wu, P., Feng, L., Wang, X., Chen, T., et al. (2018). Variation in influenza B virus epidemiology by Lineage, China. *Emerg. Infect. Dis.* 24, 1536–1540.doi: 10.3201/eid2408.180063

Yu, B., Dong, J., Wang, C., Zhan, Y., Zhang, H., Wu, J., et al. (2013). Characteristics of neutralizing antibodies to adenovirus capsid proteins in human and animal sera. *Virology* 437, 118–123. doi: 10.1016/j.virol.2012.12.014

Yu, J., Xie, Z., Zhang, T., Lu, Y., Fan, H., Yang, D., et al. (2018). Comparison of the prevalence of respiratory viruses in patients with acute respiratory infections at different hospital settings in North China, 2012-2015. *BMC Infect. Dis.* 18:72. doi: 10.1186/s12879-018-2982-3

Yuan, X., Qu, Z., Wu, X., Wang, Y., Liu, L., Wei, F., et al. (2009). Molecular modeling and epitopes mapping of human adenovirus type 3 hexon protein. *Vaccine* 27, 5103–5110. doi: 10.1016/j.vaccine.2009.06.041

Zandvliet, M. L., Falkenburg, J. H., Van Liempt, E., Veltrop-Duits, L. A., Lankester, A. C., Kalpoe, J. S., et al. (2010). Combined CD8+ and CD4+ adenovirus hexon-specific T cells associated with viral clearance after stem cell transplantation as treatment for adenovirus infection. *Haematologica* 95, 1943–1951. doi: 10.3324/haematol.2010.022947

Zhang, H. Y., Li, Z. M., Zhang, G. L., Diao, T. T., Cao, C. X., and Sun, H. Q. (2009). Respiratory viruses in hospitalized children with acute lower respiratory tract infections in harbin. *China. Jpn. J. Infect. Dis.* 62, 458–460.

Zheng, X. Y., Xu, Y. J., Guan, W. J., and Lin, L. F. (2018). Regional, age and respiratory-secretion-specific prevalence of respiratory viruses associated with asthma exacerbation: a literature review. *Arch. Virol.* 163, 845–853. doi: 10.1007/s00705-017-3700-y

Zou, L., Yi, L., Wu, J., Song, Y., Huang, G., Zhang, X., et al. (2016). Evolution and transmission of respiratory syncytial group A (RSV-A) viruses in Guangdong, China 2008-2015. *Front. Microbiol.* 7:1263. doi: 10.3389/fmicb.2016.01263

17

Adenoviromics: Mining the Human Adenovirus Species D Genome

Ashrafali M. Ismail[1], *Ji Sun Lee*[1], *Jeong Yoon Lee*[1,2], *Gurdeep Singh*[1,3], *David W. Dyer*[4], *Donald Seto*[5], *James Chodosh*[1] *and Jaya Rajaiya*[1*]

[1] Howe Laboratory, Massachusetts Eye and Ear, Harvard Medical School, Boston, MA, United States, [2] Molecular Virology Laboratory, Korea Zoonosis Research Institute, Jeonbuk National University, Jeonju, South Korea, [3] Department of Cell and Systems Biology, University of Toronto, Toronto, ON, Canada, [4] Department of Microbiology and Immunology, University of Oklahoma Health Sciences Center, Oklahoma City, OK, United States, [5] Bioinformatics and Computational Biology Program, School of Systems Biology, George Mason University, Manassas, VI, United States

***Correspondence:**
Jaya Rajaiya
jaya_rajaiya@meei.harvard.edu

Human adenovirus (HAdV) infections cause disease world-wide. Whole genome sequencing has now distinguished 90 distinct genotypes in 7 species (A-G). Over half of these 90 HAdVs fall within species D, with essentially all of the HAdV-D whole genome sequences generated in the last decade. Herein, we describe recent new findings made possible by mining of this expanded genome database, and propose future directions to elucidate new functional elements and new functions for previously known viral components.

Keywords: adenovirus, genome, evolution, transcription factor, interactome

INTRODUCTION

Human adenovirus (HAdV) infections represent a significant source of morbidity and mortality, world-wide and at all ages, through highly transmittable infections at mucosal sites, including the eye, and urinary, respiratory, and gastrointestinal tracts (Horwitz, 1996). HAdV causes fatal acute respiratory distress syndrome in healthy adults and is especially lethal in infants and the immune compromised (Bhanthumkosol, 1998; Ryu et al., 2003; Wallot et al., 2006; Engelmann et al., 2016; Tan et al., 2016; Zhang et al., 2016). No FDA-approved therapy for acute HAdV infection is available. At resolution of acute infection, persistence may develop within nasopharyngeal lymphoid tissue (Neumann et al., 1987; Garnett et al., 2002, 2009; Zhang et al., 2010; Assadian et al., 2016), as yet uncharacterized cells in the gastrointestinal tract (Roy et al., 2009), and possibly the ocular surface (Kaye et al., 2005), permitting evolution of new HAdVs through homologous recombination between two or more HAdVs infecting the same cell(s) (Lee et al., 2005, 2018; Echavarria et al., 2006; McCarthy et al., 2009; Seto et al., 2010).

HAdVs are divided phylogenetically into seven species (A-G), with a total of 90 recognized genotypes with whole genome sequences in GenBank, including the original 51 "serotypes"—determined by serum neutralization—which now all have been fully sequenced (**Table 1**) (Robinson et al., 2013a) Human adenovirus species D (HAdV-D) is the largest and most rapidly growing among all HAdV species, and contains viruses associated with epidemic keratoconjunctivitis (EKC), a severe, hyperacute ocular surface infection (Butt and Chodosh, 2006). A collaboration funded by the American Recovery and Reinvestment Act of 2009 came to fruition with the complete whole genome sequencing and analysis of all previously unsequenced HAdV-D serotypes (Robinson et al., 2013a), leading to a new understanding of adenovirus ontogeny (Jones et al., 2007; Robinson et al., 2008, 2009a,b; Robinson et al., 2011b,c; Robinson et al., 2013a,b; Walsh et al., 2009, 2010a,b; Arnold et al., 2010; Torres et al., 2010; Dehghan et al., 2011, 2013a,b; Walsh et al., 2011; Liu et al., 2011; Seto et al., 2011, 2013; Singh et al., 2012, 2013; Zhou et al., 2012)—including those

HAdV-Ds associated with EKC (Robinson et al., 2008, 2009b, 2011b; Walsh et al., 2009; Zhou et al., 2012)—and ultimately to a new typing system for HAdV based on genomics (Seto et al., 2011).

Recent published work demonstrates how genome "mining," in-depth analyses of the growing HAdV genome database, can bring about new realizations and add critical new information to prior ones. The trimeric fiber protein on adenoviruses mediates viral entry through interaction of the distal most "knob" structure on the fiber with host cell receptors. In a phylogenetic analysis of HAdV-D fiber genes, HAdV-D types associated with EKC were recently shown to form a unique clade (Ismail et al., 2016). By proteotyping, a new *in silico* methodology described in detail below, EKC virus-associated fiber knobs were uniquely shared, and signature amino acid positions distinguished EKC from non-EKC types. Remarkably, human corneal epithelial cell tropism could be predicted by the presence of a lysine or alanine at residue 240, and this amino acid residue in EKC viruses showed evidence for positive selection. These data added to the prior observation by Huang and coworkers that artificial mutation to a lysine at residue 240 in a non-EKC virus could confer infection of Chang cells, a conjunctiva derived continuous cell line (Huang et al., 1999). However, because Chang cells came later known to be contaminated by HeLa cells, the importance of residue 240 to ocular tropism was until this new observation, in some doubt.

Another recently published effort provided further evidence of the importance and potential for HAdV genome mining. Late adenoviral gene expression is initiated by the adenovirus major late promoter (Ramke et al., 2017), followed by splicing of mRNAs to the viral tripartite leader for translation (Chow et al., 1977; Akusjärvi and Pettersson, 1978; Chow and Broker, 1978; Logan and Shenk, 1984). The HAdV tripartite leader is a 200-nucleotide 5' noncoding region that circumvents the requirement for eukaryotic initiation factor 4F or cap binding protein complex (Ziff and Evans, 1978; Akusjärvi and Pettersson, 1979; Dolph et al., 1988; Zhang et al., 1989), and permits translation of HAdV mRNAs at late times in infection when cap-dependent translation is blocked due to shut down of host cellular cap-dependent mRNA translation. HAdV $5'$ untranslated regions ($5'$UTRs) are critical for cap-independent initiation, and impact mRNA localization and stability. The HAdV tripartite leader (TPL), composed of three introns (TPL 1-3), drives translation of HAdV late mRNA. The annotation of 72 HAdV genotypes for the HAdV TPL and another previously described leader, the i-leader, let to identification of newly identified polycistronic mRNAs for RID-α and RID-β within the E3 transcription unit, and a potential new open reading frame (ORF) within the i-leader sequence, with termination of this potential protein in TPL3 (Ramke et al., 2017). In addition, the authors also identified a potential new leader sequence embedded within the E3 region, tentatively named the j-leader (**Figure 1**).

STRUCTURE AND INFECTION

The HAdV is non-enveloped, icosahedral in shape, and contains a double stranded DNA genome of ~36,000 base pairs (bp)

TABLE 1 | Species and type designations for the 51 human adenovirus (HAdV) serotypes.

Type	GenBank accession no.	Genome length	Year published
HAdV-C1	AC_000017	36001	2004
HAdV-C2	AC_000007	35937	2003
HAdV-B3	AY599834	35345	2006
HAdV-E4	AY599837	35964	2006
HAdV-C5	AY601635	35931	2006
HAdV-C6	FJ349096	35758	2011
HAdV-B7	KP670856.2	35239	2016
HAdV-D8	AB448767	34980	2009
HAdV-D9	AJ854486	35083	2008
HAdV-D10	JN226746	35105	2013
HAdV-B11	AF532578	34794	2003
HAdV-A12	X73487	34125	1979
HAdV-D13	JN226747	35209	2013
HAdV-B14	JQ824845	34767	2012
HAdV-D15	KF268204	35100	2013
HAdV-B16	JN860680	35384	2011
HAdV-D17	HQ910407	35139	2011
HAdV-A18	GU191019	34177	2010
HAdV-D19	JQ326209	35153	2011
HAdV-D20	JN226749	35181	2013
HAdV-B21	AY601633	35382	2006
HAdV-D22	FJ619037	35152	2009
HAdV-D23	JN226750	35050	2013
HAdV-D24	JN226751	35166	2013
HAdV-D25	JN226752	35248	2013
HAdV-D26	EF153474	35152	2007
HAdV-D27	JN226753	35154	2013
HAdV-D28	FJ824826	35130	2010
HAdV-D29	JN226754	35214	2013
HAdV-D30	JN226755	35178	2012
HAdV-A31	AM749299	33763	2005
HAdV-D32	JN226756	35248	2013
HAdV-D33	JN226758	35131	2013
HAdV-B34	AY737797	34775	2004
HAdV-B35	AC_000019	34794	2004
HAdV-D36	GQ384080	35152	2010
HAdV-D37	AB448775	35215	2009
HAdV-D38	JN226759	35221	2013
HAdV-D39	JN226760	35152	2013
HAdV-F40	NC_001454	34214	1993
HAdV-F41	DQ315364.2	34188	2007
HAdV-D42	JN226761	35231	2013
HAdV-D43	JN226762	35012	2013
HAdV-D44	JN226763	35214	2013
HAdV-D45	JN226764	35154	2013
HAdV-D46	AY875648	35178	2006
HAdV-D47	JN226757	35106	2013
HAdV-D48	EF153473	35206	2007
HAdV-D49	DQ393829	35215	2006
HAdV-B50	AY737798	35385	2007
HAdV-D51	JN226765	35114	2013

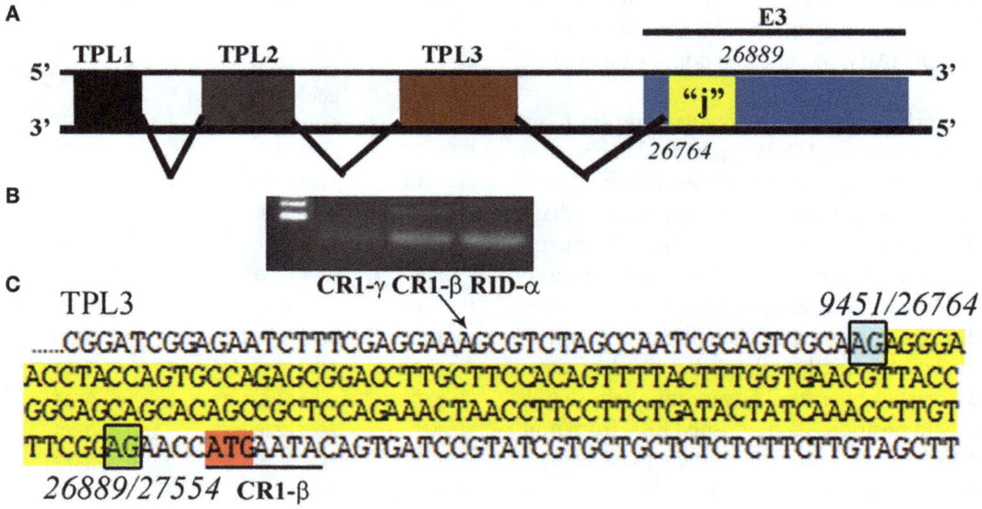

FIGURE 1 | Putative "j"-leader located within the CR1-α E3 gene. **(A)** Schematic for the location of a newly detected leader ("j"-leader) embedded within the E3 CRI-α gene, experimentally determined to be spliced to some, but not all mRNAs of the E3 genes. **(B)** Gel photomicrograph of mRNA transcripts amplified with forward primer from TPL1 and reverse primers from CR1-γ, CR1-β, and RID-α. Primers were chosen to elicit similarly sized bands to facilitate subsequent sequencing. **(C)** Nucleotide sequence of the PCR product for CR1-β. The putative j-leader sequence and splice sites are shown in yellow and green, respectively. Note an additional 4 nucleotide 5′UTR (AACC) prior to the CR1-β start site (red). The 5′UTR in **(C)** prior to the splice site for the j-leader is from TPL3. Adapted from Ramke et al. (2017) with permission.

with ~1 open reading frame (ORF) for every 1000 nucleotides. Viral DNA is associated with four (interior) core proteins including Mu, VII, V, and terminal protein. The histone-like protein (p) VII protects viral DNA from cellular DNA damage responses (Lischwe and Sung, 1977; Karen and Hearing, 2011; Avgousti et al., 2017). The outer protein coat (capsid) of the virus consists of 240 hexon capsomers and 12 penton capsomers, along with several minor capsid proteins. The latter include pVI, pIIIa, pVIII, and pIX and are important to capsid stability. Each penton capsomer contains a ring of five penton base proteins which bind and support the trimeric fiber protein with its distal fiber knob. During viral infection, the fiber knob binds to one of several host cell receptors (Nemerow, 2000; Goosney and Nemerow, 2003; Nemerow et al., 2009). The penton base protein contains two hypervariable loops. The interaction between fiber knob and a host cell receptor brings about secondary contact between the hypervariable loop 2 (HVL2) arginine-glycine-aspartic acid (RGD) motif in each penton base protein (five per penton base capsomer) with host cell integrins $\alpha_V\beta_3$, $\alpha_V\beta_5$, and $\alpha_V\beta_1$, that in turn induce endocytosis of the virus (Li et al., 1998a,b; Li et al., 2000). HAdV structural proteins can serve multiple functions. For example, the minor capsid structural protein VI (pVI) plays a critical role in at least three distinct aspects of the viral "life" cycle: endosomal escape during cell entry, nuclear assembly during viral replication, and stability of the intact, infectious virus outside the host (Wodrich et al., 2003; Wiethoff et al., 2005; Moyer et al., 2011, 2016). These findings suggest that, as with pVI, other HAdV structural proteins may have multiple functions yet to be elucidated.

GENOMICS AND EVOLUTION

The relatively large genome database for HAdV-D (over 50 unique viruses with available whole genome sequences) (**Tables 1, 2**) has permitted detailed analyses of genome relationships within this clinically important adenovirus species. HAdV-D genomes are highly conserved (>90%). However, whole genome analyses of HAdV-D have revealed specific loci of genetic hypervariability in the hexon, penton base, fiber, and E3 CR1α, β, and γ genes (**Figure 2**), dictating nonsynonymous amino acid changes in corresponding proteins (**Figure 3**). GC content confers genome stability and resistance to recombination (Gruss et al., 1991), and the genomes of HAdV-D have among the highest GC content among HAdV species (~56%). The hypervariable regions in HAdV-D were found to be sharply reduced in GC nucleotide content relative to the rest of the genome (Robinson et al., 2013a). Mutations in HAdV are relatively infrequent, with genome stability now documented in some types across decades (Hofmayer et al., 2009; Mahadevan et al., 2010; Seto et al., 2010; Dehghan et al., 2013b; Robinson et al., 2013a; Alkhalaf et al., 2015). However, those regions of the genome shown to be hypervariable and relatively low in GC content are the very same also shown to undergo homologous recombination (Robinson et al., 2009a, 2011b; Walsh et al., 2009; Zhou et al., 2012; Singh et al., 2013), driving the evolution of new genotypes.

Adenoviruses recombine specifically during viral replication (Williams et al., 1975; Meinschad and Winnacker, 1980; Munz et al., 1983), and do so by both homologous and heterologous mechanisms (Young et al., 1984; Epstein and Young, 1991; Crawford-Miksza and Schnurr, 1996). However, the evidence

TABLE 2 | Species and molecular types of human adenovirus (HAdV) genotypes 52–90.

HAdV type	#Name	GenBank accession no.	Genome length	Year published
HAdV-G52	P52H52F52/2003/USA	DQ923122.2	34250	2007
HAdV-D53	P37H22F8/2005/DEU	FJ169625	34909	2009
HAdV-D54	P54H54F8/2000/JPN	AB333801	34920	2008
HAdV-B55	P14H11F14/2006/CHN	FJ643676	34755	2010
HAdV-D56	P56H15F9/2008/FRA	HM770721	35066	2011
HAdV-C57	P1H57F6/2001/RUS	HQ003817	35818	2011
HAdV-D58	P58H58F29/1996/ARG	HQ883276	35217	2011
HAdV-D59	P64H25F56/2007/USA	JF799911	35072	2012
HAdV-D60	P60H20F60/2009/CAN	HQ007053	35050	2013
HAdV-A61	P31H31F31/2004/JPN	JF964962	33776	2011
HAdV-D62	P62H62F62/1993/GBR	JN162671	35127	2014
HAdV-D63	P30H30F29/1959/USA	JN935766	35168	2012
HAdV-D64	P22H19F37/1993/USA	EF121005	35231	2012
HAdV-D65	P58H10F9/2004/BGD	AP012285	35172	2012
HAdV-B66	P66H7F3/1987/ARG	JN860676	35080	2012
HAdV-D67	P67H9F67/2005/BGD	AP012302	35075	2013
HAdV-B68	P16H3F16/2004/ARG	JN860678	35538	Unpublished
HAdV-D69	P53H15F69/1955/SAU	JN226748	35124	2013
HAdV-D70	P70H70F29/2014/DEU	KP641339	35186	2015
HAdV-D71	P9H20F71/1987/DEU	KF268207	35192	2013
HAdV-D72	P72H30F72/1985/DEU	KF268335	34553	2013
HAdV-D73	P67H45F27/2015/DEU	KY618676	35190	2017
HAdV-D74	P70H74F51/2015/DEU	KY618677	35155	2017
HAdV-D75	P75H26F29/2015/DEU	KY618678	35104	2017
HAdV-B76	P21H21F16/DEU	KF633445	35586	2013
HAdV-B77	P35H34F7/1985/DEU	KF268328	34653	2013
HAdV-B78	P11H11F7/2000/ARG	KT970440	34881	Unpublished
HAdV-B79	P11H34F11/2015/JPN	LC177352	34779	2017
HAdV-D80	P19,23H28F22/2014/DEU	TBA	34909	Unpublished
HAdV-D81	P65H48F60/2012/JPN	AB765926.1	35198	2014
HAdV-D82	P56H15F37/2011/JPN	LC066535.1	35122	Unpublished
HAdV-D83	P83H9F15/2010/PAR	KX827426.1	35207	2017
HAdV-D84	P43H17F84/2011/PAN	MF416150	35257	2017
HAdV-D85	P37H19F8/2015/JPN	LC314153	35203	2018
HAdV-D86	P9H25F25/1978/SWE	TBA	35147	Unpublished
HAdV-D87	P9H15F25/1967/USA	MF476841	35159	Unpublished
HAdV-D88	P88H15F9/1963/USA	MF476842	35115	Unpublished
HAdV-C89	P89H2F2/2015/DEU	TBA	35998	Unpublished
HAdV-D90	P33H27F67/2017/BGD	TBA	34207*	Unpublished

#Name indicates molecular type (P, penton base; H, hexon; F, fiber)/year of isolation/country of isolation.
TBA: GenBank accession number, to be assigned.
**Metagenomics project, missing the inverted terminal repeat sequences.*

for homologous recombination as the major mechanism driving HAdV-D evolution is unassailable (Robinson et al., 2013a; Singh et al., 2013). Specifically, recombination occurs in the two penton base hypervariable regions (these code for two hypervariable loops (HVLs) on the penton base protein, separated from one another by ~125 conserved amino acids), seven hexon hypervariable regions (these are closely adjacent in the hexon gene and determine two adjacent HVLs on the hexon protein), fiber (fiber gene and protein are entirely hypervariable), and E3 CR1α, β, and γ (each also entirely hypervariable). For homologous recombination between two HAdVs to occur, at least two virus types with high nucleotide sequence homology at corresponding locations in both genomes must co-infect the same cell, and viral DNA replication should be ongoing. Co-infection by two or more HAdVs has been well documented (Lee et al., 2005; Echavarria et al., 2006; Vora et al., 2006; McCarthy et al., 2009; Halstead et al., 2010; Seto et al., 2010), as has the presence of two HAdV types in archived clinical samples (Singh et al., 2012).

"Proteotyping" is a novel approach to the study of genome evolution (Obenauer et al., 2006), and has been applied to characterize recombination among HAdV-D (Robinson et al., 2013a; Singh et al., 2013).In this method, maximum likelihood trees are used to align amino acid sequences of hypervariable, frequently recombined proteins. Each amino acid is assigned a unique, arbitrary color. Consensus residues are colored white, and gaps in the alignment are colored black. A threshold of $<10\%$ sequence divergence is used to distinguish unique proteotypes. An example of proteotyping is shown (**Figure 4**), comparing an amino acid alignment from E3 14.7K, a highly conserved gene with one distinct proteotype, with the hypervariable E3 CR1α (Singh et al., 2013), with six distinct proteotypes observed among 38 HAdV-Ds. E3 14.7K is therefore not hypervariable and not recombinant. E3 CR1α is hypervariable and recombinant.

Another way to interpret the analyses for those proteins like E3 CR1α, with more than one proteotype is that those proteotypes containing more than one HAdV type have previously recombined in nature, while those proteotypes with only one HAdV type are those that have not (yet) been shown to recombine in nature. HAdV-D37 and 29 fall within different hexon proteotypes (**Figure 5**). HAdV-D37 shares a hexon proteotype with HAdV-D13 and 30 (Robinson et al., 2013a), while HAdV-D29 shares a hexon proteotype with HAdV-D15, 56, and 69 (Singh et al., 2015). These two hexon proteotypes therefore have undergone prior homologous recombination. In contrast, the hexon proteins of HAdV-D10 and 28 are each in a proteotype with only one member; hexon recombination for these two viruses has therefore not yet been documented in nature. In sum, these data show by independent means that homologous recombination within HAdV-D is common, and confirm previously recognized patterns of homologous recombination among HAdV-D (Robinson et al., 2009a, 2011b, 2013a,b; Walsh et al., 2009, 2010a; Singh et al., 2012, 2013; Zhou et al., 2012; Gonzalez et al., 2014).

The local sequence and/or structure of DNA in regions flanking recombinogenic sites is significant for directing cellular recombination machinery to those regions. In bacteria, a signal for recombination between homologous DNA is the *c*rossover *h*otspot *i*nstigator, or Chi nucleotide sequence. This was first discovered in bacteriophage lambda, then in bacterial DNA, and later shown to mediate recombination between them (Stahl, 1998). The Chi sequence in *E. coli* (Chi_{EC}) is $5'$-GCTGGTGG-$3'$ (Smith et al., 1981; Bianco and Kowalczykowski, 1997), and its presence induces the conversion of the RecBCD enzyme from a helicase to an exonuclease, producing ssDNA that can invade homologous dsDNA during recombination (Taylor et al., 1985). The RecA enzyme of *E. coli* is loaded onto unwound ssDNA by RecBCD and promotes ssDNA exchange/recombination with homologous dsDNA (Cox, 1999; Smith, 2012). RecA has significant homology to eukaryotic Rad51 and its paralogs (Suwaki et al., 2011), enzymes that repair dsDNA breaks in human cells, facilitate homologous recombination, and during adenovirus infection, bind to the E2 DNA binding protein (Tookman et al., 2016). In our study of the region just $5'$ to HVL2 on the penton base gene, a recombination hot-spot for HAdV-D (Robinson et al., 2009a), we found Chi-like sequences (Chi_{AD}), e.g., $5'$-ACTTCTGA-$3'$ in the proteotype containing HAdV-D64, and $5'$-TCTCCTGA-$3'$ in the proteotype including HAdV-D37 (Lee et al., 2018). The putative Chi_{AD} sequences we identified in HAdV-D were found within the GC-rich component of GC/AT transition zones that precede and include HVL2, and were conserved within each proteotype. *In vitro*, *E. coli* lysates containing RecA protein increased recombination of two HAdV-D genotypes with the same penton base HVL2 proteotype. RecA was shown by ChIP to bind specifically to Chi_{AD} nucleotide sequence in the same regions, and also colocalize with adenovirus DNA within infected cell nuclei. These data suggest that Chi-like nucleotide sequences adjacent to the junction of conserved and hypervariable gene segments in HAdV-D may be an important signal for homologous recombination, and provide evidence in support of the idea that local bacterial flora might enhance natural recombination through Chi-like nucleotide sequences at HAdV-D recombination hotspots.

Another explanation for homologous recombination between HAdV, not exclusive of a role for Chi_{AD}, is the potential for GC-low (AT-rich) single stranded DNA (ssDNA) to form hairpin loops (Nagy and Bujarski, 1997; Ohshima et al., 2007), a physical nonlinearity that would facilitate binding of ssDNA of one HAdV-D type to a homologous segment of ss or dsDNA from a physically adjacent but different HAdV-D type during co-infection of the same cell. Hairpin loops and other alterations in the physical configuration of ssDNA during DNA replication might also contribute to polymerase jumping (Jennings et al., 1983; Spaan et al., 1983; Pääbo et al., 1990; Viswanathan et al., 1999), in which physical constraints to polymerization lead to translocation of the DNA polymerase to an adjacent DNA from a different virus, resulting in a recombined DNA. Polymerase jumping has been shown to occur during HAdV DNA replication (King et al., 1997; de Jong et al., 2003), although it has not been suggested previously as a mechanism for HAdV-D evolution. Analysis of 38 HAdV-D whole genome sequences identified instances of 15 nucleotide-long GC-rich sequence adjacent to 15 nucleotide-long AT-rich sequence (sometimes with a 15 or 30 nucleotide-long GC-moderate sequence intervening), located just $5'$ and $3'$ to frequently recombined gene segments, and which were shown by *in silico* analysis of their corresponding ssDNA to form hairpin loops (Robinson et al., 2013a). Taken together, these data suggest covariant effects of nucleotide sequence and ssDNA secondary structures on homologous recombination between two HAdV-Ds.

TRANSCRIPTOME

Regions of the HAdV-D genome currently thought to be "noncoding," may contain functional elements. Because viruses exist on the nano-scale, viral genomes are by necessity constrained by size, and "junk" nucleotide sequences represent an extravagance. The National Human Genome Research Institute project to identify functional elements in the human genome

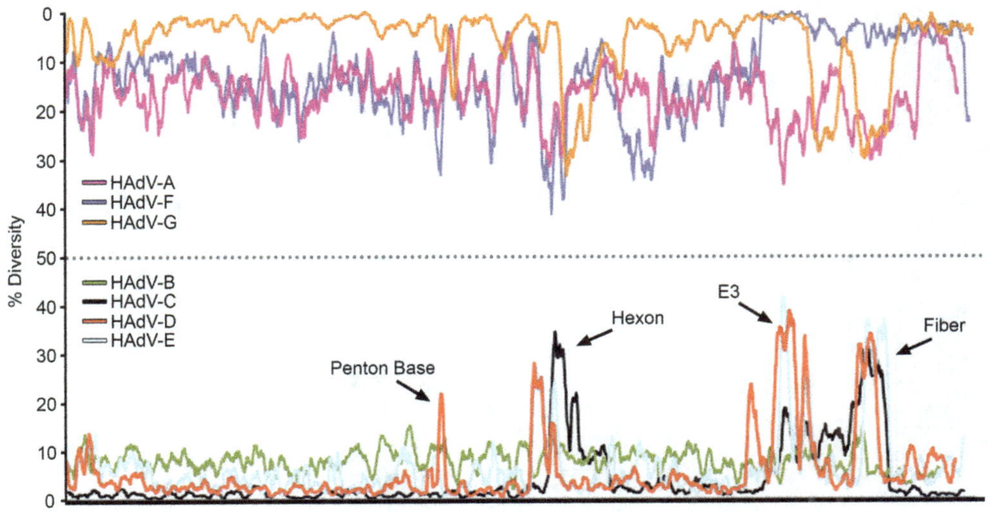

FIGURE 2 | Nucleotide diversity plots, by HAdV species, generated with DnaSP, represent the average number of nucleotide differences per site between each type in every HAdV species. The % diversity is calculated on the y-axis; the x-axis illustrates the nucleotide position on the genome. HAdV-Ds (red line on bottom half of plot) show particular diversity in the penton base, hexon, E3, and fiber coding regions, with otherwise very high conservation. From Robinson et al. (2013a) with permission.

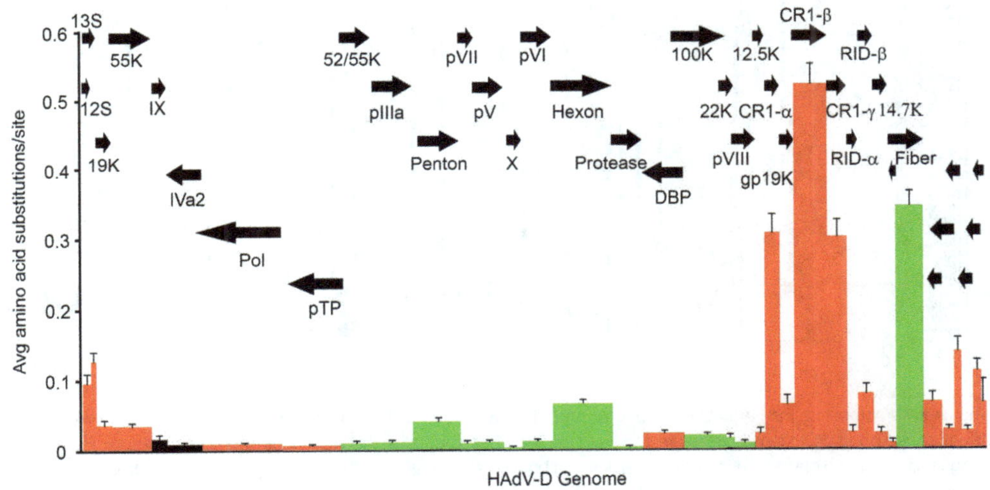

FIGURE 3 | Amino acid diversity calculated in MEGA 4.02, measuring the average amino acid substitution for each HAdV-D protein. Each bar in the graph corresponds to a protein as represented by arrows. Red = early genes. Dark green = late genes. Black = intermediate genes. The hypervariable loops of penton base and hexon proteins were also analyzed separately (light green) and showed particularly high levels of amino acid substitutions. From Robinson et al. (2013a) with permission.

(Encyclopedia of DNA Elements, or ENCODE) identified functionality in much of the human genome previously without known utility (Consortium et al., 2007; Qu and Fang, 2013; Kellis et al., 2014) The double-stranded DNA genomes of HAdV also contain regions with no known function. Transcriptional profiling of host gene expression has been studied after HAdV infection (Dorer et al., 2011) However, although viral transcriptomes have been reported for several viruses, most notably dengue, varicella zoster, and Epstein-Barr viruses (Ortmann et al., 2008; Ertl et al., 2011; Nagel et al., 2011, 2013; Arvey et al., 2013; Sujayanont et al., 2014), a *de novo* HAdV transcriptome has not been reported. Wu and coworkers used deep RNA sequencing to confirm known bat AdV transcripts (Wu et al., 2013), but did not investigate "noncoding" regions. *In silico* ORF prediction in HAdV can be difficult due to splice variants and inconsistencies in banked gene annotations (Davison et al., 2003), but in a prior annotation of HAdV-D37, ~60 new additional ORFs were predicted using in combination, the NCBI ORF finder, TIGR annotation engine, and GeneMark Heuristic model (Robinson et al., 2008) Putative genes were found within the large regions of noncoding DNA on the complementary strand opposite to established HAdV genes

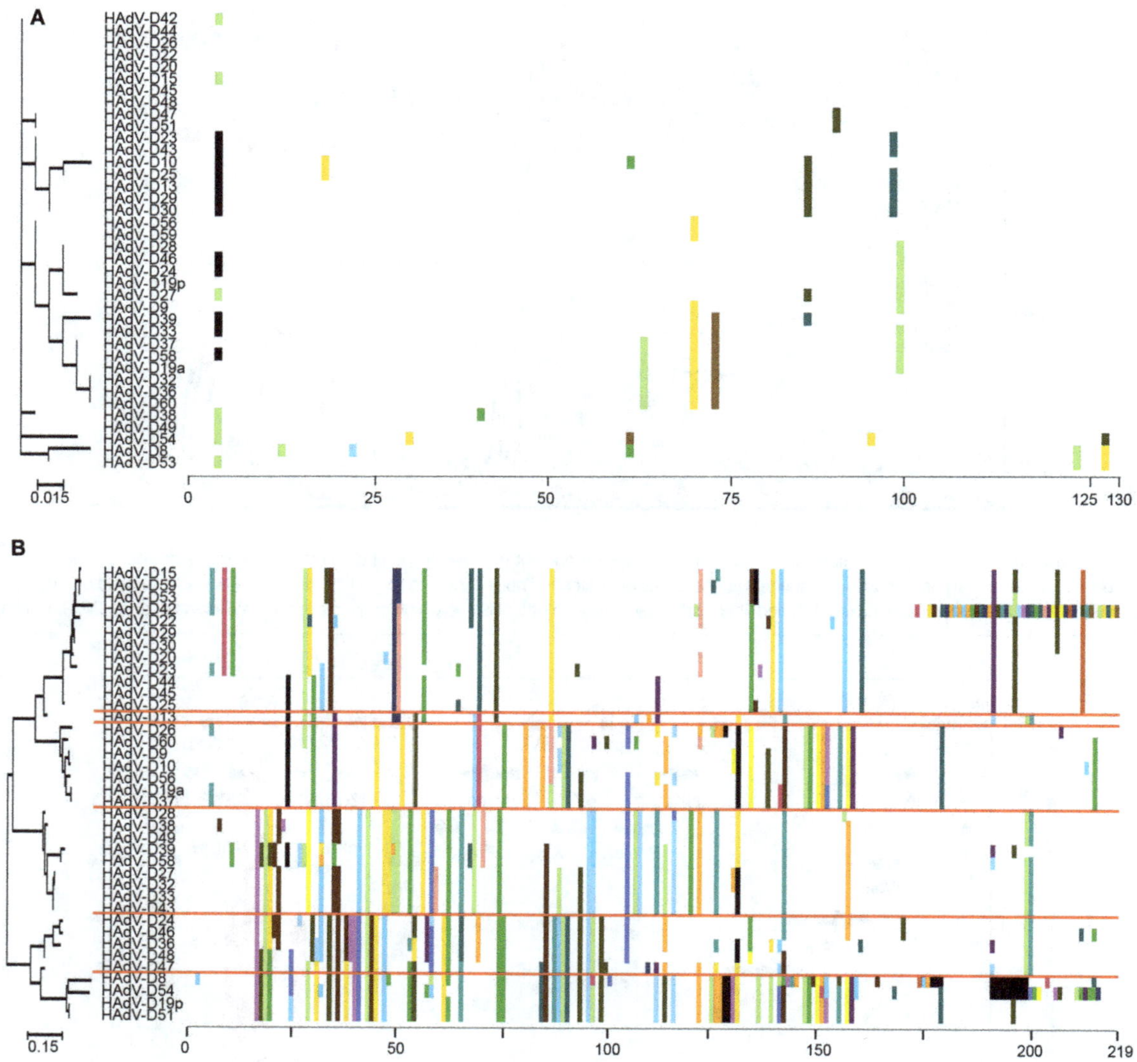

FIGURE 4 | Proteotyping analysis comparing the HAdV-D E3 14.7K **(A)** and CR1α **(B)** proteins. The 14.7K protein was conserved, while CR1α demonstrated 6 unique proteotypes. Maximum likelihood phylogenetic trees are shown to the left for each putative protein, and amino acid signatures to the right. The scale bar at the bottom left of each sub-figure denotes the phylogenetic distance reflected in horizontal dimension of the respective tree. To construct the amino acid signatures shown, each amino acid was assigned a unique color (upper right corner), consensus amino acids at each position across all 38 viruses were assigned white, and gaps in the alignment were colored black. Horizontal red lines delineate distinct proteotypes. Adapted from. Singh et al. (2013) with permission.

(**Figure 6**), in smaller regions on the coding strand within established transcription units but between confirmed genes, and overlapping or completely within established genes. Work is in progress in our laboratories to identify putative new genomic elements in HAdV by high-throughput sequencing of the viral transcriptome of HAdV-D37.

TRANSCRIPTION FACTOR BINDING SITES

HAdV uses host TFs nuclear factor I and III (NF-I and NF-III) as part of the viral DNA replication complex (Pruijn et al., 1988; Mul et al., 1990; Hatfield and Hearing, 1991, 1993) Simian AdVs typically lack the NF-I binding site, while human viruses express it. It was previously reported that HAdV-E4, originally isolated in 1952, is a product of recombination between HAdV-B16 and the simian AdV, SAdV-E26. Clinical strains of HAdV-E4 isolated recently contain a NF-I binding site in the inverted terminal repeat (Houng et al., 2006; Dehghan et al., 2013a,b) that is absent in the original isolate (Purkayastha et al., 2005), suggesting that NF-I binding may be important to viral fitness in humans. To further elucidate mechanisms of viral gene expression, we are exploring novel TF binding sites on HAdV-D DNA, using ENCODE validated methodologies (Gerstein et al., 2012; Landt et al., 2012).

PROTEIN INTERACTOMES

The major HAdV capsid structural proteins—hexon, penton base, and fiber—interact directly with extracellular mediators of host immunity (Gahéry-Ségard et al., 1998; Molinier-Frenkel

Types	Penton HVL1	Penton HVL2	Hexon	E3 CR1 α	E3 CR1 β	E3 CR1 γ	Fiber
HAdV-D56	1	8	1	3	6	6	1
HAdV-D29	6	6	1	1	1	6	5
HAdV-D15	14	10	1	1	1	1	22
HAdV-D51	10	5	2	6	10	5	17
HAdV-D19	4	5	3	6	6	8	3
HAdV-D64	6	1	3	3	4	10	3
HAdV-D25	2	6	4	1	1	1	4
HAdV-D59	8	1	4	1	6	6	1
HAdV-D9	1	8	5	3	6	6	1
HAdV-D32	11	4	5	4	14	2	13
HAdV-D54	2	9	6	6	6	5	1
HAdV-D42	14	1	7	1	1	1	22
HAdV-D20	7	10	8	1	3	5	14
HAdV-D60	14	10	8	3	10	8	20
HAdV-D10	1	8	9	3	5	7	2
HAdV-D28	9	10	10	4	9	14	9
HAdV-D27	12	3	11	4	9	3	6
HAdV-D26	1	8	12	3	8	11	8
HAdV-D45	13	1	13	1	14	2	7
HAdV-D47	2	7	14	5	8	11	15
HAdV-D36	9	6	15	5	13	8	19
HAdV-D38	14	2	16	4	14	2	18
HAdV-D24	12	3	17	5	5	12	12
HAdV-D46	3	6	18	5	5	12	12
HAdV-D49	5	4	19	4	14	2	10
HAdV-D43	6	6	20	4	11	13	9
HAdV-D39	7	8	20	4	12	15	18
HAdV-D33	9	5	21	4	11	13	13
HAdV-D58	1	4	22	4	1	6	5
HAdV-D13	6	10	23	2	11	15	18
HAdV-D30	14	5	23	1	14	6	10
HAdV-D37	14	10	23	3	4	10	3
HAdV-D23	4	5	24	1	7	9	16
HAdV-D22	14	1	25	1	2	10	21
HAdV-D53	14	10	25	1	1	1	1
HAdV-D8	1	4	26	6	6	5	1
HAdV-D44	11	4	27	1	12	4	11
HAdV-D48	4	3	28	5	12	4	11
Total proteotypes	14	10	28	6	14	15	22
Consensus nucleotide positions	14010-14075	14420-14650	18315-19320	26740-27470	27830-28990	29220-29910	31455-32660

FIGURE 5 | Proteotyping for 38 HAdV-Ds, sortec for the hexon proteotype column. Numbers and colors are arbitrary, and distinguish distinct proteotypes. Recombinants can be identified by rows. For example, HadV-D56, -D29, and -D15 fall within the same proteotype and are predicted to share highly similar nucleotide sequences for their respective hexon hypervariable regions (as confirmed by Singh et al., 2015). For HAdV-D29 and –D15, the recombination event extended through the E3 CR1β ORF gene and then ended.

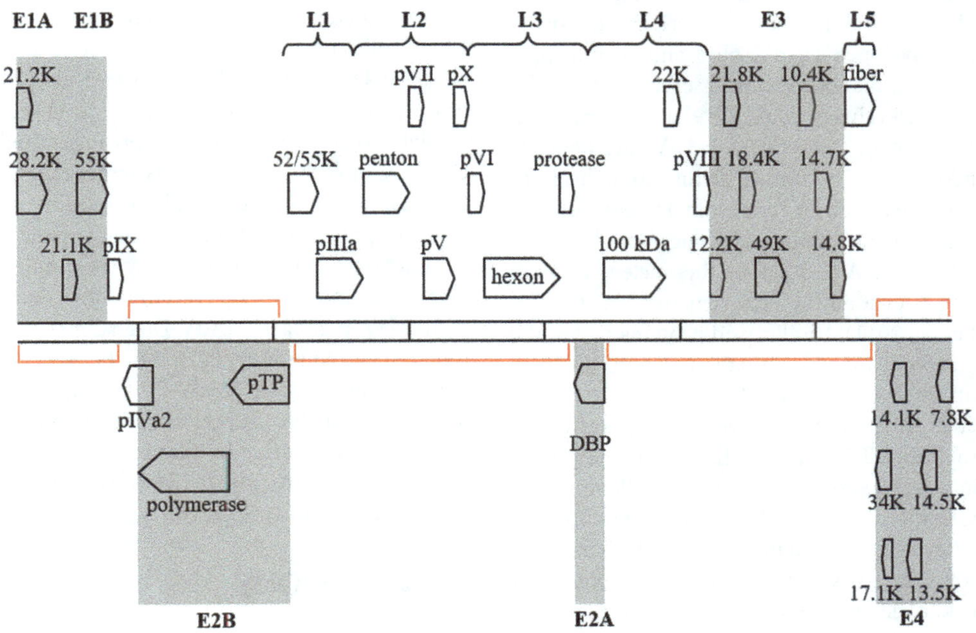

FIGURE 6 | Transcription map for HAdV-D37. Genes are divided by early (shaded) or late expression. Red brackets denote large areas of "noncoding" DNA, but many additional, smaller, potential coding regions exist between and within known genes. Adapted from Robinson et al. (2008) with permission.

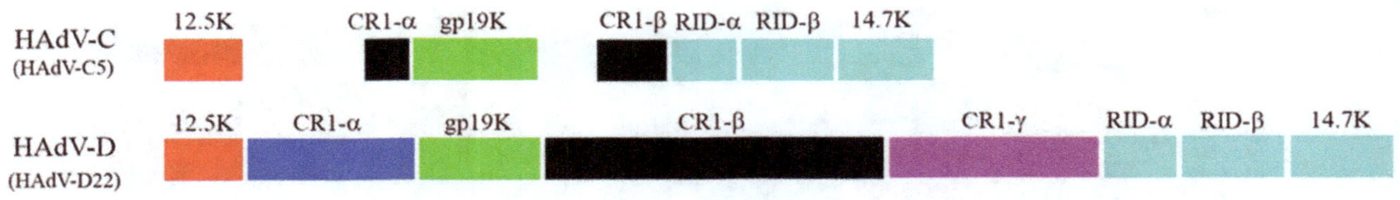

FIGURE 7 | Comparison of E3 transcription unit from HAdV-C and -D. Note in particular the difference in ORF size between CR1β of the two HAdV species. Adapted from Robinson et al. (2011c) with permission.

et al., 2002; Schoggins and Falck-Pedersen, 2006; Tamanini et al., 2006; Kalyuzhniy et al., 2008; Chintakuntlawar et al., 2010; Bradshaw et al., 2012; Flatt et al., 2013). The hexon, penton base, and fiber proteins also exhibit distinct amino acid signatures, characterizing discrete proteotypes (Robinson et al., 2013a). Gene products from the E3 transcription unit of HAdV function in viral immune evasion (Horwitz, 2004; Lichtenstein et al., 2004b; Windheim et al., 2004). In HAdV-D, the open reading frames for three of eight E3 genes—CR1α, CR1β, and CR1γ–are uniquely hypervariable compared to the other ORFs within the E3 transcription unit, and also segregate into discrete proteotypes (Singh et al., 2013). Highly conserved genes, such as DNA binding protein, DNA polymerase, and E3 14.7K, show no such variability (Robinson et al., 2013a; Singh et al., 2013).

While it may be assumed that hypervariablity in major capsid and E3 proteins is driven through evolutionary selection by the *extracellular* interactome, amino acid differences in a hypervariable protein can also lead to differences in that protein's *intracellular* interactome, the set of intrinsic host cell proteins which network with the viral protein, as was recently confirmed for E3 CR1 genes across HAdV species (Martinez-Martin et al., 2016). Viral capsid structural proteins are critical to virion stability. For the nonenveloped HAdV, fiber and penton base proteins on the external surface of the capsid serve as ligands for attachment to the host cell (Huang et al., 1999) and initiate viral entry (Wickham et al., 1993), respectively. HAdVs are typically internalized via endosomes. Endosomal acidification leads to structural instability of the capsid and endosomal release into the cytosol. HAdV capsid is then transported by microtubules to the nuclear membrane. Viral DNA then enters the nucleus through nuclear pores, leaving almost all the viral structural proteins in the cytosol (Henaff et al., 2011). Viral capsid proteins within the cell are eventually targeted for ubiquitination (Ko et al., 2010; Marvin and Wiethoff, 2012; Horan et al., 2013; Li et al., 2013) and degraded (Greber et al., 1993), but there are many opportunities for interaction with intracellular host cellular proteins during entry, trafficking, translation, assembly, and egress. Penton base HVL2, with its RGD motif, is critical to viral internalization through the interaction with host cell integrins,; (Wickham et al., 1993) but function of penton base HVL1 is unknown, and might be revealed though knowledge of its protein interactome. The closely adjacent hexon HVL1 and 2 form the epsilon epitope that determines serum neutralization, and interactions between the hexon protein and serum coagulation factor X confers liver tropism to HAdV-C5 (Sumarheni et al., 2014). However, nothing is known about potential hexon interactions with intracellular proteins during infection.

The E3 transcription unit of HAdV codes for proteins that mediate immune evasion by the virus (Horwitz, 2004). Although E3 is labeled as an early transcription region, its transcripts are expressed both early and late during viral infection (Chow et al., 1977; Chow and Broker, 1978; Bhat and Wold, 1986), and there is evidence for at least one E3 protein that late transcripts are translated (Robinson et al., 2011a). E3 gene products are not required for viral replication in cultured cells (Morin et al., 1987), but inhibit cellular and cytokine mediated host immune responses to infection (Horwitz, 2004; Lichtenstein et al., 2004b; Windheim et al., 2004). Almost all of what is known about the function of specific E3 proteins derives from studies on HAdV-C. For example, HAdV-C2 E3 CR1α directs another E3 protein (19K) to the endoplasmic reticulum of cytotoxic T cells (Wilson-Rawls et al., 1994), where 19K binds to and retains MHC class I proteins (Jefferies and Burgert, 1990), preventing presentation of viral peptides within MHC class I at the cell surface (Burgert and Kvist, 1985, 1987; Andersson et al., 1987; Burgert et al., 1987; Cox et al., 1991). CR1α, RIDα, and RIDβ proteins cooperate to evade TNFα-related apoptosis through TRAIL (Elsing and Burgert, 1998; Tollefson et al., 1998; Benedict et al., 2001; Lichtenstein et al., 2004a). CR1β (Wold et al., 1984), also called the adenovirus death protein (Tollefson et al., 1992), is required for cell lysis (Tollefson et al., 1996) and viral spread (Doronin et al., 2003). The ORF size of each E3 gene varies across HAdV species (**Figure 7**) (Robinson et al., 2011c). Similarly, immune evasion functions of E3 gene products may not be the same across HAdV species, or function similarly in all cell types (Routes and Cook, 1990). Windheim and coworkers recently showed that the CR1β protein of the eye pathogen HAdV-D64 suppresses natural killer cell function (Windheim et al., 2013). The E3 CR1 genes are uniquely hypervariable within HAdV-D, and as predicted, overlapping but distinguishable intracellular interactomes across proteotypes were recently reported by Martinez-Martin and colleagues, who used protein microarrays to identify novel CR1β binding partners (Martinez-Martin et al., 2016).

CONCLUSIONS

HAdV was critical to the dual discoveries of viral oncogenesis and RNA splicing (Berget et al., 1977; Chow et al., 1977; Whyte et al., 1988). HAdV is also a significant agent of disease for which there is no approved treatment. Recent mining of HAdV genomes has been highly productive, and there is ample evidence to suggest that further whole genome analyses will elucidate new and fundamental mechanisms in HAdV biology. In the last decade, of 27 newly identified HAdVs, 19 were HAdV-Ds, suggesting the continuing evolution of new pathogens from species D. Analyses of 38 fully sequenced HAdV-D whole genomes identified homologous recombination of specific regions within the hexon, penton base, fiber, and E3 CR1 genes as the *major* mechanism behind HAdV-D evolution, a new finding (Robinson et al., 2013a; Singh et al., 2013). Stereotypical reductions in GC content at the junction of conserved and hypervariable regions, along with Chi-like sequence motifs (also a new finding), appear likely to augment the intrinsic tendency of HAdV to undergo homologous recombination *in vivo* (Lee et al., 2018).

Recently, the whole genome sequences of 85 HAdVs from archives and current collections were determined, including both historical and circulating strains, respectively (Ismail et al., 2018). Of these, 3 novel recombinants within HAdV-B and 15 within HAdV-D were identified. Only two of the 15 HAdV-Ds were found to contain novel genes (penton base and fiber); these were subsequently typed as HAdV-D71 and 72. Isolates of HAdV-D53 and HAdV-D58, two novel genotypes recently recognized, were also identified, adding confidence in their clinical importance. Fully genotyped HAdVs now number 90, with more awaiting type numbers, and the scientific community has a 10-fold larger database of unique HAdV genomes than available only 15 years ago. Published and validated ENCODE methodologies can now be applied, and comparisons made across disparate HAdV genomes. We suggest that the HAdV genome contains previously uncharacterized functional elements, and that every HAdV protein has pleiotropic interactions. Current technologies should afford a wave of new and important discoveries that may lead to needed therapies against adenoviral diseases.

AUTHOR CONTRIBUTIONS

All authors listed have made a substantial, direct and intellectual contribution to the work, and approved it for publication.

REFERENCES

Akusjärvi, G., and Pettersson, U. (1978). Nucleotide sequence at the junction between the coding region of the adenovirus 2 hexon messenger RNA and its leader sequence. *Proc. Natl. Acad. Sci. U.S.A.* 75, 5822–5826. doi: 10.1073/pnas.75.12.5822

Akusjärvi, G., and Pettersson, U. (1979). Sequence analysis of adenovirus DNA: complete nucleotide sequence of the spliced 5' noncoding region of adenovirus 2 hexon messenger RNA. *Cell* 16, 841–850. doi: 10.1016/0092-8674(79)90099-0

Alkhalaf, M. A., Guiver, M., and Cooper, R. J. (2015). Genome stability of adenovirus types 3 and 7 during a simultaneous outbreak in Greater Manchester, UK. *J. Med. Virol.* 87, 117–124. doi: 10.1002/jmv.23969

Andersson, M., McMichael, A., and Peterson, P. A. (1987). Reduced allorecognition of adenovirus-2 infected cells. *J. Immunol.* 138, 3960–3966.

Arnold, J., Jánoska, M., Kajon, A. E., Metzgar, D., Hudson, N. R., Torres, S., et al. (2010). Genomic characterization of human adenovirus 36, a putative obesity agent. *Virus. Res.* 149, 152–161. doi: 10.1016/j.virusres.2010.01.011

Arvey, A., Tempera, I., and Lieberman, P. M. (2013). Interpreting the Epstein-Barr Virus (EBV) epigenome using high-throughput data. *Viruses* 5, 1042–1054. doi: 10.3390/v5041042

Assadian, F., Sandström, K., Bondeson, K., Laurell, G., Lidian, A., Svensson, C., et al. (2016). Distribution and molecular characterization of human adenovirus and epstein-barr virus infections in tonsillar lymphocytes isolated from patients diagnosed with tonsillar diseases. *PLoS ONE* 11:e0154814. doi: 10.1371/journal.pone.0154814

Avgousti, D. C., Della Fera, A. N., Otter, C. J., Herrmann, C., Pancholi, N. J., and Weitzman, M. D. (2017). Adenovirus core protein VII down-regulates the DNA damage response on the host genome. *J Virol.* 91:e01089-17. doi: 10.1128/JVI.01089-17

Benedict, C. A., Norris, P. S., Prigozy, T. I., Bodmer, J. L., Mahr, J. A., Garnett, C. T., et al. (2001). Three adenovirus E3 proteins cooperate to evade apoptosis by tumor necrosis factor-related apoptosis-inducing ligand receptor-1 and−2. *J. Biol. Chem.* 276, 3270–3278. doi: 10.1074/jbc.M008218200

Berget, S. M., Moore, C., and Sharp, P. A. (1977). Spliced segments at the 5' terminus of adenovirus 2 late mRNA. *Proc. Natl. Acad. Sci. U. S. A.* 74, 3171–3175. doi: 10.1073/pnas.74.8.3171

Bhanthumkosol, D. (1998). Fatal adenovirus infections in infants probably infected with HIV. *J. Med. Assoc. Thai.* 81, 214–222.

Bhat, B. M., and Wold, W. S. (1986). Genetic analysis of mRNA synthesis in adenovirus region E3 at different stages of productive infection by RNA-processing mutants. *J. Virol.* 60, 54–63.

Bianco, P. R., and Kowalczykowski, S. C. (1997). The recombination hotspot Chi is recognized by the translocating RecBCD enzyme as the single strand of DNA containing the sequence 5'-GCTGGTGG-3'. *Proc. Natl. Acad. Sci. U. S. A.* 94, 6706–6711. doi: 10.1073/pnas.94.13.6706

Bradshaw, A. C., Coughlan, L., Miller, A. M., Alba, R., van Rooijen, N., Nicklin, S. A., et al. (2012). Biodistribution and inflammatory profiles of novel penton and hexon double-mutant serotype 5 adenoviruses. *J Control Release* 164, 394–402. doi: 10.1016/j.jconrel.2012.05.025

Burgert, H. G., and Kvist, S. (1985). An adenovirus type 2 glycoprotein blocks cell surface expression of human histocompatibility class I antigens. *Cell* 41, 987–997. doi: 10.1016/S0092-8674(85)80079-9

Burgert, H. G., and Kvist, S. (1987). The E3/19K protein of adenovirus type 2 binds to the domains of histocompatibility antigens required for CTL recognition. *EMBO J.* 6, 2019–2026.

Burgert, H. G., Maryanski, J. L., and Kvist, S. (1987). "E3/19K" protein of adenovirus type 2 inhibits lysis of cytolytic T lymphocytes by blocking cell-surface expression of histocompatibility class I antigens. *Proc. Natl. Acad. Sci. U.S.A.* 84, 1356–1360. doi: 10.1073/pnas.84.5.1356

Butt, A. L., and Chodosh, J. (2006). Adenoviral keratoconjunctivitis in a tertiary care eye clinic. *Cornea* 25, 199–202. doi: 10.1097/01.ico.0000170693.13326.fb

Chintakuntlawar, A. V., Zhou, X., Rajaiya, J., and Chodosh, J. (2010). Viral capsid is a pathogen-associated molecular pattern in adenovirus keratitis. *PLoS Pathog.* 6:e1000841. doi: 10.1371/journal.ppat.1000841

Chow, L. T., and Broker, T. R. (1978). The spliced structures of adenovirus 2 fiber message and the other late mRNAs. *Cell* 15, 497–510. doi: 10.1016/0092-8674(78)90019-3

Chow, L. T., Gelinas, R. E., Broker, T. R., and Roberts, R. J. (1977). An amazing sequence arrangement at the 5' ends of adenovirus 2 messenger RNA. *Cell* 12, 1–8. doi: 10.1016/0092-8674(77)90180-5

Consortium, E. P., Birney, E., Stamatoyannopoulos, J. A., Dutta, A., Guig,ó, R., Gingeras, T. R., et al. (2007). Identification and analysis of functional elements in 1% of the human genome by the ENCODE pilot project. *Nature* 447, 799–816. doi: 10.1038/nature05874

Cox, J. H., Bennink, J. R., and Yewdell, J. W. (1991). Retention of adenovirus E19 glycoprotein in the endoplasmic reticulum is essential to its ability to block antigen presentation. *J. Exp. Med.* 174, 1629–1637. doi: 10.1084/jem.174.6.1629

Cox, M. M. (1999). Recombinational DNA repair in bacteria and the RecA protein. *Prog. Nucleic Acid Res. Mol. Biol.* 63, 311–366. doi: 10.1016/S0079-6603(08)60726-6

Crawford-Miksza, L. K., and Schnurr, D. P. (1996). Adenovirus serotype evolution is driven by illegitimate recombination in the hypervariable regions of the hexon protein. *Virology* 224, 357–367. doi: 10.1006/viro.1996.0543

Davison, A. J., Benko, M., and Harrach, B. (2003). Genetic content and evolution of adenoviruses. *J. Gen. Virol.* 84, 2895–2908. doi: 10.1099/vir.0.19497-0

de Jong, R. N., van der Vliet, P. C., and Brenkman, A. B. (2003). Adenovirus DNA replication: protein priming, jumping back and the role of the DNA binding protein DBP. *Curr. Top. Microbiol. Immunol.* 272, 187–211. doi: 10.1007/978-3-662-05597-7_7

Dehghan, S., Seto, J., Hudson, N. R., Robinson, C. M., Jones, M. S., Dyer, D. W., et al. (2011). Complete genome sequence of human adenovirus prototype 17. *J. Virol.* 85, 11540–11541. doi: 10.1128/JVI.06051-11

Dehghan, S., Seto, J., Jones, M. S., Dyer, D. W., Chodosh, J., and Seto, D. (2013a). Simian adenovirus type 35 has a recombinant genome comprising human and simian adenovirus sequences, which predicts its potential emergence as a human respiratory pathogen. *Virology* 447, 265–273. doi: 10.1016/j.virol.2013.09.009

Dehghan, S., Seto, J., Liu, E. B., Walsh, M. P., Dyer, D. W., Chodosh, J., et al. (2013b). Computational analysis of four human adenovirus type 4 genomes reveals molecular evolution through two interspecies recombination events. *Virology* 443, 197–207. doi: 10.1016/j.virol.2013.05.014

Dolph, P. J., Racaniello, V., Villamarin, A., Palladino, F., and Schneider, R. J. (1988). The adenovirus tripartite leader may eliminate the requirement for cap-binding protein complex during translation initiation. *J. Virol.* 62, 2059–2066.

Dorer, D. E., Holtrup, F., Fellenberg, K., Kaufmann, J. K., Engelhardt, S., Hoheiselet, J. D., al. (2011). Replication and virus-induced transcriptome of HAdV-5 in normal host cells versus cancer cells–differences of relevance for adenoviral oncolysis. *PLoS ONE* 6, e27934. doi: 10.1371/journal.pone.0027934

Doronin, K., Toth, K., Kuppuswamy, M., Krajcsi, P., Tollefson, A. E., and Wold, W. S. (2003). Overexpression of the ADP (E3-11.6K) protein increases cell lysis and spread of adenovirus. *Virology* 305, 378–387. doi: 10.1006/viro.20 02.1772

Echavarria, M., Maldonado, D., Elbert, G., Videla, C., Rappaport, R., and Carballal, G. (2006). Use of PCR to demonstrate presence of adenovirus species B, C, or F as well as coinfection with two adenovirus species in children with flu-like symptoms. *J. Clin. Microbiol.* 44, 625–627. doi: 10.1128/JCM.44.2.625-627.2006

Elsing, A., and Burgert, H. G. (1998). The adenovirus E3/10.4K-14.5K proteins down-modulate the apoptosis receptor Fas/Apo-1 by inducing its internalization. *Proc. Natl. Acad. Sci. U.S.A.* 95, 10072–10077. doi: 10.1073/pnas.95.17.10072

Engelmann, I., Coiteux, V., Heim, A., Magro, L., Dewilde, A., Dulery, R., et al. (2016). Severe adenovirus pneumonia followed by bacterial septicaemia: relevance of co-infections in allogeneic hematopoietic stem cell transplantation. *Infect Disord Drug Targets* 16, 69–76. doi: 10.2174/1871526516666160407114623

Epstein, L. H., and Young, C. S. (1991). Adenovirus homologous recombination does not require expression of the immediate-early E1a gene. *J. Virol.* 65, 4475–4479.

Ertl, R., Birzele, F., Hildebrandt, T., and Klein, D. (2011). Viral transcriptome analysis of feline immunodeficiency virus infected cells using second generation sequencing technology. *Vet. Immunol. Immunopathol.* 143, 314–324. doi: 10.1016/j.vetimm.2011.06.010

Flatt, J. W., Kim, R., Smith, J. G., Nemerow, G. R., and Stewart, P. L. (2013). An intrinsically disordered region of the adenovirus capsid is implicated in neutralization by human alpha defensin 5. *PLoS ONE* 8:e61571. doi: 10.1371/journal.pone.0061571

Gahéry-Ségard, H., Farace, F., Godfrin, D., Gaston, J., Lengagne, R., Tursz, T., et al. (1998). Immune response to recombinant capsid proteins of adenovirus in humans: antifiber and anti-penton base antibodies have a synergistic effect on neutralizing activity. *J. Virol.* 72, 2388–2397.

Garnett, C. T., Erdman,D., Xu, W., Gooding, L. R. (2002). Prevalence and quantitation of species C adenovirus DNA in human mucosal lymphocytes. *J. Virol.* 76, 10608–16. doi: 10.1128/JVI.76.21.10608-10616.2002

Garnett, C. T., Talekar, G., Mahr, J. A., Huang, W., Zhang, Y., Ornelles, D. A., et al. (2009). Latent species C adenoviruses in human tonsil tissues. *J. Virol.* 83, 2417–2428. doi: 10.1128/JVI.02392-08

Gerstein, M. B., Kundaje, A., Hariharan, M., Landt, S. G., Yan, K. K., Cheng, C., et al. (2012). Architecture of the human regulatory network derived from ENCODE data. *Nature* 489, 91–100. doi: 10.1038/nature11245

Gonzalez, G., Koyanagi, K. O., Aoki, K., Kitaichi, N., Ohno, S., Kaneko, H., et al. (2014). Intertypic modular exchanges of genomic segments by homologous recombination at universally conserved segments in human adenovirus species D. *Gene* 547, 10–17. doi: 10.1016/j.gene.2014.04.018

Goosney, D. L., and Nemerow, G. R. (2003). Adenovirus infection: taking the back roads to viral entry. *Curr. Biol.* 13, R99–R100. doi: 10.1016/S0960-9822(03)00037-X

Greber, U. F., Willetts, M., Webster, P., and Helenius, A. (1993). Stepwise dismantling of adenovirus 2 during entry into cells. *Cell* 75, 477–486. doi: 10.1016/0092-8674(93)90382-Z

Gruss, A., Moretto, V., Ehrlich, S. D., Duwat, P., and Dabert, P. (1991). GC-rich DNA sequences block homologous recombination *in vitro*. *J. Biol. Chem.* 266, 6667–6669.

Halstead, D. C., Gray, G. C., Meyer, K. S., Stanciu, S. R., and Gorospe, W. C. (2010). Recombinant adenovirus (AdV) Type 3 and Type 14 isolated from a fatal case of pneumonia. *Rev. Med. Microbiol.* 21, 28–30. doi: 10.1097/MRM.0b013e3283393523

Hatfield, L., and Hearing, P. (1991). Redundant elements in the adenovirus type 5 inverted terminal repeat promote bidirectional transcription *in vitro* and are important for virus growth *in vivo*. *Virology* 184, 265–276. doi: 10.1016/0042-6822(91)90843-Z

Hatfield, L., and Hearing, P. (1993). The NFIII/OCT-1 binding site stimulates adenovirus DNA replication *in vivo* and is functionally redundant with adjacent sequences. *J. Virol.* 67, 3931–3939.

Henaff, D., Salinas, S., and Kremer, E. J. (2011). An adenovirus traffic update: from receptor engagement to the nuclear pore. *Future Microbiol.* 6, 179–192. doi: 10.2217/fmb.10.162

Hofmayer, S., Madisch, I., Darr, S., Rehren, F., and Heim, A. (2009). Unique sequence features of the human adenovirus 31 complete genomic sequence are conserved in clinical isolates. *BMC Genom.* 10:557. doi: 10.1186/1471-2164-10-557

Horan, K. A., Hansen, K., Jakobsen, M. R., Holm, C. K., Søby, S., Unterholzner, L., et al. (2013). Proteasomal degradation of herpes simplex virus capsids in macrophages releases DNA to the cytosol for recognition by DNA sensors. *J. Immunol.* 190, 2311–2319. doi: 10.4049/jimmunol.12 02749

Horwitz, M. S. (1996). "Adenoviruses," in *Fields Virology*, eds B. N. Fields, D. M. Knipe, P. M. Howley (Philadelphia, PA: Lippincott-Raven), 2149–2171

Horwitz, M. S. (2004). Function of adenovirus E3 proteins and their interactions with immunoregulatory cell proteins. *J. Gene. Med.* 6 (Suppl 1), S172–S183. doi: 10.1002/jgm.495

Houng, H. S., Clavio, S., Graham, K., Kuschner, R., Sun, W., Russell, K. L., et al. (2006). Emergence of a new human adenovirus type 4 (Ad4) genotype: identification of a novel inverted terminal repeated (ITR) sequence from majority of Ad4 isolates from US military recruits. *J. Clin. Virol.* 35, 381–387. doi: 10.1016/j.jcv.2005.11.008

Huang, S., Reddy, V., Dasgupta, N., and Nemerow, G. R. (1999). A single amino acid in the adenovirus type 37 fiber confers binding to human conjunctival cells. *J. Virol.* 73, 2798–2802.

Ismail, A. M., Cui, T., Dommaraju, K., Singh, G., Dehghan, S., Seto, J., et al. (2018). Genomic analysis of a large set of currently-and historically-important human adenovirus pathogens. *Emerg. Microbes Infect.* 7:10. doi: 10.1038/s41426-017-0004-y

Ismail, A. M., Lee, J. S., Dyer, D. W., Seto, D., Rajaiya, J., and Chodosh, J. (2016). Selection pressure in the human adenovirus fiber knob drives cell specificity in epidemic keratoconjunctivitis. *J. Virol.* 90, 9598–9607. doi: 10.1128/JVI.01010-16

Jefferies, W. A., and Burgert, H. G. (1990). E3/19K from adenovirus 2 is an immunosubversive protein that binds to a structural motif regulating the intracellular transport of major histocompatibility complex class I proteins. *J. Exp. Med.* 172, 1653–1664. doi: 10.1084/jem.172.6.1653

Jennings, P. A., Finch, J. T., Winter, G., and Robertson, J. S. (1983). Does the higher order structure of the influenza virus ribonucleoprotein guide sequence rearrangements in influenza viral RNA? *Cell* 34, 619–627. doi: 10.1016/0092-8674(83)90394-X

Jones, M. S., Harrach, B., Ganac, R. D., Gozum, M. M., Dela Cruz, W. P., Riedel, B., et al. (2007). New adenovirus species found in a patient presenting with gastroenteritis. *J. Virol.* 81, 5978–5984. doi: 10.1128/JVI.02650-06

Kalyuzhniy, O., Di Paolo, N. C., Silvestry, M., Hofherr, S. E., Barry, M. A., Stewart, P. L., et al. (2008). Adenovirus serotype 5 hexon is critical for virus infection of hepatocytes *in vivo*. *Proc. Natl. Acad. Sci. U.S.A.* 105, 5483–5488. doi: 10.1073/pnas.0711757105

Karen, K. A., and Hearing, P. (2011). Adenovirus core protein VII protects the viral genome from a DNA damage response at early times after infection. *J. Virol.* 85, 4135–4142. doi: 10.1128/JVI.02540-10

Kaye, S. B., Lloyd, M., Williams, H., Yuen, C., Scott, J. A., O'Donnell, N., et al. (2005). Evidence for persistence of adenovirus in the tear film a decade following conjunctivitis. *J. Med. Virol.* 77, 227–231. doi: 10.1002/jmv.20440

Kellis, M., Wold B., Snyder, M. P., Bernstein, B. E., Kundaje, A., Marinov, G. K., et al. (2014). Defining functional DNA elements in the human genome. *Proc. Natl. Acad. Sci. U.S.A.* 111, 6131–6138. doi: 10.1073/pnas.1318948111

King, A. J., Teertstra, W. R., and van der Vliet, P. C. (1997). Dissociation of the protein primer and DNA polymerase after initiation of adenovirus DNA replication. *J. Biol. Chem.* 272, 24617–24623. doi: 10.1074/jbc.272.39.24617

Ko, A., Lee, E. W., Yeh, J. Y., Yang, M. R., Oh, W., Moon, J. S., et al. (2010). MKRN1 induces degradation of West Nile virus capsid protein by functioning as an E3 ligase. *J. Virol* 84, 426–436. doi: 10.1128/JVI.00725-09

Landt, S. G., Marinov, G. K., Kundaje, A., Kheradpour, P., Pauli, F., Batzoglou, S., et al. (2012). ChIP-seq guidelines and practices of the ENCODE and modENCODE consortia. *Genome Res.* 22, 1813–1831. doi: 10.1101/gr.136184.111

Lee, J. A., Kim, N. H., Kim, S. J., Choi, E. H., and Lee, H. J. (2005). Rapid identification of human adenovirus types 3 and 7 from respiratory specimens via multiplex type-specific PCR. *J. Clin. Microbiol.* 43, 5509–5514. doi: 10.1128/JCM.43.11.5509-5514.2005

Lee, J. Y., Lee, J. S., Materne, E. C., Rajala, R., Ismail, A. M., Seto, D et al. (2018). Bacterial RecA protein promotes adenoviral recombination during *in vitro* infection. *mSphere* 3:e00105-18. doi: 10.1128/mSphere.00105-18

Li, C., He, Y., Nicolson, S., Hirsch, M., Weinberg, M. S., Zhang, P., et al. (2013). Adeno-associated virus capsid antigen presentation is dependent on endosomal escape. *J. Clin Invest.* 123, 1390–1401. doi: 10.1172/JCI66611

Li, E., Stupack, D., Bokoch, G. M., and Nemerow, G. R. (1998a). Adenovirus endocytosis requires actin cytoskeleton reorganization mediated by Rho family GTPases. *J. Virol.* 72, 8806–8812.

Li, E., Stupack, D., Klemke, R., Cheresh, D. A., and Nemerow, G. R. (1998b). Adenovirus endocytosis via alpha(v) integrins requires phosphoinositide-3-OH kinase. *J. Virol.* 72, 2055–2061.

Li, E., Stupack, D. G., Brown, S. L., Klemke, R., Schlaepfer, D. D., and Nemerow, G. R. (2000). Association of p130CAS with phosphatidylinositol-3-OH kinase mediates adenovirus cell entry. *J. Biol. Chem.* 275, 14729–14735. doi: 10.1074/jbc.275.19.14729

Lichtenstein, D. L., Doronin, K., Toth, K., Kuppuswamy, M., Wold, W. S., and Tollefson, A. E. (2004a). Adenovirus E3-6.7K protein is required in conjunction with the E3-RID protein complex for the internalization and degradation of TRAIL receptor 2. *J. Virol.* 78, 12297–12307. doi: 10.1128/JVI.78.22.12297-12307.2004

Lichtenstein, D. L., Toth, K., Doronin, K., Tollefson, A. E., and Wold, W. S. (2004b). Functions and mechanisms of action of the adenovirus E3 proteins. *Int. Rev. Immunol.* 23, 75–111. doi: 10.1080/08830180490265556

Lischwe, M. A., and Sung, M. T. (1977). A histone-like protein from adenovirus chromatin. *Nature* 267, 552–554. doi: 10.1038/267552a0

Liu, E. B., Ferreyra, L., Fischer, S. L., Pavan, J. V., Nates, S. V., Hudson, N. R., et al. (2011). Genetic analysis of a novel human adenovirus with a serologically unique hexon and a recombinant fiber gene. *PLoS ONE* 6:e24491. doi: 10.1371/journal.pone.0024491

Logan, J., and Shenk, T. (1984). Adenovirus tripartite leader sequence enhances translation of mRNAs late after infection. *Proc. Natl. Acad. Sci. U.S.A.* 81, 3655–3659. doi: 10.1073/pnas.81.12.3655

Mahadevan, P., Seto, J., Tibbetts, C., and Seto, D. (2010). Natural variants of human adenovirus type 3 provide evidence for relative genome stability across time and geographic space. *Virology* 397, 113–118. doi: 10.1016/j.virol.2009.10.052

Martinez-Martin, N., Ramani, S. R., Hackney, J. A., Tom, I., Wranik, B. J., Chan, M., et al. (2016). The extracellular interactome of the human adenovirus family reveals diverse strategies for immunomodulation. *Nat. Commun.* 7:11473. doi: 10.1038/ncomms11473

Marvin, S. A., and Wiethoff, C. M. (2012). Emerging roles for ubiquitin in adenovirus cell entry. *Biol. Cell* 104, 188–198. doi: 10.1111/boc.201100096

McCarthy, T., Lebeck, M. G., Capuano, A. W., Schnurr, D. P., and Gray, G. C. (2009). Molecular typing of clinical adenovirus specimens by an algorithm which permits detection of adenovirus coinfections and intermediate adenovirus strains. *J. Clin. Virol.* 46, 80–84. doi: 10.1016/j.jcv.2009.06.008

Meinschad, C., and Winnacker, E. L. (1980). Recombination in adenovirus. I. Analysis of recombinant viruses under non-selective conditions. *J. Gen. Virol.* 48, 219–224. doi: 10.1099/0022-1317-48-1-219

Molinier-Frenkel, V., Lengagne, R., Gaden, F., Hong, S. S., Choppin, J., Gahery-Ségard, H., et al. (2002). Adenovirus hexon protein is a potent adjuvant for activation of a cellular immune response. *J. Virol.* 76, 127–135. doi: 10.1128/JVI.76.1.127-135.2002

Morin, J. E., Lubeck, M. D., Barton, J. E., Conley, A. J., Davis, A. R., and Hung, P. P. (1987). Recombinant adenovirus induces antibody response to hepatitis B virus surface antigen in hamsters. *Proc. Natl. Acad. Sci. U.S.A.* 84, 4626–4630. doi: 10.1073/pnas.84.13.4626

Moyer, C. L., Besser, E. S., and Nemerow, G. R. (2016). A single maturation cleavage site in adenovirus impacts cell entry and capsid assembly. *J. Virol.* 90, 521–532. doi: 10.1128/JVI.02014-15

Moyer, C. L., Wiethoff, C. M., Maier, O., Smith, J. G., and Nemerow, G. R. (2011). Functional genetic and biophysical analyses of membrane disruption by human adenovirus. *J. Virol.* 85, 2631–2641. doi: 10.1128/JVI.02321-10

Mul, Y. M., Verrijzer, C. P., and van der Vliet, P. C. (1990). Transcription factors NFI and NFIII/oct-1 function independently, employing different mechanisms to enhance adenovirus DNA replication. *J. Virol.* 64, 5510–5518.

Munz, P. L., Young, C., and Young, C. S. (1983). The genetic analysis of adenovirus recombination in triparental and superinfection crosses. *Virology* 126, 576–586. doi: 10.1016/S0042-6822(83)80014-2

Nagel, M. A., Choe, A., Gilden, D., Traina-Dorge, V., Cohrs, R. J., and Mahalingam, R. (2013). GeXPS multiplex PCR analysis of the simian varicella virus transcriptome in productively infected cells in culture and acutely infected ganglia. *J. Virol. Methods* 193, 151–158. doi: 10.1016/j.jviromet.2013.05.020

Nagel, M. A., Choe, A., Traktinskiy, I., Cordery-Cotter, R., Gilden, D., and Cohrs, R. J. (2011). Varicella-zoster virus transcriptome in latently infected human ganglia. *J. Virol.* 85, 2276–2287. doi: 10.1128/JVI.01862-10

Nagy, P. D., and Bujarski, J. J. (1997). Engineering of homologous recombination hotspots with AU-rich sequences in brome mosaic virus. *J. Virol.* 71, 3799–3810.

Nemerow, G. R. (2000). Cell receptors involved in adenovirus entry. *Virology* 274, 1–4. doi: 10.1006/viro.2000.0468

Nemerow, G. R., Pache, L., Reddy, V., and Stewart, P. L. (2009). Insights into adenovirus host cell interactions from structural studies. *Virology* 384, 380–388. doi: 10.1016/j.virol.2008.10.016

Neumann, R., Genersch, E., and Eggers, H. J. (1987). Detection of adenovirus nucleic acid sequences in human tonsils in the absence of infectious virus. *Virus Res.* 7, 93–97. doi: 10.1016/0168-1702(87)90060-8

Obenauer, J. C., Denson, J., Mehta, P. K., Su, X., Mukatira, S., Finkelstein, D. B., et al. (2006). Large-scale sequence analysis of avian influenza isolates. *Science* 311, 1576–1580. doi: 10.1126/science.1121586

Ohshima, K., Tomitaka, Y., Wood, J. T., Minematsu, Y., Kajiyama, H., Tomimura, K., et al. (2007). Patterns of recombination in turnip mosaic virus genomic sequences indicate hotspots of recombination. *J. Gen. Virol.* 88, 298–315. doi: 10.1099/vir.0.82335-0

Ortmann, A. C., Brumfield, S. K., Walther, J., McInnerney, K., Brouns, S. J., van de Werken, H. J., et al. (2008). Transcriptome analysis of infection of the archaeon Sulfolobus solfataricus with Sulfolobus turreted icosahedral virus. *J. Virol.* 82, 4874–4883. doi: 10.1128/JVI.02583-07

Pääbo, S., Irwin, D. M., and Wilson, A. C. (1990). DNA damage promotes jumping between templates during enzymatic amplification. *J. Biol. Chem.* 265, 4718–4721.

Pruijn, G. J., van Miltenburg, R. T., Claessens, J. A., and van der Vliet, P. C. (1988). Interaction between the octamer-binding protein nuclear factor III and the adenovirus origin of DNA replication. *J. Virol.* 62, 3092–3102.

Purkayastha, A., Su, J., McGraw, J., Ditty, S. E., Hadfield, T. L., Seto, J., et al. (2005). Genomic and bioinformatics analyses of HAdV-4vac and HAdV-7vac, two human adenovirus (HAdV) strains that constituted original prophylaxis against HAdV-related acute respiratory disease, a reemerging epidemic disease. *J. Clin. Microbiol.* 43, 3083–3094. doi: 10.1128/JCM.43.7.3083-3094.2005

Qu, H., and Fang, X. (2013). A brief review on the human encyclopedia of DNA elements (ENCODE) project. *Genomics Proteomics Bioinformatics* 11, 135–141. doi: 10.1016/j.gpb.2013.05.001

Ramke, M., Lee, J. Y., Dyer, D. W., Seto, D., Rajaiya, J., and Chodosh, J. (2017). The 5'UTR in human adenoviruses: leader diversity in late gene expression. *Sci. Rep.* 7:618. doi: 10.1038/s41598-017-00747-y

Robinson, C. M., Rajaiya, J., Walsh, M. P., Seto, D., Dyer, D. W., Jones, M. S., et al. (2009a). Computational analysis of human adenovirus type 22 provides evidence for recombination among species D human adenoviruses in the penton base gene. *J. Virol.* 83, 8980–8985. doi: 10.1128/JVI.00786-09

Robinson, C. M., Rajaiya, J., Zhou, X., Singh, G., Dyer, D. W., and Chodosh, J. (2011a). The E3 CR1-gamma gene in human adenoviruses associated with epidemic keratoconjunctivitis. *Virus Res.* 160, 120–127. doi: 10.1016/j.virusres.2011.05.022

Robinson, C. M., Seto, D., Jones, M. S., Dyer, D. W., and Chodosh, J. (2011c). Molecular evolution of human species D adenoviruses. *Infect. Genet. Evol.* 11, 1208–1217. doi: 10.1016/j.meegid.2011.04.031

Robinson, C. M., Shariati, F., Gillaspy, A. F., Dyer, D. W., and Chodosh, J. (2008). Genomic and bioinformatics analysis of human adenovirus type 37: new insights into corneal tropism. *BMC Genom.* 9:213. doi: 10.1186/1471-2164-9-213

Robinson, C. M., Shariati, F., Zaitshik, J., Gillaspy, A. F., Dyer, D. W., and Chodosh, J. (2009b). Human adenovirus type 19: genomic and bioinformatics analysis of a keratoconjunctivitis isolate. *Virus Res.* 139, 122–126. doi: 10.1016/j.virusres.2008.10.001

Robinson, C. M., Singh, G., Henquell, C., Walsh, M. P., Peigue-Lafeuille, H., Seto, D., et al. (2011b). Computational analysis and identification of an emergent human adenovirus pathogen implicated in a respiratory fatality. *Virology* 409, 141–147. doi: 10.1016/j.virol.2010.10.020

Robinson, C. M., Singh, G., Lee, J. Y., Dehghan, S., Rajaiya, J., Liu, E. B., et al. (2013a). Molecular evolution of human adenoviruses. *Sci. Rep.* 3:1812. doi: 10.1038/srep01812

Robinson, C. M., Zhou, X., Rajaiya, J., Yousuf, M. A., Singh, G., DeSerres, J. J., et al. (2013b). Predicting the next eye pathogen: analysis of a novel adenovirus. *MBio* 4, e00595–e00512. doi: 10.1128/mBio.00595-12

Routes, J. M., and Cook, J. L. (1990). Resistance of human cells to the adenovirus E3 effect on class I MHC antigen expression. Implications for antiviral immunity. *J. Immunol.* 144, 2763–2770.

Roy, S., Vandenberghe, L. H., Kryazhimskiy, S., Grant, R., Calcedo, R., Yuan, X., et al. (2009). Isolation and characterization of adenoviruses persistently shed from the gastrointestinal tract of non-human primates. *PLoS Pathog.* 5:e1000503. doi: 10.1371/journal.ppat.1000503

Ryu, J. S., Cho, J. H., Han, H. S., Jung, M. H., Yoon, Y. H., Song, E. S., et al. (2003). Acute respiratory distress syndrome induced by adenovirus in an otherwise healthy woman. *Yonsei Med. J.* 44, 732–735. doi: 10.3349/ymj.2003.44.4.732

Schoggins, J. W., and Falck-Pedersen, E. (2006). Fiber and penton base capsid modifications yield diminished adenovirus type 5 transduction and proinflammatory gene expression with retention of antigen-specific humoral immunity. *J. Virol.* 80, 10634–10644. doi: 10.1128/JVI.01359-06

Seto, D., Chodosh, J., Brister, J. R., Jones, M. S., and Members of the Adenovirus Research, C. (2011). Using the whole-genome sequence to characterize and name human adenoviruses. *J. Virol.* 85, 5701–5702. doi: 10.1128/JVI.00354-11

Seto, D., Jones, M. S., Dyer, D. W., and Chodosh, J. (2013). Characterizing, typing, and naming human adenovirus type 55 in the era of whole genome data. *J. Clin. Virol.* 58, 741–742. doi: 10.1016/j.jcv.2013.09.025

Seto, J., Walsh, M. P., Metzgar, D., and Seto, D. (2010). Computational analysis of adenovirus serotype 5 (HAdV-C5) from an HAdV coinfection shows genome stability after 45 years of circulation. *Virology* 404, 180–186. doi: 10.1016/j.virol.2010.05.010

Singh, G., Robinson, C. M., Dehghan, S., Jones, M. S., Dyer, D. W., Seto, D., et al. (2013). Homologous recombination in E3 genes of human adenovirus species D. *J. Virol.* 87, 12481–12488. doi: 10.1128/JVI.01927-13

Singh, G., Robinson, C. M., Dehghan, S., Schmidt, T., Seto, D., Jones, M. S., et al. (2012). Overreliance on the hexon gene, leading to misclassification of human adenoviruses. *J. Virol.* 86, 4693–4695. doi: 10.1128/JVI.06969-11

Singh, G., Zhou, X., Lee, J. Y., Yousuf, M. A., Ramke, M., et al. (2015). Recombination of the epsilon determinant and corneal tropism: human adenovirus species D types 15, 29, 56, and 69. *Virology* 485, 452–459. doi: 10.1016/j.virol.2015.08.018

Smith, G. R. (2012). How RecBCD enzyme and Chi promote DNA break repair and recombination: a molecular biologist's view. *Microbiol. Mol. Biol. Rev.* 76, 217–228. doi: 10.1128/MMBR.05026-11

Smith, G. R., Kunes, S. M., Schultz, D. W., Taylor, A., and Triman, K. L. (1981). Structure of chi hotspots of generalized recombination. *Cell* 24, 429–436. doi: 10.1016/0092-8674(81)90333-0

Spaan, W., Delius, H., Skinner, M., Armstrong, J., Rottier, P., Smeekens, S., et al. (1983). Coronavirus mRNA synthesis involves fusion of non-contiguous sequences. *EMBO J.* 2, 1839–1844.

Stahl, F. W. (1998). Recombination in phage lambda: one geneticist's historical perspective. *Gene* 223, 95–102. doi: 10.1016/S0378-1119(98)00246-7

Sujayanont, P., Chininmanu, K., Tassaneetrithep, B., Tangthawornchaikul, N., Malasit, P., and Suriyaphol, P. (2014). Comparison of phi29-based whole genome amplification and whole transcriptome amplification in dengue virus. *J. Virol. Methods* 195, 141–147. doi: 10.1016/j.jviromet.2013.10.005

Sumarheni, S., Hong, S. S., Josserand, V., Coll, J. L., Boulanger, P., Schoehn, G., et al. (2014). Human full-length coagulation factor X and a GLA domain-derived 40-mer polypeptide bind to different regions of the adenovirus serotype 5 hexon capsomer. *Hum. Gene. Ther.* 25, 339–349. doi: 10.1089/hum.2013.222

Suwaki, N., Klare, K., and Tarsounas, M. (2011). RAD51 paralogs: roles in DNA damage signalling, recombinational repair and tumorigenesis. *Semin. Cell Dev. Biol.* 22, 898–905. doi: 10.1016/j.semcdb.2011.07.019

Tamanini, A., Nicolis, E., Bonizzato, A., Bezzerri, V., Melotti, P., Assael, B. M., et al. (2006). Interaction of adenovirus type 5 fiber with the coxsackievirus and adenovirus receptor activates inflammatory response in human respiratory cells. *J. Virol.* 80, 11241–11254. doi: 10.1128/JVI.00721-06

Tan, D., Zhu, H., Fu, Y., Tong, F., Yao, D., Walline, J., et al. (2016). Severe community-acquired pneumonia caused by human adenovirus in immunocompetent adults: a multicenter case series. *PLoS ONE* 11:e0151199. doi: 10.1371/journal.pone.0151199

Taylor, A. F., Schultz, D. W., Ponticelli, A. S., and Smith, G. R. (1985). RecBC enzyme nicking at Chi sites during DNA unwinding: location and orientation-dependence of the cutting. *Cell* 41, 153–163. doi: 10.1016/0092-8674(85)90070-4

Tollefson, A. E., Hermiston, T. W., Lichtenstein, D. L., Colle, C. F., Tripp, R. A., Dimitrov, T., et al. (1998). Forced degradation of Fas inhibits apoptosis in adenovirus-infected cells. *Nature* 392, 726–730. doi: 10.1038/33712

Tollefson, A. E., Scaria, A., Hermiston, T. W., Ryerse, J. S., Wold, L. J., and Wold, W. S. (1996). The adenovirus death protein (E3-11.6K) is required at very late stages of infection for efficient cell lysis and release of adenovirus from infected cells. *J. Virol.* 70, 2296–2306.

Tollefson, A. E., Scaria, A., Saha, S. K., and Wold, W. S. (1992). The 11,600-MW protein encoded by region E3 of adenovirus is expressed early but is greatly amplified at late stages of infection. *J. Virol.* 66, 3633–3642.

Tookman, L. A., Browne, A. K., Connell, C. M., Bridge, G., Ingemarsdotter, C. K., Dowson, S., et al. (2016). RAD51 and BRCA2 enhance oncolytic adenovirus Type 5 activity in ovarian cancer. *Mol. Cancer Res.* 14, 44–55. doi: 10.1158/1541-7786.MCR-15-0188-T

Torres, S., Chodosh, J., Seto, D., and Jones, M. S. (2010). The revolution in viral genomics as exemplified by the bioinformatic analysis of human adenoviruses. *Viruses* 2, 1367–1381. doi: 10.3390/v2071367

Viswanathan, V. K., Krcmarik, K., and Cianciotto, N. P. (1999). Template secondary structure promotes polymerase jumping during PCR amplification. *Biotechniques* 27, 508–511. doi: 10.2144/99273st04

Vora, G. J., Lin, B., Gratwick, K., Meador, C., Hansen, C., Tibbetts, C., et al. (2006). Co-infections of adenovirus species in previously vaccinated patients. *Emerg. Infect. Dis.* 12, 921–930. doi: 10.3201/eid1206.050245

Wallot, M. A., Dohna-Schwake, C., Auth, M., Nadalin, S., Fiedler, M., Malagó, M., et al. (2006). Disseminated adenovirus infection with respiratory failure in pediatric liver transplant recipients: impact of intravenous cidofovir and inhaled nitric oxide. *Pediatr. Transplant.* 10, 121–127. doi: 10.1111/j.1399-3046.2005.00411.x

Walsh, M. P., Chintakuntlawar, A., Robinson, C. M., Madisch, I., Harrach, B., Hudson, N. R., et al. (2009). Evidence of molecular evolution driven by recombination events influencing tropism in a novel human adenovirus that causes epidemic keratoconjunctivitis. *PLoS ONE* 4:e5635. doi: 10.1371/journal.pone.0005635

Walsh, M. P., Seto, J., Jones, M. S., Chodosh, J., Xu, W., and Seto, D. (2010a). Computational analysis identifies human adenovirus type 55 as a re-emergent acute respiratory disease pathogen. *J. Clin. Microbiol.* 48, 991–993. doi: 10.1128/JCM.01694-09

Walsh, M. P., Seto, J., Liu, E. B., Dehghan, S., Hudson, N. R., Lukashev, A. N., et al. (2011). Computational analysis of two species C human adenoviruses provides evidence of a novel virus. *J. Clin. Microbiol.* 49, 3482–3490. doi: 10.1128/JCM.00156-11

Walsh, M. P., Seto, J., Tirado, D., Chodosh, J., Schnurr, D., Seto, D., et al. (2010b). Computational analysis of human adenovirus serotype 18. *Virology* 404, 284–292. doi: 10.1016/j.virol.2010.05.013

Whyte, P., Buchkovich, K. J., Horowitz, J. M., Friend, S. H., Raybuck, M., Weinberg, R. A., et al. (1988). Association between an oncogene and an anti-oncogene: the adenovirus E1A proteins bind to the retinoblastoma gene product. *Nature* 334, 124–129. doi: 10.1038/334124a0

Wickham, T. J., Mathias, P., Cheresh, D. A., and Nemerow, G. R. (1993). Integrins alpha v beta 3 and alpha v beta 5 promote adenovirus internalization but not virus attachment. *Cell* 73, 309–319. doi: 10.1016/0092-8674(93)90231-E

Wiethoff, C. M., Wodrich, H., Gerace, L., and Nemerow, G. R. (2005). Adenovirus protein VI mediates membrane disruption following capsid disassembly. *J. Virol.* 79, 1992–2000. doi: 10.1128/JVI.79.4.1992-2000.2005

Williams, J., Grodzicker, T., Sharp, P., and Sambrook, J. (1975). Adenovirus recombination: physical mapping of crossover events. *Cell* 4, 113–119. doi: 10.1016/0092-8674(75)90117-8

Wilson-Rawls, J., Deutscher, S. L., and Wold, W. S. (1994). The signal-anchor domain of adenovirus E3-6.7K, a type III integral membrane protein, can direct adenovirus E3-gp19K, a type I integral membrane protein, into the membrane of the endoplasmic reticulum. *Virology* 201, 66–76. doi: 10.1006/viro.1994.1266

Windheim, M., Hilgendorf, A., and Burgert, H. G. (2004). Immune evasion by adenovirus E3 proteins: exploitation of intracellular trafficking pathways. *Curr. Top. Microbiol. Immunol.* 273, 29–85. doi: 10.1007/978-3-662-05599-1_2

Windheim, M., Southcombe, J. H., Kremmer, E., Chaplin, L., Urlaub, D., Falk, C. S., et al. (2013). A unique secreted adenovirus E3 protein binds to the leukocyte common antigen CD45 and modulates leukocyte functions. *Proc. Natl. Acad. Sci. U.S.A.* 110, E4884–E4893. doi: 10.1073/pnas.1312420110

Wodrich, H., Guan, T., Cingolani, G., Von Seggern, D., Nemerow, G., and Gerace, L. (2003). Switch from capsid protein import to adenovirus assembly by cleavage of nuclear transport signals. *EMBO J.* 22, 6245–6255. doi: 10.1093/emboj/cdg614

Wold, W. S., Cladaras, C., Magie, S. C., and Yacoub, N. (1984). Mapping a new gene that encodes an 11,600-molecular-weight protein in the E3 transcription unit of adenovirus 2. *J. Virol.* 52:307–313.

Wu, L., Zhou, P., Ge, X., Wang, L. F., Baker, M. L., and Shi, Z. (2013). Deep RNA sequencing reveals complex transcriptional landscape of a bat adenovirus. *J. Virol.* 87, 503–511. doi: 10.1128/JVI.02332-12

Young, C. S., Cachianes, G., Munz, P., and Silverstein, S. (1984). Replication and recombination in adenovirus-infected cells are temporally and functionally related. *J. Virol.* 51, 571–577.

Zhang, S. Y., Luo, Y. P., Huang, D. D., Fan, H., Lu, Q. B., Wo, Y., et al. (2016). Fatal pneumonia cases caused by human adenovirus 55 in immunocompetent adults. *Infect Dis. (Lond).* 48, 40–47. doi: 10.3109/23744235.2015.1055585

Zhang, Y., Dolph, P. J., and Schneider, R. J. (1989). Secondary structure analysis of adenovirus tripartite leader. *J. Biol. Chem.* 264, 10679–10684.

Zhang, Y., Huang, W., Ornelles, D. A., and Gooding, L. R. (2010). Modeling adenovirus latency in human lymphocyte cell lines. *J. Virol.* 84, 8799–8810. doi: 10.1128/JVI.00562-10

Zhou, X., Robinson, C. M., Rajaiya, J., Dehghan, S., Seto, D., Jones, M. S., et al. (2012). Analysis of human adenovirus type 19 associated with epidemic keratoconjunctivitis and its reclassification as adenovirus type 64. *Invest. Ophthalmol. Vis. Sci.* 53, 2804–2811. doi: 10.1167/iovs.12-9656

Ziff, E. B., and Evans, R. M. (1978). Coincidence of the promoter and capped 5' terminus of RNA from the adenovirus 2 major late transcription unit. *Cell* 15, 1463–1475. doi: 10.1016/0092-8674(78)90070-3

18

Respiratory Viral Infections in Patients with Cancer or Undergoing Hematopoietic Cell Transplant

Diego R. Hijano[1], Gabriela Maron[1] and Randall T. Hayden[2]*

[1] Department of Infectious Diseases, St Jude Children's Research Hospital, Memphis, TN, United States, [2] Department of Pathology, St Jude Children's Research Hospital, Memphis, TN, United States

***Correspondence:**
Randall T. Hayden
Randall.Hayden@stjude.org

Survival rates for pediatric cancer have steadily improved over time but it remains a significant cause of morbidity and mortality among children. Infections are a major complication of cancer and its treatment. Community acquired respiratory viral infections (CRV) in these patients increase morbidity, mortality and can lead to delay in chemotherapy. These are the result of infections with a heterogeneous group of viruses including RNA viruses, such as respiratory syncytial virus (RSV), influenza virus (IV), parainfluenza virus (PIV), metapneumovirus (HMPV), rhinovirus (RhV), and coronavirus (CoV). These infections maintain a similar seasonal pattern to those of immunocompetent patients. Clinical manifestations vary significantly depending on the type of virus and the type and degree of immunosuppression, ranging from asymptomatic or mild disease to rapidly progressive fatal pneumonia Infections in this population are characterized by a high rate of progression from upper to lower respiratory tract infection and prolonged viral shedding. Use of corticosteroids and immunosuppressive therapy are risk factors for severe disease. The clinical course is often difficult to predict, and clinical signs are unreliable. Accurate prognostic viral and immune markers, which have become part of the standard of care for systemic viral infections, are currently lacking; and management of CRV infections remains controversial. Defining effective prophylactic and therapeutic strategies is challenging, especially considering, the spectrum of immunocompromised patients, the variety of respiratory viruses, and the presence of other opportunistic infections and medical problems. Prevention remains one of the most important strategies against these viruses. Early diagnosis, supportive care and antivirals at an early stage, when available and indicated, have proven beneficial. However, with the exception of neuraminidase inhibitors for influenza infection, there are no accepted treatments. In high-risk patients, pre-emptive treatment with antivirals for upper respiratory tract infection (URTI) to decrease progression to LRTI is a common strategy. In the future, viral load and immune markers may prove beneficial in predicting severe disease, supporting decision making and monitor treatment in this population.

Keywords: respiratory infection, virus, cancer, immunocompromised, hematopoietic cell transplant, RSV, influenza, child

INTRODUCTION

Respiratory viruses represent the most common infections in children (Tregoning and Schwarze, 2010; Meissner, 2016; Kou et al., 2018). In healthy children, they usually cause upper respiratory tract infections (URTI) with a benign, self-limited course (Tregoning and Schwarze, 2010; Meissner, 2016). However, immunocompromised hosts, particularly those undergoing transplant are particularly vulnerable to severe infections (Whimbey et al., 1996, 1997; Couch et al., 1997; Englund et al., 1999, 2011; Englund, 2001; Kim et al., 2007; Campbell et al., 2015). Furthermore, the spectrum of immunocompromised patients has expanded over the past decade owing to prolonged survival of those with various malignancies and to advances in hematopoietic cell transplantation (HCT) (Englund, 2001; Englund et al., 2011; Fisher et al., 2017). As diagnostic test improve and virus are detected more rapidly, the burden of these infections and their clinical outcomes have been progressively recognized (Englund et al., 1996, 1999; Englund, 2001). Although respiratory infections can be due to opportunistic infections, uncommon or atypical organisms, community respiratory virus are usually the cause of hospitalization in these patients (Englund et al., 1999, 2011; Fisher et al., 2017).

Respiratory viral infections include RNA viruses such as paramyxoviruses (RSV, parainfluenza, HMPV), orthomyxoviruses (influenza), picornaviruses (rhinovirus), and coronaviruses, as well as DNA viruses such as adenovirus, bocavirus, and polyomaviruses (Whimbey et al., 1996, 1997; Englund et al., 1999; Kim et al., 2007). These RNA viruses are among the most common causes of respiratory infection in immunocompromised patients (Whimbey et al., 1997; Hirsch et al., 2013) (**Table 1**). Although the annual activity of these viruses is variable, distinct patterns have been described. They cause seasonal outbreaks, and most are predominantly seen during the winter (Whimbey et al., 1996, 1997; Kim et al., 2007).

Clinical presentation can range from asymptomatic viral shedding to severe respiratory distress (Hakim et al., 2016b; Fisher et al., 2017). Severity of disease depends on intrinsic viral factors, as well on patient characteristics including underlying diagnosis and treatment, with myelosuppression and HCT bearing the highest morbidity and mortality (Kim et al., 2007; Hakim et al., 2016b; Fisher et al., 2017). Adverse outcomes are far more likely in immunocompromised patients than in non-immunocompromised individuals and include progression to pneumonia, respiratory failure, and increased mortality rates (Kim et al., 2014). In immunocompromised adults with cancer, progression to LRTI ranges from 30 to 50%, and for those who develop pneumonia, mortality can be as high as 75% (Hirsch et al., 2013; Renaud et al., 2013; Chemaly et al., 2014; Campbell et al., 2015; Hutspardol et al., 2015; Chu et al., 2016). Mortality associated with respiratory viruses in children undergoing HCT varies, usually ranging between 10 and 14% but can be as high as 30% (Ljungman et al., 2001; Luján-Zilbermann et al., 2001; Hutspardol et al., 2015). Although significantly lower than in adults, mortality remains considerably higher than that for the general population. Long term complications associated with respiratory viral infections, such as airflow obstruction and bronchiolitis obliterans, have developed in HCT and lung transplant recipients (Campbell et al., 2015; Chu et al., 2016).

A focus of interest has been to determine and assess risk factors for progression to LRTI with the goal to detect patients who might benefit from interventions that could prevent clinical progression. Age, lymphopenia, high-dose total body irradiation and presence of co-pathogens are significant risk factors for progression to LRTI (El Saleeby et al., 2008; Waghmare et al., 2013; Kim et al., 2014). Clinical scores have been developed for adults undergoing HCT and in healthy children with RSV infection to better predict severity (Shah et al., 2014; Caserta et al., 2017). However, the former has not been validated in children and the latter lacks important features surrounding this particular sub group of patients.

DIAGNOSTIC

Diagnostic testing for respiratory viruses has evolved tremendously in the past several years. This is equally true for HCT patients as it has been for immunocompetent patients, where the same testing modalities are utilized. Molecular amplification techniques have largely supplanted cell culture as the primary means of detecting and identifying viruses in clinical diagnostic samples (Mahony, 2008; Mahony et al., 2011). Antigen-based detection is used in some acute care settings, but typically shows inferior sensitivity and specificity compared to molecular methods. PCR is the most common amplification technique, with FDA cleared or approved *in vitro* diagnostic tests available commercially to detect all common respiratory viral pathogens (Caliendo, 2011) (**Table 2**). These are marketed as single analyte assays (such as tests that detect only influenza A), as assays detecting only a small number of analytes (for example, detecting only influenza and RSV), and as broad-panel test (detecting 12–20 different pathogens) (Rand et al., 2011; Hammond et al., 2012; Hayden et al., 2012; Popowitch et al., 2013; Salez et al., 2015). Often the latter also include some common bacterial agents of infection. Such molecular tests generally have a high degree of sensitivity and specificity, with a much more rapid time to result compared to culture. Larger, multiplexed panels can be advantageous in an immunocompromised population as even the detection of pathogens without available specific antiviral therapies can have important implications for infection control and potentially for decisions surrounding the time of transplant. Furthermore, symptoms can be atypical, making it difficult to predict the most likely agents of infection with any degree of clinical certainty. Such highly sensitive tests raise numerous questions, however. Despite uncertain clinical significance, the incidence of detectable multi-viral infections tends to be increased using these methods, sometimes with four or more agents detected simultaneously. The advent of molecular testing has also increased the time of detectable viral shedding which is often lengthened in immunocompromised patients, and the risk of spread or recurrence during periods of asymptomatic shedding is unknown. Quantitative methods (as noted elsewhere in this work) may shed light, both on viral

TABLE 1 | Taxonomy and virologic properties of the major human respiratory RNA viruses[a].

Virus	Family	Size (nm)	RNA genome	Envelope	Genetic or antigenic types
Respiratory syncytial virus	*Paramyxoviridae*	120–200	Linear ss(–)	Yes	Antigenic subgroups A and B with 10 A genotypes and 13 B genotypes
Influenza virus	*Orthomyxoviridae*	80–120	Segmented ss(–)	Yes	3 antigenic types (A, B, C); A has 3 HA and 2 NA human subtypes
Parainfluenza virus	*Paramyxoviridae*	120–180	Linear ss(–)	Yes	4 serotypes (1, 2, 3, 4); subtypes 4a and 4b
Metapneumovirus	*Paramyxoviridae*	120–180	Linear ss(–)	Yes	Subtypes A and B; subgroups A1/A2 and B1/B2, respectively
Rhinoviruses	*Picornaviridae*	20–27	Linear ss(+)	No	>100 antigenic types
Coronaviruses	*Coronaviridae*	80–160	Linear ss(+)	Yes	6 genotypes (229E, OC43, NL63, HKU1, SARS-CoV, MERS-CoV)

[a]*ss(–), single-stranded negative-sense RNA; ss(+), single-stranded positive-sense RNA; HA, hemagglutinin; NA, neuraminidase; SARS-CoV, severe acute respiratory syndrome-coronavirus; MERS-CoV, Middle East respiratory syndrome-coronavirus. Reproduced from Hodinka (2016).*

TABLE 2 | Laboratory methods for diagnosis of the major human respiratory RNA viruses[a].

Methods	Sensitivity	Specificity	Test time	Clinical usefulness
VIRUS CULTURE SYSTEMS				
Conventional tube	Low-moderate	High	3–14 d	Capable of growing any virus; involves considerable time, labor, and resources
Shell vial or microwell plate	Low-moderate	High	1–3 d	Rapid centrifugation-assisted cultures for select viruses; less sensitive than tube cultures
DIRECT ANTIGEN DETECTION TESTS				
Immunofluorescence	Moderate	Moderate-high	1–2 h	Rapid, multianalyte detection; moderately complex and subjective reading
Immunoassays	Low-moderate	Moderate-high	≤15 min	Fast and simple to use; amenable to point-of-care testing
Nucleic acid amplification tests	High	High	15 min–8 h	New reference standard; superior performance characteristics
Serology	NA	NA	NA	Not useful for diagnosis; used for research and epidemiologic studies

[a]*d, days; h, hours; min, minutes. Reproduced from Hodinka (2016).*

dynamics and on the clinical implications of asymptomatic shedding. Such information awaits increased availability of these tests, together with publication of more studies in this high-risk population.

Several authors have studied the yield and correlation of respiratory samples from upper airway and lower airway in the setting of LRTI. Hakki et al. analyzed 72 paired nasopharyngeal (NP) and bronchoalveolar lavage fluid specimens from immunocompromised adult patients for respiratory viruses. NP samples had a positive and negative predictive value of 86.4 and 94% respectively. In three sets the NP sample was negative and the BAL was positive (Hakki et al., 2014). Azadeh et al. report that 20% of patients with an initial negative NP wash had a positive BAL sample, suggesting that a BAL may be valuable when there are concerns for LRTI and the NP wash is negative (Azadeh et al., 2015). This has been particularly reported by several groups in the setting of severe pandemic H1N1 influenza infection (Mulrennan et al., 2010; Yeh et al., 2010; Lee et al., 2011).

Susceptibility testing is limited to influenza. Emergence of universal resistance of IV A H1N1 and IV A H3N2 to adamantanes, as well as rapid emergence of oseltamivir resistant IV A H1N1 led to increased efforts to closely monitor drug resistance (Renaud et al., 2010, 2011a,b; Okomo-Adhiambo et al., 2014, 2015). Both phenotypic and genotypic assays have developed, but genotypic methods are most commonly used for routine testing to detect neuraminidase inhibitor resistance of influenza viruses in clinical specimens (Hirsch et al., 2013; Marjuki et al., 2013; Okomo-Adhiambo et al., 2013; Laplante and St George, 2014; Tamura et al., 2015).

ISOLATION CONTROL PRACTICES

Several strategies have been suggested to decrease the risk of hospital transmission of respiratory viruses. Hand hygiene, screening visitors for respiratory symptoms, education of healthcare personal to avoid caring for patients if they are sick and isolation of patients with respiratory symptoms are among the most widely strategies implemented across institutions (Dykewicz, 2001; Tomblyn et al., 2009; Engelhard et al., 2013; Hirsch et al., 2013). Molecular testing has allowed for more rapid detection of viral etiology becoming an important tool to guide prevention practices. Whole genome sequencing—next generation sequencing is emerging as a potent tool to further enhance outbreak investigation and has been successfully applied in rhinovirus, influenza, and RSV (Gilchrist et al., 2015; Greninger et al., 2017; Kothari et al., 2017; Zhu Y. et al., 2017; Houlihan et al., 2018). A particular challenge in this population is the high proportion of asymptomatic patients with respiratory viral infections and whether isolation in the absence of symptoms is indicated (Raad et al., 1997; Waghmare et al., 2016). Quantitative methods may aid useful information on determining the infectious risk in these patients.

Patients with respiratory symptoms should be put immediately on contact and droplet isolation. At St Jude we use clinical symptoms and viral etiology to determine isolation strategies. We stop isolation in patients with infections due to rhinovirus, enterovirus, coronavirus, or unidentified etiology after 48 h of resolution of symptoms with no retesting needed. Patients with respiratory infection due to RSV, influenza, HMPV, or HPIV require both resolution of symptoms and a negative test to be taken off isolation.

TREATMENT

Although advances in the treatment of respiratory infections have been made, management of viral infections in this population remains a challenge (Ljungman et al., 2001; Casper et al., 2010; Chemaly et al., 2014; Waghmare et al., 2016; Shahani et al., 2017). Treatment is primarily supportive and includes, fluid replacement, oxygen for hypoxia and mechanical ventilation if necessary (Meissner, 2016; Kou et al., 2018). Bronchodilators may provide some benefit (Meissner, 2016; Kou et al., 2018). Given the significant mortality rate in immunocompromised host, antiviral therapy should be considered when available (Casper et al., 2010; Renaud and Englund, 2012; Hirsch et al., 2013; Waghmare et al., 2016; Shahani et al., 2017). However, antiviral options are scarce and limited to influenza and, to a lesser extent, RSV (**Table 3**) (Casper et al., 2010; Chemaly et al., 2014; Waghmare et al., 2016; Jorquera and Tripp, 2017; Shahani et al., 2017). In addition, adjunctive therapy such as intravenous immunoglobulin (IVIG) or monoclonal antibodies, such as palivizumab, have shown mixed results (Ghosh et al., 2000; de Fontbrune et al., 2007; Hirsch et al., 2013; Falsey et al., 2017). Several antivirals and monoclonal antibodies are at different stages of development for the treatment of respiratory viruses (**Table 4**).

RSV

RSV is a single stranded, negative-sense RNA virus within the family *Paramyxoviridae*. Its genome transcribes to produce 11 proteins: NS1, NS2, N, P, M, SH, G, F, M2-1, M2-2, and L (Papenburg and Boivin, 2010; Tregoning and Schwarze, 2010). The attachment glycoprotein (G) and the fusion (F) glycoprotein are the two major glycoproteins on the surface of RSV. They control the initial phases of infection (McLellan et al., 2013). F protein is the main target for antiviral development. However, both G and F glycoproteins are targeted by neutralizing antibodies during natural infection (Capella et al., 2017; Melero et al., 2017; Tian et al., 2017). There is a single antigenic type of RSV, divided into two subgroups, A and B. Usually one of these groups predominates on an epidemic. The significant of the variants and its role on disease severity is not well-understood (Hall et al., 1990; Walsh et al., 1997, 2018; Devincenzo, 2004).

Respiratory syncytial virus (RSV) is the most common cause of lower respiratory tract infection in children. Premature infants, infants with cardiac disease, and severely immunocompromised patients experience increased morbidity and mortality (Domachowske and Rosenberg, 1999; DeVincenzo et al., 2003; Devincenzo, 2004; Hall et al., 2009, 2013). RSV infections resembles the same seasonal pattern in patients with HCT and/or other hematological diseases and its occurrence is a result of increased risk of infection from the community, household contacts, and nosocomial transmission (Hall, 2001; Hall et al., 2009, 2013). In a single center study, Hakim and colleagues determined the epidemiology of respiratory viruses on children with acute lymphoblastic leukemia. They reported that RSV was the second most common respiratory accounting for 31% of all episodes of respiratory viral infections (Hakim et al., 2016b). Hirsch et al. described that RSV infection in pediatric patients with acute myeloid leukemia can be up to 2.2% (Hirsch et al., 2013). Fisher et al found that RSV was the third most common respiratory viral infection in pediatric patients undergoing HCT after RhV and PIV, with an all cause fatality rate of 10% (Fisher et al., 2017).

RSV LRTI is associated with increased rate of hospitalization and mortality. Several risk factors have been described for RSV LRTI (Seo et al., 2013; Chemaly et al., 2014; Kim et al., 2014). El-Saleeby and colleagues found that younger age and lymphopenia were significantly associated with RSV LRTI in children (El Saleeby et al., 2008). In Hakim's study a lower nadir ALC also associated with RSV LTRI (Hakim et al., 2016b). In fact, RSV, as compared to other virus, was more likely to be associated with LRTI, accounting for 58% of all viral episodes of LRTI (Hakim et al., 2016b). Age, neutropenia, lymphocytopenia, graft-vs.-host disease, use of myeloablative conditioning regimens, use of corticosteroids, a recent HCT, and pre-engraftment are the most significant risk factors included in an index developed by investigators at University of Texas MD Anderson Cancer Center to categorize patients into prognostic risk groups (Shah et al., 2014). Waghmare et al. explored several risk factors for RSV mortality in patients undergoing HCT with RSV infection, including the presence of RSV viremia. This was present in one third of the patients after development of LRTI. While neutropenia and mechanical ventilation were significantly associated with RSV viremia, no effect from lymphopenia or steroids use was observed. In this cohort viremia was independently associated with mortality. Treatment with aerosolized ribavirin was associated with improved outcomes, including decrease overall mortality and mortality due to respiratory failure (Waghmare et al., 2013).

Attempts to correlate viral load with RSV disease severity have yielded mixed results (Devincenzo, 2004; DeVincenzo et al., 2005; Gerna et al., 2008; Franz et al., 2010; El Saleeby et al., 2011; Walsh et al., 2018). On one hand, DeVincenzo et al. noted that patients that were intubated had higher viral load than those who were not, and that higher viral load was associated with longer stayed in the hospital (Buckingham et al., 2000; DeVincenzo and Buckingham, 2002; DeVincenzo et al., 2005). However, other studies have not found such association (Gerna et al., 2008; Franz et al., 2010; Lukens et al., 2010). Fuller et al. reported an association of viral load and disease severity in patients under 5 years of age but not in older patients (Fuller et al., 2013). The inconsistency of results may be due to technical difficulties of precisely quantifying virus load at a mucosal surface, or perhaps optimal analysis may require sampling over several days. At St.

TABLE 3 | Current approved antivirals for treatment of the major human respiratory RNA viruses.

Virus	Antiviral	Drug class	Dose/Duration		Side effects	Resistance
Respiratory syncytial virus	Ribavirin	Nucleoside analog	Children/Adults: Inhaled Oral	2 grams over 2 h TID Loading dose of 600 mg 200 mg TID on day 1 400 mg TID on day 2 Then maximum 30/mg/kg/day	Bronchospasm Hemolysis, liver and renal toxicity	None reported
Influenza virus	Oseltamivir	NAI	Adults Children ≥ 12 months >40 kg 24–40 kg 16–23 kg 15 kg or less	75 mg PO twice per day 75 mg PO twice per day 60 mg PO twice per day 45 mg PO twice per day 30 mg PO twice per day	Nausea, vomiting	Influenza A(H1N1) virus strains H275Y substitution leads to resistance
			Children < 12 months	3 mg/kg/dose PO twice per day		
			Longer duration (10 days) for immunocompromised individuals			
	Zanamivir	NAI	Adults	Two 5-mg inhalations (10 mg total) twice per day	Bronchospasm, diarrhea, nausea, headache, dizziness	Influenza A (H1N1) with both an H275Y and E119D or E119G. NA substitution lead to resistance
			Children (age, 7 years or older)	Two 5-mg inhalations (10 mg total) twice per day		
	Peramivir	NAI	Adults	600 mg single dose (IV)	Neutropenia, diarrhea	Influenza A(H1N1) virus strains with H275Y substitution leads to resistance
			Children (age, 29 days of life or older)	N/A		
			Longer duration (5 days) for immunocompromised individuals			
	Amantadine*	M2 inhibitors	≥10 years and ≥40 kg ≥10 years and <40 kg 1–9 years.	100 mg PO twice daily 5 mg/kg/day PO in 2 doses 5 mg/kg/day PO in 2 doses	Cardiac, neurologic and gastrointestinal events; neutropenia	High prevalence of resistance in all Influenza A (H3N2) and (H1N1) pdm09 Not active against Influenza B
	Rimantadine*	M2 inhibitors	≥10 years/Adolescents 1 – 9 years	5 mg/kg/day PO in 2 doses 6.6 mg/kg/day PO in 2 doses	Neurological and cardiac events	Same as for Amantadine
	Baloxavir marboxil	Endonuclease inhibitor	≥ 12 years and ≥80 kg ≥12 years and <80 kg.	80 mg PO once 40 mg PO once	Diarrhea, bronchitis	Influenza A (H3N2) and (H1N1) with substitutions I38F/M/F show reduced susceptibility.
Parainfluenza virus	None licensed					
Metapneumovirus	None licensed					
Rhinovirus	None licensed					
Coronavirus	None licensed					

**Not recommended given high prevalence of resistance for influenza A strains. Adapted from Englund et al. (1990, 1994), Knight et al. (1991), Boeckh et al. (2007), Casper et al. (2010), Renaud et al. (2010, 2011a,c), Hirsch et al. (2013), Waghmare et al. (2016), Shahani et al. (2017), AAP (2018), and Hayden et al. (2018).*

Jude, we have developed a droplet digital PCR assay to quantify RSA A and RSV B in respiratory specimens. Initial clinical validation was performed with 73 samples from 19 patients with RSV infection. RSV viral load was significantly higher in febrile patients <5 years old, whereas no statistical difference was noted with older patients. Patients who presented with either cough

TABLE 4 | Antivirals and monoclonal antibodies on the pipeline for treatment of the major human respiratory RNA viruses.

Virus	Antiviral	Drug class/mechanism of action	Route of administration	Company
Respiratory syncytial virus	ALS-8176 (a.k.a Lumicitabine)	Nucleoside analog RNA-dependent RNA-polymerase (RdRp)	Orally	Alios BioPharma
	GS-5806 (a.k.a Presatovir)	Fusion inhibitor*	Orally	Gilead
	VP-14637 (aka MDT-637)	Fusion inhibitor*	Inhaled	ViroPharma
	JNJ-53718678	Fusion inhibitor	Orally	Johnson & Johnson
	BTA-C585 (a.k.a Enzaplatovir)	Fusion inhibitor*	Orally	Vaxart
	AK-0529	Fusion inhibitor	Orally	Ark Biosciences
	RSV604	Nucleoprotein inhibitor	Orally	Astra Zeneca
	ALN-RSV01	Nucleoprotein inhibitor	Orally	AlnylamPharmaceuticals
	Palivizumab (Synagis)	Monoclonal antibody	Intramuscular	MedImmune
	REGN2222 (a.k.a Suptavumab)	Monoclonal antibody	Intramuscular	RegeneronPharmaceuticals
	MEDI8897	Monoclonal antibody	Intramuscular	MedImmune
	ALX-0171	Monoclonal antibody	Inhaled	Ablynx
Influenza virus	DAS181 (a.k.a.Fludase)	Targets the Viral Receptor (Sialic Acid)	Inhaled	Ansun BioPharma
	Laninamivir (CS-8958)	Long-acting neuraminidase inhibitors	Inhaled	Biota
	Favipiravir (T705)	Nucleotide analog RNA polymerase	Orally	Toyama Chemical
	JNJ-63623872 (a.k.a VX-787)	Nonnucleoside inhibitor	Orally	Janssen
	Nitazoxanide (a.k.a NT-300)	Thiazolides Inhibits the maturation of influenza virus HA	Orally	Romark Laboratories
	MEDI8852	Monoclonal antibody	Intravenous	AstraZeneca
	VIS410	Monoclonal antibody	Intravenous	Visterra
Parainfluenza virus	DAS181 (a.k.a.Paradase)	Targets the Viral Receptor (Sialic Acid)	Inhaled	Ansun BioPharma
Human Metapneumovirus	MAb 338	Monoclonal antibody	Intravenous	Medimmune
Human Rhinovirus	Vapendavir	Binds to the RhV VP1 capsid	Orally	Aviragen Therapeutics

**inhibit RSV fusion through a similar mechanism, and RSV variants exhibiting drug resistance have displayed cross-resistance to these inhibitors. Adapted from (Douglas et al. (2005); Triana-Baltzer et al. (2009b); Boeckh and Englund (2010); Kiso et al. (2010); Sleeman et al. (2010); Watanabe et al. (2010); Guzmán-Suarez et al. (2012); Moss et al. (2012); Adedeji et al. (2013); Matz (2013); Clark et al. (2014); DeVincenzo et al. (2014, 2015); Rossignol (2014); Byrn et al. (2015); Battles et al. (2016); Waghmare et al. (2016); Coates et al. (2017); Heylen et al. (2017); Jorquera and Tripp (2017); Kim et al. (2017); Koszalka et al. (2017); Mejias et al. (2017); Roymans et al. (2017); Shahani et al. (2017); Heo (2018); Omoto et al. (2018); Rossey et al. (2018), and Stevens et al. (2018).*

or nasal congestion had significantly higher viral load when compared to those who did not. Patients presenting with all 3 signs and symptoms had higher viral load when compared to those that only presented with one symptom. Eight patients with RSV infection were treated with Ribavirin. Seven of them received inhaled ribavirin and one received IV ribavirin since the patient was on mechanical ventilation. Viral load upon completion of treatment was significantly reduced (Data not published). Viral load testing for RSV is not widely available for clinical diagnostic use, and no FDA-approved methodology is currently on the market.

Ribavirin is a nucleoside analog that resembles guanosine and acts by inhibiting the dehydrogenase enzyme impairing the synthesis of guanosine triphosphate leading to reduce cellular deposits of guanidine necessary for viral growth (Shahani et al., 2017). Initiation and elongation of RNA is hampered impeding viral protein synthesis (Knight et al., 1991; Chemaly et al., 2014, 2016). Aerosolized ribavirin is the only FDA-approved treatment of severe RSV-LRTIs in hospitalized infants and young children with underlying compromising conditions (prematurity, cardiopulmonary disease, or immunosuppression) (Chemaly et al., 2014, 2016; Waghmare et al., 2016). Furthermore, ribavirin-based antiviral therapy is recommended by European guidelines for leukemia patients and HCT recipients at high risk of complications (Hirsch et al., 2013).

Shah et al. performed a systematic review based mainly on retrospective studies and found that ribavirin-based therapy was associated with a significant decrease in progression from URTIs to LRTIs. Furthermore, ribavirin alone or in combination with immunomodulatory therapy improved mortality rates when compared to no therapy in adult HCT recipients (Shah and Chemaly, 2011). This topic has recently gained a lot of interest given the increase in price of inhaled ribavirin from \$6105 per day in January 2013 to \$29,953 per day, based on average whole- sale price (Chemaly et al., 2016). As a consequence of this rise, a 5-day and a 10-day treatment course would cost \$149,765 and \$299,530 respectively. However, the oral formulation is ~\$25 per day depending on dosing strategy (Chemaly et al., 2016; Waghmare et al., 2016). Some authors suggest that the oral formulation is not effective given low achievable plasma concentrations (Waghmare et al., 2016). Other studies show benefit of using oral ribavirin for adult patients with RSV infection (Damlaj et al., 2015; Foolad et al., 2017, 2018; Pasikhova et al., 2018). These unanswered questions are important given the difference in cost between the two formulations (Shah et al., 2016a).

Adjuvant therapy for RSV infection has also been controversial. Various other therapies such as intravenous immunoglobulin (IVIG), RSV hyperimmunoglobulin, and palivizumab, have been used for treatment (Shah and Chemaly, 2011; Shah et al., 2012; Waghmare et al., 2016; Shahani et al., 2017). Animal models and initial studies showed benefits of ribavirin plus RSV hyperimmunoglobulin compared to ribavirin alone (Gruber et al., 1987; Whimbey et al., 1995; Ottolini et al., 1999; Ghosh et al., 2000; Falsey et al., 2017). However, production of RSV IVIG has since been discontinued. In adult HCT recipients with RSV pneumonia, uncontrolled studies suggested that use of combination therapy with ribavirin and IVIG improved survival (Whimbey et al., 1995; Ghosh et al., 2000). However, combined use of ribavirin and IVIG has not been supported by a randomized trial. In forty allogenic HCT recipients with RSV infection, palivizumab failed to reduce progression to LRTI or mortality (de Fontbrune et al., 2007). Given the questionable efficacy and high cost of palivizumab (Ambrose and McLaurin, 2015), routine use has been discouraged; and practices vary widely among institutions.

At our institution, ribavirin is recommended for treatment of RSV URTI or LRTI in patients <2 years old with ALC below 300, or in patients of any age with an ALC below 100 who have a diagnosis of AML or relapsed or high risk ALL, those undergoing HCT or have pre-existing severe heart or lung disease (**Figure 1**). We do not use palivizumab as part of treatment, and only consider IVIG if total Ig is below 400 mg/dl. Other antivirals against RSV are at different stages of development (**Table 4**) (Jorquera and Tripp, 2017).

Palivizumab has been proven effective in reducing severe RSV infection in premature infants and children with chronic lung disease (AAP, 2014a,b). Although efficacy of palivizumab has not been assess in randomized trials in immunocompromised, prudent use of palivizumab in these population may be indicated. Kassis et al. described successfully control of a nosocomial outbreak of RSV in a bone marrow transplant unit where use of palivizumab reduced transmission of RSV in high risk group patients (Kassis et al., 2010).

At St. Jude, Palivizumab is administered in 5 monthly doses (November-March) to all patients with AML, SCID, or HCT recipients (including pre-HCT conditioning) who are ≤ 24 months of age and patients ≤ 12 months of age with a diagnosis of acute lymphoblastic leukemia. Other patients ≤ 24 months of age who are receiving intensive, immunosuppressive chemotherapy during the RSV season are considered for prophylaxis on a case by case basis.

INFLUENZA

Human influenza viruses (IVs) are members of the family *Orthomyxoviridae* and belong to three genera that contain single antigenically distinct species of the same name: influenza A, influenza B, and influenza C. They have a segmented, single stranded, negative sense RNA genome (Nicholson et al., 2003). The three IVs types are distinguished by antigenic differences in their nucleoprotein and matrix protein. The two main surface glycoproteins, hemagglutinin (HA) and neuraminidase (NA) are critical in the replication cycle and pathogenesis of IVS (Nicholson et al., 2003).

The seasonal prevalence of influenza infections in immunocompromised patients, closely parallels the community wide prevalence (Appiah et al., 2015; Bednarska et al., 2015). The incidence of influenza in transplant recipients is low. However, influenza infection remains a significant cause of morbidity and mortality in these patients (Weigt et al., 2011). The incidence in HCT recipients ranges from 1 to 3% (Nichols et al., 2004). Hakim et al. found that influenza was the most common virus pediatric patients with acute lymphoblastic leukemia (ALL), accounting for 38% of respiratory infections. In this cohort, the majority of patients presented with URTI, and only 6 had evidence of progression to LRTI. Of those, 3 had 2009 pandemic H1N1 influenza A virus, and one had RSV and influenza B virus co-infection, while the remaining 2 patients had influenza A virus that was not subtyped (Hakim et al., 2016b).

The clinical presentation of influenza does not differ considerably from that described in the general population. URTI symptoms consist of rhinitis and cough. Fever is usually seen in patients with pneumonia (Chemaly et al., 2006; Kumar et al., 2018). Less frequently, patients can present with gastrointestinal and neurological symptoms (Ison and Hayden, 2002; Peck et al., 2007). Risk factors associated with severity of infection and progression to LRTI have been described, including lymphopenia, steroids use, and delayed antiviral therapy (Ljungman et al., 2001, 2011; Martino et al., 2005; Chemaly et al., 2006; Khanna et al., 2009; Choi et al., 2011). Initiation of antiviral treatment within 48 h of symptoms has been associated with improved outcomes (Nichols et al., 2004; Choi et al., 2011; Espinosa-Aguilar et al., 2011). Tantawi et al. reported 90 children and adolescents with different cancer types who presented with LRTIs necessitating hospital admission. Respiratory viruses were identified in 37.7% of the patients, the majority with hematological malignancies. Influenza were the most common virus associated with hospital admission (influenza A 47%, influenza B 12%). All patients admitted to the ICU had bacterial co-infection. Those who received oseltamivir had a less severe clinical picture (Tantawy et al., 2015).

Respiratory complications, such as mechanical ventilation are associated with mortality in immunocompromised patients with influenza infection. The latter ranges from 6 to 28% and can be related to direct viral pathogenesis or to superimposed bacterial infections (Ljungman et al., 2001; Nichols et al., 2004; Choi et al., 2011; Renaud and Campbell, 2011; Fisher et al., 2017).

In pediatric cancer patients, antiviral treatment should be initiated as early as possible, even if patients have been symptomatic for over 48 h, since there may be benefits even with delayed therapy (AAP, 2018). While Influenza B is inherently resistant to M2 inhibitors (amantadine and rimantadine), influenza A has become resistant overtime. Hence, their use is

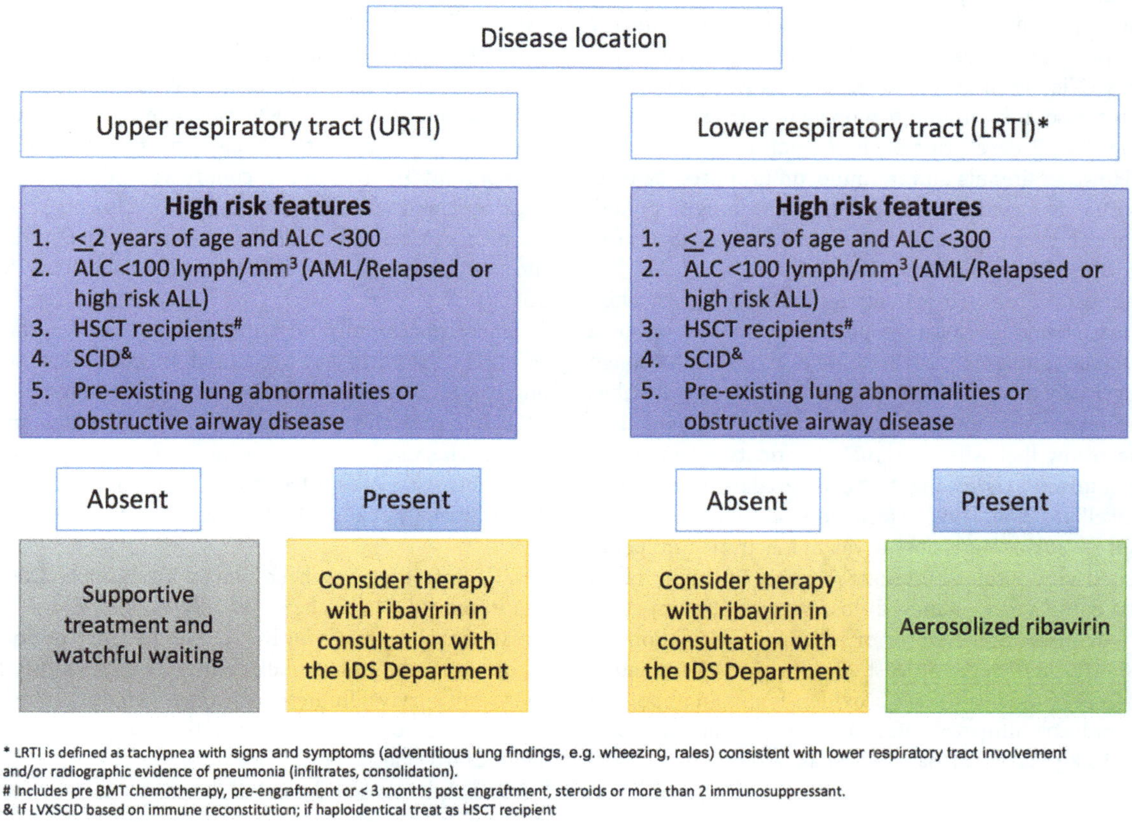

FIGURE 1 | Institutional decision tree used at St Jude for inhaled Ribavirin therapy based on risk factors of patients infected with RSV.

limited. Neuraminidase inhibitors (NAIs), such as oseltamivir, zanamivir, and peramivir are now first line for prophylaxis and treatment of influenza A and B (Casper et al., 2010; Fiore et al., 2011; Chemaly et al., 2014). Oseltamivir is given by mouth, and its main side effects are nausea, vomiting and diarrhea. Inhaled zanamivir can cause bronchospasm, so it should be used cautiously in in patients with chronic lung disease. Intravenous zanamivir is available for compassionate use only. Peramivir is the only NAI approved for IV use (Ison and Hayden, 2002; Louie et al., 2012a,b; Ison, 2014). Studies comparing oseltamivir to peramivir have shown similar outcomes. However, the efficacy and safety of peramivir in immunocompromised patients needs further assessment (de Jong et al., 2014).

Most mutations conferring resistance to NAIs, such as H275Y in pandemic influenza A H1N1, do not lead to resistance in zanamivir, and its inhaled formulation has been successfully used to treat these patients (Renaud et al., 2011a; Fraaij et al., 2015; Waghmare et al., 2016). This is especially important, since immunocompromised patients are at increased risk of developing resistant mutants (Couturier et al., 2010; Renaud et al., 2010, 2011a,c; Carr et al., 2011b; Hamada et al., 2012; Fraaij et al., 2015). Combination therapy has poorly been studied and has not shown benefits. Some experts have recommended increased dosing of oseltamivir due to concerns of poor absorption in patients with mucositis or graft vs. host disease. However, the benefits of such intervention have not been conclusively demonstrated (Casper et al., 2010; Watcharananan et al., 2010). Length of therapy remains controversial. Given the median time to progression to LRTI and the potential for recurrence, longer treatment courses (10 days) have been suggested in this population (Khanna et al., 2009; Waghmare et al., 2016).

Endonuclease inhibitors are a new class of antiviral drugs (Clark et al., 2014; Byrn et al., 2015). Phase III development of Baloxavir marboxil (Xofluza, Shionogi & Co Ltd) is underway in the USA, EU and other countries (Heo, 2018; Omoto et al., 2018). Xofluza was approved in Japan on February 2018 and has recently been approved in the USA as single oral dose for the treatment of influenza A or B virus infection of patients 12 years of age and older (FDA, 2018). The main side effects described have been diarrhea and bronchitis. Amino acid substitutions to the endonuclease active site (I38F/T) have shown reduce susceptibility for Influenza A (H3N2) and (H1N1) strains (Hayden et al., 2018). Further studies need to be done to determine whether a single dose would be appropriate for immunocompromised patients.

Early diagnosis and isolation precautions are critical in preventing transmission. Post-exposure antiviral chemoprophylaxis should be given to any immunocompromised patient who comes in close contact with proven or suspected cases during the infectious period of the case (Fiore et al., 2011). The infectious period for persons with influenza is estimated to range from 1 day before up to 7 days after development of symptoms (Nicholson et al., 2003). If a patient comes into contact with a case in an immunocompetent host whose illness started more than 7 days prior, then chemoprophylaxis is not necessary. However, infants and immunocompromised patients shed the virus and remain contagious for a longer period. Post-exposure chemoprophylaxis should last up to 7 days after the last known exposure to influenza.

All immunocompromised patients 6 months of age or older should be vaccinated as soon as possible with the seasonal influenza vaccine (Ljungman, 2012; Rubin et al., 2014). Although its immunogenicity in immunocompromised patients is variable, and vaccine response is lower than in the general population, some studies show that when vaccinated patients get influenza the severity of infection is less that that compared to unvaccinated patients (Engelhard et al., 1993; Machado et al., 2005; Issa et al., 2011; Beck et al., 2012). High-dose trivalent inactivated influenza vaccine elicited a more robust immune response in children with cancer when compared to standard-dose vaccine (Hakim et al., 2016a). At our institution 2 doses of influenza vaccination are recommended, administered at least 28 days apart. Vaccination of family members and health care providers is also an important measure to prevent influenza infection in these patients (Carr et al., 2011a; Hakim et al., 2016a; Sykes et al., 2017).

PARAINFLUENZA

Parainfluenza viruses (PIVs) belong to the family *Paramyxoviridae* and have a structure similar to that of RSV with a negative sense, single-stranded RNA genome that encodes six common viral proteins. Hemagglutinin-neuraminidase (HN) and F glycoprotein promote viral attachment and fusion of the viral and host cell membranes (Hall, 2001; Henrickson, 2003). At present, 5 serotypes of Human PIVs (HPIVs) have been recognized: HPIV-1, HPIV-2, HPIV-3, HPIV-4a, and HPIV-4b. They differ in their frequency of occurrence, spectrum of clinical disease and epidemic patterns (Henrickson, 2003). PIV3 is the most common serotype producing infections. Infections can occur at any time during the year. However, during spring and summer there is a peak of activity (Hall, 2001; Henrickson, 2003).

A recent multicenter study aiming to define the epidemiology and outcomes of respiratory virus infection in pediatric HCT recipients showed PIV as the second most common virus. In this cohort RVI was associated with an all-cause case fatality rate of 11 and 8% of patients with HPIV infection died (Fisher et al., 2017). A large retrospective study of 1,554 children diagnosed with cancer found that PIV was the most common respiratory virus with an incidence of 54% (74/137). Median age was 3.9 years and 30% of the patients were HCT recipients (Maeng et al., 2012). Most of the patients presented with URTI and 20% of them progressed to LRTI with a median of 4 days from onset of symptoms (Maeng et al., 2012). Hakim et al found that HPIV was the third most common viral infections in patients with ALL. Unlike RSV, patients with HPIV in this cohort were more likely to present with URTI (Hakim et al., 2016b). Neutropenia, lymphopenia, coinfection, and use of steroids have been described as risks factors for progression (Srinivasan et al., 2011a,b; Ustun et al., 2012; Seo et al., 2014). LRTI was significantly associated with mortality, between 5 to 31 days from initial diagnosis. The overall mortality rate in this cohort was 23% and no differences were observed when comparing HCT recipients with non-HCT recipients (Maeng et al., 2012). However, other studies reported mortality rates up to 46% (Nichols et al., 2001; Shah et al., 2016b).

There is currently no antiviral approved for the treatment of HPIV. Ribavirin has been used anecdotical in several cases and has not impacted clinical outcomes, including progression to LRTI and mortality (Chemaly et al., 2012; Renaud and Englund, 2012). The use of IVIG has not improved survival of HCT recipients with PIVs infections (Knight et al., 1991; Shah et al., 2012; Chemaly et al., 2014; Waghmare et al., 2016; Shahani et al., 2017).

PIV infection has been linked to bronchiolitis obliterans syndrome (BOS) (Vilchez et al., 2001, 2003; Erard et al., 2006). Treatment alternatives for BOS are limited, in part due to the lack of understanding of its pathogenesis. Furthermore, BOS limits long term survival in these patients, highlighting the importance of prevention of PIVs infection in these patients (Chaparro et al., 1997; Erard et al., 2006).

Although several hospital outbreaks have been reported, nosocomial transmission has been significantly reduced by implementing isolation, hand hygiene, and disinfection of surfaces. There are currently no licensed vaccines for PIVs. Live attenuated PIV vaccines are under development and preliminary results from phase 1 trials suggest that they are safe and immunogenic (Karron et al., 1995a,b; Adderson et al., 2015).

HMPV

Human metapneumovirus (HMPV) is a single stranded, negative sense RNA enveloped virus from the family *Paramyxoviridae*. The genomic organization is similar to that of RSV with the exception that there is no NS-1 or NS-2. The virus attaches to and enters the host cell through the G and F protein. There are two major subtypes (A and B) composed of subgroups A1/A2 and B1/B2 (Papenburg and Boivin, 2010; Schildgen et al., 2011).

MPV incidence in immunocompromised hosts has been reported to be as high as 40%. The incidence in those with hematological malignancies did not differ compared to HCT recipients. Although no specific risk factor was described in the included studies, incidence in adult patients was slightly higher than in children (Shah et al., 2016c). Hakim et al. found that 10% of all acute respiratory infections with an identified virus in children with ALL was due to HMPV. Of these, only one patient developed LRTI (Hakim et al., 2016b).

HMPV may cause URTI or LRTI in immunocompromised patients. Asymptomatic viral shedding has been described. Patients usually present with nasal congestion, cough, sore throat, or fever. However, once LRTI develops, patients can present with progressive pneumonia, hypotension, and shock (Kamboj et al., 2008; Hoppe et al., 2016; Samuel et al., 2016; Seo et al., 2016; El Chaer et al., 2017).

A recent article of 181 HMPV infections reported that the vast majority of infections are in patients with hematological malignancies or recipients of HCT. Most of the patients had a community acquired infection and 61% presented with URTI. Of those who presented with LRTI, 25% had progression from URTI. The incidence of LRTI in this review was 34% (El Chaer et al., 2017). Risk factors associated with LRTI were use of steroids, low lymphocyte count and, early onset of infection after HCT. LRTI was significantly associated with mortality, which ranged from 0 to 17% in most studies, but can be as high as 43% (Renaud et al., 2013; Shah et al., 2016c; Pasikhova et al., 2018).

There is currently no approved antiviral therapy for HMPV. Several attempts have been made to evaluate the role of antiviral therapy with ribavirin for HMPV infections. Considering the limitations on study design given the low number of patients, most of these studies showed no benefits from antiviral therapy with similar mortality rates when compared patients who did not get antiviral treatment (Hoppe et al., 2016; Shah et al., 2016c; Pasikhova et al., 2018). Fusion inhibitors and monoclonal antibodies are under development but have not yet reached clinical trials (**Table 4**) (Ulbrandt et al., 2006; Deffrasnes et al., 2008).

RHINOVIRUS

The RhVs belong to the genus *Enterovirus* within the family *Picornaviridae.* They include three genetically distinct groups: A, B, and C. They are single-stranded, positive sense, RNA viruses. The genome encodes one polypeptide that is cleaved in four structural proteins (VP1-4) and 7 non-structural proteins. RhVs are antigenically diverse with over 100 serotypes identified to date (Greenberg, 2011; Jacobs et al., 2013).

Rhinovirus has been described as the most common respiratory pathogen isolated in immunocompromised children undergoing HCT (Loria et al., 2015; Fisher et al., 2017), with an incidence as high as 22.3% by day 100 (Milano et al., 2010).

The median time for a first positive tests has been reported at 44 days following HCT but can be as early as 2 days and as late as 93 days. There is no apparent seasonality for RhV detection. Prolonged viral shedding is common with a median of 3 weeks (Milano et al., 2010). Higher viral load at initial presentation has been significantly associated with prolonged viral shedding (Ogimi et al., 2018b). In the former study, thirteen percent of patients with RhV infection had no respiratory symptoms at the time of diagnosis. The remaining patients had URT symptoms. Four patients underwent a BAL for concerns of progression to LRTI, of these two died of respiratory failure (Milano et al., 2010). These results agreed with a study from Seo et al looking at 697 transplant recipients with rhinovirus infection. In this cohort, eighty one percent of patients presented with URTI. Patients with low monocyte count, oxygen use and steroid dose > 1 mg/kg/day had significantly increased risk of LRTI. Mortality was higher in those with LRTI (41 vs. 6%) (Seo et al., 2017). A multicenter study of respiratory viral infections in pediatric HCT recipient reported an all cause fatality rate of 10% in those patients with RhV infection (Fisher et al., 2017).

Pre-transplant rhinovirus detection has been significantly associated with increased mortality at day 100 (Campbell et al., 2015). However, Abandhe et al. did not find any differences in ICU admission, length of hospitalization or mortality (Abandeh et al., 2013). Currently, treatment of RhV infection consists of supportive care. Antiviral medications for RhV are under investigation (**Table 4**).

CORONAVIRUS

CoVs are enveloped, positive sense, single stranded RNA viruses belonging to the family *Coronaviridae.* There are six coronaviruses divided in two genera that can infect humans. CoV 229E and NL63 belong to the genus alphacoronavirus and OC43, HKU1, severe acute respiratory syndrome (SARS)-CoV, and Middle East respiratory syndrome (MERS)-CoV are members of the genus betacoronavirus. The genome codes for two non-structural proteins and four structural proteins (van der Hoek, 2007; Greenberg, 2011).

While CoVs are an important cause of the common cold in the general population, there is limited information on the clinical manifestations in immunocompromised hosts. Milano et al. described the epidemiology and risk factors of CoVs infection among HCT recipients. The cumulative incidence estimated at day 100 was 11.1%. The median time of first detection was 53 days (range, 2–93 days). Seasonal outbreaks were common in the winter with 13 of 22 cases first detected in December through March. The median time of shedding was over 3 weeks (Milano et al., 2010).

Ogimi et al. described several risks factors related to prolonged viral shedding, such as higher viral load, use of steroids, and myeloablative conditioning (Ogimi et al., 2017a). Univariate analysis of potential risk factors showed no significant association of acquisition with patient age, gender, underlying disease risk, stem cell source, CMV serostatus, donor type, acute GVHD, conditioning regimen, or engraftment status. Infection with coronaviruses was not associated with mortality in this cohort (Milano et al., 2010). However, another group reported similar mortality rates in HCT recipients to those observed with other viruses such as RSV, influenza virus, and PIV (Ogimi et al., 2017b).

A recent article from Seattle Children's Hospital looked at 85 immunocompromised and 1152 non-immunocompromised children with HCoV infection. Other than median age which was significantly higher for immunocompromised patients, demographic characteristics were similar. Viral co-infection was most commonly seen in non-immunocompromised patients, mostly due to detection of RSV. CoVs strains did not differed between the two groups. The most common clinical presentation was URTI. Younger age, male sex, presence of an underlying pulmonary disorder, and detection of a respiratory co-pathogen, particularly RSV, were associated with an increased likelihood of LRTD or severe LRTD. However, lymphopenia was not associated with more severe disease in this cohort (Ogimi et al., 2018a).

There is currently no treatment available for coronaviruses. However, current *in vitro* evaluation of HCoV therapy includes investigation of antiviral, as well as human monoclonal antibodies (Pyrc et al., 2007; Adedeji et al., 2013) (**Table 4**).

NEW DEVELOPMENTS IN THERAPEUTICS

RSV

Nucleoside analogs contain a base, or a base analog linked to a ribose-like moiety that can be incorporated by viral polymerases stopping polymerization and inhibiting replication (Jorquera and Tripp, 2017). ALS-8176 (a.k.a lumicitabine; Alios BioPharma/Janssen) is a nucleoside analog that inhibits the polymerization function of the L protein by causing immediate chain termination of RNA synthesis (Jorquera and Tripp, 2017). In RSV experimentally infected healthy adults, ALS-8176 was significantly associated with more rapid viral clearance, greater reduction of viral load and improvement of clinical symptoms (DeVincenzo et al., 2015). Several fusion inhibitors under development are directed at glycoprotein F with the goal of blocking viral entry into cells lining the respiratory tract (Battles et al., 2016; Jorquera and Tripp, 2017). GS-5806 (a.k.a. Presatovir; Gilead Sciences) is an oral RSV entry inhibitor and functions as an allosteric blocker of the F protein preventing RSV entry by blocking the virus–cell fusion process. Experiments with healthy volunteers with RSV infection showed that treatment with GS-5806 resulted in a reduction of mucus weight, symptom score and viral load (DeVincenzo et al., 2014). Similar results were observed with JNJ-53718678 (Johnson & Johnson) (Stevens et al., 2018). Finally, targeting the nucleoprotein has gained interest given that is highly conserved and essential for virus assembly (Jorquera and Tripp, 2017). RNA interference is a process in which small interfering RNAs (siRNAs) decrease protein production by degrading specific mRNA. Healthy adult volunteers experimentally infected with RSV who received intranasal ALN-RSV01 (Alnylam Pharmaceuticals) showed significant reduction of RSV replication when compared to placebo (DeVincenzo et al., 2010).

Monoclonal (mAbs) have been used for prophylaxis of RSV-related hospital admissions in pediatric populations. There are several mAbs targeting different epitopes of F protein under development (Rossey et al., 2018). REGN2222 (Suptavumab; Regeneron Pharmaceuticals) is a fully human mAb IgG1 that has proven safety and tolerability in healthy adults. In a recent phase III clinical trial REGN222 failed to prevent RSV infections in infants and the company has discontinued further development.. MEDI8897 (MedImmune) is a recombinant human IgG1κ mAb with a modified Fc region that extends more than 3-fold its half-life to 85–117 days after one single dose (Zhu Q. et al., 2017). Finally, ALX-0171 (Ablynx) is an inhaled trimeric nanobody that binds the antigenic site II of the F protein and neutralizes RSV A and B. It has shown significant reduction of viral load in infants hospitalized with RSV, when compared to placebo (Ablynx, 2016).

Influenza

Fludase (DAS181, Ansun BioPharma), a novel sialidase fusion protein, has shown *in vitro* activity toward all influenza strains isolated to date, such as H5N1, H1N1, H7N9 including those that have shown oseltamivir resistance (Triana-Baltzer et al., 2009a,b; Moss et al., 2010). A phase II clinical trial on healthy volunteers showed safety, tolerability, and effectivity in reducing viral load in the groups receiving DAS181 compared to placebo (Moss et al., 2012).

Laninamivir (CS-8958; Biota Pharmaceuticals, Alpharetta, GA, USA) is a long-acting NAI administered via a dry-powder inhaler for the treatment of influenza (Shahani et al., 2017). A double-blind, randomized controlled trial in healthy adults demonstrated that a single inhalation of lanimavir octonate is effective for the treatment of influenza. Importantly, lanimavir remains active against oseltamivir-resistant virus (Watanabe et al., 2010).

Favipiravir (T705; Toyama Chemical, Tokyo, Japan) is an investigational nucleotide analog that inhibits the viral RNA polymerase of most influenza strains (Kiso et al., 2010; Sleeman et al., 2010). Two phase 3 studies on adults with uncomplicated influenza have been completed and results are pending (NCT02026349 and NCT02008344).

JNJ-63623872 (VX-787; Janssen Pharma, Titusville, USA) inhibits influenza A replication by a novel mechanism that involves blocking the activity of the polymerase complex.

Nitazoxanide (NT-300; Romark Laboratories, Florida, USA), an antiparasitic agent, has shown broad activity toward influenza A including A(pH1N1) and H7N9, as well as influenza B and strains resistant to oseltamivir (Rossignol, 2014; Tilmanis et al., 2017). A Phase 2b/3 clinical trial comparing nitazoxanide vs. placebo, showed reduction of clinical symptoms and viral shedding in patients with uncomplicated influenza infection (Haffizulla et al., 2014). There are several ongoing trials including a phase 3 to evaluate the role of nitazoxanide for children 12 year of age or older and adults with uncomplicated influenza infection (NCT03336619). mAbs directed toward the highly conserved HA stalk of influenza virus are being developed for both prophylaxis and treatment (Shahani et al., 2017).

Parainfluenza

Paradase (DAS181, Ansun BioPharma) is a novel sialidase fusion protein that prevents viral propagation by cleaving sialic acid from respiratory epithelial cells leading to impair entry of the virus to the cells (Guzmán-Suarez et al., 2012; Chalkias et al., 2014; Chemaly et al., 2014). DAS181 has been given for compassionate use in immunocompromised patients, and has been associated with benefits (Chen et al., 2011; Drozd et al., 2013; Waghmare et al., 2015). Ansun Biopharma has completed a multi-site phase II study comparing DAS181 with placebo in immunocompromised patients with Parainfluenza LRTI requiring oxygen (NCT01644877). In 2017 the U.S. Food and Drug Administration (FDA) has granted Breakthrough

Therapy Designation to DAS181 for the treatment of lower respiratory tract PIV infection in immunocompromised patients (Biopharma, 2017). Phase 3 trials are currently being planned.

Metapneumovirus

Fusion inhibitors targeting the F protein have demonstrated viral inhibition *in vitro* and in animal models (Deffrasnes et al., 2008). A phase 2b study to evaluate the safety, tolerability and pharmacokintetics of ALS-8176 (a.k.a lumicitabine; Alios BioPharma/Janssen) in hospitalized adults with metapneumovirus infection is being planned (NCT03502694). Two mAbs, MAb 338 (Medimmune, Gaithersburg, MD, USA) and human Fab DS7, have prophylactic and therapeutic potential (Ulbrandt et al., 2006). However, clinical studies have not yet been performed.

Rhinovirus

Vapendavir (Aviragen Therapeutics, Alpharetta, GA, USA) is an oral antiviral that attaches to the viral capsid preventing release of RNA into the cells. It has activity against RhV type A and B (Shahani et al., 2017).Vapendavir has reduced clinical symptoms in asthmatic adults. It was well-tolerated and there were no serious adverse events reported (Matz, 2013).

Coronavirus

Treatment of coronavirus will require broadly active compounds designed to quickly respond to new zoonotic epidemics of pathogenic coronaviruses. There are several steps in coronavirus life cycle where antiviral agents could be implemented (Pyrc et al., 2007). Adedeji et al. reported different strategies under development to block viral entry of SARS-CoV (Adedeji et al., 2013).

Adoptive T Cell Therapy

Adoptive transfer of specific T cells is a promising approach as technologies for isolation and expansion become widely available (Englund et al., 2011; Gerdemann et al., 2012; Heslop and Leen, 2013; Leen et al., 2014; Baugh et al., 2018). There are two main limitations to immunotherapy strategies for respiratory viruses. One is that, with the exception of influenza, knowledge of viral immunology is less complete than for CMV and EBV. A second limitation is logistic in that these viruses cause the greatest morbidity in the early post transplantation period, and it may not be feasible to generate CTLs in time to cover this period of high risk. However, Aguayo-Hiraldo et al. successfully expanded and use PIV specific T cells (Aguayo-Hiraldo et al., 2017).The same group generated HMPV specific T cells for adoptive transfer in patients after allogeneic HCT (Tzannou et al., 2017). Finally, multivirus-specific lymphocytes for the RSV and Influenza have shown promising results (Gerdemann et al., 2012).

CONCLUSION

Immunocompromised patients remain vulnerable to respiratory viral infections. Risk of severe LRTI and increased mortality are a common characteristic. Hematological malignancies and HCT recipients bear most of the burden of these viruses. Age, baseline diagnosis, use of steroids, lymphopenia, and early onset after transplant are shared risk factors for LRTI and mortality. Higher viral load has been associated with risk of LRTI in some studies. Early diagnosis can help prevent further spread of these viruses and prompt supportive measures and antivirals when indicated. However, management of these infections remains challenging. Clinical symptoms are not always reliable and progression to LRTI can happen within days of onset of symptoms. In addition, most patients have prolonged viral shedding, making both clinical evolution and molecular testing insufficient to guide length of therapy. Persistently positive tests often lead to concerns of resistant viral strains given the high within host viral diversification that occurs in these patients. There are limited antiviral options available mostly for influenza and to some extent RSV. These problems highlight the need for objective biomarkers that could help guide therapy. Standardization of valid assays to assess viral load will provide unbiased and reproducible measures that could be universally applied to the management of respiratory viral infections in immunocompromised patients. Immune monitoring assays assessing IFN-γ producing T cells against specific antigens are gaining interest in the field of systemic viral infection. A set of objective and validated tools related to the host-viral interaction (such as viral load and specific immune response) could lead to parameters that will significantly impact decision making on how to approach and monitor therapeutic options in immunocompromised patients with respiratory viral infections. Having early objective predictors of adverse outcomes could identify children at highest risk for LRTI and death, directing treatment more specifically and in a timelier manner than is currently possible with potential benefits of increased pediatric survival.

AUTHOR CONTRIBUTIONS

DH performed the search and literature review. DH, GM, and RH wrote the manuscript. All authors approved the final version of the manuscript.

REFERENCES

AAP (2014a). Updated guidance for palivizumab prophylaxis among infants and young children at increased risk of hospitalization for respiratory syncytial virus infection. *Pediatrics* 134, e620–e638. doi: 10.1542/peds.2014-1666

AAP (2014b). Updated guidance for palivizumab prophylaxis among infants and young children at increased risk of hospitalization for respiratory syncytial virus infection. *Pediatrics* 134, 415–420. doi: 10.1542/peds.2014-1665

AAP (2018). Recommendations for prevention and control of influenza in children, 2018–2019. *Pediatrics* 140:e20172550. doi: 10.1542/peds.2017-2550

Abandeh, F. I., Lustberg, M., Devine, S., Elder, P., Andritsos, L., and Martin, S. I. (2013). Outcomes of hematopoietic stem cell transplant recipients with rhinovirus infection: a matched, case-control study. *Bone Marrow Transplant.* 48, 1554–1557. doi: 10.1038/bmt.2013.100

Ablynx (2016). *Inhaled ALX-0171: Phase I/IIa Study in 53 hospitalised RSV-Infected Children [Online].* Available online at: http://www.ablynx.com/uploads/data/files/ablynx_alx-0171_first-in-infant%20study%20results_webcast%20presentation.pdf [Accessed].

Adderson, E., Branum, K., Sealy, R. E., Jones, B. G., Surman, S. L., Penkert, R., et al. (2015). Safety and immunogenicity of an intranasal Sendai virus-based human parainfluenza virus type 1 vaccine in 3- to 6-year-old children. *Clin. Vaccine Immunol.* 22, 298–303. doi: 10.1128/cvi.00618-14

Adedeji, A. O., Severson, W., Jonsson, C., Singh, K., Weiss, S. R., and Sarafianos, S. G. (2013). Novel inhibitors of severe acute respiratory syndrome coronavirus entry that act by three distinct mechanisms. *J. Virol.* 87, 8017–8028. doi: 10.1128/jvi.00998-13

Aguayo-Hiraldo, P. I., Arasaratnam, R. J., Tzannou, I., Kuvalekar, M., Lulla, P., Naik, S., et al. (2017). Characterizing the cellular immune response to parainfluenza virus 3. *J. Infect. Dis.* 216, 153–161. doi: 10.1093/infdis/jix203

Ambrose, C. S., and McLaurin, K. K. (2015). The medicaid cost of palivizumab. *J. Pediatr. Infect. Dis. Soc.* 4, 83–84. doi: 10.1093/jpids/piu025

Appiah, G. D., Blanton, L., D'Mello, T., Kniss, K., Smith, S., Mustaquim, D., et al. (2015). Influenza activity - United States, 2014-15 season and composition of the 2015-16 influenza vaccine. *MMWR Morb. Mortal. Wkly. Rep.* 64, 583–590.

Azadeh, N., Sakata, K. K., Brighton, A. M., Vikram, H. R., and Grys, T. E. (2015). FilmArray respiratory panel assay: comparison of nasopharyngeal swabs and bronchoalveolar lavage samples. *J. Clin. Microbiol.* 53, 3784–3787. doi: 10.1128/jcm.01516-15

Battles, M. B., Langedijk, J. P., Furmanova-Hollenstein, P., Chaiwatpongsakorn, S., Costello, H. M., Kwanten, L., et al. (2016). Molecular mechanism of respiratory syncytial virus fusion inhibitors. *Nat. Chem. Biol.* 12, 87–93. doi: 10.1038/nchembio.1982

Baugh, K. A., Tzannou, I., and Leen, A. M. (2018). Infusion of cytotoxic T lymphocytes for the treatment of viral infections in hematopoetic stem cell transplant patients. *Curr. Opin. Infect. Dis.* 31, 292–300. doi: 10.1097/qco.0000000000000456

Beck, C. R., McKenzie, B. C., Hashim, A. B., Harris, R. C., and Nguyen-Van-Tam, J. S. (2012). Influenza vaccination for immunocompromised patients: systematic review and meta-analysis by etiology. *J. Infect. Dis.* 206, 1250–1259. doi: 10.1093/infdis/jis487

Bednarska, K., Hallmann-Szelinska, E., Kondratiuk, K., and Brydak, L. B. (2015). Evaluation of the activity of influenza and influenza-like viruses in the epidemic season 2013/2014. *Adv. Exp. Med. Biol.* 857, 1–7. doi: 10.1007/5584_2015_116

Biopharma, A. (2017). *Ansun BioPharma Announces Breakthrough Designation for Its Experimental Drug DAS181 [Online].* Available online at: http://www.ansunbiopharma.com/news/ (Accessed September 3, 2018).

Boeckh, M., Englund, J., Li, Y., Miller, C., Cross, A., Fernandez, H., et al. (2007). Randomized controlled multicenter trial of aerosolized ribavirin for respiratory syncytial virus upper respiratory tract infection in hematopoietic cell transplant recipients. *Clin. Infect. Dis.* 44, 245–249. doi: 10.1086/509930

Boeckh, M., and Englund, J. A. (2010). Evaluation of therapeutics for RSV: an important step forward. *Am. J. Respir. Crit. Care Med.* 182, 1217–1219. doi: 10.1164/rccm.201008-1230ED

Buckingham, S. C., Bush, A. J., and Devincenzo, J. P. (2000). Nasal quantity of respiratory syncytical virus correlates with disease severity in hospitalized infants. *Pediatr. Infect. Dis. J.* 19, 113–117. doi: 10.1097/00006454-200002000-00006

Byrn, R. A., Jones, S. M., Bennett, H. B., Bral, C., Clark, M. P., Jacobs, M. D., et al. (2015). Preclinical activity of VX-787, a first-in-class, orally bioavailable inhibitor of the influenza virus polymerase PB2 subunit. *Antimicrob. Agents Chemother.* 59, 1569–1582. doi: 10.1128/aac.04623-14

Caliendo, A. M. (2011). Multiplex PCR and emerging technologies for the detection of respiratory pathogens. *Clin. Infect. Dis.* 52(Suppl. 4), S326–S330. doi: 10.1093/cid/cir047

Campbell, A. P., Guthrie, K. A., Englund, J. A., Farney, R. M., Minerich, E. L., Kuypers, J., et al. (2015). Clinical outcomes associated with respiratory virus detection before allogeneic hematopoietic stem cell transplant. *Clin. Infect. Dis.* 61, 192–202. doi: 10.1093/cid/civ272

Capella, C., Chaiwatpongsakorn, S., Gorrell, E., Risch, Z. A., Ye, F., Mertz, S. E., et al. (2017). Prefusion F, postfusion F, G antibodies, and disease severity in infants and young children with acute respiratory syncytial virus infection. *J. Infect. Dis.* 216, 1398–1406. doi: 10.1093/infdis/jix489

Carr, S., Allison, K. J., Van De Velde, L. A., Zhang, K., English, E. Y., Iverson, A., et al. (2011a). Safety and immunogenicity of live attenuated and inactivated influenza vaccines in children with cancer. *J. Infect. Dis.* 204, 1475–1482. doi: 10.1093/infdis/jir561

Carr, S., Ilyushina, N. A., Franks, J., Adderson, E. E., Caniza, M., Govorkova, E. A., et al. (2011b). Oseltamivir-resistant influenza A and B viruses pre- and postantiviral therapy in children and young adults with cancer. *Pediatr. Infect. Dis. J.* 30, 284–288. doi: 10.1097/INF.0b013e3181ff863b

Caserta, M. T., Qiu, X., Tesini, B., Wang, L., Murphy, A., Corbett, A., et al. (2017). Development of a global respiratory severity score for respiratory syncytial virus infection in infants. *J. Infect. Dis.* 215, 750–756. doi: 10.1093/infdis/jiw624

Casper, C., Englund, J., and Boeckh, M. (2010). How I treat influenza in patients with hematologic malignancies. *Blood* 115, 1331–1342. doi: 10.1182/blood-2009-11-255455

Chalkias, S., Mackenzie, M. R., Gay, C., Dooley, C., Marty, F. M., Moss, R. B., et al. (2014). DAS181 treatment of hematopoietic stem cell transplant patients with parainfluenza virus lung disease requiring mechanical ventilation. *Transpl. Infect. Dis.* 16, 141–144. doi: 10.1111/tid.12177

Chaparro, C., Scavuzzo, M., Winton, T., Keshavjee, S., and Kesten, S. (1997). Status of lung transplant recipients surviving beyond five years. *J. Heart Lung Transplant.* 16, 511–516.

Chemaly, R. F., Aitken, S. L., Wolfe, C. R., Jain, R., and Boeckh, M. J. (2016). Aerosolized ribavirin: the most expensive drug for pneumonia. *Transpl. Infect. Dis.* 18, 634–636. doi: 10.1111/tid.12551

Chemaly, R. F., Ghosh, S., Bodey, G. P., Rohatgi, N., Safdar, A., Keating, M. J., et al. (2006). Respiratory viral infections in adults with hematologic malignancies and human stem cell transplantation recipients: a retrospective study at a major cancer center. *Medicine* 85, 278–287. doi: 10.1097/01.md.0000232560.22098.4e

Chemaly, R. F., Hanmod, S. S., Rathod, D. B., Ghantoji, S. S., Jiang, Y., Doshi, A., et al. (2012). The characteristics and outcomes of parainfluenza virus infections in 200 patients with leukemia or recipients of hematopoietic stem cell transplantation. *Blood* 119, 2738–2745; quiz 2969. doi: 10.1182/blood-2011-08-371112

Chemaly, R. F., Shah, D. P., and Boeckh, M. J. (2014). Management of respiratory viral infections in hematopoietic cell transplant recipients and patients with hematologic malignancies. *Clin. Infect. Dis.* 59(Suppl. 5), S344–S351. doi: 10.1093/cid/ciu623

Chen, Y. B., Driscoll, J. P., McAfee, S. L., Spitzer, T. R., Rosenberg, E. S., Sanders, R., et al. (2011). Treatment of parainfluenza 3 infection with DAS181 in a patient after allogeneic stem cell transplantation. *Clin. Infect. Dis.* 53, e77–e80. doi: 10.1093/cid/cir501

Choi, S. M., Boudreault, A. A., Xie, H., Englund, J. A., Corey, L., and Boeckh, M. (2011). Differences in clinical outcomes after 2009 influenza A/H1N1 and seasonal influenza among hematopoietic cell transplant recipients. *Blood* 117, 5050–5056. doi: 10.1182/blood-2010-11-319186

Chu, H. Y., Chin, J., Pollard, J., Zerr, D. M., and Englund, J. A. (2016). Clinical outcomes in outpatient respiratory syncytial virus infection in immunocompromised children. *Influenza Other Respir. Viruses* 10, 205–210. doi: 10.1111/irv.12375

Clark, M. P., Ledeboer, M. W., Davies, I., Byrn, R. A., Jones, S. M., Perola, E., et al. (2014). Discovery of a novel, first-in-class, orally bioavailable azaindole inhibitor (VX-787) of influenza PB2. *J. Med. Chem.* 57, 6668–6678. doi: 10.1021/jm5007275

Coates, M., Brookes, D., Kim, Y. I., Allen, H., Fordyce, E. A. F., Meals, E. A., et al. (2017). Preclinical characterization of PC786, an inhaled small-molecule respiratory syncytial virus L protein polymerase inhibitor. *Antimicrob. Agents Chemother.* 61:e00737-17. doi: 10.1128/aac.00737-17

Couch, R. B., Englund, J. A., and Whimbey, E. (1997). Respiratory viral infections in immunocompetent and immunocompromised persons. *Am. J. Med.* 102, 2–9; discussion 25–26.

Couturier, B. A., Bender, J. M., Schwarz, M. A., Pavia, A. T., Hanson, K. E., and She, R. C. (2010). Oseltamivir-resistant influenza A 2009 H1N1 virus in immunocompromised patients. *Influenza Other Respir. Viruses* 4, 199–204. doi: 10.1111/j.1750-2659.2010.00144.x

Damlaj, M., Bartoo, G., Gijima, D., Hashmi, S., Litzow, M. R., Hogan, W., et al. (2015). Oral ribavirin for the treatment of respiratory syncytial virus infection in allogeneic stem cell transplant recipients-utility of the immunodeficiency scoring index for risk stratification. *Biol. Blood Marrow Transplant.* 21, S173–S174. doi: 10.1016/j.bbmt.2014.11.255

de Fontbrune, F. S., Robin, M., Porcher, R., Scieux, C., de Latour, R. P., Ferry, C., et al. (2007). Palivizumab treatment of respiratory syncytial virus infection after allogeneic hematopoietic stem cell transplantation. *Clin. Infect. Dis.* 45, 1019–1024. doi: 10.1086/521912

de Jong, M. D., Ison, M. G., Monto, A. S., Metev, H., Clark, C., O'Neil, B., et al. (2014). Evaluation of intravenous peramivir for treatment of influenza in hospitalized patients. *Clin. Infect. Dis.* 59, e172–e185. doi: 10.1093/cid/ciu632

Deffrasnes, C., Hamelin, M. E., Prince, G. A., and Boivin, G. (2008). Identification and evaluation of a highly effective fusion inhibitor for human metapneumovirus. *Antimicrob. Agents Chemother.* 52, 279–287. doi: 10.1128/aac.00793-07

DeVincenzo, J., Lambkin-Williams, R., Wilkinson, T., Cehelsky, J., Nochur, S., Walsh, E., et al. (2010). A randomized, double-blind, placebo-controlled study of an RNAi-based therapy directed against respiratory syncytial virus. *Proc. Natl. Acad. Sci. U.S.A.* 107, 8800–8805. doi: 10.1073/pnas.0912186107

Devincenzo, J. P. (2004). Natural infection of infants with respiratory syncytial virus subgroups A and B: a study of frequency, disease severity, and viral load. *Pediatr. Res.* 56, 914–917. doi: 10.1203/01.Pdr.0000145255.86117.6a

DeVincenzo, J. P., Aitken, J., and Harrison, L. (2003). Respiratory syncytial virus (RSV) loads in premature infants with and without prophylactic RSV fusion protein monoclonal antibody *J. Pediatr.* 143, 123–126. doi: 10.1016/s0022-3476(03)00213-0

DeVincenzo, J. P., and Buckingham, S. C. (2002). Relationship between respiratory syncytial virus load and illness severity in children. *J. Infect. Dis.* 186, 1376–1377; author reply 1377. doi: 10.1086/344331

DeVincenzo, J. P., El Saleeby, C. M., and Bush, A. J. (2005). Respiratory syncytial virus load predicts disease severity in previously healthy infants. *J. Infect. Dis.* 191, 1861–1868. doi: 10.1086/430008

DeVincenzo, J. P., McClure, M. W., Symons, J. A., Fathi, H., Westland, C., Chanda, S., et al. (2015). Activity of oral ALS-008176 in a respiratory syncytial virus challenge study. *N. Engl. J. Med.* 373, 2048–2058 doi: 10.1056/NEJMoa1413275

DeVincenzo, J. P., Whitley, R. J., Mackman, R. L., Scaglioni-Weinlich, C., Harrison, L., Farrell, E., et al. (2014). Oral GS-5806 activity in a respiratory syncytial virus challenge study. *N. Engl. J. Med.* 371, 711–722. doi: 10.1056/NEJMoa1401184

Domachowske, J. B., and Rosenberg, H. F. (1999). Respiratory syncytial virus infection: immune response, immunopathogenesis, and treatment. *Clin. Microbiol. Rev.* 12, 298–309.

Douglas, J. L., Panis, M. L., Ho, E., Lin, K. Y., Krawczyk, S. H., Grant, D. M., et al. (2005). Small molecules VP-14637 and JNJ-2408068 inhibit respiratory syncytial virus fusion by similar mechanisms. *Antimicrob. Agents Chemother.* 49, 2460–2466. doi: 10.1128/aac.49.6.2460-2466.2005

Drozd, D. R., Limaye, A. P., Moss, R. B., Sanders, R. L., Hansen, C., Edelman, J. D., et al. (2013). DAS181 treatment of severe parainfluenza type 3 pneumonia in a lung transplant recipient. *Transpl. Infect. Dis.* 15, E28–32. doi: 10.1111/tid.12045

Dykewicz, C. A. (2001). Guidelines for preventing opportunistic infections among hematopoietic stem cell transplant recipients: focus on community respiratory virus infections. *Biol. Blood Marrow Transplant.* 7(Suppl.), 19s–22s. doi: 10.1053/bbmt.2001.v7.pm11777100

El Chaer, F., Shah, D. P., Kmeid, J., Ariza-Heredia, E. J., Hosing, C. M., Mulanovich, V. E., et al. (2017). Burden of human metapneumovirus infections in patients with cancer: risk factors and outcomes. *Cancer* 123, 2329–2337. doi: 10.1002/cncr.30599

El Saleeby, C. M., Bush, A. J., Harrison, L. M., Aitken, J. A., and Devincenzo, J. P. (2011). Respiratory syncytial virus load, viral dynamics, and disease severity in previously healthy naturally infected children. *J. Infect. Dis.* 204, 996–1002. doi: 10.1093/infdis/jir494

El Saleeby, C. M., Somes, G. W., DeVincenzo, J. P., and Gaur, A. H. (2008). Risk factors for severe respiratory syncytial virus disease in children with cancer: the importance of lymphopenia and young age. *Pediatrics* 121, 235–243. doi: 10.1542/peds.2007-1102

Engelhard, D., Mohty, B., de la Camara, R., Cordonnier, C., and Ljungman, P. (2013). European guidelines for prevention and management of influenza in hematopoietic stem cell transplantation and leukemia patients: summary of ECIL-4 (2011), on behalf of ECIL, a joint venture of EBMT, EORTC, ICHS, and ELN. *Transpl. Infect. Dis.* 15, 219–232. doi: 10.1111/tid.12054

Engelhard, D., Nagler, A., Hardan, I., Morag, A., Aker, M., Baciu, H., et al. (1993). Antibody response to a two-dose regimen of influenza vaccine in allogeneic T cell-depleted and autologous BMT recipients. *Bone Marrow Transplant.* 11, 1–5.

Englund, J., Feuchtinger, T., and Ljungman, P. (2011). Viral infections in immunocompromised patients. *Biol. Blood Marrow Transplant.* 17, S2–S5. doi: 10.1016/j.bbmt.2010.11.008

Englund, J. A. (2001). Diagnosis and epidemiology of community-acquired respiratory virus infections in the immunocompromised host. *Biol. Blood Marrow Transplant.* 7(Suppl.), 2s–4s. doi: 10.1053/bbmt.2001.v7.pm11777101

Englund, J. A., Piedra, P. A., Ahn, Y. M., Gilbert, B. E., and Hiatt, P. (1994). High-dose, short-duration ribavirin aerosol therapy compared with standard ribavirin therapy in children with suspected respiratory syncytial virus infection. *J. Pediatr.* 125, 635–641.

Englund, J. A., Piedra, P. A., Jefferson, L. S., Wilson, S. Z., Taber, L. H., and Gilbert, B. E. (1990). High-dose, short-duration ribavirin aerosol therapy in children with suspected respiratory syncytial virus infection. *J. Pediatr.* 117(2 Pt 1), 313–320.

Englund, J. A., Piedra, P. A., Jewell, A., Patel, K., Baxter, B. B., and Whimbey, E. (1996). Rapid diagnosis of respiratory syncytial virus infections in immunocompromised adults. *J. Clin. Microbiol.* 34, 1649–1653.

Englund, J. A., Whimbey, E., and Atmar, R. L. (1999). Diagnosis of respiratory viruses in cancer and transplant patients. *Curr. Clin. Top. Infect. Dis.* 19, 30–59.

Erard, V., Chien, J. W., Kim, H. W., Nichols, W. G., Flowers, M. E., Martin, P. J., et al. (2006). Airflow decline after myeloablative allogeneic hematopoietic cell transplantation: the role of community respiratory viruses. *J. Infect. Dis.* 193, 1619–1625. doi: 10.1086/504268

Espinosa-Aguilar, L., Green, J. S., Forrest, G. N., Ball, E. D., Maziarz, R. T., Strasfeld, L., et al. (2011). Novel H1N1 influenza in hematopoietic stem cell transplantation recipients: two centers' experiences. *Biol. Blood Marrow Transplant.* 17, 566–573. doi: 10.1016/j.bbmt.2010.07.018

Falsey, A. R., Koval, C., DeVincenzo, J. P., and Walsh, E. E. (2017). Compassionate use experience with high-titer respiratory syncytical virus (RSV) immunoglobulin in RSV-infected immunocompromised persons. *Transpl. Infect. Dis.* 19:e12657. doi: 10.1111/tid.12657

FDA (2018). *FDA Approves New Drug to Treat Influenza* [Online]. U.S. Food and Drug Administration. Available online at: https://www.fda.gov/NewsEvents/Newsroom/PressAnnouncements/ucm624226.htm (Accessed October 25, 2018).

Fiore, A. E., Fry, A., Shay, D., Gubareva, L., Bresee, J. S., and Uyeki, T. M. (2011). Antiviral agents for the treatment and chemoprophylaxis of influenza — recommendations of the Advisory Committee on Immunization Practices (ACIP). *MMWR Recomm. Rep.* 60, 1–24.

Fisher, B. T., Danziger-Isakov, L., Sweet, L. R., Munoz, F. M., Maron, G., Tuomanen, E., et al. (2017). A multicenter consortium to define the epidemiology and outcomes of inpatient respiratory viral infections in pediatric hematopoietic stem cell transplant recipients. *J. Pediatric Infect. Dis. Soc.* 7, 275–282. doi: 10.1093/jpids/pix051

Foolad, F., Aitken, S. L., Shigle, T. L., Prayag, A., Ghantoji, S. S., Ariza-Heredia, E. J., et al. (2018). Impact of ribavirin formulation and host risk factors on 90-day mortality in Hematopoietic Cell Transplant (HCT) patients with RSV infection. *Biol. Blood Marrow Transplant.* 24, S369–S370. doi: 10.1016/j.bbmt.2017.12.451

Foolad, F., Prayag, A., Ghantoji, S. S., Ariza-Heredia, E. J., and Chemaly, R. F. (2017). Use of oral ribavirin for the treatment of RSV infections in Hematopoietic Cell Transplant (HCT) recipients. *Biol. Blood Marrow Transplant.* 23: S189. doi: 10.1016/j.bbmt.2016.12.367

Fraaij, P. L., Schutten, M., Javouhey, E., Burleigh, L., Outlaw, R., Kumar, D., et al. (2015). Viral shedding and susceptibility to oseltamivir in hospitalized immunocompromised patients with influenza in the Influenza Resistance Information Study (IRIS). *Antivir. Ther.* 20, 633–642. doi: 10.3851/imp2957

Franz, A., Adams, O., Willems, R., Bonzel, L., Neuhausen, N., Schweizer-Krantz, S., et al. (2010). Correlation of viral load of respiratory pathogens and co-infections with disease severity in children hospitalized for lower respiratory tract infection. *J. Clin. Virol.* 48, 239–245. doi: 10.1016/j.jcv.2010.05.007

Fuller, J. A., Njenga, M. K., Bigogo, G., Aura, B., Ope, M. O., Nderitu, L., et al. (2013). Association of the CT values of real-time PCR of viral upper respiratory tract infection with clinical severity, Kenya. *J. Med. Virol.* 85, 924–932. doi: 10.1002/jmv.23455

Gerdemann, U., Keirnan, J. M., Katari, U. L., Yanagisawa, R., Christin, A. S., Huye, L. E., et al. (2012). Rapidly generated multivirus-specific cytotoxic T lymphocytes for the prophylaxis and treatment of viral infections. *Mol. Ther.* 20, 1622–1632. doi: 10.1038/mt.2012.130

Gerna, G., Campanini, G., Rognoni, V., Marchi, A., Rovida, F., Piralla, A., et al. (2008). Correlation of viral load as determined by real-time RT-PCR and clinical characteristics of respiratory syncytial virus lower respiratory tract infections in early infancy. *J. Clin. Virol.* 41, 45–48. doi: 10.1016/j.jcv.2007.10.018

Ghosh, S., Champlin, R. E., Englund, J., Giralt, S. A., Rolston, K., Raad, I., et al. (2000). Respiratory syncytial virus upper respiratory tract illnesses in adult blood and marrow transplant recipients: combination therapy with aerosolized ribavirin and intravenous immunoglobulin. *Bone Marrow Transplant.* 25, 751–755. doi: 10.1038/sj.bmt.1702228

Gilchrist, C. A., Turner, S. D., Riley, M. F., Petri, W. A. Jr., and Hewlett, E. L. (2015). Whole-genome sequencing in outbreak analysis. *Clin. Microbiol. Rev.* 28, 541–563. doi: 10.1128/cmr.00075-13

Greenberg, S. B. (2011). Update on rhinovirus and coronavirus infections. *Semin. Respir. Crit. Care Med.* 32, 433–446. doi: 10.1055/s-0031-1283283

Greninger, A. L., Zerr, D. M., Qin, X., Adler, A. L., Sampoleo, R., Kuypers, J. M., et al. (2017). Rapid metagenomic next-generation sequencing during an investigation of hospital-acquired human parainfluenza virus 3 infections. *J. Clin. Microbiol.* 55, 177–182. doi: 10.1128/jcm.01881-16

Gruber, W. C., Wilson, S. Z., Throop, B. J., and Wyde, P. R. (1987). Immunoglobulin administration and ribavirin therapy: efficacy in respiratory syncytial virus infection of the cotton rat. *Pediatr. Res.* 21, 270–274. doi: 10.1203/00006450-198703000-00013

Guzmán-Suarez, B. B., Buckley, M. W., Gilmore, E. T., Vocca, E., Moss, R., Marty, F. M., et al. (2012). Clinical potential of DAS181 for treatment of parainfluenza-3 infections in transplant recipients. *Transpl. Infect. Dis.* 14, 427–433. doi: 10.1111/j.1399-3062.2012.00718.x

Haffizulla, J., Hartman, A., Hoppers, M., Resnick, H., Samudrala, S., Ginocchio, C., et al. (2014). Effect of nitazoxanide in adults and adolescents with acute uncomplicated influenza: a double-blind, randomised, placebo-controlled, phase 2b/3 trial. *Lancet Infect. Dis.* 14, 609–618. doi: 10.1016/s1473-3099(14)70717-0

Hakim, H., Allison, K. J., Van de Velde, L. A., Tang, L., Sun, Y., Flynn, P. M., et al. (2016a). Immunogenicity and safety of high-dose trivalent inactivated influenza vaccine compared to standard-dose vaccine in children and young adults with cancer or HIV infection. *Vaccine* 34, 3141–3148. doi: 10.1016/j.vaccine.2016.04.053

Hakim, H., Dallas, R., Zhou, Y., Pei, D., Cheng, C., Flynn, P. M., et al. (2016b). Acute respiratory infections in children and adolescents with acute lymphoblastic leukemia. *Cancer* 122, 798–805. doi: 10.1002/cncr.29833

Hakki, M., Strasfeld, L. M., and Townes, J. M. (2014). Predictive value of testing nasopharyngeal samples for respiratory viruses in the setting of lower respiratory tract disease. *J. Clin. Microbiol.* 52, 4020–4022. doi: 10.1128/jcm.01944-14

Hall, C. B. (2001). Respiratory syncytial virus and parainfluenza virus. *N. Engl. J. Med.* 344, 1917–1928. doi: 10.1056/nejm200106213442507

Hall, C. B., Simoes, E. A., and Anderson, L. J. (2013). Clinical and epidemiologic features of respiratory syncytial virus. *Curr. Top. Microbiol. Immunol.* 372, 39–57. doi: 10.1007/978-3-642-38919-1_2

Hall, C. B., Walsh, E. E., Schnabel, K. C., Long, C. E., McConnochie, K. M., Hildreth, S. W., et al. (1990). Occurrence of groups A and B of respiratory syncytial virus over 15 years: associated epidemiologic and clinical characteristics in hospitalized and ambulatory children. *J. Infect. Dis.* 162, 1283–1290.

Hall, C. B., Weinberg, G. A., Iwane, M. K., Blumkin, A. K., Edwards, K. M., Staat, M. A., et al. (2009). The burden of respiratory syncytial virus infection in young children. *N. Engl. J. Med.* 360, 588–598. doi: 10.1056/NEJMoa0804877

Hamada, N., Imamura, Y., Hara, K., Kashiwagi, T., Imamura, Y., Nakazono, Y., et al. (2012). Intrahost emergent dynamics of oseltamivir-resistant virus of pandemic influenza A (H1N1) 2009 in a fatally immunocompromised patient. *J. Infect. Chemother.* 18, 865–871. doi: 10.1007/s10156-012-0429-0

Hammond, S. P., Gagne, L. S., Stock, S. R., Marty, F. M., Gelman, R. S., Marasco, W. A., et al. (2012). Respiratory virus detection in immunocompromised patients with FilmArray respiratory panel compared to conventional methods. *J. Clin. Microbiol.* 50, 3216–3221. doi: 10.1128/jcm.00538-12

Hayden, F. G., Sugaya, N., Hirotsu, N., Lee, N., de Jong, M. D., Hurt, A. C., et al. (2018). Baloxavir marboxil for uncomplicated influenza in adults and adolescents. *N. Engl. J. Med.* 379, 913–923. doi: 10.1056/NEJMoa1716197

Hayden, R. T., Gu, Z., Rodriguez, A., Tanioka, L., Ying, C., Morgenstern, M., et al. (2012). Comparison of two broadly multiplexed PCR systems for viral detection in clinical respiratory tract specimens from immunocompromised children. *J. Clin. Virol.* 53, 308–313. doi: 10.1016/j.jcv.2011.12.020

Henrickson, K. J. (2003). Parainfluenza viruses. *Clin. Microbiol. Rev.* 16, 242–264. doi: 10.1128/CMR.16.2.242-264.2003

Heo, Y. A. (2018). Baloxavir: first global approval. *Drugs* 78, 693–697. doi: 10.1007/s40265-018-0899-1

Heslop, H. E., and Leen, A. M. (2013). T-cell therapy for viral infections. *Hematol. Am. Soc. Hematol. Educ. Program* 2013, 342–347. doi: 10.1182/asheducation-2013.1.342

Heylen, E., Neyts, J., and Jochmans, D. (2017). Drug candidates and model systems in respiratory syncytial virus antiviral drug discovery. *Biochem. Pharmacol.* 127, 1–12. doi: 10.1016/j.bcp.2016.09.014

Hirsch, H. H., Martino, R., Ward, K. N., Boeckh, M., Einsele, H., and Ljungman, P. (2013). Fourth European Conference on Infections in Leukaemia (ECIL-4): guidelines for diagnosis and treatment of human respiratory syncytial virus, parainfluenza virus, metapneumovirus, rhinovirus, and coronavirus. *Clin. Infect. Dis.* 56, 258–266. doi: 10.1093/cid/cis844

Hodinka, R. L. (2016). "Respiratory RNA Viruses," in *Diagnostic Microbiology of the Immunocompromised Host, 2nd Edn,* eds R. T. Hayden, D. M. Wolk, K. C. Carroll, and Y.-W. Tang (Washington, DC: American Society of Microbiology), 233–271.

Hoppe, B. P., de Jongh, E., Griffioen-Keijzer, A., Zijlstra-Baalbergen, J. M., IJzerman, E. P., and Baboe, F. (2016). Human metapneumovirus in haematopoietic stem cell transplantation recipients: a case series and review of the diagnostic and therapeutic approach. *Neth. J. Med.* 74, 336–341.

Houlihan, C. F., Frampton, D., Ferns, R. B., Raffle, J., Grant, P., Reidy, M., et al. (2018). Use of whole-genome sequencing in the investigation of a nosocomial influenza virus outbreak. *J. Infect. Dis.* 218, 1485–1489. doi: 10.1093/infdis/jiy335

Hutspardol, S., Essa, M., Richardson, S., Schechter, T., Ali, M., Krueger, J., et al. (2015). Significant transplantation-related mortality from respiratory virus infections within the first one hundred days in children after hematopoietic stem cell transplantation. *Biol. Blood Marrow Transplant.* 21, 1802–1807. doi: 10.1016/j.bbmt.2015.06.015

Ison, M. G. (2014). Optimum timing of oseltamivir: lessons from Bangladesh. *Lancet Infect. Dis.* 14, 88–89. doi: 10.1016/s1473-3099(13)70287-1

Ison, M. G., and Hayden, F. G. (2002). Viral infections in immunocompromised patients: what's new with respiratory viruses? *Curr. Opin. Infect. Dis.* 15, 355–367. doi: 10.1097/00001432-200208000-00002

Issa, N. C., Marty, F. M., Gagne, L. S., Koo, S., Verrill, K. A., Alyea, E. P., et al. (2011). Seroprotective titers against 2009 H1N1 influenza A virus after vaccination in allogeneic hematopoietic stem cell transplantation recipients. *Biol. Blood Marrow Transplant.* 17, 434–438. doi: 10.1016/j.bbmt.2010.10.002

Jacobs, S. E., Lamson, D. M., St George, K., and Walsh, T. J. (2013). Human rhinoviruses. *Clin. Microbiol. Rev.* 26, 135–162. doi: 10.1128/cmr.00077-12

Jorquera, P. A., and Tripp, R. A. (2017). Respiratory syncytial virus: prospects for new and emerging therapeutics. *Expert Rev. Respir. Med.* 11, 609–615. doi: 10.1080/17476348.2017.1338567

Kamboj, M., Gerbin, M., Huang, C. K., Brennan, C., Stiles, J., Balashov, S., et al. (2008). Clinical characterization of human metapneumovirus infection among patients with cancer. *J. Infect.* 57, 464–471. doi: 10.1016/j.jinf.2008.10.003

Karron, R. A., Wright, P. F., Hall, S. L., Makhene, M., Thompson, J., Burns, B. A., et al. (1995a). A live attenuated bovine parainfluenza virus type 3 vaccine is safe, infectious, immunogenic, and phenotypically stable in infants and children. *J. Infect. Dis.* 171, 1107–1114.

Karron, R. A., Wright, P. F., Newman, F. K., Makhene, M., Thompson, J., Samorodin, R., et al. (1995b). A live human parainfluenza type 3 virus vaccine is attenuated and immunogenic in healthy infants and children. *J. Infect. Dis.* 172, 1445–1450.

Kassis, C., Champlin, R. E., Hachem, R. Y., Hosing, C., Tarrand, J. J., Perego, C. A., et al. (2010) Detection and control of a nosocomial respiratory syncytial virus outbreak in a stem cell transplantation unit: the role of palivizumab. *Biol. Blood Marrow Transplant.* 16, 1265–1271. doi: 10.1016/j.bbmt.2010.03.011

Khanna, N., Steffen, I., Studt, J. D., Schreiber, A., Lehmann, T., Weisser, M., et al. (2009). Outcome of influenza infections in outpatients after allogeneic hematopoietic stem cell transplantation. *Transpl. Infect. Dis.* 11, 100–105. doi: 10.1111/j.1399-3062.2008.00362.x

Kim, Y. I., Pareek, R., Murphy, R., Harrison, L., Farrell, E., Cook, R., et al. (2017). The antiviral effects of RSV fusion inhibitor, MDT-637, on clinical isolates, vs its achievable concentrations in the human respiratory tract and comparison to ribavirin. *Influenza Other Respir. Viruses* 11, 525–530. doi: 10.1111/irv.12503

Kim, Y. J., Boeckh, M., and Englund, J. A. (2007). Community respiratory virus infections in immunocompromised patients: hematopoietic stem cell and solid organ transplant recipients, and individuals with human immunodeficiency virus infection. *Semin. Respir. Crit. Care Med.* 28, 222–242. doi: 10.1055/s-2007-976494

Kim, Y. J., Guthrie, K. A., Waghmare, A., Walsh, E. E., Falsey, A. R., Kuypers, J., et al. (2014). Respiratory syncytial virus in hematopoietic cell transplant recipients: factors determining progression to lower respiratory tract disease. *J. Infect. Dis.* 209, 1195–1204. doi: 10.1093/infdis/jit832

Kiso, M., Takahashi, K., Sakai-Tagawa, Y., Shinya, K., Sakabe, S., Le, Q. M., et al. (2010). T-705 (favipiravir) activity against lethal H5N1 influenza A viruses. *Proc. Natl. Acad. Sci. U.S.A.* 107, 882–887. doi: 10.1073/pnas.0909603107

Knight, V., Gilbert, B. E., Wyde, P. R., and Englund, J. A. (1991). High dose-short duration ribavirin aerosol treatment–a review. *Bull. Int. Union Tuberc. Lung Dis.* 66, 97–101.

Koszalka, P., Tilmanis, D., and Hurt, A. C. (2017). Influenza antivirals currently in late-phase clinical trial. *Influenza Other Respir. Viruses* 11, 240–246. doi: 10.1111/irv.12446

Kothari, A., Burgess, M. J., Crescencio, J. C. R., Kennedy, J. L., Denson, J. L., Schwalm, K. C., et al. (2017). The role of next generation sequencing in infection prevention in human parainfluenza virus 3 infections in immunocompromised patients. *J. Clin. Virol.* 92, 53–55. doi: 10.1016/j.jcv.2017.05.010

Kou, M., Hwang, V., and Ramkellawan, N. (2018). Bronchiolitis: From practice guideline to clinical practice. *Emerg. Med. Clin. North Am.* 36, 275–286. doi: 10.1016/j.emc.2017.12.006

Kumar, D., Ferreira, V. H., Blumberg, E., Silveira, F., Cordero, E., Perez-Romero, P., et al. (2018). A five-year prospective multi-center evaluation of influenza infection in transplant recipients. *Clin. Infect. Dis.* 67, 1322–1329. doi: 10.1093/cid/ciy294

Laplante, J., and St George, K. (2014). Antiviral resistance in influenza viruses: laboratory testing. *Clin. Lab. Med.* 34, 387–408. doi: 10.1016/j.cll.2014.02.010

Lee, N., Chan, P. K., Wong, C. K., Wong, K. T., Choi, K. W., Joynt, G. M., et al. (2011). Viral clearance and inflammatory response patterns in adults hospitalized for pandemic 2009 influenza A(H1N1) virus pneumonia. *Antivir. Ther.* 16, 237–247. doi: 10.3851/imp1722

Leen, A. M., Heslop, H. E., and Brenner, M. K. (2014). Antiviral T-cell therapy. *Immunol. Rev.* 258, 12–29. doi: 10.1111/imr.12138

Ljungman, P. (2012). Vaccination of immunocompromised patients. *Clin. Microbiol. Infect.* 18(Suppl. 5), 93–99. doi: 10.1111/j.1469-0691.2012.03971.x

Ljungman, P., de la Camara, R., Perez-Bercoff, L., Abecasis, M., Nieto Campuzano, J. B., Cannata-Ortiz, M. J., et al. (2011). Outcome of pandemic H1N1 infections in hematopoietic stem cell transplant recipients. *Haematologica* 96, 1231–1235. doi: 10.3324/haematol.2011.041913

Ljungman, P., Ward, K. N., Crooks, B. N., Parker, A., Martino, R., Shaw, P. J., et al. (2001). Respiratory virus infections after stem cell transplantation: a prospective study from the Infectious Diseases Working Party of the European Group for Blood and Marrow Transplantation. *Bone Marrow Transplant.* 28, 479–484. doi: 10.1038/sj.bmt.1703139

Loria, C., Domm, J. A., Halasa, N. B., Heitman, E., Miller, E. K., Xu, M., et al. (2015). Human rhinovirus C infections in pediatric hematology and oncology patients. *Pediatr. Transplant.* 19, 94–100. doi: 10.1111/petr.12383

Louie, J. K., Yang, S., Acosta, M., Yen, C., Samuel, M. C., Schechter, R., et al. (2012a). Treatment with neuraminidase inhibitors for critically ill patients with influenza A (H1N1)pdm09. *Clin. Infect. Dis.* 55, 1198–1204. doi: 10.1093/cid/cis636

Louie, J. K., Yang, S., Yen, C., Acosta, M., Schechter, R., and Uyeki, T. M. (2012b). Use of intravenous peramivir for treatment of severe influenza A(H1N1)pdm09. *PLoS ONE* 7:e40261. doi: 10.1371/journal.pone.0040261

Luján-Zilbermann, J., Benaim, E., Tong, X., Srivastava, D. K., Patrick, C. C., and DeVincenzo, J. P. (2001). Respiratory virus infections in pediatric hematopoietic stem cell transplantation. *Clin. Infect. Dis.* 33, 962–968. doi: 10.1086/322628

Lukens, M. V., van de Pol, A. C., Coenjaerts, F. E., Jansen, N. J., Kamp, V. M., Kimpen, J. L., et al. (2010). A systemic neutrophil response precedes robust CD8(+) T-cell activation during natural respiratory syncytial virus infection in infants. *J. Virol.* 84, 2374–2383. doi: 10.1128/jvi.01807-09

Machado, C. M., Cardoso, M. R., da Rocha, I. F., Boas, L. S., Dulley, F. L., and Pannuti, C. S. (2005). The benefit of influenza vaccination after bone marrow transplantation. *Bone Marrow Transplant.* 36, 897–900. doi: 10.1038/sj.bmt.1705159

Maeng, S. H., Yoo, H. S., Choi, S. H., Yoo, K. H., Kim, Y. J., Sung, K. W., et al. (2012). Impact of parainfluenza virus infection in pediatric cancer patients. *Pediatr. Blood Cancer* 59, 708–710. doi: 10.1002/pbc.23390

Mahony, J. B. (2008). Detection of respiratory viruses by molecular methods. *Clin. Microbiol. Rev.* 21, 716–747. doi: 10.1128/cmr.00037-07

Mahony, J. B., Petrich, A., and Smieja, M. (2011). Molecular diagnosis of respiratory virus infections. *Crit. Rev. Clin. Lab. Sci.* 48, 217–249. doi: 10.3109/10408363.2011.640976

Marjuki, H., Mishin, V. P., Sleeman, K., Okomo-Adhiambo, M., Sheu, T. G., Guo, L., et al. (2013). Bioluminescence-based neuraminidase inhibition assay for monitoring influenza virus drug susceptibility in clinical specimens. *Antimicrob. Agents Chemother.* 57, 5209–5215. doi: 10.1128/aac.01086-13

Martino, R., Porras, R. P., Rabella, N., Williams, J. V., Ramila, E., Margall, N., et al. (2005). Prospective study of the incidence, clinical features, and outcome of symptomatic upper and lower respiratory tract infections by respiratory viruses in adult recipients of hematopoietic stem cell transplants for hematologic malignancies. *Biol. Blood Marrow Transplant.* 11, 781–796. doi: 10.1016/j.bbmt.2005.07.007

Matz, J. (2013). Vapendavir significantly improves upper respiratory symptoms of naturally acquired rhinovirus infection in asthmatic adults: Results of a phase 2 clinical trial. *Eur. Respir. J.* 42(Suppl 57), 1493.

McLellan, J. S., Ray, W. C., and Peeples, M. E. (2013). Structure and function of respiratory syncytial virus surface glycoproteins. *Curr. Top. Microbiol. Immunol.* 372, 83–104. doi: 10.1007/978-3-642-38919-1_4

Meissner, H. C. (2016). Viral bronchiolitis in children. *N. Engl. J. Med.* 374, 62–72. doi: 10.1056/NEJMra1413456

Mejias, A., Garcia-Maurino, C., Rodriguez-Fernandez, R., Peeples, M. E., and Ramilo, O. (2017). Development and clinical applications of novel antibodies for prevention and treatment of respiratory syncytial virus infection. *Vaccine* 35, 496–502. doi: 10.1016/j.vaccine.2016.09.026

Melero, J. A., Mas, V., and McLellan, J. S. (2017). Structural, antigenic and immunogenic features of respiratory syncytial virus glycoproteins relevant for vaccine development. *Vaccine* 35, 461–468. doi: 10.1016/j.vaccine.2016.09.045

Milano, F., Campbell, A. P., Guthrie, K. A., Kuypers, J., Englund, J. A., Corey, L., et al. (2010). Human rhinovirus and coronavirus detection among allogeneic hematopoietic stem cell transplantation recipients. *Blood* 115, 2088–2094. doi: 10.1182/blood-2009-09-244152

Moss, R. B., Davey, R. T., Steigbigel, R. T., and Fang, F. (2010). Targeting pandemic influenza: a primer on influenza antivirals and drug resistance. *J. Antimicrob. Chemother.* 65, 1086–1093. doi: 10.1093/jac/dkq100

Moss, R. B., Hansen, C., Sanders, R. L., Hawley, S., Li, T., and Steigbigel, R. T. (2012). A phase II study of DAS181, a novel host directed antiviral for the treatment of influenza infection. *J. Infect. Dis.* 206, 1844–1851. doi: 10.1093/infdis/jis622

Mulrennan, S., Tempone, S. S., Ling, I. T., Williams, S. H., Gan, G. C., Murray, R. J., et al. (2010). Pandemic influenza (H1N1) 2009 pneumonia: CURB-65 score for predicting severity and nasopharyngeal sampling for diagnosis are unreliable. *PLoS ONE* 5:e12849. doi: 10.1371/journal.pone.0012849

Nichols, W. G., Corey, L., Gooley, T., Davis, C., and Boeckh, M. (2001). Parainfluenza virus infections after hematopoietic stem cell transplantation: risk factors, response to antiviral therapy, and effect on transplant outcome. *Blood* 98, 573–578. doi: 10.1182/blood.v98.3.573

Nichols, W. G., Guthrie, K. A., Corey, L., and Boeckh, M. (2004). Influenza infections after hematopoietic stem cell transplantation: risk factors, mortality, and the effect of antiviral therapy. *Clin. Infect. Dis.* 39, 1300–1306. doi: 10.1086/425004

Nicholson, K. G., Wood, J. M., and Zambon, M. (2003). Influenza. *Lancet* 362, 1733–1745. doi: 10.1016/s0140-6736(03)14854-4

Ogimi, C., Englund, J. A., Bradford, M. C., Qin, X., Boeckh, M., and Waghmare, A. (2018a). Characteristics and outcomes of coronavirus infection in children: the role of viral factors and an immunocompromised state. *J. Pediatric Infect. Dis. Soc.* pix093. doi: 10.1093/jpids/pix093

Ogimi, C., Greninger, A. L., Waghmare, A. A., Kuypers, J. M., Shean, R. C., Xie, H., et al. (2017a). Prolonged shedding of human coronavirus in hematopoietic cell transplant recipients: risk factors and viral genome evolution. *J. Infect. Dis.* 216, 203–209. doi: 10.1093/infdis/jix264

Ogimi, C., Waghmare, A. A., Kuypers, J. M., Xie, H., Yeung, C. C., Leisenring, W. M., et al. (2017b). Clinical significance of human coronavirus in bronchoalveolar lavage samples from hematopoietic cell transplant recipients and patients with hematologic malignancies. *Clin. Infect. Dis.* 64, 1532–1539. doi: 10.1093/cid/cix160

Ogimi, C., Xie, H., Leisenring, W. M., Kuypers, J. M., Jerome, K. R., Campbell, A. P., et al. (2018b). Initial high viral load is associated with prolonged shedding of human rhinovirus in allogeneic hematopoietic cell transplant recipients. *Biol. Blood Marrow Transplant.* 24, 2160–2163. doi: 10.1016/j.bbmt.2018.07.006

Okomo-Adhiambo, M., Fry, A. M., Su, S., Nguyen, H. T., Elal, A. A., Negron, E., et al. (2015). Oseltamivir-resistant influenza A(H1N1)pdm09 viruses, United States, 2013-14. *Emerging Infect. Dis.* 21, 136–141. doi: 10.3201/eid2101.141006

Okomo-Adhiambo, M., Nguyen, H. T., Abd Elal, A., Sleeman, K., Fry, A. M., and Gubareva, L. V. (2014). Drug susceptibility surveillance of influenza viruses circulating in the United States in 2011-2012: application of the WHO antiviral working group criteria. *Influenza Other Respir. Viruses* 8, 258–265. doi: 10.1111/irv.12215

Okomo-Adhiambo, M., Sheu, T. G., and Gubareva, L. V. (2013). Assays for monitoring susceptibility of influenza viruses to neuraminidase inhibitors. *Influenza Other Respir. Viruses* 7(Suppl. 1), 44–49. doi: 10.1111/irv.12051

Omoto, S., Speranzini, V., Hashimoto, T., Noshi, T., Yamaguchi, H., Kawai, M., et al. (2018). Characterization of influenza virus variants induced by treatment with the endonuclease inhibitor baloxavir marboxil. *Sci. Rep.* 8, 9633. doi: 10.1038/s41598-018-27890-4

Ottolini, M. G., Porter, D. D., Hemming, V. G., Zimmerman, M. N., Schwab, N. M., and Prince, G. A. (1999). Effectiveness of RSVIG prophylaxis and therapy of respiratory syncytial virus in an immunosuppressed animal model. *Bone Marrow Transplant.* 24, 41–45. doi: 10.1038/sj.bmt.1701813

Papenburg, J., and Boivin, G. (2010). The distinguishing features of human metapneumovirus and respiratory syncytial virus. *Rev. Med. Virol.* 20, 245–260. doi: 10.1002/rmv.651

Pasikhova, Y., Hayne, J., and Baluch, A. (2018). Oral Ribavirin for the Treatment of Respiratory Syncytial Virus (RSV) and Human Metapneumovirus (hMPV) Infections in Hematology Patients and Stem Cell Transplant (SCT) Recipients at a Nci-Designated Cancer Center. *Biol. Blood Marrow Transplant.* 24: S383. doi: 10.1016/j.bbmt.2017.12.471

Peck, A. J., Englund, J. A., Kuypers, J., Guthrie, K. A., Corey, L., Morrow, R., et al. (2007). Respiratory virus infection among hematopoietic cell transplant recipients: evidence for asymptomatic parainfluenza virus infection. *Blood* 110, 1681–1688. doi: 10.1182/blood-2006-12-060343

Popowitch, E. B., O'Neill, S. S., and Miller, M. B. (2013). Comparison of the Biofire FilmArray RP, Genmark eSensor RVP, Luminex xTAG RVPv1, and Luminex xTAG RVP fast multiplex assays for detection of respiratory viruses. *J. Clin. Microbiol.* 51, 1528–1533. doi: 10.1128/jcm.03368-12

Pyrc, K., Berkhout, B., and van der Hoek, L. (2007). Antiviral strategies against human coronaviruses. *Infect. Disord. Drug Targets* 7, 59–66. doi: 10.2174/187152607780090757

Raad, I., Abbas, J., and Whimbey, E. (1997). Infection control of nosocomial respiratory viral disease in the immunocompromised host. *Am. J. Med.* 102, 48–52; discussion 53–44.

Rand, K. H., Rampersaud, H., and Houck, H. J. (2011). Comparison of two multiplex methods for detection of respiratory viruses: filmArray RP and xTAG RVP. *J. Clin. Microbiol.* 49, 2449–2453. doi: 10.1128/jcm.02582-10

Renaud, C., Boudreault, A. A., Kuypers, J., Lofy, K. H., Corey, L., Boeckh, M. J., et al. (2011a). H275Y mutant pandemic (H1N1) 2009 virus in immunocompromised patients. *Emerg. Infect. Dis.* 17, 653–660; quiz 765. doi: 10.3201/eid1704.101429

Renaud, C., and Campbell, A. P. (2011). Changing epidemiology of respiratory viral infections in hematopoietic cell transplant recipients and solid organ transplant recipients. *Curr. Opin. Infect. Dis.* 24, 333–343. doi: 10.1097/QCO.0b013e3283480440

Renaud, C., and Englund, J. A. (2012). Antiviral therapy of respiratory viruses in haematopoietic stem cell transplant recipients. *Antivir. Ther.* 17, 175–191. doi: 10.3851/imp2060

Renaud, C., Kuypers, J., Aspesberro, F., Rosenfeld, M., and Englund, J. A. (2011c). Emergence of oseltamivir-resistant pandemic H1N1 in an immunocompetent child with severe status asthmaticus. *J. Asthma* 48, 572–575. doi: 10.3109/02770903.2011.582660

Renaud, C., Kuypers, J., and Englund, J. A. (2011b). Emerging oseltamivir resistance in seasonal and pandemic influenza A/H1N1. *J. Clin. Virol.* 52, 70–78. doi: 10.1016/j.jcv.2011.05.019

Renaud, C., Pergam, S. A., Polyak, C., Jain, R., Kuypers, J., Englund, J. A., et al. (2010). Early emergence of an H275Y mutation in a hematopoietic cell transplant recipient treated with intravenous peramivir. *Transpl. Infect. Dis.* 12, 513–517. doi: 10.1111/j.1399-3062.2010.00582.x

Renaud, C., Xie, H., Seo, S., Kuypers, J., Cent, A., Corey, L., et al. (2013). Mortality rates of human metapneumovirus and respiratory syncytial virus lower respiratory tract infections in hematopoietic cell transplantation recipients. *Biol. Blood Marrow Transplant.* 19, 1220–1226. doi: 10.1016/j.bbmt.2013.05.005

Rossey, I., McLellan, J. S., Saelens, X., and Schepens, B. (2018). Clinical potential of prefusion RSV F-specific antibodies. *Trends Microbiol.* 26, 209–219. doi: 10.1016/j.tim.2017.09.009

Rossignol, J. F. (2014). Nitazoxanide: a first-in-class broad-spectrum antiviral agent. *Antiviral Res.* 110, 94–103. doi: 10.1016/j.antiviral.2014.07.014

Roymans, D., Alnajjar, S. S., Battles, M. B., Sitthicharoenchai, P., Furmanova-Hollenstein, P., Rigaux, P., et al. (2017). Therapeutic efficacy of a respiratory syncytial virus fusion inhibitor. *Nat. Commun.* 8: 167. doi: 10.1038/s41467-017-00170-x

Rubin, L. G., Levin, M. J., Ljungman, P., Davies, E. G., Avery, R., Tomblyn, M., et al. (2014). 2013 IDSA clinical practice guideline for vaccination of the immunocompromised host. *Clin. Infect. Dis.* 58, 309–318. doi: 10.1093/cid/cit816

Salez, N., Vabret, A., Leruez-Ville, M., Andreoletti, L., Carrat, F., Renois, F., et al. (2015). Evaluation of four commercial multiplex molecular tests for the diagnosis of acute respiratory infections. *PLoS ONE* 10:e0130378. doi: 10.1371/journal.pone.0130378

Samuel, S., Nanjappa, S., Cooper, C. D., and Greene, J. N. (2016). Human metapneumovirus infection in immunocompromised patients. *Cancer Control* 23, 442–445. doi: 10.1177/107327481602300416

Schildgen, V., van den Hoogen, B., Fouchier, R., Tripp, R. A., Alvarez, R., Manoha, C., et al. (2011). Human metapneumovirus: lessons learned over the first decade. *Clin. Microbiol. Rev.* 24, 734–754. doi: 10.1128/cmr.00015-11

Seo, S., Campbell, A. P., Xie, H., Chien, J. W., Leisenring, W. M., Englund, J. A., et al. (2013). Outcome of respiratory syncytial virus lower respiratory tract disease in hematopoietic cell transplant recipients receiving aerosolized ribavirin: significance of stem cell source and oxygen requirement. *Biol. Blood Marrow Transplant.* 19, 589–596. doi: 10.1016/j.bbmt.2012.12.019

Seo, S., Gooley, T. A., Kuypers, J. M., Stednick, Z., Jerome, K. R., Englund, J. A., et al. (2016). Human metapneumovirus infections following hematopoietic cell transplantation: factors associated with disease progression. *Clin. Infect. Dis.* 63, 178–185. doi: 10.1093/cid/ciw284

Seo, S., Waghmare, A., Scott, E. M., Xie, H., Kuypers, J. M., Hackman, R. C., et al. (2017). Human rhinovirus detection in the lower respiratory tract of hematopoietic cell transplant recipients: association with mortality. *Haematologica* 102, 1120–1130. doi: 10.3324/haematol.2016.153767

Seo, S., Xie, H., Campbell, A. P., Kuypers, J. M., Leisenring, W. M., Englund, J. A., et al. (2014). Parainfluenza virus lower respiratory tract disease after hematopoietic cell transplant: viral detection in the lung predicts outcome. *Clin. Infect. Dis.* 58, 1357–1368. doi: 10.1093/cid/ciu134

Shah, D. P., Ghantoji, S. S., Ariza-Heredia, E. J., Shah, J. N., El Taoum, K. K., Shah, P. K., et al. (2014). Immunodeficiency scoring index to predict poor outcomes in hematopoietic cell transplant recipients with RSV infections. *Blood* 123, 3263–3268. doi: 10.1182/blood-2013-12-541359

Shah, D. P., Ghantoji, S. S., Azzi, J., Avadhanula, V., Kmeid, J., El Chaer, F., et al. (2016a). An open label, block-randomized, ribavirin efficacy trial for management of RSV infections in Hematopoietic Cell Transplant (HCT) recipients: clinical and economic implications. *Biol. Blood Marrow Transplant.* 22, S52–S53. doi: 10.1016/j.bbmt.2015.11.338

Shah, D. P., Ghantoji, S. S., Mulanovich, V. E., Ariza-heredia, E. J., and Chemaly, R. F. (2012). Management of respiratory viral infections in hematopoietic cell transplant recipients. *Am. J. Blood Res.* 2, 203–218.

Shah, D. P., Shah, P. K., Azzi, J. M., and Chemaly, R. F. (2016b). Parainfluenza virus infections in hematopoietic cell transplant recipients and hematologic malignancy patients: a systematic review. *Cancer Lett.* 370, 358–364. doi: 10.1016/j.canlet.2015.11.014

Shah, D. P., Shah, P. K., Azzi, J. M., El Chaer, F., and Chemaly, R. F. (2016c). Human metapneumovirus infections in hematopoietic cell transplant recipients and hematologic malignancy patients: a systematic review. *Cancer Lett.* 379, 100–106. doi: 10.1016/j.canlet.2016.05.035

Shah, J. N., and Chemaly, R. F. (2011). Management of RSV infections in adult recipients of hematopoietic stem cell transplantation. *Blood* 117, 2755–2763. doi: 10.1182/blood-2010-08-263400

Shahani, L., Ariza-Heredia, E. J., and Chemaly, R. F. (2017). Antiviral therapy for respiratory viral infections in immunocompromised patients. *Expert Rev. Anti Infect. Ther.* 15, 401–415. doi: 10.1080/14787210.2017.1279970

Sleeman, K., Mishin, V. P., Deyde, V. M., Furuta, Y., Klimov, A. I., and Gubareva, L. V. (2010). In vitro antiviral activity of favipiravir (T-705) against drug-resistant influenza and 2009 A(H1N1) viruses. *Antimicrob. Agents Chemother.* 54, 2517–2524. doi: 10.1128/aac.01739-09

Srinivasan, A., Wang, C., Yang, J., Inaba, H., Shenep, J. L., Leung, W. H., et al. (2011a). Parainfluenza virus infections in children with hematologic malignancies. *Pediatr. Infect. Dis. J.* 30, 855–859. doi: 10.1097/INF.0b013e31821d190f

Srinivasan, A., Wang, C., Yang, J., Shenep, J. L., Leung, W. H., and Hayden, R. T. (2011b). Symptomatic parainfluenza virus infections in children undergoing hematopoietic stem cell transplantation. *Biol. Blood Marrow Transplant.* 17, 1520–1527. doi: 10.1016/j.bbmt.2011.03.001

Stevens, M., Rusch, S., DeVincenzo, J., Kim, Y. I., Harrison, L., Meals, E. A., et al. (2018). Antiviral activity of oral JNJ-53718678 in healthy adult volunteers challenged with respiratory syncytial virus: a placebo-controlled study. *J. Infect. Dis.* 218, 748–756. doi: 10.1093/infdis/jiy227

Sykes, A., Gerhardt, E., Tang, L., and Adderson, E. E. (2017). The effectiveness of trivalent inactivated influenza vaccine in children with acute leukemia. *J. Pediatr.* 191, 218–224.e211. doi: 10.1016/j.jpeds.2017.08.071

Tamura, D., Okomo-Adhiambo, M., Mishin, V. P., Guo, Z., Xu, X., Villanueva, J., et al. (2015). Application of a seven-target pyrosequencing assay to improve the detection of neuraminidase inhibitor-resistant Influenza A(H3N2) viruses. *Antimicrob. Agents Chemother.* 59, 2374–2379. doi: 10.1128/aac.04939-14

Tantawy, A. A., Barakat, M. M., Adly, A. A., Ebeid, F. S., Shamaa, M. F., and Yassin, M. (2015). One-year prospective study of community acquired influenza and parainfluenza viral infections in hospitalized egyptian children with malignancy: single center experience. *Pediatr. Hematol. Oncol.* 32, 304–314. doi: 10.3109/08880018.2015.1013230

Tian, D., Battles, M. B., Moin, S. M., Chen, M., Modjarrad, K., Kumar, A., et al. (2017). Structural basis of respiratory syncytial virus subtype-dependent neutralization by an antibody targeting the fusion glycoprotein. *Nat. Commun.* 8, 1877. doi: 10.1038/s41467-017-01858-w

Tilmanis, D., van Baalen, C., Oh, D. Y., Rossignol, J. F., and Hurt, A. C. (2017). The susceptibility of circulating human influenza viruses to tizoxanide, the active metabolite of nitazoxanide. *Antiviral Res.* 147, 142–148. doi: 10.1016/j.antiviral.2017.10.002

Tomblyn, M., Chiller, T., Einsele, H., Gress, R., Sepkowitz, K., Storek, J., et al. (2009). Guidelines for preventing infectious complications among hematopoietic cell transplantation recipients: a global perspective. *Biol. Blood Marrow Transplant.* 15, 1143–1238. doi: 10.1016/j.bbmt.2009.06.019

Tregoning, J. S., and Schwarze, J. (2010). Respiratory viral infections in infants: causes, clinical symptoms, virology, and immunology. *Clin. Microbiol. Rev.* 23, 74–98. doi: 10.1128/cmr.00032-09

Triana-Baltzer, G. B., Gubareva, L. V., Klimov, A. I., Wurtman, D. F., Moss, R. B., Hedlund, M., et al. (2009a). Inhibition of neuraminidase inhibitor-resistant influenza virus by DAS181, a novel sialidase fusion protein. *PLoS ONE* 4:e7838. doi: 10.1371/journal.pone.0007838

Triana-Baltzer, G. B., Gubareva, L. V., Nicholls, J. M., Pearce, M. B., Mishin, V. P., Belser, J. A., et al. (2009b). Novel pandemic influenza A(H1N1) viruses are potently inhibited by DAS181, a sialidase fusion protein. *PLoS ONE* 4:e7788. doi: 10.1371/journal.pone.0007788

Tzannou, I., Nicholas, S. K., Lulla, P., Aguayo-Hiraldo, P. I., Misra, A., Martinez, C. A., et al. (2017). Immunologic profiling of human metapneumovirus for the development of targeted immunotherapy. *J. Infect. Dis.* 216, 678–687. doi: 10.1093/infdis/jix358

Ulbrandt, N. D., Ji, H., Patel, N. K., Riggs, J. M., Brewah, Y. A., Ready, S., et al. (2006). Isolation and characterization of monoclonal antibodies which neutralize human metapneumovirus *in vitro* and *in vivo*. *J. Virol.* 80, 7799–7806. doi: 10.1128/jvi.00318-06

Ustun, C., Slaby, J., Shanley, R. M., Vydra, J., Smith, A. R., Wagner, J. E., et al. (2012). Human parainfluenza virus infection after hematopoietic stem cell transplantation: risk factors, management, mortality, and changes over time. *Biol. Blood Marrow Transplant.* 18, 1580–1588. doi: 10.1016/j.bbmt.2012.04.012

van der Hoek, L. (2007). Human coronaviruses: what do they cause? *Antivir. Ther.* 12(4 Pt B), 651–658.

Vilchez, R. A., Dauber, J., McCurry, K., Iacono, A., and Kusne, S. (2003). Parainfluenza virus infection in adult lung transplant recipients: an emergent clinical syndrome with implications on allograft function. *Am. J. Transplant* 3, 116–120. doi: 10.1034/j.1600-6143.2003.00024.x

Vilchez, R. A., McCurry, K., Dauber, J., Iacono, A., Keenan, R., Zeevi, A., et al. (2001). The epidemiology of parainfluenza virus infection in lung transplant recipients. *Clin. Infect. Dis.* 33, 2004–2008. doi: 10.1086/324348

Waghmare, A., Campbell, A. P., Xie, H., Seo, S., Kuypers, J., Leisenring, W., et al. (2013). Respiratory syncytial virus lower respiratory disease in hematopoietic cell transplant recipients: viral RNA detection in blood, antiviral treatment, and clinical outcomes. *Clin. Infect. Dis.* 57, 1731–1741. doi: 10.1093/cid/cit639

Waghmare, A., Englund, J. A., and Boeckh, M. (2016). How I treat respiratory viral infections in the setting of intensive chemotherapy or hematopoietic cell transplantation. *Blood* 127, 2682–2692. doi: 10.1182/blood-2016-01-634873

Waghmare, A., Wagner, T., Andrews, R., Smith, S., Kuypers, J., Boeckh, M., et al. (2015). Successful treatment of parainfluenza virus respiratory tract infection with DAS181 in 4 immunocompromised children. *J. Pediatric Infect. Dis. Soc.* 4, 114–118. doi: 10.1093/jpids/piu039

Walsh, E. E., McConnochie, K. M., Long, C. E., and Hall, C. B. (1997). Severity of respiratory syncytial virus infection is related to virus strain. *J. Infect. Dis.* 175, 814–820.

Walsh, E. E., Wang, L., Falsey, A. R., Qiu, X., Corbett, A., Holden-Wiltse, J., et al. (2018). Virus-specific antibody, viral load, and disease severity in respiratory syncytial virus infection. *J. Infect. Dis.* 218, 208–217. doi: 10.1093/infdis/jiy106

Watanabe, A., Chang, S. C., Kim, M. J., Chu, D. W., and Ohashi, Y. (2010). Long-acting neuraminidase inhibitor laninamivir octanoate versus oseltamivir for treatment of influenza: a double-blind, randomized, noninferiority clinical trial. *Clin. Infect. Dis.* 51, 1167–1175. doi: 10.1086/656802

Watcharananan, S. P., Suwatanapongched, T., Wacharawanichkul, P., Chantratitaya, W., Mavichak, V., and Mossad, S. B. (2010). Influenza A/H1N1 2009 pneumonia in kidney transplant recipients: characteristics and outcomes following high-dose oseltamivir exposure. *Transpl. Infect. Dis.* 12, 127–131. doi: 10.1111/j.1399-3062.2010.00493.x

Weigt, S. S., Gregson, A. L., Deng, J. C., Lynch, J. P. 3rd, and Belperio, J. A. (2011). Respiratory viral infections in hematopoietic stem cell and solid organ transplant recipients. *Semin. Respir. Crit. Care Med.* 32, 471–493. doi: 10.1055/s-0031-1283286

Whimbey, E., Champlin, R. E., Couch, R. B., Englund, J. A., Goodrich, J. M., Raad, I., et al. (1996). Community respiratory virus infections among hospitalized adult bone marrow transplant recipients. *Clin. Infect. Dis.* 22, 778–782.

Whimbey, E., Champlin, R. E., Englund, J. A., Mirza, N. Q., Piedra, P. A., Goodrich, J. M., et al. (1995). Combination therapy with aerosolized ribavirin and intravenous immunoglobulin for respiratory syncytial virus disease in adult bone marrow transplant recipients. *Bone Marrow Transplant.* 16, 393–399.

Whimbey, E., Englund, J. A., and Couch, R. B. (1997). Community respiratory virus infections in immunocompromised patients with cancer. *Am. J. Med.* 102, 10–18; discussion 25–16.

Yeh, E., Luo, R. F., Dyner, L., Hong, D. K., Banaei, N., Baron, E. J., et al. (2010). Preferential lower respiratory tract infection in swine-origin 2009 A(H1N1) influenza. *Clin. Infect. Dis.* 50, 391–394. doi: 10.1086649875

Zhu, Q., McLellan, J. S., Kallewaard, N. L., Ulbrandt, N. D., Palaszynski, S., Zhang, J., et al. (2017). A highly potent extended half-life antibody as a potential RSV vaccine surrogate for all infants. *Sci. Transl. Med.* 9:eaaj1928. doi: 10.1126/scitranslmed.aaj1928

Zhu, Y., Zembower, T. R., Metzger, K. E., Lei, Z., Green, S. J., and Qi, C. (2017). Investigation of respiratory syncytial virus outbreak on an adult stem cell transplant unit by use of whole-genome sequencing. *J. Clin. Microbiol.* 55, 2956–2963. doi: 10.1128/jcm.00360-17

19

Secondary Bacterial Infections during Pulmonary Viral Disease: Phage Therapeutics as Alternatives to Antibiotics?

Prasanth Manohar[1,2†], Belinda Loh[1†], Sudarsanan Athira[3], Ramesh Nachimuthu[3], Xiaoting Hua[4,5], Susan C. Welburn[1,6] and Sebastian Leptihn[1,4,6]*

[1] Zhejiang University-University of Edinburgh Institute, Zhejiang University, Haining, China, [2] The Second Affiliated Hospital, School of Medicine, Zhejiang University, Hangzhou, China, [3] Antibiotic Resistance and Phage Therapy Laboratory, School of Biosciences and Technology, Vellore Institute of Technology, Vellore, India, [4] Department of Infectious Diseases, Sir Run Run Shaw Hospital, School of Medicine, Zhejiang University, Hangzhou, China, [5] Key Laboratory of Microbial Technology and Bioinformatics of Zhejiang Province, Hangzhou, China, [6] Infection Medicine, Biomedical Sciences, Edinburgh Medical School, College of Medicine and Veterinary Medicine, The University of Edinburgh, Edinburgh, United Kingdom

***Correspondence:**
Sebastian Leptihn
Leptihn@intl.zju.edu.cn

† These authors have contributed equally to this work

Secondary bacterial infections manifest during or after a viral infection(s) and can lead to negative outcomes and sometimes fatal clinical complications. Research and development of clinical interventions is largely focused on the primary pathogen, with research on any secondary infection(s) being neglected. Here we highlight the impact of secondary bacterial infections and in particular those caused by antibiotic-resistant strains, on disease outcomes. We describe possible non-antibiotic treatment options, when small molecule drugs have no effect on the bacterial pathogen and explore the potential of phage therapy and phage-derived therapeutic proteins and strategies in treating secondary bacterial infections, including their application in combination with chemical antibiotics.

Keywords: secondary bacterial infection, pulmonary viruses, SARS-CoV-2, COVID-19, phage therapy, phage endolysins

INTRODUCTION

The past two decades have seen the emergence of four severe viral outbreaks including the 2002 Severe Acute Respiratory Syndrome (SARS) Coronavirus (CoV) epidemic, the 2009 influenza A H1N1 pandemic, 2012 Middle East Respiratory Syndrome (MERS) outbreak, and most recently the COVID-19 pandemic. Emergence of novel lethal CoV strains in human populations are becoming more frequent and are of increasing global concern; SARS-CoV-2, a novel CoV that caused a first major outbreak in China in 2019 has now infected almost 8 million people globally and resulted in 434,000 deaths (as of June 15, 2020), a far greater disease burden than SARS and MERS (Guarner, 2020; Kannan et al., 2020). The spectrum of clinical presentations of COVID-19 is highly variable; infections range from being asymptomatic to severe viral pneumonia with respiratory failure, often leading to death (Li et al., 2020). During an epidemic, or pandemic, early development and roll-out of antiviral treatments that can reduce morbidity and mortality is critical. However, even with many potential repurposed and new anti-viral drug candidates able to inhibit replication or attachment of the virus, a major consequence of disease progression in patients at later stages of infection, are secondary bacterial infections. At least one in seven COVID-19 patients was found to be additionally infected with a secondary bacterial infection with 50% of the fatalities during the SARS-CoV-2 epidemic caused by untreated or untreatable secondary bacterial infections, in most cases in the lung (Zhou et al., 2020). While antibiotics do not have impact on the virus itself, almost all seriously ill patients are treated with antibiotics to attempt to prevent the occurrence of secondary bacterial infections. Any surge in antibiotic use during the COVID-19 pandemic will have a detrimental effect on antibiotic resistance rates for nosocomial bacterial pathogens, fueling global growth of antibiotic resistant bacterial pathogens (Reardon, 2020).

Secondary Bacterial Infections

Secondary bacterial infections develop in patients during or after initial infection with an infective pathogen, often a virus (Morris et al., 2017; Wang et al., 2018) and are associated with high morbidity and mortality rates (**Figure 1**) (Mallia et al., 2012). Co-infections, secondary infections, or "superinfections" occur during viral epidemics; around 50 million deaths were ascribed to bacterial co-infections during the 1918–1919 Spanish Flu pandemic; although clinical records often do now record such infection complications (Kash and Taubenberger, 2015; MacIntyre et al., 2018). While secondary infections occur in succession to the primary infection, co-infections are caused by multiple pathogens of viral, bacterial, or fungal origin and occur simultaneously at the same time. There tends to be a strong focus on a single pathogen rather than a combination of pathogens, especially for the viral–bacterial infections most commonly observed in patients (Jamieson et al., 2010). *Staphylococcus aureus*, *Streptococcus pneumoniae*, *Neisseria meningitides*, *Haemophilus influenzae*, *Klebsiella pneumoniae*, and members of the genus *Proteus*, *Enterobacter*, and *Citrobacter* spp., are some of the most commonly isolated bacteria during secondary infections (Handel et al., 2009). Hospitals are a common source of the pathogens that cause secondary infections, these so-called nosocomial pathogen infections are acquired from an environment in which antibiotics are commonplace, and as such; many have acquired resistance to a broad range of antibiotics. Decades of misuse and, over-prescribing of antibiotics has resulted in selection of pathogens that show multi-drug resistance (MDR). MDR is a global health challenge as in many cases no (chemical) antibiotics exist to treat such infections, including secondary infections. Secondary bacterial infections are facilitated by the exposure to a pathogen together with an immune system that is inapt to appropriately react to both pathogen types, as a consequence of the primary viral infection. For such patients, the only option is to support their immune system and prevent progression of the infection that could lead to the death of the patient such as septic shock. Antibiotics therapies deployed as a "last resort" or the use of exceptionally high doses of antibiotics often have negative consequences. Many key human pathogens are showing resistance to antibiotics including Methicillin-resistant *S. aureus* (MRSA), multidrug-resistant *Streptococcus*, Vancomycin-resistant *Enterococci* (VRE), resistant *Mycobacterium*, Carbapenem-resistant *Enterobacteriaceae* (CRE), Colistin-resistant *Klebsiella*, Carbapenem-resistant *Pseudomonas aeruginosa*, and Carbapenem-resistant *Acinetobacter baumannii* (Kumar and Chordia, 2017). The problem is exacerbated by the discontinuation by big pharma of chemical antibiotics discovery programs in the search for chemical antibiotics (Loh and Leptihn, 2020). Other options to treat MDR infections would be beneficial.

Molecular Basis of Manifestation of Secondary Bacterial Infections

There are several hypotheses why secondary infections quickly establish in patients with a pulmonary viral infection, including immunological host changes, mechanical damage and diffusion, and removal of mucus within the lungs. Much of how secondary infections manifest themselves and what role the immune response to a virus influences the defense against a prokaryotic pathogen, is poorly understood. The prevalence of secondary bacterial infections during a primary virus disease is due to the altered immune response to one pathogen (here: the virus) that often changes the response of the system to the other infectious agent (here: the bacterium), resulting in increased morbidity (Hendaus et al., 2015). Severe viral infections initiate changes in the immune response of the host that persist for a prolonged period of time. These immune alterations termed "trained immunity," "innate imprinting," or "immune paralysis," change the inflammatory response of immune cells (Williams et al., 2004; Bordon, 2014; Cheng et al., 2014; Roquilly et al., 2017; Morgan et al., 2018). In addition, viral infections of the respiratory system can lead to immune responses that alter the microbiome of the host. This change in the microbiome has been suggested to possibly modulate immune cell priming against secondary bacterial challenge (Hanada et al., 2018).

In most cases, epithelial cells are damaged during the primary viral infection, impeding mucociliary clearance that leads to an accumulation of mucus (Perry et al., 2005). Bacteria are able to diffuse into the mucus but thickened dense mucus impedes penetration of host immune cells. Secondary bacterial infections are also facilitated by the immune response of the host to a viral attack. One of the more important factors seems to be the immunosuppression of the host innate immune response initiated by the viral infection which facilitates opportunistic bacteria, like *Streptococcus* to infect the host (Kim et al., 2011). Cells of a host suffering from a viral infection are more susceptible to bacterial attachment and colonization (Pittet et al., 2010; Nyangacha et al., 2017). Many viruses, including influenza virus, rhinovirus, and respiratory syncytial virus (RSV), have detrimental effects on the mucosal layer facilitating bacterial adherence of, e.g., *S. pneumoniae*, *P. aeruginosa*, and *H. influenzae*, as well as biofilm formation on the linings of the lungs (Morris, 2007). For some pulmonary viruses such as influenza, Toll-like receptor (TLR) pathways are altered, possibly from sustained de-sensitization, which results in an increase of attachment of bacteria to epithelial cells (Kurt-Jones et al., 2000; Haynes et al., 2001). TLR and RIG-I-like receptor activation results in the production of Type I Interferon, changing the inflammatory response to TLR ligands,

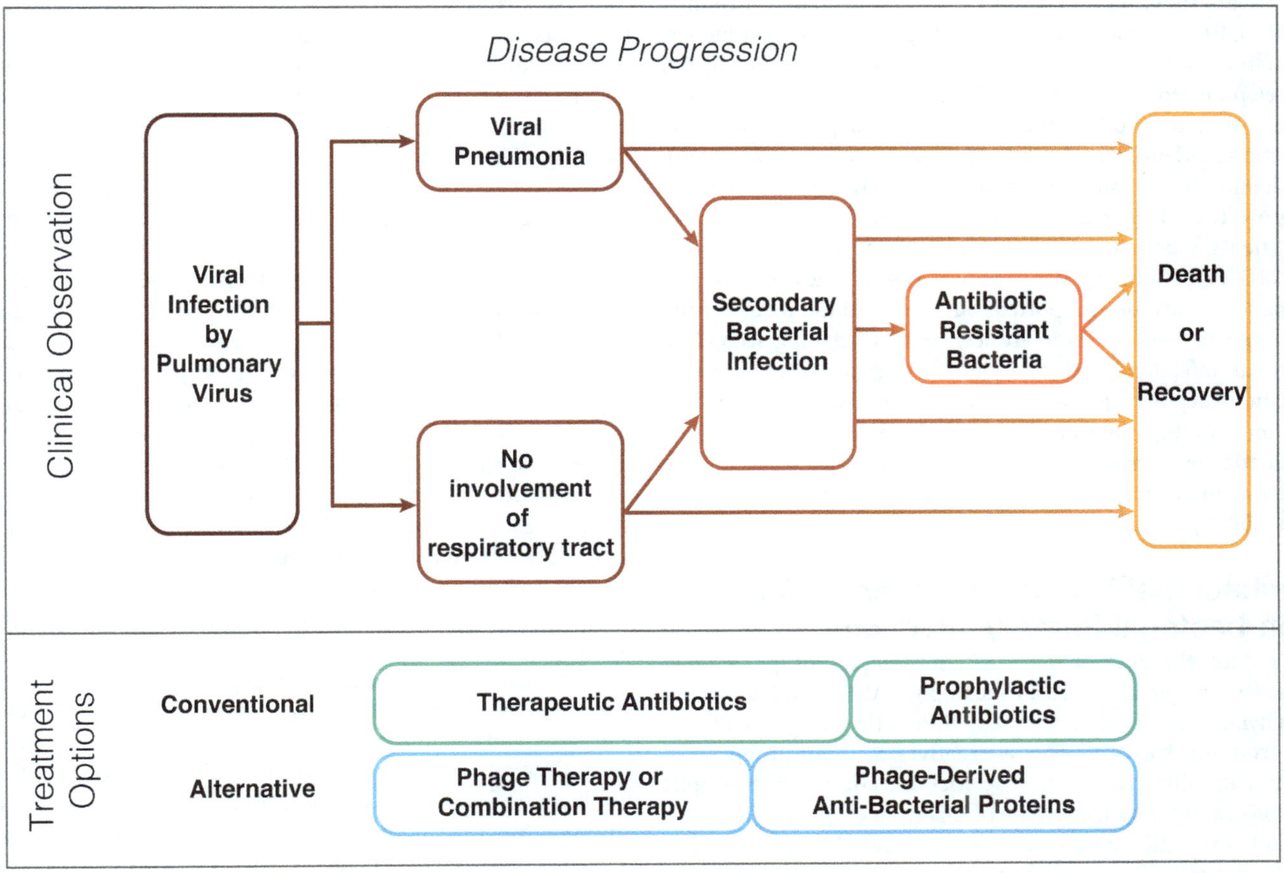

FIGURE 1 | Possible clinical progression of patients with a pulmonary virus infection and prophylaxis or treatment options for bacterial secondary infections.

e.g., bacterial lipopolysaccharide (Doughty et al., 2001; Nansen and Thomsen, 2001). Polymicrobial, viral–bacterial co-infections can develop as a result of an altered immune response combined with accessible routes of entry for the bacterial pathogen(s).

For patients with viral–bacterial infections, the availability of therapeutic options for both infectious agents is crucial. Antivirals are deployed to combat the virus, which have no effect on the bacterial pathogens (McCullers, 2011), and bacterial infections are treated with antibiotics, or such small-molecule compounds to try and prevent secondary infections. Broad-spectrum antibiotic may result in undesirable inflammatory responses in the afflicted person (Brook, 1995, 2002; Mahar et al., 2014). To prevent complications caused by secondary bacterial infections and to eliminate bacterial pathogens, alternative antibacterial therapies are needed.

Coronavirus, Pneumonia, Antibiotics, and Antibiotic Resistance

Some of the most significant outbreaks, epidemics, and global pandemics, with high morbidities and mortality are from viral respiratory infections caused by influenza virus or CoV species; for which treatment is compromised by secondary bacterial infections (Yang et al., 2020; Zhou et al., 2020). While a viral infection alone can be detrimental to a patient, the pathogen that exasperates disease progression is most commonly of bacterial origin (Yang et al., 2020). During the 2009 H1N1 influenza pandemic, between 29 and 55% of fatal cases were caused by secondary bacterial infections (Center for Disease Control and Prevention, 2012). During the ongoing COVID-19 pandemic, around 15% of hospital cases have been associated with secondary bacterial pathogens, and 50% of patients died (Zhou et al., 2020). Clinical cases of COVID-19 have developed high rates of up to 50% of secondary bacterial infections leading to secondary bacterial pneumonia. Half of COVID-19 fatalities experienced some form of secondary infection (pulmonary or other) that may have contributed to their death. During severe COVID-19 disease with pneumonia, the air sacs of the lungs fill with pus and fluids, nutritious substrates for pathogens including *P. aeruginosa* and *S. aureus*. Tissues are breached by the cytolytic activity of the virus and bacteria invade deeper into the tissue, continuing to secrete toxins that further destroying surrounding cells. The frequency (30–40%) of complications due to bacterial involvement was significantly higher in fatal COVID-19 patients than for COVID-19 survivors (Zhou et al., 2020). In fatal COVID-19 cases, death is most frequently a result of respiratory failure from severe pneumonia, caused either by SARS-CoV-2 itself or as a result of a secondary bacterial infection (Tetro, 2020).

Patients suffering of a pulmonary virus infection, including COVID-19, are often administered prophylactic antibiotics, including azithromycin, moxifloxacin, ceftriaxone, vancomycin, or cefepime, to reduce the risk of secondary infections; often in addition to another antibiotic that is deployed once the infection is identified (Holshue et al., 2020; Wang et al., 2020). As the numbers of antibiotic-resistant bacterial strains continue to grow, there is increased the risk of superinfection in severely ill patients, especially in intensive care units (ICUs). During the COVID-19 pandemic, many clinical case studies of COVID-19 patients have been reported, but mainly these focus on the viral infection itself. There are few reports detailing secondary bacterial infections and even less describing AMR. Until a vaccine is deployed globally, bacterial secondary infections will continue to be important in COVID-19 clinical care. New antibiotics or alternative treatments targeted against secondary bacterial infections need to be developed for COVID-19 and subsequent pandemics.

Antibacterial Therapy in Patients With Non-bacterial Primary Infections

To reduce the risk of superinfections, cases of pneumonia caused by respiratory viruses including SARS-CoV-2 are often prophylactically treated with antibiotics that target a broad-spectrum of bacteria. The alternative, i.e., no prophylactic treatment, often results in bacterial infections, in principle, demonstrating the effectiveness of this strategy. Prophylactic use of antibiotics, however, contributes to the AMR crisis and is ineffective when patients acquire antibiotic-resistant strains—nosocomial hospital-acquired infections are commonly observed for ICU patients infected with a respiratory virus (Zhou et al., 2020). Nosocomial infections are becoming more common due to the rise of resistant bacterial pathogens. Alternative antibacterial therapeutic strategies are needed; such as phage therapy or phage-derived therapeutic proteins.

Phage Therapy and Phage-Based Strategies During Viral Epidemics

An alternative approach to treating secondary bacterial infections, especially AMR pathogens, is the application of phage therapy; using microbial viruses to kill their host, ideally clearing the bacterial infection (Altamirano and Barr, 2019). Bacteriophages are naturally occurring viruses that use bacteria as hosts after employing the host machinery for propagation, including genome replication, protein synthesis, and phage assembly (**Figure 2**). Lysogenic bacteriophages undergo a "dormant" state as non-replicative, genome-integrated phages (Monteiro et al., 2019; Hampton et al., 2020). Some filamentous phages allow the host to continue to grow and divide while the phages are being produced (Loh et al., 2017, 2019; Kuhn and Leptihn, 2019). Phage therapy was discovered before antibiotics but the opportunities from the "dawn of the antibiotic era" delayed pursuit of commercial therapeutic phage strategies (Pirisi, 2000; Housby and Mann, 2009; Manohar et al., 2019c). With increasing AMR, and depletion of antibiotic resources, phage therapy has once more piqued the interest of the scientific community and pharmaceutical industry (Seguin et al., 2006; Nyangacha et al., 2017; Manohar et al., 2019c; Loh and Leptihn, 2020). Phages and phage-derived therapeutic proteins have advantages and disadvantages as compared with antibiotic therapies (**Figure 3**).

A major advantage of phages is that they exhibit bacterial host specificity (Seguin et al., 2006) and selectively target pathogenic bacteria without adverse effects on the normal microflora (Brüssow, 2005). Phages may be genus- or species-specific, and even strain-specific, infecting and killing their target bacterium. As most secondary bacterial infections are caused by one bacterial genus, species or strain, phage therapy offers a promising treatment option. Clinical studies using phages have demonstrated success at eliminating resistant bacterial strains (Capparelli et al., 2007; Kutter et al., 2010; Chan et al., 2013). Intact phage particles do not adversely interact with human cells and are not able to cause infections in humans (Barr, 2019; Van Belleghem et al., 2019). The self-replicating nature of phages enables them to function as "active and self-replicating" drugs once administered to the patient so dosage is less important to reach therapeutic levels; however—in practice—a large quantity of phages are being deployed (Barr, 2019). Phages show low toxicity; being mainly composed of protein and DNA and eventually undergo degradation inside a patient's body. Degradation of phage particles does not result in the production of toxic molecules, unlike antibiotics that could apply strain on the liver and might result in organ failure. Since most secondary bacterial infections occur in immunocompromised or immunodeficient patients, it is necessary to study the efficacy of phage therapy under such conditions. Previous studies on cancer patients and renal allograft patients showed that phage therapy can be effective in treating secondary bacterial infections and co-infections (Weber-Dabrowska et al., 2001; Międzybrodzki et al., 2012). Phages often do not cause an immune response, in contrast to human-pathogenic viruses (Manohar et al., 2019a). The levels to which administered phages can induce immune responses have been well studied and no adverse side effects have been observed (Borysowski and Górski, 2008; Ahmadi et al., 2016; Jault et al., 2019; Voelker, 2019). While there is a lack of evidence showing the efficacy of phage therapy during viral infections, bacteriophages have been shown to be effective prophylactic agents (Ahmadi et al., 2016).

Synergistic Effects of Phages and Antibiotics

A number of factors can result in phage resistance in bacteria, such as the alteration in phage receptors on the bacterial cell surface; degradation of phage DNA by restriction endonuclease produced by the host bacteria; emergence of mechanisms inhibiting the penetration of phage DNA into the bacterial host, among others (Jo et al., 2016b; Valério et al., 2017). Under certain conditions, such as low phage to bacterium ratios, or when using a single phage to treat an infection, phage-resistant bacteria can emerge. This selection of resistant mutants is a shortcoming of phage therapy. Clinical applications often make

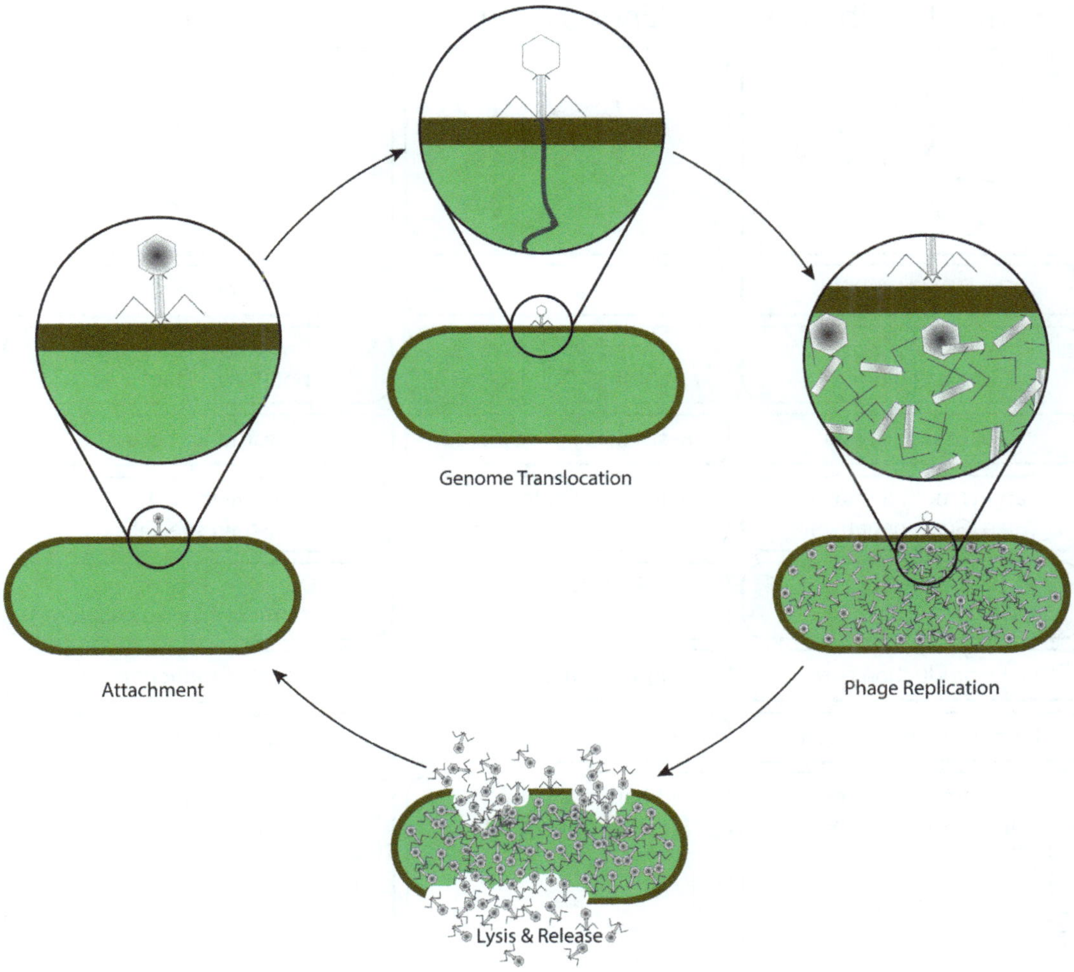

FIGURE 2 | Life cycle of a lytic phage, commonly used in phage therapy. After specific recognition and attachment to the host cell (attachment), phage proteins insert into the envelope of the cell, forming a channel through which the viral genome is translocated into the cytoplasm of the bacterium (genome translocation). The host machinery replicates the genomic information, and synthesizes phage proteins which self-assemble to form the virus structure (phage replication). Later in the life cycle, specific phage proteins such as holins and endolysins are synthesized. Enzymatic activity of endolysins leads to a disintegration of the host envelope, resulting in host cell lysis and release of phage progeny (lysis and release). The new phages are now able to attach and infect new host cells again, continuing the life cycle.

use of multiple phages, making the occurrence of multiple resistance mechanisms unlikely (Summers, 2001; Lin et al., 2017).

Another solution to overcome such limitations is to conduct combination therapy. The combined use of phages and antibiotics is expected to provide stronger suppression of bacterial growth and is expected to help reduce bacterial resistance against phages and antibiotics (different targets are used by the two agents). Recent *in vitro* and *in vivo* studies have shown improved efficacy in controlling the growth of bacterial pathogens such as *Pseudomonas fluorescens*, *Pseudomonas aeruginosa*, *Escherichia coli*, and *S. aureus* using combinations of phages and antibiotics (Torres-Barceló et al., 2016; Chaudhry et al., 2017). Phage-antibiotic therapy is reported to have higher success rates in preventing the emergence of bacterial resistance as bacteria that become non-susceptible to one agent can still be killed by the other and *vice versa*. Phage-antibiotic therapy can prevent the emergence of double resistant bacterial mutants, as a bacterium is unlikely to acquire phage and antibiotic resistance simultaneously. For the success of combination therapies, it is essential to carefully choose the dosage as well as the point of administration of each antibacterial agent. Administration of antibiotics prior to the phage resulted in the decreased evolution of phage resistance due to antibiotic stress (Torres-Barceló, 2018; Tagliaferri et al., 2019). Phage-antibiotic combinations that have different bacterial targets can assist in enhanced bacterial inactivation.

The use of sub-lethal concentrations (concentration of antibiotics lower than minimal inhibitory concentrations) of antibiotics can enhance phage productivity mediating phage induced bacterial decline (Tagliaferri et al., 2019), known as phage-antibiotic synergy. One factor proposed responsible for phage-antibiotic synergy is bacterial elongation or filamentation induced by sub-lethal concentrations of antibiotics (Kim et al., 2018). While different antibiotics exhibit different inhibitory

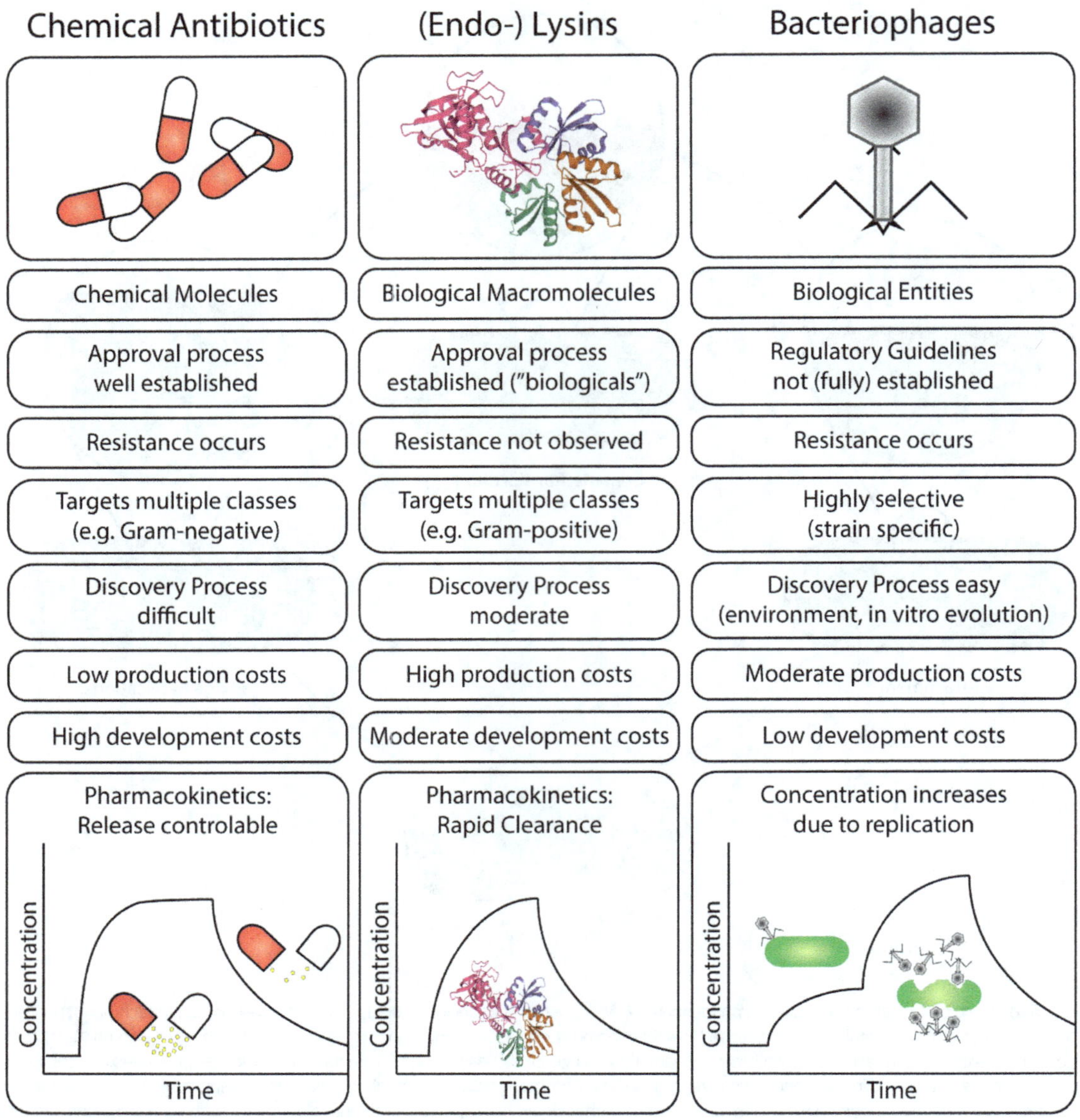

FIGURE 3 | Comparison of scientific, clinical, and pharmaceutical characteristics of chemical antibiotics, endolysins, and bacteriophages in the treatment of bacterial infections.

mechanisms, they often result in the blocking of bacterial cell division causing elongation of the bacterial cell, as a large bacterial surface area is available for phage attachment, bacterial cells are vulnerable toward phage infection, increasing the efficacy of phage lytic activity (Comeau et al., 2007; Kim et al., 2018). Antibiotic-induced morphological changes in the host bacterium can permit faster phage assembly due to altered or abundant precursors required for phage maturation, which ultimately can result in an acceleration of cell lysis (Nouraldin et al., 2016). Beta-lactam antibiotics and quinolones can stimulate virulent phage production, together with the changes induced in bacterial membrane proteins by antibiotics and may enhance the lytic activity of phages and increase phage burst size observed in phage-antibiotic studies (Jo et al., 2016a). A further advantage of using sub-inhibitory concentrations of antibiotics is avoidance of side effects from administration of otherwise necessary higher doses of the antibiotic (Knezevic et al., 2013).

Infections caused by biofilm-forming bacteria, especially nosocomial infections, are difficult to treat using antibiotics (Pires et al., 2017). The emergence of ventilator-associated secondary pneumonia is often due to biofilm forming bacteria such as *Pseudomonas* and *Staphylococcus* (Zhou et al., 2020). Phage-antibiotic therapy has shown promise for biofilms and in embedded bacteria; phages can enzymatically penetrate the microenvironment created by biofilm-forming cells to infect and kill target bacteria (Pires et al., 2017). Phages, when administered in combination with an antibiotic, can increase the susceptibility of bacteria and reduce plasmid-borne bacterial resistance by targeting plasmid bearing bacteria in the biofilm (Łusiak-Szelachowska et al., 2020). Combined phage and antibiotic therapy with a sequential approach of administering the antibiotic after phage treatment of the biofilm has shown success; initial treatment of the biofilm with phages caused biofilm disintegration, while later administration of the antibiotic prevented biofilm regrowth as well as the emergence of phage-resistant mutants. Phages can enable antibiotics to penetrate biofilm layers by degrading the biofilm matrix; phages penetrate into deeper layers of the biofilm, replicating in the lower layers and facilitating the destruction of the biofilm (Łusiak-Szelachowska et al., 2020). Antibiotics administered following biofilm treatment by phages enhance bacterial reduction Akturk et al., 2019.

Phage Endolysins as Antibacterial Agents

Phage proteins can be extracted and also engineered for deployment as an alternative to whole phage therapeutic applications. Endolysins are phage-encoded enzymes produced at the end of the bacteriophage lytic lifecycle that facilitate release of phage progeny into the environment, degrading the peptidoglycan layer of the host bacterial cell wall (Imanishi et al., 2019). The ability of endolysins to digest the bacterial cell wall when applied exogenously offers the opportunity for their deployment as potential antibacterial agents, to target and kill pathogenic bacteria, potentially without harming the normal microflora due to specificity of enzyme activity (Haddad Kashani et al., 2017). The chances of bacteria developing resistance toward endolysins are low since endolysins target cell wall molecules essential for bacterial viability (Łusiak-Szelachowska et al., 2020). Phage-derived endolysins are promising candidates for treating secondary bacterial infections or multi-drug resistant infections (Imanishi et al., 2019; Kim et al., 2020). There are five main classes of endolysins based on their enzymatic specificity (**Figure 4**) (Schmelcher et al., 2012). Several applications for endolysins have been reported, including use in biocontrol agents against bacterial

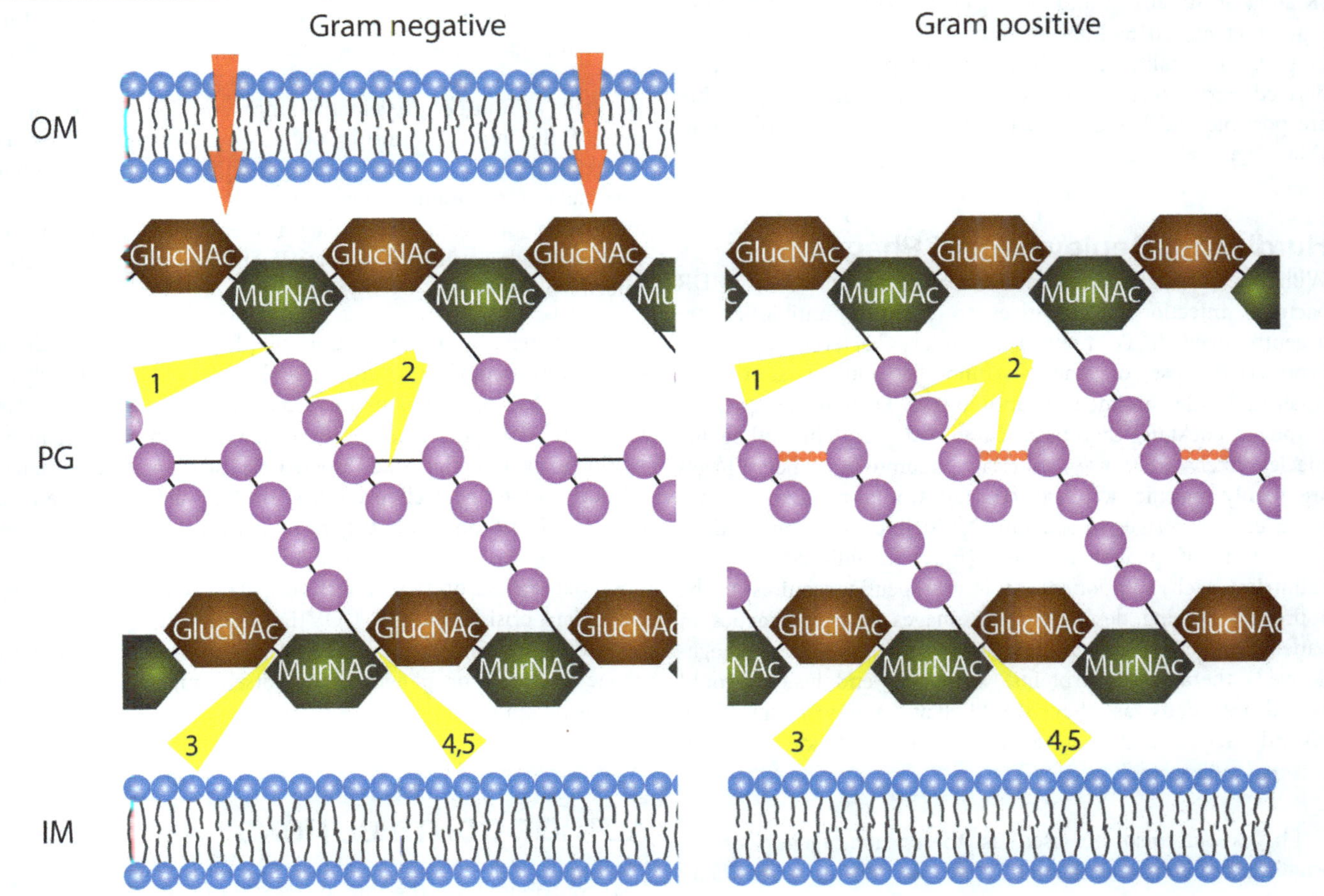

FIGURE 4 | Illustration of phage endolysins classified by their enzymatic activity. In order to reach the peptidoglycan (PG) layer, in the case of Gram-negative bacteria, the outer membrane (OM) has to be traversed (red arrows, details in text).The PG layer is represented with alternate repeating sugar units, *N*-acetylglucosamine (GlucNAc), and *N*-acetylmuramic acid (MurNAc). In Gram-negative bacteria, tetrapeptide chains (purple spheres) extend from each MurNAc of the long sugar chains and are directly cross-linked by short interpeptide bridges (black solid line) via the third residue to D-Ala of another peptide chain. In Gram-positive bacteria, the tetrapeptide chains (purples spheres) are linked via pentapeptide bridges (red spheres). All residues are purple spheres. IM, inner membrane. Depending on the organism, residues at position 3 are either L603 Lysine (mainly Gram-positive bacteria) or meso-diaminopimelic acid (Gram-negative bacteria and Gram-positive bacilli). Endolysin cleavage sites are indicated by yellow triangles: 1, *N*-acetylmuramoyl-L-alanine amidases; 2, endopeptidases; 3, endo-*N*-acetyl606 glucosaminidases; 4, *N*-acetyl muramidases; 5, lytic transglycosylases.

pathogens in food and agricultural industries (Matamp and Bhat, 2019) and as strong antibacterial agents for human pathogens in animal models (Guo et al., 2017; Haddad Kashani et al., 2017; de Wit et al., 2019). Most naturally occurring endolysins have limited effect on Gram-negative bacteria as the outer membrane (OM) protects the peptidoglycan layer from being attacked by the enzyme. However, efficient endolysin-mediated inactivation of Gram-negative pathogens can be achieved by either chemical/physical permeabilization of the OM (such as pressure or chelation of divalent ions), or by creating endolysin-peptide-fusions that have the ability to permeabilize the OM (Briers and Lavigne, 2015).

The application of bacteriophages in therapy has been successful in treating: (i) MDR *A. baumannii* infections (Schooley et al., 2017); (ii) against Mycobacterial infections (Dedrick et al., 2019); (iii) burn-wound infections caused by *P. aeruginosa* (Jault et al., 2019); (iv) infections caused by *S. aureus* (Fabijan et al., 2020); (v) Enterococcal infections (Khalifa et al., 2016); and (vi) against MDR *E. coli* infections (Sarker et al., 2016; Kakasis and Panitsa, 2019). Preparations of phage cocktails, phage banks, phage powders, and phage-derived endolysins as part of phage therapeutic approaches are possible and bring strategies closer to clinical applications (Manohar et al., 2019b,c).

Hurdles for Deployment of Phages

With the looming crisis of increasing numbers of MDR bacterial infections, alternatives to chemical antibiotics are urgently needed. To prevent secondary bacterial infections, prophylactic use of phages could be applied similar to small-molecule broadband antibiotics. This would require a "phage cocktail" that targets a broad range of pathogenic species likely to cause bacterial pneumonia. Since phages are highly specific, a phage cocktail would need to contain a variety of phages. Regulatory guidelines for the medical application of phages are not (fully) established in most countries; each component of a therapeutic requires to be approved, making deployment of phages as prophylactics in patients infected with pulmonary viruses, complex. Phage-derived therapeutic proteins such as endolysins would be advantageous as they would have a lower specificity toward bacteria and be able to inactivate a broader range of bacterial pathogens.

Phages can also be used as therapeutic agents for an established bacterial infection. Due to the high specificity of phages, phage therapy can be considered a personalized medicine (Loh and Leptihn, 2020). However, a phage to which the causative pathogen is susceptible would need to be rapidly identified. To treat multi-drug resistant pathogens, and to be prepared for the next pandemic where such infections, especially nosocomial ones, have a major impact on patient survival, phage libraries, and rapid on-site (hospital) screening platforms should be made available for use.

While phage therapy is unlikely to replace chemical antibiotics in clinical practice, it offers a potential solution to be used in combination with antibiotics or alone. Limitations of phage therapy in treating secondary bacterial infections include: the preparation of therapeutic cGMP (Good Manufacturing Practice) phages; a lack of proper clinical trials or guidelines to treat patients in different clinical conditions; a lack of regulatory guidelines to prepare and administer phages; patient acceptance, and possibly, adverse immune responses leading to primary treatment failure.

CONCLUSION

Secondary bacterial infections play a critical role in the morbidity and mortality rates of patients initially falling ill with pulmonary viral diseases. Evidence from the current SARS-CoV-2 pandemic shows that the antibiotic-resistant bacterial infections are a significant threat to hospitalized COVID-19 patients. Nosocomial infections including ventilator-associated infections are often unavoidable and especially so during a pandemic, and the use of broad-spectrum antibiotics is often a routine preventative measure. Phage therapy is one of the most promising options for treating secondary bacterial infections. Phage therapy either as a stand-alone treatment or in combination with antibiotics may offer a valuable alternative for treating secondary bacterial infections. Clinical studies should evaluate the efficacy of phage therapy in virus infected patients.

The potential for application of phage products, such as endolysins, should be investigated. Pulmonary CoVs will likely be a clinical challenge for many years to come. Viral pandemics from CoVs and emerging pathogens are inevitable in our globalized world with interconnected societies, travel, and commerce. We require to be well prepared for long-term management of COVID-19 and for the next pandemic, exploring and establishing new avenues to treat bacterial pathogens commonly observed in secondary infections. To avert an emerging healthcare crisis due from COVID-1 and antibiotic-resistance of secondary infections; medical interventions employing phage products or phage therapy itself might be our most promising options.

AUTHOR CONTRIBUTIONS

PM contributed to the initial idea. PM, BL, SW, and SL contributed to the concept and writing. BL and SL prepared the figures. SA, RN, and XH contributed to the review and comments.

REFERENCES

Ahmadi, M., Karimi Torshizi, M. A., Rahimi, S., and Dennehy, J. J. (2016). Prophylactic bacteriophage administration more effective than post-infection administration in reducing *Salmonella enterica* serovar Enteritidis shedding in quail. *Front. Microbiol.* 7:1253. doi: 10.3389/fmicb.2016.01253

Akturk, E., Oliveira, H., Santos, S. B., Costa, S., Kuyumcu, S., Melo, L. D., et al. (2019). Synergistic action of phage and antibiotics: parameters to enhance the killing efficacy against mono and dual-species biofilms. *Antibiotics* 8:103. doi: 10.3390/antibiotics8030103

Altamirano, F. L., and Barr, J. J. (2019). Phage therapy in the postantibiotic era. *Clin. Microbiol. Rev.* 32:e00066-18.

Barr, J. J. (2019). Missing a phage: unraveling tripartite symbioses within the human gut. *mSystems* 4:e00105-19.

Bordon, Y. (2014). Macrophages: innate memory training. *Nat. Rev. Immunol.* 14:713. doi: 10.1038/nri3759

Borysowski, J., and Górski, A. (2008). Is phage therapy acceptable in the immunocompromised host? *Int. J. Infect. Dis.* 12, 466–471. doi: 10.1016/j.ijid.2008.01.006

Briers, Y., and Lavigne, R. (2015). Breaking barriers: expansion of the use of endolysins as novel antibacterials against Gram-negative bacteria. *Future Microbiol.* 10, 377–390. doi: 10.2217/fmb.15.8

Brook, I. (1995). Microbiology of secondary bacterial infection in scabies lesions. *J. Clin. Microbiol.* 33, 2139–2140. doi: 10.1128/jcm.33.8.2139-2140.1995

Brook, I. (2002). Secondary bacterial infections complicating skin lesions. *J. Med. Microbiol.* 51, 808–812. doi: 10.1099/0022-1317-51-10-808

Brüssow, H. (2005). Phage therapy: the *Escherichia coli* experience. *Microbiol* 151, 2133–2140. doi: 10.1099/mic.0.27849-0

Capparelli, R., Parlato, M., Borriello, G., Salvatore, P., and Iannelli, D. (2007). Experimental phage therapy against *Staphylococcus aureus* in mice. *Antimicrob. Agents Chemother.* 51, 2765–2773. doi: 10.1128/aac.01513-06

Center for Disease Control and Prevention (2012). Available online at: https://www.cdc.gov/flu/spotlights/pandemic-global-estimates.htm (accessed June 15, 2020).

Chan, B. K., and Abedon, S. T. (2012). Phage therapy pharmacology: phage cocktails. *Adv. Appl. Microbiol.* 78, 1–23.

Chan, B. K., Abedon, S. T., and Loc-Carrillo, C. (2013). Phage cocktails and the future of phage therapy. *Future Microbiol.* 8, 769–783. doi: 10.2217/fmb.13.47

Chaudhry, W. N., Concepcion-Acevedo, J., Park, T., Andleeb, S., Bull, J. J., and Levin, B. R. (2017). Synergy and order effects of antibiotics and phages in killing *Pseudomonas aeruginosa* biofilms. *PLoS One* 12:e0168615. doi: 10.1371/journal.pone.0168615

Cheng, S. C., Quintin, J., Cramer, R. A., Shepardson, K. M., Saeed, S., Kumar, V., et al. (2014). mTOR-and HIF-1α–mediated aerobic glycolysis as metabolic basis for trained immunity. *Science* 345:1250684. doi: 10.1126/science.1250684

Comeau, A. M., Tétart, F., Trojet, S. N., Prere, M. F., and Krisch, H. M. (2007). Phage-antibiotic synergy (PAS): β-lactam and quinolone antibiotics stimulate virulent phage growth. *PLoS One* 2:e799. doi: 10.1371/journal.pone.0000799

de Wit, J., Totté, J. E., van Mierlo, M. M., van Veldhuizen, J., van Doorn, M. B., Schuren, F. H., et al. (2019). Endolysin treatment against *Staphylococcus aureus* in adults with atopic dermatitis: a randomized controlled trial. *J. Allergy Clin. Immunol.* 144, 860–863. doi: 10.1016/j.jaci.2019.05.020

Dedrick, R. M., Guerrero-Bustamante, C. A., Garlena, R. A., Russell, D. A., Ford, K., Harris, K., et al. (2019). Engineered bacteriophages for treatment of a patient with a disseminated drug-resistant *Mycobacterium abscessus*. *Nat. Med.* 25, 730–733. doi: 10.1038/s41591-019-0437-z

Doughty, L. A., Nguyen, K. B., Durbin, J. E., and Biron, C. A. (2001). A role for IFN-αβ in virus infection-induced sensitization to endotoxin. *J. Immunol.* 166, 2658–2664. doi: 10.4049/jimmunol.166.4.2658

Fabijan, A. P., Lin, R. C., Ho, J., Maddocks, S., Zakour, N. L., and Iredell, J. R. (2020). Safety of bacteriophage therapy in severe *Staphylococcus aureus* infection. *Nat. Microbiol.* 5, 465–472. doi: 10.1038/s41564-019-0634-z

Guarner, J. (2020). Three emerging coronaviruses in two decades. *Am. J. Clin. Pathol.* 153, 420–421. doi: 10.1093/ajcp/aqaa029

Guo, M., Feng, C., Ren, J., Zhuang, X., Zhang, Y., Zhu, Y., et al. (2017). A novel antimicrobial endolysin, LysPA26, against *Pseudomonas aeruginosa*. *Front. Microbiol.* 8:293. doi: 10.3389/fmicb.2017.00293

Haddad Kashani, H., Fahimi, H., Dasteh Goli, Y., and Moniri, R. (2017). A novel chimeric endolysin with antibacterial activity against methicillin-resistant *Staphylococcus aureus*. *Front. Cell. Infect. Microbiol.* 7:290. doi: 10.3389/fcimb.2017.00290

Hampton, H. G., Watson, B. N., and Fineran, P. C. (2020). The arms race between bacteria and their phage foes. *Nature* 577, 327–336. doi: 10.1038/s41586-019-1894-8

Hanada, S., Pirzadeh, M., Carver, K. Y., and Deng, J. C. (2018). Respiratory viral infection-induced Microbiome alterations and secondary bacterial pneumonia. *Front. Immunol.* 9:2640. doi: 10.3389/fimmu.2018.02640

Handel, A., Longini, I. M., and Antia, R. (2009). Intervention strategies for an influenza pandemic taking into account secondary bacterial infections. *Epidem* 1, 185–195. doi: 10.1016/j.epidem.2009.09.001

Haynes, L. M., Moore, D. D., Kurt-Jones, E. A., Finberg, R. W., Anderson, L. J., and Tripp, R. A. (2001). Involvement of toll-like receptor 4 in innate immunity to respiratory syncytial virus. *J. Virol.* 75, 10730–10737. doi: 10.1128/jvi.75.22.10730-10737.2001

Hendaus, M. A., Jomha, F. A., and Alhammadi, A. H. (2015). Virus-induced secondary bacterial infection: a concise review. *Ther. Clin. Risk Manag.* 11, 1265–1271.

Holshue, M. L., DeBolt, C., Lindquist, S., Lofy, K. H., Wiesman, J., Bruce, H., et al. (2020). First case of 2019 novel coronavirus in the United States. *N. Engl. J. Med.* 382, 929–936.

Housby, J. N., and Mann, N. H. (2009). Phage therapy. *Drug Discov. Today* 14, 536–540.

Imanishi, I., Uchiyama, J., Tsukui, T., Hisatsune, J., Ide, K., Matsuzaki, S., et al. (2019). Therapeutic potential of an endolysin derived from kayvirus S25-3 for staphylococcal impetigo. *Viruses* 11:769. doi: 10.3390/v11090769

Jamieson, A. M., Yu, S., Annicelli, C. H., and Medzhitov, R. (2010). Article influenza virus-induced glucocorticoids compromise innate host defense against a secondary bacterial infection. *Cell Host Microbe* 7, 103–114. doi: 10.1016/j.chom.2010.01.010

Jault, P., Leclerc, T., Jennes, S., Pirnay, J. P., Que, Y. A., Resch, G., et al. (2019). Efficacy and tolerability of a cocktail of bacteriophages to treat burn wounds infected by *Pseudomonas aeruginosa* (PhagoBurn): a randomised, controlled, double-blind phase 1/2 trial. *Lancet Infect. Dis.* 19, 35–45. doi: 10.1016/s1473-3099(18)30482-1

Jo, A., Ding, T., and Ahn, J. (2016a). Synergistic antimicrobial activity of bacteriophages and antibiotics against *Staphylococcus aureus*. *Food Sci. Biotechnol.* 25, 935–940. doi: 10.1007/s10068-016-0153-0

Jo, A., Kim, J., Ding, T., and Ahn, J. (2016b). Role of phage-antibiotic combination in reducing antibiotic resistance in *Staphylococcus aureus*. *Food Sci Biotechnol.* 25, 1211–1215. doi: 10.1007/s10068-016-0192-6

Kakasis, A., and Panitsa, G. (2019). Bacteriophage therapy as an alternative treatment for human infections. A comprehensive review. *Int. J. Antimicrob. Agents* 53, 16–21. doi: 10.1016/j.ijantimicag.2018.09.004

Kannan, S., Shaik Syed Ali, P., Sheeza, A., and Hemalatha, K. (2020). COVID-19 (Novel Coronavirus 2019) - recent trends. *Eur. Rev. Med. Pharmacol. Sci.* 24, 2006–2011.

Kash, J. C., and Taubenberger, J. K. (2015). Infectious disease theme issue the role of viral, host, and secondary bacterial factors in influenza pathogenesis. *Am. J. Pathol.* 185, 1528–1536. doi: 10.1016/j.ajpath.2014.08.030

Khalifa, L., Shlezinger, M., Beyth, S., Houri-Haddad, Y., Coppenhagen-Glazer, S., Beyth, N., et al. (2016). Phage therapy against *Enterococcus faecalis* in dental root canals. *J. Oral Microbiol.* 8:32157.

Kim, M., Jo, Y., Hwang, Y. J., Hong, H. W., Hong, S. S., Park, K., et al. (2018). Phage-antibiotic synergy via delayed lysis. *Appl. Environ. Microbiol.* 84: e02085-18.

Kim, S., Lee, D. W., Jin, J. S., and Kim, J. (2020). Antimicrobial activity of LysSS, a novel phage endolysin, against *Acinetobacter baumannii* and *Pseudomonas aeruginosa*. *J. Glob. Antimicrob. Res.* doi: 10.1016/j.jgar.2020.01.005 [Epub ahead of print].

Kim, Y. G., Park, J. H., Reimer, T., Baker, D. P., Kawai, T., Kumar, H., et al. (2011). Viral infection augments Nod1/2 signaling to potentiate lethality associated with secondary bacterial infections. *Cell Host Microbe* 9, 496–507. doi: 10.1016/j.chom.2011.05.006

Knezevic, P., Curcin, S., Aleksic, V., Petrusic, M., and Vlaski, L. (2013). Phage-antibiotic synergism : a possible approach to combatting *Pseudomonas aeruginosa*. *Res. Microbiol.* 164, 55–60. doi: 10.1016/j.resmic.2012.08.008

Kuhn, A., and Leptihn, S. (2019). "Helical and filamentous phages," in *Reference Module in Life Sciences* ed. M. G. Feiss (Amsterdam: Elsevier). doi: 10.1016/B978-0-12-809633-8.20986-2

Kumar, A., and Chordia, N. (2017). "Bacterial resistance against antibiotics," in *Drug Resistance in Bacteria, Fungi, Malaria, and Cancer*, eds G. Arora, A. Sajid, and V. Kalia (Cham: Springer), 171–192. doi: 10.1007/978-3-319-48683-3_7

Kurt-Jones, E. A., Popova, L., Kwinn, L., Haynes, L. M., Jones, L. P., Tripp, R. A., et al. (2000). Pattern recognition receptors TLR4 and CD14 mediate response to respiratory syncytial virus. *Nat. Immunol.* 1, 398–401. doi: 10.1038/80833

Kutter, E., De Vos, D., Gvasalia, G., Alavidze, Z., Gogokhia, L., Kuhl, S., et al. (2010). Phage therapy in clinical practice: treatment of human infections. *Curr. Pharm. Biotechnol.* 11, 69–86. doi: 10.2174/138920110790725401

Li, X., Geng, M., Peng, Y., Meng, L., and Lu, S. (2020). Molecular immune pathogenesis and diagnosis of COVID-19. *J. Pharm. Anal.* 10, 102–108. doi: 10.1016/j.jpha.2020.03.001

Lin, D. M., Koskella, B., and Lin, H. C. (2017). Phage therapy: an alternative to antibiotics in the age of multi-drug resistance. *World J. Gastrointest. Pharmacol. Ther.* 8, 162–173.

Loh, B., Haase, M., Mueller, L., Kuhn, A., and Leptihn, S. (2017). The transmembrane morphogenesis protein gp1 of filamentous phages contains walker A and walker B motifs essential for phage assembly. *Viruses* 9:73. doi: 10.3390/v9040073

Loh, B., Kuhn, A., and Leptihn, S. (2019). The fascinating biology behind phage display: filamentous phage assembly. *Mol. Microbiol.* 111, 1132–1138. doi: 10.1111/mmi.14187

Loh, B., and Leptihn, S. (2020). A call for a multidisciplinary future of phage therapy to combat multi-drug resistant bacterial infections. *Infect. Microbes Dis.* 2, 1–2. doi: 10.1097/im9.0000000000000018

Łusiak-Szelachowska, M., Weber-Dąbrowska, B., and Górski, A. (2020). Bacteriophages and lysins in biofilm control. *Virol. Sin.* 35, 125–133. doi: 10.1007/s12250-019-00192-3

MacIntyre, C. R., Chughtai, A. A., Barnes, M., Ridda, I., Seale, H., Toms, R., et al. (2018). The role of pneumonia and secondary bacterial infection in fatal and serious outcomes of pandemic influenza a (H1N1) pdm09. *BMC Infect. Dis.* 18:637. doi: 10.1186/s12879-018-3548-0

Mahar, P. D., Wasiak, J., Cleland, H., Paul, E., Gin, D., Watters, D. A., et al. (2014). Secondary bacterial infection and empirical antibiotic use in toxic epidermal necrolysis patients. *J. Burn Care Res.* 35, 518–524. doi: 10.1097/bcr.0000000000000062

Mallia, P., Footitt, J., Sotero, R., Jepson, A., Contoli, M., Trujillo-Torralbo, M. B., et al. (2012). Rhinovirus infection induces degradation of antimicrobial peptides and secondary bacterial infection in chronic obstructive pulmonary disease. *Am. J. Respir. Crit. Care Med.* 186, 1117–1124. doi: 10.1164/rccm.201205-0806oc

Manohar, P., Tamhankar, A. J., Leptihn, S., and Ramesh, N. (2019a). Pharmacological and immunological aspects of phage therapy. *Infect. Microbes Dis.* 1, 34–42. doi: 10.1097/im9.0000000000000013

Manohar, P., Tamhankar, A. J., Leptihn, S., and Ramesh, N. (2019b). Improved lyophilization conditions for long-term storage of bacteriophages. *Sci. Rep.* 9:15242.

Manohar, P., Tamhankar, A. J., Lundborg, C. S, and Nachimuthu, R. (2019c). Therapeutic characterization and efficacy of bacteriophage cocktails infecting *Escherichia coli*, *Klebsiella pneumoniae* and *Enterobacter* species. *Front. Microbiol.* 10:574. doi: 10.3389/fmicb.2019.00574

Matamp, N., and Bhat, S. G. (2019). Phage endolysins as potential antimicrobials against multidrug resistant *Vibrio alginolyticus* and *Vibrio parahaemolyticus*: current status of research and challenges ahead. *Microorganisms* 7:84. doi: 10.3390/microorganisms7030084

McCullers, J. A. (2011). Preventing and treating secondary bacterial infections with antiviral agents. *Antivir. Ther.* 16, 123–135. doi: 10.3851/imp1730

Międzybrodzki, R., Borysowski, J., Weber-Dąbrowska, B., Fortuna, W., Letkiewicz, S., Szufnarowski, K., et al. (2012). Clinical aspects of phage therapy. *Adv. Virus Res.* 83, 73–121.

Monteiro, R., Pires, D. P., Costa, A. R., and Azeredo, J. (2019). Phage therapy: going temperate? *Trends Microbiol.* 27, 368–378. doi: 10.1016/j.tim.2018.10.008

Morgan, D. J., Casulli, J., Chew, C., Connolly, E., Lui, S., Brand, O. J., et al. (2018). Innate immune cell suppression and the link with secondary lung bacterial pneumonia. *Front. Immunol.* 9:2943. doi: 10.3389/fimmu.2018.02943

Morris, D. E., Cleary, D. W., and Clarke, S. C. (2017). Secondary bacterial infections associated with influenza pandemics. *Front. Microbiol.* 8:1041. doi: 10.3389/fmicb.2017.01041

Morris, D. P. (2007). Bacterial biofilm in upper respiratory tract infections. *Curr. Infect. Dis. Rep.* 9, 186–192. doi: 10.1007/s11908-007-0030-3

Nansen, A., and Thomsen, A. R. (2001). Viral infection causes rapid sensitization to lipopolysaccharide: central role of IFN-αβ. *J. Immunol.* 166, 982–988. doi: 10.4049/jimmunol.166.2.982

Nouraldin, A. A., Baddour, M. M., Harfoush, R. A., and Essa, S. A. (2016). Bacteriophage-antibiotic synergism to control planktonic and biofilm producing clinical isolates of *Pseudomonas aeruginosa*. *Alexandria J. Med.* 52, 99–105. doi: 10.1016/j.ajme.2015.05.002

Nyangacha, R. M., Odongo, D., Oyieke, F., Ochwoto, M., Korir, R., Ngetich, R. K., et al. (2017). Secondary bacterial infections and antibiotic resistance among tungiasis patients in Western, Kenya. *PLoS Negl. Trop. Dis.* 11, e0005901. doi: 10.1371/journal.pntd.0005901

Perry, A. K., Gang, C. H., Zheng, D., Hong, T. A., and Cheng, G. (2005). The host type I interferon response to viral and bacterial infections. *Cell Res.* 15, 407–422. doi: 10.1038/sj.cr.7290309

Pires, D. P., Melo, L. D., Boas, D. V., Sillankorva, S., and Azeredo, J. (2017). Phage therapy as an alternative or complementary strategy to prevent and control biofilm-related infections. *Curr. Opin. Microbiol.* 39, 48–56. doi: 10.1016/j.mib.2017.09.004

Pirisi, A. (2000). Phage therapy-advantages over antibiotics? *Lancet* 356:1418. doi: 10.1016/s0140-6736(05)74059-9

Pittet, L. A., Hall-Stoodley, L., Rutkowski, M. R., and Harmsen, A. G. (2010). Influenza virus infection decreases tracheal mucociliary velocity and clearance of Streptococcus pneumoniae. *Am. J. Respir. Cell Mol.* 42, 450–460. doi: 10.1165/rcmb.2007-0417oc

Reardon, S. (2020). *Antibiotic Treatment for COVID-19 Complications Could Fuel Resistant Bacteria*. Available online at: https://www.sciencemag.org/news/2020/04/antibiotic-treatment-covid-19-complications-could-fuel-resistant-bacteria (accessed June 15, 2020).

Roquilly, A., McWilliam, H. E., Jacqueline, C., Tian, Z., Cinotti, R., Rimbert, M., et al. (2017). Local modulation of antigen-presenting cell development after resolution of pneumonia induces long-term susceptibility to secondary infections. *Immunity* 47, 135–147.

Sarker, S. A., Sultana, S., Reuteler, G., Moine, D., Descombes, P., Charton, F., et al. (2016). Oral phage therapy of acute bacterial diarrhea with two coliphage preparations: a randomized trial in children from Bangladesh. *EBioMedicine* 4, 124–137. doi: 10.1016/j.ebiom.2015.12.023

Schmelcher, M., Donovan, D. M., and Loessner, M. J. (2012). Bacteriophage endolysins as novel antimicrobials. *Future Microbiol.* 7, 1147–1171. doi: 10.2217/fmb.12.97

Schooley, R. T., Biswas, B., Gill, J. J., Hernandez-Morales, A., Lancaster, J., Lessor, L., et al. (2017). Development and use of personalized bacteriophage-based therapeutic cocktails to treat a patient with a disseminated resistant *Acinetobacter baumannii* infection. *Antimicrob. Agents Chemother.* 61: e00954-17.

Seguin, P., Laviolle, B., Chanavaz, C., Donnio, P. Y., Gautier-Lerestif, A. L., Campion, J. P., et al. (2006). Factors associated with multidrug-resistant bacteria in secondary peritonitis: impact on antibiotic therapy. *Clin. Microbiol. Infect.* 12, 980–985. doi: 10.1111/j.1469-0691.2006.01507.x

Summers, W. C. (2001). Bacteriophage therapy. *Annu. Rev. Microbiol.* 55, 437–451.

Tagliaferri, T. L., Jansen, M., and Horz, H. P. (2019). Fighting pathogenic bacteria on two fronts: phages and antibiotics as combined strategy. *Front. Cell. Infect. Microbiol.* 9:22. doi: 10.3389/fcimb.2019.00022

Tetro, J. A. (2020). Is COVID-19 receiving ADE from other coronaviruses? *Microb. Infect.* 22, 72–73. doi: 10.1016/j.micinf.2020.02.006

Torres-Barceló, C. (2018). The disparate effects of bacteriophages on antibiotic-resistant bacteria. *Emerg. Microbes Infect.* 7, 1–2.

Torres-Barceló, C., Franzon, B., Vasse, M., and Hochberg, M. E. (2016). Long-term effects of single and combined introductions of antibiotics and bacteriophages on populations of *Pseudomonas aeruginosa*. *Evol. Appl.* 9, 583–595. doi: 10.1111/eva.12364

Valério, N., Oliveira, C., Jesus, V., Branco, T., Pereira, C., Moreirinha, C., et al. (2017). Effects of single and combined use of bacteriophages and antibiotics to inactivate *Escherichia coli*. *Virus Res.* 240, 8–17. doi: 10.1016/j.virusres.2017.07.015

Van Belleghem, J. D., Dąbrowska, K., Vaneechoutte, M., and Barr, J. J. (2019). "Phage interaction with the mammalian immune system," in *Phage Therapy: A Practical Approach*, eds (Cham: Springer), 91–122. doi: 10.1007/978-3-030-26736-0_4

Voelker, R. (2019). FDA approves bacteriophage trial. *JAMA* 321, 638–638.

Wang, D., Hu, B., Hu, C., Zhu, F., Liu, X., Zhang, J., et al. (2020). Clinical characteristics of 138 hospitalized patients with 2019 novel coronavirus-infected pneumonia in Wuhan, China. *JAMA* 323, 1061–1069.

Wang, H., Anthony, D., Selemidis, S., Vlahos, R., and Bozinovski, S. (2018). Resolving viral-induced secondary bacterial infection in COPD: A concise review. *Front. Immunol.* 9:2345. doi: 10.3389/fimmu.2018.02345

Weber-Dabrowska, B., Mulczyk, M., and Górski, A. (2001). Bacteriophage therapy for infections in cancer patients. *Clin. Appl. Immunol. Rev.* 1, 131–134. doi: 10.1016/s1529-1049(01)00015-0

Williams, A. E., Edwards, L., Humphreys, I. R., Snelgrove, R., Rae, A., Rappuoli, R., et al. (2004). Innate imprinting by the modified heat-labile toxin of *Escherichia coli* (LTK63) provides generic protection against lung infectious disease. *J. Immunol.* 173, 7435–7443. doi: 10.4049/jimmunol.173.12.7435

Yang, X., Yu, Y., Xu, J., Shu, H., Liu, H., Wu, Y., et al. (2020). Clinical course and outcomes of critically ill patients with SARS-CoV-2 pneumonia in Wuhan, China: a single-centered, retrospective, observational study. *Lancet Respir. Med.* 8, 475–481. doi: 10.1016/s2213-2600(20)30079-5

Zhou, F., Yu, T., Du, R., Fan, G., Liu, Y., Liu, Z., et al. (2020). Clinical course and risk factors for mortality of adult inpatients with COVID-19 in Wuhan, China: a retrospective cohort study. *Lancet* 395, 1054–1062. doi: 10.1016/s0140-6736(20)30566-3

20

In Vitro Modelling of Respiratory Virus Infections in Human Airway Epithelial Cells

Laurine C. Rijsbergen[1], Laura L. A. van Dijk[1], Maarten F. M. Engel[2], Rory D. de Vries[1] and Rik L. de Swart[1]*

[1] *Department of Viroscience, Postgraduate School of Molecular Medicine, Erasmus MC, University Medical Centre Rotterdam, Rotterdam, Netherlands,* [2] *Medical Library, Erasmus MC, University Medical Centre Rotterdam, Rotterdam, Netherlands*

***Correspondence:**
Rik L. de Swart
r.deswart@erasmusmc.nl

Respiratory tract infections (RTI) are a major cause of morbidity and mortality in humans. A large number of RTIs is caused by viruses, often resulting in more severe disease in infants, elderly and the immunocompromised. Upon viral infection, most individuals experience common cold-like symptoms associated with an upper RTI. However, in some cases a severe and sometimes life-threatening lower RTI may develop. Reproducible and scalable *in vitro* culture models that accurately reflect the human respiratory tract are needed to study interactions between respiratory viruses and the host, and to test novel therapeutic interventions. Multiple *in vitro* respiratory cell culture systems have been described, but the majority of these are based on immortalized cell lines. Although useful for studying certain aspects of viral infections, such monomorphic, unicellular systems fall short in creating an understanding of the processes that occur at an integrated tissue level. Novel *in vitro* models involving primary human airway epithelial cells and, more recently, human airway organoids, are now in use. In this review, we describe the evolution of *in vitro* cell culture systems and their characteristics in the context of viral RTIs, starting from advances after immortalized cell cultures to more recently developed organoid systems. Furthermore, we describe how these models are used in studying virus-host interactions, e.g. tropism and receptor studies as well as interactions with the innate immune system. Finally, we provide an outlook for future developments in this field, including co-factors that mimic the microenvironment in the respiratory tract.

Keywords: respiratory viral diseases, primary airway epithelium culture, organoid culture, co-culture, airway modeling

INTRODUCTION

Respiratory tract infections (RTIs) are a major source of morbidity and mortality in humans (1). Almost 300 million episodes of lower RTIs (e.g. pneumoniae and bronchitis) occurred in 2015 and about 3 million people die each year. This places RTIs amongst the leading causes of death worldwide (2, 3). A large fraction of RTIs is caused by viruses (50 to 90%) (4). Respiratory viruses include human rhinovirus (HRV), influenza A and B virus (IAV and IBV), human respiratory syncytial virus (HRSV), human metapneumovirus (HMPV), human coronavirus (HCoV), human parainfluenzavirus (HPIV), and human adenovirus (HAdV). Most respiratory viruses have single-stranded RNA genomes, with the exception of adenoviruses that have double-stranded DNA genomes. The highest morbidity and mortality due to RTIs is seen in infants, elderly and immunocompromised individuals, but also healthy individuals without underlying risk factors can be affected (5). Furthermore, RTIs have been associated with exacerbations of asthma or chronic obstructive pulmonary disease (COPD) (6, 7).

Recently, severe acute respiratory syndrome coronavirus 2 (SARS-CoV-2) has captured global headlines as the causative agent in the coronavirus disease 2019 (COVID-19) pandemic (8), highlighting the impact of respiratory viruses on global health. As this pandemic has shown, options for prophylaxis and treatment of viral respiratory infections are limited. For some viruses, such as influenza virus or adenovirus, vaccines are available but both efficacy and coverage are suboptimal. Antiviral drugs against acute respiratory virus infections often have limited efficacy. Therefore, development of novel and improved antiviral drugs and vaccines remains of high priority to improve global health.

The human respiratory tract (RT) is the primary site where respiratory viruses enter, replicate, disseminate and cause disease. These viruses are transmitted by aerosols and/or droplets. RTIs in most cases start by infection of airway epithelial cells in the upper respiratory tract (URT) (nasal cavity, pharynx, larynx), and are associated with common cold-like symptoms, including rhinitis, sore throat, runny nose, and nasal congestion. During the course of infection, the lower respiratory tract (LRT) (trachea, primary bronchi, lungs) can become involved, causing more severe disease, such as pneumonia or bronchitis (9). How severe lower RTIs develop and why only some individuals are affected could be a stochastic process related to dose and route of the inoculum. However, the development of severe LRTIs remains a black box and is an important topic of investigation. Many of these studies are performed *in vivo*, which provides important data on the pathogenesis of respiratory viruses [reviewed elsewhere (10–14)] but has some downsides, such as differences between animal or human host factors, ethical concerns and practical challenges. *In vitro* models have as advantages that they originate from the relevant host species, express the relevant host factors, are of less ethical concern and easier to work with than animal models. Therefore, a reproducible and scalable *in vitro* culture system that accurately represents the human RT would be valuable to study respiratory virus infections and test new treatments. Here we investigate the differences between commonly used *in vitro* primary airway cell culture models and how these models are used for studying respiratory virus infections. The first part of this review describes several characteristics of the RT, then we will review the evolution of *in vitro* cell culture systems in the context of viral RTIs, starting from advances after immortalized cell lines to recently developed stem cell (SC)-based organoid cultures. Finally, an outlook is provided for future developments in this field.

METHODOLOGY AND STUDY DESIGN

This systematic review was prepared in accordance with PRISMA (Preferred Reporting Items for Systematic Reviews and Meta-analyses) guidelines (15). A systematic literature search, on the 21st of January of 2021, was conducted using title, abstract, index term and author keyword fields for respiratory viruses and human airway epithelial cells (HAEC) or their variations. Of note, primary olfactory epithelial cells were not included, since there are described previously (16). Embase, Medline (Ovid), and Web of Science Core Collection databases (**Supplementary Material 1**) were searched from inception until 21st January 2021. Search results were restricted to English and excluded case-reports. Articles were imported and deduplicated in EndNote™. Two researchers independently screened title and abstract for study eligibility criteria (17). Consensus was achieved after discussion upon disagreement. The electronic search was performed in Embase, Medline and WoS (**Supplementary Material 2**).

RESULTS

943 references were obtained and screened on basis of title and abstract (**Figure 1**). After the first screening, studies using only animal material, material of diseased patients, or immortalized cell lines were excluded. In addition, studies performed with respiratory bacteria (e.g. *Heamophilus influenzae*) and where adenoviruses were used as a vector were excluded. For the second screening full-text articles were assessed for eligibility and divided into seven topics: pathogenesis (N=165), signal transduction (N=93), co-cultures (N=21), zoonosis (N=11), reviews (N=32), drug/molecule testing (N=145), and disease (e.g. cystic fibrosis and chronic obstructive pulmonary disease) (N=28). Studies regarding signal transduction, drug/molecule testing and diseases such as chronic obstructive pulmonary disease and cystic fibrosis were excluded at this stage (n=504). Finally, 151 studies were selected for this systematic review. To provide sufficient background information we also included 69 additional papers based on relevant content for this review, resulting in a final selection of 220 papers.

DISCUSSION

The Respiratory Tract

The RT can be divided into separate sections, either based on physiology (URT *versus* LRT, **Figure 2A**) or the type of respiratory epithelium (**Figure 2B**). The URT includes the nasal cavity, mouth, larynx and pharynx (throat), and beginning of the trachea (18). In the nasal cavity inspired air is

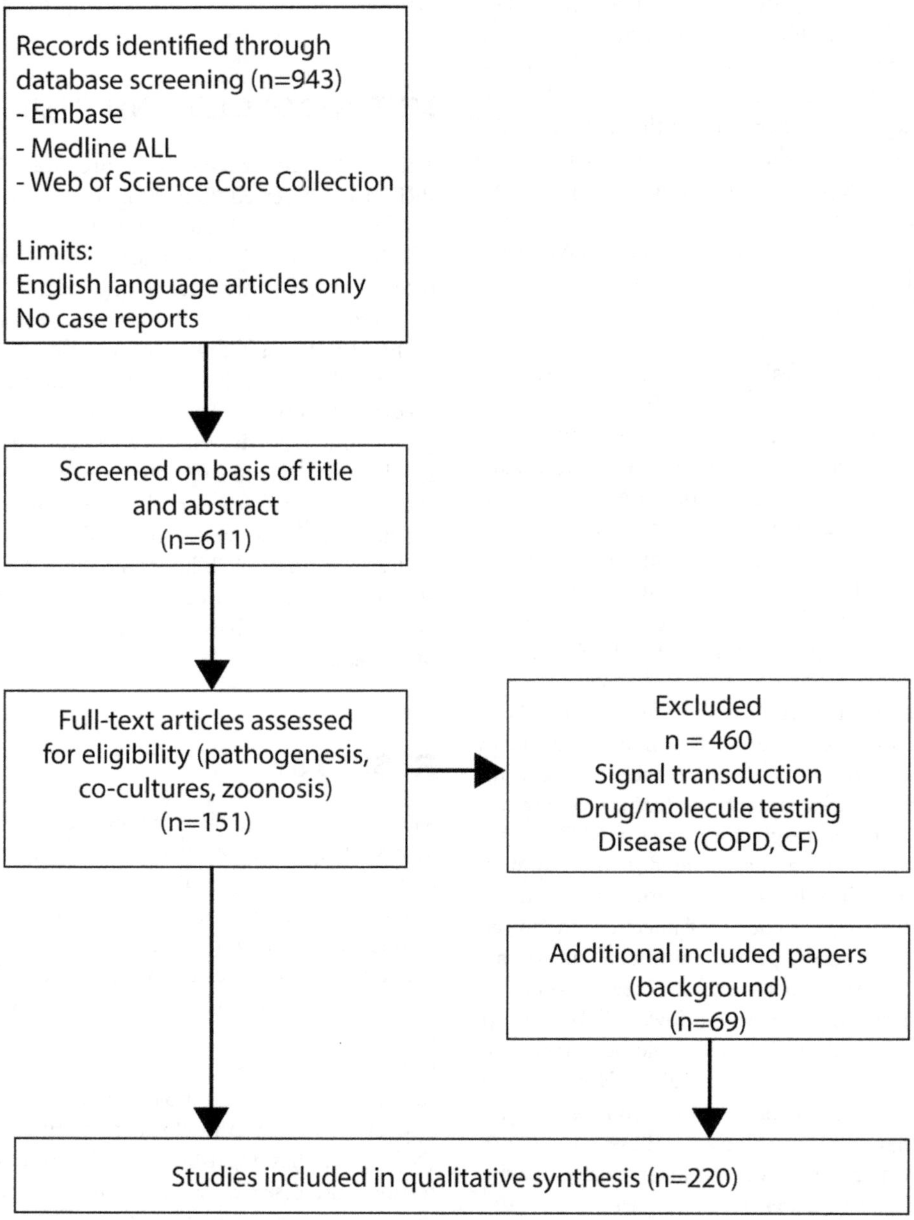

FIGURE 1 | PRISMA flow diagram of the study selection process.

warmed and humidified before it travels down the RT. Additionally, the nasal cavity houses the olfactory receptors that bind molecules resulting in impulses to the brain that enable smell. The nasal cavities drain into the nasopharynx that is in turn attached to the trachea (19). The trachea connects the throat to the LRT, starting at the primary bronchial branches (20, 21). The two bronchial branches bifurcate further into smaller tubes called the bronchi and bronchioles, which end in the alveoli; tiny air sacs facilitating gas exchange (22, 23). The entire RT is covered by epithelium and it is estimated that an adult of 176 cm or an infant of 60 cm have a lung epithelial surface of 78 m^2 or 4 m^2, respectively (24).

The airway epithelium has a crucial barrier and immune functions. The mucus covering the airway epithelium is the first barrier that respiratory viruses have to pass to reach the airway epithelial cells. The airway epithelium itself has essential inflammatory, immune and regenerative capacities to combat these viruses.

The airway epithelium is composed of several cell types held together by tight junctions and adherens junctions that form a barrier against invading pathogens. The nasal cavity is lined with two distinct kinds of epithelium: the olfactory epithelium (1-2% of the nasal epithelium) and the respiratory epithelium (>98% of the nasal epithelium) (19). The neurons in the olfactory

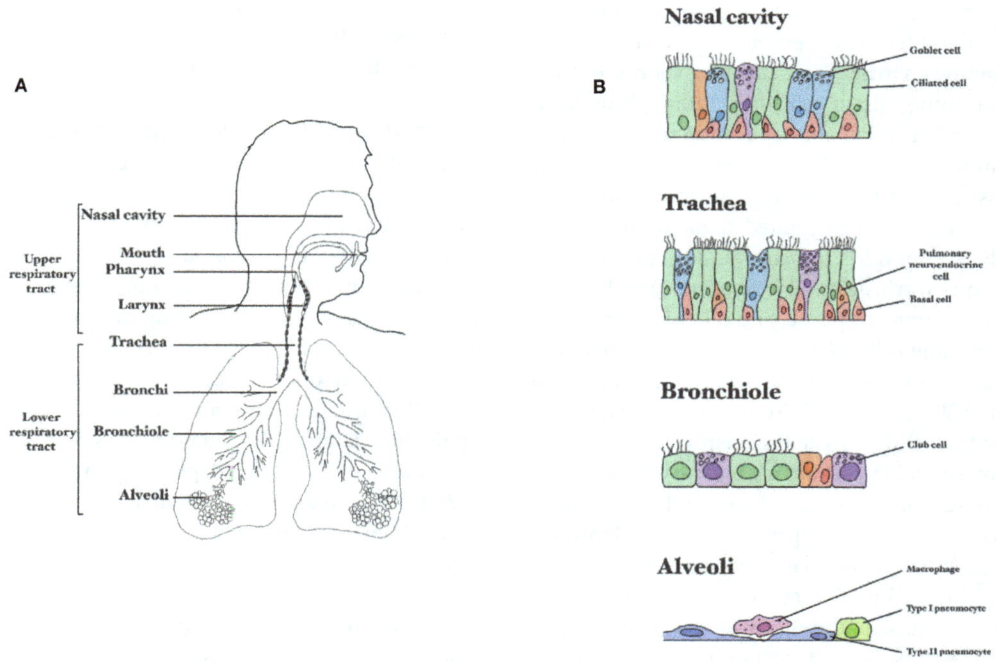

FIGURE 2 | Composition of the respiratory tract. **(A)** Division between the upper and lower respiratory tract. **(B)** Schematic representation of epithelial layer in the different parts of the respiratory tract.

epithelium in the nose are directly connected to the central nervous system *via* the olfactory nerve. Viruses that infect the olfactory epithelium can use this nerve as a shortcut to reach the central nervous system (25). The epithelial layer in the nasal atrium consists of multi-layered keratinized squamous epithelium and further down the nose this becomes multi-row cylindrical epithelium. Many respiratory epithelial cells are also ciliated, facilitating mucus transport towards the pharynx and trachea (19). From the trachea downwards, the RT is lined with ciliated pseudostratified columnar epithelium (20). In the bronchioles, the epithelium gradually changes from pseudostratified into simple cuboidal and in the alveolar ducts and alveoli there is simple squamous epithelium (mainly type alveolar type I cells) (20).

Ciliated cells account for 50% to 80% of the airway epithelial cells, and have 200-300 motile cilia on their surface to displace mucus, enabling muco-ciliary clearance (26). The cells producing mucus are goblet cells, comprising around 9% of the respiratory epithelial cells (27). Next to goblet cells there are club cells; cuboidal non-ciliated non-mucous secretory cells. Club cells secrete extracellular matrix components, and can serve as progenitor cells for themselves and for ciliated cells (28). These cells are not very abundant in the URT, but in the terminal bronchioles account for approximately 11-22% of the cells (28). Epithelial and mucus-producing cells are supported by airway basal cells. Whereas the epithelial and mucus-producing cells are terminally differentiated and cannot renew, basal cells possess stem-cell like properties (29, 30). Basal cells occupy 31% of the respiratory epithelial cell population, the density of basal cells decreases when descending into the small airways (31). Another important cell type of the airways is the pulmonary neuroendocrine cell, comprising 1 out of 2500 epithelial cells from the trachea onto the alveolar ducts (32), forming the lung self-renewing SC niche relevant in airway epithelial regeneration (33). The alveolar epithelium consists mostly of two cell types, alveolar type I and type II cells (ATI and ATII). ATI are very thin, squamous cells, accounting for over 90% of the surface area in the lungs and provide an efficient barrier for air exchange (34). About 7% of the surface area comprises ATII, which are smaller and cuboidal, and function mostly in the production and uptake of lung surfactant (35). ATIIs can differentiate into ATI (36). In addition to ATI and ATII, also immune cells, like alveolar macrophages, are present in the alveoli.

Besides a barrier function, respiratory epithelial cells have inherent innate immunity functions. They recognize respiratory viruses via pattern recognition receptors, eventually leading to the production of cytokines and chemokines that render the cells and their neighboring cells in an antiviral state (37). The bridge between this innate response and adaptive immunity is formed by dendritic cells (DCs). There are tissue-resident DCs, that form an integrated network within the respiratory epithelium. Upon activation, for instance by a virus infection, they can travel to the lymph nodes to initiate an adaptive immune response. There are also migratory DCs that can be attracted to the site of infection and aid here in the local immune response. Besides DCs, natural killer cells, innate lymphoid cells, T cells and B cells orchestrate the immune response in the respiratory epithelium (38). Eventually, all elements contribute to an effective integrated immune response.

In Vitro Models

Multiple *in vitro* respiratory cell culture systems have been developed to study the interaction between the different airway cell types and respiratory viruses. To date, the majority of these models is based on immortalized cell lines. Although useful in the study of direct viral infection and replication mechanisms at a cellular and molecular level, such monomorphic and unicellular systems fall short in creating an understanding of the processes that occur at an integrated tissue level (39, 40). We need more advanced models to better understand infection dynamics in relation to intrinsic cellular resistance mechanisms, including the innate immune response, and other factors such as microbiome and immune cells. New *in vitro* models have been proposed and used for some time, especially involving the use of primary HAEC. HAEC are derived from surgical material or brushings (nose or throat) that are subsequently cultured in the laboratory. More recently, 3D-cultures such as airway organoids (AO), formed from SCs, have been developed and hold promise as a useful tool to study host-pathogen interactions. However, this technique is still in its infancy, laborious and expensive. To perform in-depth studies into interactions between the host airway and respiratory viruses, the ultimate goal is to create a reproducible, scalable, feasible and economic *in vitro* culture system that faithfully recapitulates the architecture of the RT as well as the dynamics of infection.

Primary Respiratory Epithelial Cells

HAEC are obtained from human respiratory tissue, which can originate from different anatomical sites of the RT (41). Respiratory tissue is now obtained in different ways: during lung transplantation, during tissue resection in cancer patients, during other surgical procedures (e.g. turbinoplasty/-ectomy or nasal polypectomy) or from cadaveric explants (41). In addition, nasal and bronchial brushings, which are less invasive, can be performed to obtain HAEC (42). HAEC from healthy donors are now commercially available (43). Additionally, material from, for instance, COPD patients and/or smokers is also available (44, 45). Acquiring HAEC from various donors allows us to study and compare the RT of both healthy and diseased individuals.

Undifferentiated Primary Respiratory Epithelial Cells

Primary undifferentiated HAEC ($HAEC_{un}$) are relatively easy to culture, but can only be passaged a few times. After obtaining tissue, the primary airway epithelial cells are directly isolated and cultured. For the isolation of primary airway epithelial cells from lung transplants or biopsies, the tissue is cut into smaller pieces and then dissociated *via* the addition of a protease-containing digestion cocktail, followed by generation of uniform single-cell suspensions (46, 47). Tissue obtained from brushings can be cultured directly (47). After isolation, HAEC can be used in this undifferentiated form for experiments. In addition to normal culture flasks or plates, HAEC can also be seeded on a collagen-coated semi-permeable membrane (transwell) (48). In this transwell system, medium is present on both the apical and the basolateral side. When a 100% confluent monolayer has formed to separate the apical and basolateral compartments, the $HAEC_{un}$ can be used for experiments. These $HAEC_{un}$ are not polarized and these cultures do not have ciliated cells or goblet cells, and therefore lack important characteristics of the airways.

Differentiated Primary Respiratory Epithelial Cells

Although more challenging to culture, differentiated HAEC ($HAEC_{dif}$) represent the RT more faithfully than their undifferentiated counterparts. To differentiate primary respiratory epithelial cells in the transwell system, medium is removed from the apical compartment after the confluent monolayer has formed, creating an air-liquid interface (ALI). This, in combination with specific growth factors, induces differentiation of these cells over a timeframe of 3-4 weeks (48). Eventually, a polarized, pseudostratified respiratory epithelium is formed, containing basal cells, ciliated cells, and goblet cells or club cells (depending on the anatomical location) (48, 49). These $HAEC_{dif}$ resemble the human RT anatomically (50, 51) but a continuous airflow, blood flow, and the presence of immune cells are still lacking.

Considerations for Use of Primary Cells

Comparing studies using primary HAEC is difficult, because of differences in donor variability **(1)**, anatomic source of the cells **(2)**, culture methods (e.g. medium and growth factors) **(3)** and the use of undifferentiated *versus* differentiated cells **(4)** (**Figure 3**).

1. Variability in culturability, morphology and phenotype between primary HAEC obtained from different donors has been described. This donor variability can depend on multiple factors, like age, gender, smoking history, or obesity (52–56). Variation in infection and replication levels of viruses between donors was regularly observed (57–60). Explanations could be differences in: receptor presence or distribution, cytokine responses, donors and environmental factors (61, 62). It is dependent on the research question how important these dissimilarities are.
2. In addition to donor variability, the source of the cells (ranging from nose to alveoli) can make comparison of studies difficult (63, 64), because of variations in susceptibility to viral infections and virus-host interactions (9). The preferential anatomical site should be determined by the research question (e.g. study URT or LRT) and comparing cells of multiple regions of the RT for susceptibility, virus replication and host responses.
3. The importance of culture medium is highlighted in a HRSV infection study, where two different media for differentiation of pediatric HAEC (nasal) were used: PneumaCult^{TM} and Promocell^{TM}. The former led to an overall greater total number of cells, but the proportion of ciliated and goblet cells was similar. The replication kinetics of HRSV was similar in both cultures, but in the culture with PneumoCultTM more ciliated cells were infected. HRSV infection of the PneumoCultTM cultures led to a higher IFNλ secretion, which could be due to the increased infection of ciliated cells (65).

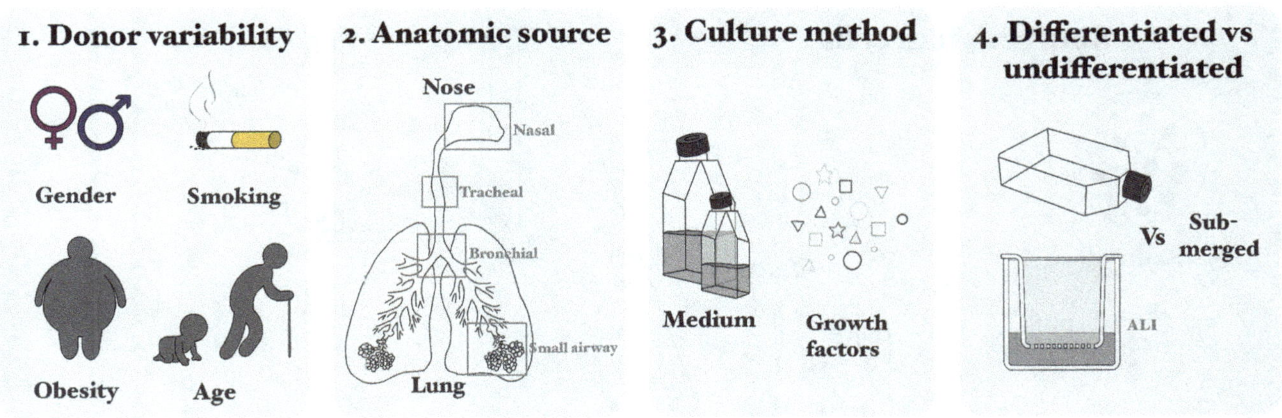

FIGURE 3 | Considerations for using primary cells: differences in donor variability **(1)**, anatomic source of the cells **(2)**, culture methods (e.g. medium and growth factors) **(3)** and the use of undifferentiated *versus* differentiated cells **(4)**.

4. Several studies describe different expression patterns of cellular receptors that can mediate virus entry, resulting in varying infection percentages or different immune response between $HAEC_{un}$ and $HAEC_{dif}$ (66–69).

$HAEC_{un}$ can be passaged approximately three times prior to differentiation, after which loss of epithelial integrity, differential gene expression, or senescence occurs (70–72). This restricts the number of experiments that can be performed. That is why immortalized variants of HAEC have been created. Jonsdottir and colleagues (2019) described that insertion of the Rho-associated protein kinase (ROCK) inhibitor Y-27632 *via* a lentiviral vector increased the longevity of the primary respiratory epithelial cells (73). Alternatively, exogenous induction of human telomerase reverse transcriptase (hTERT) can be used to prolong primary cell life (74). Immortalization resolves the issue of the restricted number of experiments, but it remains unknown if all the characteristics of the respiratory epithelial cells remain the same. And, even in these immortalized variants, senescence can occur after a few passages (75, 76). Genetic engineering of HAEC is challenging and may compromise translational aspects of the model.

In conclusion, primary HAEC can be extracted from all parts of the airways and differentiated into a pseudostratified monolayer resembling the *in vivo* situation. Although several variables and parameters must be considered, primary HAEC are a promising culture system to study RTIs.

Stem Cell-Based Models

SC-based models have the potential to overcome the problems associated with the limited lifespan of primary HAEC. SCs can be used to make organoids, which are three dimensional cultures that can self-organize and renew (77). Organoid culture is a novel and innovative technology and was first described in 2009 with organoids from the gut (78). In 2012, the technique to culture AO was developed (79). Until now, human AO are mostly made from SCs obtained from adult lungs. Adults tissues are more accessible than embryonic SCs or induced pluripotent (iPSCs) and have less ethical restraints. Nevertheless, AO from embryonic SCs are also used (80, 81). Although most studies describe AO obtained from the lung, AO can be made from almost all parts of the RT, and are thus a suitable alternative to primary HAEC (82). Additionally, genetic modifications are also more feasible in AO than in primary HAEC.

Different SCs can be used to generate AO. First, embryonic SCs obtained from the inner cell mass of an early staged embryo have the potential to form every cell of the human body (83). However, the use of these cells remains ethically controversial. Second, iPSCs can also differentiate into almost every cell type of the human body (84). To obtain these iPSCs, somatic cells (for example skin cells) are reprogrammed to the progenitor state by addition of several transcription factors. However, specific factors, including growth factors and cytokines, are needed for differentiation into respiratory epithelial cells (85), which has so far not been successful. The challenges to find the optimal factors to differentiate these iPSCs into airway epithelial cells can be overcome by using organ-specific adult SCs. These cells can differentiate into the cell types of the respective organ (86). In this case, airway epithelial SCs can be isolated from tissue or URT brushings (87). The isolated basal cells can subsequently be used for the formation of 3D undifferentiated AO, using Matrigel and medium with specific growth factors. These AO, cultured either in 3D in matrigel or on transwell filters at ALI, can then be differentiated into cultures that represent the cells of the RT, such as basal cells, goblet cells, ciliated cells or alveolar cells (81, 87–92) (**Figure 4A**). In a differentiated spheroid AO, the basal cells are on the outside of the sphere, the goblet cells excrete their mucus into the lumen while the cilia move the mucus around (see **Figure 4B**). Similar to primary cell cultures, there are indications that culture medium influences organoid morphology and behavior, which is something that has to be studied in more detail (92, 93).

AO appear to be a promising model mimicking the human RT and once established can be maintained for a long period of

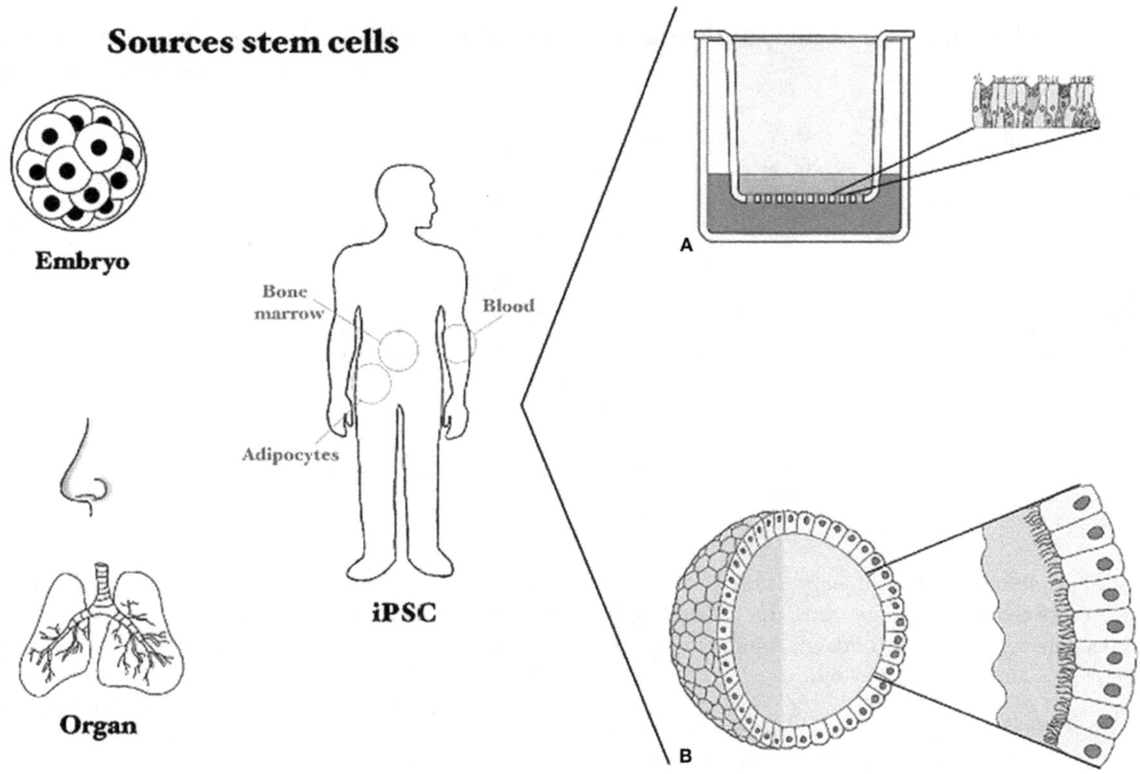

FIGURE 4 | Sources of stem cells and culture methods. Several sources for stem cells are shown: embryonic stem cells, induced pluripotent stem cells (iPSC) and organ-derived or nasal brushing-derived. **(A)** Shows a Transwell system on which primary cells or stem-cell based cells can be cultured, **(B)** shows an airway organoid sphere with cilia and mucus on the inside.

time. Limited studies have been performed with AO and respiratory viruses so far due to the novelty of the technique. However, the studies that have been performed show great promise for studying virus-host interaction and drug screening studies in this model.

Studying Respiratory Virus Infections

To understand the pathogenesis of respiratory virus infections, it is important to study (1) tropism, (2) receptor usage, (3) immune response, (4) cytopathic effects and damage, and (5) tissue regeneration after clearance. Primary cell culture models are crucial in these studies, because viruses rapidly adapt to culture in immortalized cell lines (81, 94, 95). In this second part of the review, we summarize how these properties of respiratory viruses have been investigated in light of the advantages of using primary HAEC and AO (**Table 1**).

Receptor Studies

One of the mechanisms by which viruses enter a host cell is receptor-mediated entry; the appropriate receptor needs to be present on the cell for the virus to enter. Immortalized cell lines are often used to identify such a cellular receptor, for example by genomic- and interactome- based approaches (141, 142). Primary HAEC mimic the natural targets cells of respiratory viruses better than continuous cell lines and are thus important for receptor identification, as illustrated in the following examples.

For most HCoVs, receptors were initially identified in cell lines, followed by confirmation and verification of these receptors in primary HAEC (58, 66, 91, 105–107, 143–148). An example of the importance of using primary HAEC was seen in the search for a model for HCoV-HKU1. This virus only replicates in primary differentiated tracheobronchial epithelial cells. Through studies in these cells, the HCoV-HKU1 receptor (O-acetylated sialic acid) was ultimately identified (108, 149). Differential binding of avian and human influenza viruses to their receptors was investigated in primary $HAEC_{dif}$ (bronchial), which express both α-2,3- and α-2,6-linked oligosaccharides. Infections with avian and human influenza viruses confirmed that viruses with avian origin preferably bind to α-2,3-linked oligosaccharides, whereas viruses from human origin bind to α-2,6-linked oligosaccharides (133). For most HRV subtypes their receptor was identified in immortalized cell lines and validated in HAEC, except for HRV-C (96–99, 150–153). For HRV-C the receptor was found in primary differentiated bronchial epithelial cells and in *ex vivo* organ transplants, since this HRV subtype does not replicate in continuous cell lines (101, 154).

Many HRSV receptor candidates have been proposed in literature, but arguably the relevant *in vivo* receptor has not yet

TABLE 1 | Summary table of the studies on respiratory viruses performed in primary respiratory epithelial cells and stem cell-based models.

Virus family		Characteristics (receptor, tropism, innate immune response)	Cell culture model	References
Rhinovirus				
Receptor		Major group: ICAM-1Minor group: LDL-RHRV-C CDHR3	$HAEC_{un/dif}$ (bronchial and tracheal)	(96–101)
Tropism		Ciliated epithelial cells	$HAEC_{dif}$ (bronchial)	(101)
Cytokines		TNF-α, IL-6, IL-8, and IP-10, IL-17C, type I IFN, type III IFN, CCL5, IL-1α, IL-1β, IL-1Ra, CXCL10	$HAEC_{dif}$ (bronchial)	(102–104)
Coronavirus				
Receptor		HCoV-229E: CD13HCoV-HKU1: O-acetylated sialic acidSARS-CoV/SARS-CoV-2: ACE2, SXLMERS-CoV: DPP4	$HAEC_{dif}$ (bronchial)Stem cell-based alveolospheres	(58, 66, 91, 105–108)
Tropism		Sars-CoV/SARS-CoV-2: ciliated epithelial cells, type III pneumocytes, club cellsMERS-CoV/HcoV-229: non-ciliated epithelial cellsHCoV-HKU1: Type I pneumocytes	$HAEC_{un/dif}$ (bronchial)AOATIATIIStem cell-based alveolospheres	(57, 88–91, 105, 107, 109–111)
Cytokines		Type I IFN, type III IFN, CCL20, IL-33, CXCL5, CXCL6, CXCL8, CXCL20, IL-6, CXCL2, CXCL3, CXCL10, CXCL11, IL-17, IL-18, IL-1β, CCL4, CCL5, IL-8, IL-1α, IP-10, MIP-1β	$HAEC_{un/dif}$ (bronchial)AOATIATIIStem cell-based alveolospheres	(90, 91, 110–114)
Influenza virus				
Receptor		Avian influenza viruses: α-2,3-linked oligosaccharidesHuman influenza viruses: α-2,6-linked oligosaccharides	$HAEC_{un/dif}$AO	(93, 115)
Tropism		Ciliated cells, sometimes basal cells	$HAEC_{un/dif}$ (nasal, bronchial, tracheobronchial) AO	(93, 115)
Cytokines		IL-1b, IL-6, IP-10, CCL2, CCL5, CXCL11, and IL-8, IL-1α, CXCL10, type I IFN, type III IFN	$HAEC_{un/dif}$ (nasal, bronchial, tracheobronchial)	(116–118)
Pneumovirus				
Receptor		HRSV: CXCR3, IGFR1, nucleolin, HMPV: heparan sulfate	$HAEC_{dif}$ (nasal and bronchial)	(119–121)
Tropism		Ciliated epithelial cells, type II pneumocytes, sometimes goblet cells and basal cells	$HAEC_{dif}$ (nasal, tracheobronchial, bronchiolar) AO	(87, 122–125)
Cytokines		IL-6, IL-8, RANTES, type I IFN, type III IFN, CXCL-1, IP10, TFN-α, IL-10, CXCL-8, TRAIL, CXCL1	Primary (un)differentiated nasal and small airway epithelial cellshTERT-NECsAirway organoids	(126–132)
Parainfluenza virus				
Receptor		HPIV-1: α-2,3-linked sialic acid residuesHPIV-3: α-2,6-linked sialic acid residues	$HAEC_{dif}$ (tracheobronchial)	(133–135)
Tropism		Ciliated epithelial cells	$HAEC_{dif}$ (tracheobronchial)	(134, 136)
Cytokines		CXCL10 and CXCL11	$HAEC_{dif}$ (tracheobronchial)	(137)
Adenovirus				
Receptor		HAdV-B type 14: Desmoglein 2HAdV-c type 5: CAR	$HAEC_{dif}$ (bronchial)	(138)
Tropism		Lung parenchyma	AO	(139)
Cytokines		Meyer-Berg 2020 Stem cell research & therapy	$HAEC_{dif}$ (bronchial)	(140)

HAECun, undifferentiated human airway epithelial cells; HAECdif, differentiated human airway epithelial cells; ATI, type I alveolar cells; ATII, type II alveolar cells; AO, airway organoids.

been identified. Ciliated epithelial cells are the main target cell of HRSV (155), therefore primary $HAEC_{dif}$ are the most suitable model to perform receptor studies. CXC3R1, insulin-like growth factor-1 (IGFR1) and nucleolin have been identified as potential cellular receptors for HRSV. CXC3R1 would probably not have been found if it were not for primary HAEC, since this receptor is absent (unless transfected) on immortalized cell lines (119, 120). The other two receptors have been confirmed and validated in primary HAEC (121, 156). Although closely related to HRSV, the proposed receptors for HMPV are not the same as for HRSV, but studies with primary respiratory epithelial cells from different locations in the RT have proposed integrins and heparin sulfate as receptors (126, 127, 157, 158).

Lastly, using primary $HAEC_{dif}$ (tracheobronchial), it was confirmed that HPIV-3 uses α-2,6-linked sialic acid residues and HPIV-1 uses α-2,3-linked sialic acid residues as cellular receptors (133, 134). Primary HAEC have also been used to identify or verify the receptors for HAdV (138, 159).

All the above-mentioned examples clearly illustrate that HAEC are important for identifying the cellular entry receptor for respiratory viruses. Although initially the receptor is often found in cell lines, primary cell models are essential in confirming and validating this receptor and these results translate better to the *in vivo* situation.

Tropism

Regarding viral tropism, *in vivo* models and *ex vivo* culture models provide valuable information. However, it has to be kept in mind that in *in vivo* studies the animal is often not the natural host of the virus, introducing a possible bias. Human post-mortem material from either healthy or infected individuals is also useful for binding studies, but this material is not always available. Cell lines are immortalized and often express unique gene expression patterns that are not representative of *in vivo* cell types. Primary airway models can overcome these hurdles and are a thus powerful tool to investigate viral tropism, since most cell types from the RT are represented in these models.

In the SARS-CoV-2 pandemic, differentiated AO (AO_{dif}) and primary HAEC rapidly helped elucidate that SARS-CoV-2 mainly infects ciliated cells, club cells and ATII, but not goblet cells (88–91, 109, 110). For other coronaviruses, similar models were used to determine their respective tropism, for instance HCoV-229E and MERS-CoV infect non-ciliated cells and HCoV-HKU1 predominantly infects ATII (105, 107, 160, 161). Multiple studies have been performed with influenza viruses in HAEC or AO. It was found that, for example, seasonal H1N1 was able to infect ciliated cells, goblet cells and alveolar cells, whereas pandemic H1N1 was also able to infect club cells (89, 93, 115). HRV is a common cause of respiratory infections in humans and both HRV-A and HRV-B can be cultured in conventional cell models, while this is not the case for HRV-C. However, by using 3D Matrigel cultures with primary $HAEC_{dif}$ HRV-C can be propagated (159). For all three HRV subtypes the tropism could be determined in primary $HAEC_{dif}$ (bronchial): HRV-A and HRV-B infect basal cells and HRV-C infects ciliated epithelial cells (101, 162). It was also confirmed that HRV can replicate in cells from both the URT (adenoids) and LRT (bronchus) (163). Clinical characteristics of HRV are also recapitulated in primary airway models. For instance, HRV-B infections are associated with less severe infections and studies in primary $HAEC_{dif}$ (nasal and bronchial) reported that HRV-B replicates slower and leads to less cytotoxicity than HRV-A and HRV-C (164, 165). For both HRSV and HMPV it was confirmed in $HAEC_{dif}$ and AO_{dif} mainly targets the ciliated epithelial cells (122, 123, 128, 166–168). One study showed that basal cells could also be infected by HRSV after epithelial injury, using commercially obtained primary $HAEC_{dif}$ (bronchial) (124).

In conclusion, with primary airway cultures or SC-based cultures it is possible to culture viruses that are difficult to culture in immortalized cell lines and these models can provide reliable information on the viral tropism.

Disease Modelling

Studying pathogenesis is challenging *in vitro*, both in continuous and primary cell lines. A single or limited number of cell types are present in *in vitro* cultures, not resembling a full organism. As alternative, cytopathic effect (CPE) can be studied. CPE in primary $HAEC_{dif}$ often resembles the natural situation more closely compared to continuous cells. HRSV offers a good example: in continuous cell lines it forms big syncytia (hence the name), but in primary HAEC HRSV forms little to no syncytia, which is in line with observations *in vivo* (both animal models and humans) (48, 122, 129, 168–170). A clinical observation in HRSV disease is neutrophil inflammation, which is involved in severe HRSV disease. This clinical phenomenon has been mimicked in HRSV-infected primary $HAEC_{dif}$ (nasal) that were co-cultured with neutrophils (171). AO have significantly improved disease modelling opportunities. HRSV, HMPV and HPIV have been investigated in AO_{dif}, and for example for HRSV epithelial cell sloughing was shown, which was absent in HPIV infections. These observations both fit with clinical observations. Other hallmarks of HRSV and HMPV disease, such as infection of ciliated epithelial cells and mucus production were also recapitulated in AO and in primary HAEC (80, 87, 125, 155, 172). These hallmarks are impossible to mimic in 2D cell lines and thus highlight the usefulness of 3D AO to study respiratory virus pathogenesis.

Innate Immune Responses

When a virus enters a cell, this cell will directly mount an innate immune response, both in the infected cell and in surrounding cells. This usually includes the production of several cytokines and chemokines to attract more immune cells and activate the adaptive immune system. Studying the innate immune system in primary HAEC has as an advantage over continuous cell lines, because they potentially produce more clinically relevant cytokines that would also be produced by the natural target cells. For instance, for SARS-CoV it was described that ATII are less susceptible than ATI, which was linked to a robust innate immune response (161). This pronounced innate immune response was not found in primary $HAEC_{dif}$ (bronchial, chemically differentiated) after MERS-CoV, SARS-CoV or HCoV-229E infection, indicating immune evasion (173). It appears that each corona-virus induces specific innate immune responses, with few cytokines and ISGs overlapping (90, 91, 110, 112–114). In response to influenza virus infection, similar cytokines, mainly IL-1β, IL-6 and IL-8, were produced in $HAEC_{dif}$ from different parts of the RT (114, 116–118). For HRSV and HMPV infections it has also been shown that similar cytokines, predominantly type I and/or type III IFN, are produced in $HAEC_{dif}$ (nasal, bronchial and small airway) (123, 126–132, 168).

Different subtypes of HPIV are associated with certain clinical observations: HPIV1 can stay undetected for days, whereas HPIV2 is associated with mild disease and HPIV3 with more severe respiratory disease. These clinical observations have been linked to cytokine profiles that were found in primary $HAEC_{dif}$ (tracheobronchial). It was shown that for HPIV1 there was no early innate immune response, whereas for HPIV2 innate cytokines were produced at early time points and for HPIV3 cytokines increased overtime (61).

It was observed that HRV induced an innate immune response in 3D matrigel cultures with primary $HAEC_{dif}$ that inhibited viral replication, but that this was only short-lived because a second peak of viral replication was measured. This correlated with the production of the cytokines TNF-α, IL-6, Il-8, and IP-10. Based on these results, the authors postulated that the second peak appeared due to the production of new virus, after the eclipse caused by the innate immune system (102). Similar replication kinetics and cytokines were seen in other studies, including type I and type III IFN (103, 104, 174, 175). In one study it was shown that upon HRV infection IL-17C was produced in the basolateral compartment and induced CXLC1, which is a neutrophil attractant and may contribute to exacerbations of lower airway disease (103).

To summarize, many studies underline the importance of using primary HAEC and AO when studying innate immune responses. Although these models seem to be a good proxy for clinically relevant cytokines *in vivo*, studies directly comparing the innate cytokine responses between continuous cell lines and primary cell models are lacking. Nevertheless, complex cell systems that mimic the *in vivo* target cells of viruses probably model the antiviral innate immune response better than cell lines.

Other Applications of Primary Respiratory Epithelial Cells

Primary HAEC can mimic host factors related to lifestyle, such as smoking history and obesity. Smoking history might predispose to more severe SARS-CoV-2 disease, possibly to the upregulation of the ACE2 receptor, which was found in formalin-fixed paraffin-embedded human lung tissues and in brushings of the airway epithelium (176–178). This difference was not observed in primary $HAEC_{dif}$ (bronchial), but the number of donors was limited (179). Obesity is related to more severe influenza symptoms, which has been shown in primary ATII, where cells from obese donors were more susceptible to a pandemic IAV than non-obese donors (52).

Primary HAEC are also useful for studying stability of viruses under environmental conditions. For example, primary $HAEC_{dif}$ (bronchial) were used to study the impact of relative humidity on the stability of a pandemic influenza A virus in aerosols and droplets. Aerosols and droplets were created and supplemented with extracellular matrix material harvested from the apical surface of the HAEC and then the amount of virus was determined in MDKC cells (180). None of the experimental humidity conditions affected the stability of IAV H1N1 when aerosols and droplets were supplemented with extracellular matrix, but without supplementation, a humidity-dependent decay of virus infectivity was observed (180). This provided evidence that extracellular matrix can protect influenza viruses from decay and thereby promote spreading (181, 182).

Primary $HAEC_{dif}$ have also been proposed as a screening model for evaluating and monitoring the infectivity, pathogenicity and antigenicity of virus variants, for instance during an outbreak. In the current SARS-CoV-2 pandemic many new, and supposedly more infectious, variants are arising. Information on these variants is important, so that interventions can be tailored. Using primary HAEC, it was found that SARS-CoV-2 variant (D614G) replicates better than the original wild-type strain in the nasal and proximal airways, which was not observed in VeroE6 cells. Increased replication in the URT might lead to more transmission (183). During influenza seasons of 2013-2014 and 2015-2016 the vaccine effectiveness against the circulating influenza strains was reduced. The reason for this was a reduction in sustained multi-cycle replication. This was found in primary $HAEC_{dif}$ (nasal), but not in MDCK cells (182). These important data regarding novel virus variants would not have been available without primary airway models and are important for managing pandemics and developing interventions.

In this section, we illustrated that primary cell models may serve as an authentic model for *in vitro* respiratory viral pathogenesis studies, recapitulating viral infection in the host. They are useful for identifying viral receptors, determining viral tropism, mimicking disease and assessing innate immune responses in respiratory epithelial cells. Additionally, some viruses that are difficult to culture can be propagated in primary HAEC and often not in cell lines (184). Although continuous cell lines can give seminal insights into virus-host interactions, they also render selective pressure on viruses, leading to culture adaptations. One of the advantages of continuous cell lines is the possibility for genetic modification, which is thus far impossible in primary respiratory cell cultures. This hurdle can be overcome in the future by using AO derived from human SCs, which could be engineered to express desired host features.

Co-Cultures

As described above, *in vitro* primary cell models can be used to investigate different aspects of virus-host interactions. However, still a big part of the micro-environment of the cells is not reflected in these models. (1) The lungs fill up with air and deflate during breathing, creating an airflow and stretching of the epithelium. (2) To supply the lungs with sufficient nutrients and to take up incoming oxygen, endothelial blood vessels are connected to the respiratory epithelial cells. (3) The airways are also normally colonized with all different kinds of micro-organisms, referred to as the microbiome. (4) Also, several types of immune cells are present to fight potential pathogens. These four features are usually not recapitulated in HAEs nor AOs, but are important for an integrated *in vitro* airway model.

Endothelial Cells

Endothelial blood vessels are connected to the airway epithelial cells *in vivo* and therefore important to also include in an *in vitro* airway model. Co-cultures with endothelium have been performed, with primary HAEC placed on a chip and microvascular endothelial cells on the opposite side of the porous membrane, with a fluid flow underneath (185). This small airway-on-a-chip model recapitulates tissue-tissue interactions, physicochemical microenvironments, and vascular perfusion of the RT (185, 186). Unfortunately, these models are costly and often not compatible with a biosafety level (BSL)-II or BSL-III laboratory environment required for performing pathogenic virus infections. A way to mimic air flow has been addressed by applying mechanical forces to the airway-on-a-chip model, recreating a breathing movement (187). In another study, primary HAEC were cultured at the apical side of transwell filters and primary microvascular endothelial cells at the basolateral side to create an alveolar-capillary system. This system was used to study influenza virus and staphylococcus aureus (SA) co-infections (188). Thus, although progress is being made, the use of transwell filters and airway-on-a-chip models to model the epithelial-endothelial barrier to study respiratory virus pathogenesis is still limited.

Microbiome

Next to co-cultures with endothelial cells, co-culture models with bacteria and/or viruses to mimic co-infections or the microbiome are being developed. One option is an infection with a bacterium preceding viral infection. In $HAEC_{dif}$ (alveolar), co-cultured with primary microvascular endothelial cells, it was found that methicillin-resistant SA (MRSA) dysregulated the host immune response and decreased the barrier function (188). Another option is a viral infection preceding an infection with a bacterium, for instance initial IAV infection resulted in increased replication of *S. pneumonia* in primary $HAEC_{dif}$ (bronchial). In contrast, in primary HAEC it was then found that pre-exposure to HRV reduced the viral titers of subsequent influenza virus exposure, which was supported by clinical data (189). Co-culturing cells with bacteria poses a challenge, since these micro-organisms replicate fast and rapidly overgrow the respiratory epithelial cells, often leading to cell death. In some of these studies, bacteria were inactivated to overcome this problem, but it is questionable if this still mimics the real-life situation since several features of the bacteria are lost (190). However, it has been shown that inactivated bacteria can influence respiratory virus infections. For instance, UV-inactivated *nontypable Heamophilus influenzae* (NTHI) enhanced the susceptibility of human bronchial epithelial cells to HPIV, likely due to upregulation of ICAM-1, a cellular receptor for HPIV (191, 192). Another way around the toxicity problem could be only co-culturing bacteria for a short time. Obviously, this does not mimic the microbiome or a co-infection (193–196). Nonetheless, this still allowed investigation of bacterial adherence to the (infected) primary HAEC or transmigration of bacteria. Alternatively, co-cultures could be regularly washed. Using this method researchers were able to culture NTHI with commercially available primary HAEC for 10 days (197). Combining co-cultures of bacteria and AO have, to our knowledge, not been described yet, but lessons can be learned from co-cultures of bacteria and intestinal organoids or skin organoids (197, 198).

It is important to study the effect of bacteria and viruses on the innate immune state of the HAEC. Certain innate immune profiles influence the outcome of viral infections, for instance for HRSV. It was described, in humans, that neutrophilic inflammation at the time of viral challenge predisposed individuals to symptomatic HRSV infection (199). These data suggest that co-cultures with, for instance, neutrophils might be required to fully mimic the microenvironment of the RT. In conclusion, although there is only limited data available on this topic, more studies are being performed and we are confident it is feasible to create an *in vitro* airway model combined with the microbiome.

Immune Cells

Another important feature of the airways is the (intra-epithelial) presence of immune cells that are often involved in the defense against respiratory virus infections. Co-cultures of neutrophils with primary $HAEC_{un}$ (trachea) that were infected with HPIV were already performed in the 1990s (200, 201). These studies showed enhanced adhesion of neutrophils to HPIV-infected cells. This has later been shown in AO infected with HRSV, where it was even possible to visualize the preferential neutrophil movement to the infected AO. Co-cultures of primary HAEC (nasal or bronchial) with DCs or T cells have also been described, either with virus present prior to adding the cells, or after. In these studies, researchers investigated both the effect on the immune responses as well as viral replication (87, 202, 203). They showed that the presence of DCs or T cells enhanced antiviral and inflammatory responses and inhibited viral replication. A triple co-culture has also been described, in which primary $HAEC_{dif}$ (bronchial) were co-cultured with monocyte-derived DCs (moDCs) and macrophages (204). Here, the moDCs were infected with HRSV and added apically to a layer of HAEC in a transwell system. Uninfected moDCs were simultaneously added to the basolateral membrane of the insert. This led to the transmission of HRSV to the HAEC, but not to the moDCs located basolaterally. However, when macrophages were added to the apical surface of this co-culture, the basolateral moDCs were infected too, indicating some type of trans-epithelial transport mechanism. This study shows the importance of having multiple factors in a culture to understand the infection process (205). All in all, combining primary $HAEC_{dif}$ with endothelial cells, airflow, the microbiome and immune cells would be an ideal model to mimic our RT.

CONCLUSION AND FUTURE DIRECTIONS

We need scalable, feasible, affordable and reproducible *in vitro* models that adequately reflect the complexity of our RT and the cascade of events that occur during viral infections. We illustrated in this review that primary HAEC and AO are promising models for the RT and for studying respiratory viral pathogenesis. Since the field of primary epithelial cell models and AO is rapidly progressing, future applications of these models are endless. Currently these models are used for testing and developing effective treatments for SARS-CoV-2 (206). Another potential future application of primary HAEC is using species-specific cells to study the zoonotic potential of viruses. With these models it is possible to test the infectivity of the viruses isolated from the natural hosts in primary human respiratory epithelial cells and vice versa (207–210).

Furthermore, primary HAEC and AO can be used for drug screening studies, to test the potential of a drug, small molecule or antibody to inhibit virus replication in the context of a more representative tissue environment. There are many papers describing drug studies performed in HAEC (211). In the future, the use of AO for drug screening studies can be of great value as well (212).

The ultimate goal is to design a model that reflects the respiratory environment in all critical aspects to understand respiratory virus infections and host interaction in detail. Therefore, the usage of self-organized AO models would be preferable over the use of primary HAEC, either in 2D at ALI or 3D. Although initially more expensive and laborious to set up, such AO cultures can be maintained for long periods and are expected to generate the most reproducible results. However, primary HAEC are still a good model to use, especially for rapid screening of inter-individual variation of different donors in response to respiratory virus infections, or fast initial drug screening.

A state-of-the-art development is the lung-on-a-chip model. This model allows co-culture of primary respiratory epithelial cells, for instance primary HAEC or AO, with endothelial cells and mimics breathing by using an airflow and stretching. This model might recapitulate the human airways most faithfully, but there are still many challenges to be overcome before this can be used widely. This model is expensive, and requires specific expertise and equipment. One of the biggest hurdles is using the lung-on-a-chip model in a BSL-II or higher laboratory environment. However, the first study using a lung-on-a-chip model in combination with a respiratory virus (Influenza A) has been published recently showing the potential of this model (213).

In conclusion, primary HAEC are better suited for investigating basic virus-host interactions, such as receptor use and tropism of a respiratory virus than cell lines. However, for investigating the more complex interplay between virus, target cells and immune responses, AO appear to be more suitable. Further improving this model by introducing additional system factors, such endothelium and airflow (as has been done for lung-on-a-chip models), commensal bacteria and immune cells are required to even more closely mimic the micro-environment present in the RT. This culture system will help us understand viral respiratory infections and host responses, and to develop effective therapies to cure these infections.

AUTHOR CONTRIBUTIONS

LR, LD, RV, and RS have been involved in conceptualization, project administration, and visualization. ME was responsible for the methodology with direct involvement of LR and LD. LR and LD were responsible for data curation, investigation, formal analysis, and wrote the original manuscript. All authors contributed to the article and approved the submitted version. RV and RS have been responsible for the supervision. In addition to RV and RS, ME was also involved in providing the resources.

REFERENCES

GBD 2016 Lower Respiratory Infections Collaborators. Estimates of the Global, Regional, and National Morbidity, Mortality, and Aetiologies of Lower Respiratory Infections in 195 Countries, 1990-2016: A Systematic Analysis for the Global Burden of Disease Study 2016. *Lancet Infect Dis* (2018) 18(11):1191–210. doi: 10.1016/S1473-3099(18)30310-4

Shi T, McAllister DA, O'Brien KL, Simoes EAF, Madhi SA, Gessner BD, et al. Global, Regional, and National Disease Burden Estimates of Acute Lower Respiratory Infections Due to Respiratory Syncytial Virus in Young Children in 2015: A Systematic Review and Modelling Study. *Lancet* (2017) 390(10098):946–58. doi: 10.1016/S0140-6736(17)30938-8

Who. *The Top 10 Causes of Death* (2018). Available at: https://www.who.int/ news-room/fact-sheets/detail/the-top-10-causes-of-death.

Henrickson KJ. Viral Pneumonia in Children. *Semin Pediatr Infect Dis* (1998) 9(3):217–33. doi: 10.1016/S1045-1870(98)80035-6

Greenberg SB. Respiratory Viral Infections in Adults. *Curr Opin Pulm Med* (2002) 8(3):201–8. doi: 10.1097/00063198-200205000-00009

Busse WW, Lemanske RF, Gern JE. Role of Viral Respiratory Infections in Asthma and Asthma Exacerbations. *Lancet* (2010) 376(9743):826–34. doi: 10.1016/ S0140-6736(10)61380-3

Nicholson KG, Kent J, Ireland DC. Respiratory Viruses and Exacerbations of Asthma in Adults. *Bmj* (1993) 307(6910):982–6. doi: 10.1136/bmj.307. 6910.982

Zheng J. SARS-CoV-2: An Emerging Coronavirus That Causes a Global Threat. *Int J Biol Sci* (2020) 16(10):1678–85. doi: 10.7150/ijbs.45053

Dasaraju PV, Liu C. Chapter 93 Infections of the Respiratory System. *Med Microbiol* (1996) 1.

Altamirano-Lagos MJ, Dıaz FE, Mansilla MA, Rivera-Pérez D, Soto D, McGill JL, et al. Current Animal Models for Understanding the Pathology Caused by the Respiratory Syncytial Virus. *Front Microbiol* (2019) 10:873. doi: 10.3389/ fmicb.2019.00873

X M, P NG. Cellular and Animals Models for Rhinovirus Infection in Asthma. *Contrib Microbiol* (2007) 14:33–41. doi: 10.1159/000107053

Muñoz-Fontela C, Dowling WE, Funnell SGP, Gsell P-S, Riveros-Balta AX, Albrecht RA, et al. Animal Models for COVID-19. *Nat* (2020) 586 (7830):509–15. doi: 10.1159/000107053

N TQ, R R, C YK. Animal Models for Influenza Research: Strengths and Weaknesses. *Viruses* (2021) 13(6):1011. doi: 10.3390/ v13061011

MacPhail M, Schickli JH, Tang RS, Kaur J, Robinson C, Fouchier RAM, et al. Identification of Small-Animal and Primate Models for Evaluation of

Vaccine Candidates for Human Metapneumovirus (hMPV) and Implications for hMPV Vaccine Design. *J Gen Virol* (2004) 85(6):1655–63. doi: 10.1099/ vir.0.79805-0

Moher D, Liberati A, Tetzlaff J, Altman DG. *Preferred Reporting Items for Systematic Reviews and Meta-Analyses: The PRISMA Statement. Vol. 339, BMJ.* Tavistock Square, London, UK: British Medical Journal Publishing Group (2009). p. 332–6.

Rawson NE, Ozdener MH. Primary Culture of the Human Olfactory Neuroepithelium. *Methods Mol Biol* (2013) 945:81–93. doi: 10.1007/978-1-62703-125-7_6

Bramer WM, Milic J, Mast F. *Reviewing Retrieved References for Inclusion in Systematic Reviews Using Endnote. Vol. 105, Journal of the Medical Library Association.* Erasmus MC, Rotterdam, The Netherlands: Medical Library Association (2017). p. 84–7.

Morris IR. Functional Anatomy of the Upper Airway. *Emerg Med Clin North Am* (1988) 6(4):639–69. doi: 10.1016/S0733-8627(20)30518-6

Scherzad A, Hagen R, Hackenberg S. Current Understanding of Nasal Epithelial Cell Mis-Differentiation. *J Inflammation Res* (2019) 12:309–17. doi: 10.2147/JIR. S180853

Breeze R, Turk M. Cellular Structure, Function and Organization in theLower Respiratory Tract. *Env Heal Perspect* (1984) 55:3–24. doi: 10.1289/ ehp.84553

Brand-Saberi BEM, Schäfer T. Trachea: Anatomy and Physiology. *Thorac Surg Clin* (2014) 24(1):1–5. doi: 10.1016/j.thorsurg.2013.09.004

Davies A, Moores C. Structure of the Respiratory System, Related to Function. *Respir Syst* (2010) 11–28. doi: 10.1016/B978-0-7020-3370- 4.00002-5

Ranga V, Kleinerman J. Structure and Function of Small Airways in Health and Disease. *Arch Pathol Lab Med* (1978) 102(12):609–17.

Guha S, Hariharan P, Myers MR. Enhancement of ICRP's Lung Deposition Model for Pathogenic Bioaerosols. *Aerosol Sci Technol* (2014) 48(12):1226– 35. doi: 10.1080/02786826.2014.975334

Riel DV, Verdijk R, Kuiken T. The Olfactory Nerve: A Shortcut for Influenza and Other Viral Diseases Into the Central Nervous System. *J Pathol* (2015) 235(2):277–87. doi: 10.1002/path.4461

Yaghi A, Dolovich MB. Airway Epithelial Cell Cilia and Obstructive Lung Disease. *Cells* (2016) 5(4):40. doi: 10.3390/cells5040040

Harkema JR, Plopper CG, Pinkerton KE. Comparative Structure of the Respiratory Tract: Airway Architecture in Humans and Animals. In: MD Cohen, JT Zelikoff and RB Schlesinger, editors. *Pulmonary Immunotoxicology.* Boston, MA: Springer US (2000). p. 1–59.

Rokicki W, Rokicki M, Wojtacha J, Dżeljijli A. The Role and Importance of Club Cells (Clara Cells) in the Pathogenesis of Some Respiratory Diseases. *Kardiochir Torakochirurgia Pol* (2016) 13(1):26–30. doi: 10.5114/ kitp.2016.58961

Hajj R, Baranek T, Le Naour R, Lesimple P, Puchelle E, Coraux C. Basal Cells of the Human Adult Airway Surface Epithelium Retain Transit-Amplifying Cell Properties. *Stem Cells* (2007) 25(1):139–48. doi: 10.1634/stemcells.2006- 0288

Hong KU, Reynolds SD, Watkins S, Fuchs E, Stripp BR. *In Vivo* Differentiation Potential of Tracheal Basal Cells: 666evidence for Multipotent and Unipotent Subpopulations. *Am J Physiol Lung Cell Mol Physiol* (2004) 286(4):L643–9. doi: 10.1152/ajplung.00155.2003

Boers JE, Ambergen AW, Thunnissen FB. Number and Proliferation of Basal and Parabasal Cells in Normal Human Airway Epithelium. *Am J Respir Crit Care Med* (1998) 157:2000–6. doi: 10.1164/ajrccm.157.6.9707011

Gosney JR, Sissons MC, Allibone RO. Neuroendocrine Cell Populations in Normal Human Lungs: A Quantitative Study. *Thorax* (1988) 43(11):878–82. doi: 10.1136/thx.43.11.878

Cutz E, Yeger H, Pan J. Pulmonary Neuroendocrine Cell System in Pediatric Lung Disease-Recent Advances. *Pediatr Dev Pathol* (2007) 10(6):419–35. doi: 10.2350/07-04-0267.1

Crapo JD, Barry BE, Gehr P, Bachofen M, Weibel ER. Cell Number and Cell Characteristics of the Normal Human Lung. *Am Rev Respir Dis* (1982) 126 (2):332–7.

Daniels CB, Orgeig S. Pulmonary Surfactant: The Key to the Evolution of Air Breathing. *News Physiol Sci* (2003) 18:151–7. doi: 10.1152/nips.01438.2003

Adamson IY, Bowden DH. The Type 2 Cell as Progenitor of Alveolar Epithelial Regeneration. A Cytodynamic Study in Mice After Exposure to Oxygen. *Lab Invest* (1974) 30(1):35–42.

Vareille M, Kieninger E, Edwards MR, Regamey N. The Airway Epithelium:Soldier in the Fight Against Respiratory Viruses. *Clin Microbiol Rev* (2011) 24(1):210–29. doi: 10.1128/CMR.00014-10

Zhang JM, An J. Cytokines, Inflammation, and Pain. *Int Anesth Clin* (2007) 45(2):27–37. doi: 10.1097/AIA.0b013e318034194e

Ferreira Lopes S, Vacher G, Ciarlo E, Savova-Bianchi D, Roger T, Niculita- Hirzel H. Primary and Immortalized Human Respiratory Cells Display Different Patterns of Cytotoxicity and Cytokine Release Upon Exposure to Deoxynivalenol, Nivalenol and Fusarenon-X. *Toxins (Basel)* (2017) 9 (11):337. doi: 10.3390/toxins9110337

Swain RJ, Kemp SJ, Goldstraw P, Tetley TD, Stevens MM. Assessment of Cell Line Models of Primary Human Cells by Raman Spectral Phenotyping. *Biophys J* (2010) 98(8):1703–11. doi: 10.1016/j.bpj.2009.12.4289

Forrest IA, Murphy DM, Ward C, Jones D, Johnson GE, Archer L, et al. Primary Airway Epithelial Cell Culture From Lung Transplant Recipients. *Eur Respir J* (2005) 26(6):1080–5. doi: 10.1183/09031936.05.00141404

Lopez-Souza N, Avila PC, Widdicombe JH. Polarized Cultures of Human Airway Epithelium From Nasal Scrapings and Bronchial Brushings. *Vitr Cell Dev Biol - Anim* (2003) 39(7):266–9. doi: 10.1290/1543-706X(2003)039<0266:PCOHAE>2.0.CO;2

Müller L, Brighton LE, Carson JL, Fischer 2WA, Jaspers I. Culturing of Human Nasal Epithelial Cells at the Air Liquid Interface. *J Vis Exp* (2013) 80):50646. doi: 10.3791/50646

Awatade NT, Wong SL, Hewson CK, Fawcett LK, Kicic A, Jaffe A, et al. Human Primary Epithelial Cell Models: Promising Tools in the Era of Cystic Fibrosis Personalized Medicine. *Front Pharmacol* (2018) 9:1429. doi: 10.3389/fphar.2018.01429

Horvath KM, Brighton LE, Zhang W, Carson JL, Jaspers I. Epithelial Cells From Smokers Modify Dendritic Cell Responses in the Context of Influenza Infection. *Am J Respir Cell Mol Biol* (2011) 45(2):237–45. doi: 10.1165/ rcmb.2010-0190OC

Bandyopadhyay G, Huyck HL, Misra RS, Bhattacharya S, Wang Q, Mereness J, et al. Dissociation, Cellular Isolation, and Initial Molecular Characterization of Neonatal and Pediatric Human Lung Tissues. *Am J Physiol Lung Cell Mol Physiol* (2018) 315(4):L576–l583. doi: 10.1152/ ajplung.00041.2018

Gowers KHC, Hynds RE, Thakrar RM, Carroll B, Birchall MA, Janes SM. Optimized Isolation and Expansion of Human Airway Epithelial Basal Cells From Endobronchial Biopsy Samples. *J Tissue Eng Regener Med* (2018) 12 (1):e313–7. doi: 10.1002/term.2466

Villenave R, Shields MD, Power UF. Respiratory Syncytial Virus Interaction With Human Airway Epithelium. *Trends Microbiol* (2013) 21(5):238–44. doi: 10.1016/j.tim.2013.02.004

Broadbent L, Villenave R, Guo-Parke H, Douglas I, Shields MD, Power UF. In Vitro Modeling of RSV Infection and Cytopathogenesis in Well- Differentiated Human Primary Airway Epithelial Cells (WD-PAECs). *Methods Mol Biol* (2016) 1442:119–39. doi: 10.1007/978-1-4939-3687-8_9

Pezzulo AA, Starner TD, Scheetz TE, Traver GL, Tilley AE, Harvey BG, et al. The Air-Liquid Interface and Use of Primary Cell Cultures are Important to Recapitulate the Transcriptional Profile of *In Vivo* Airway Epithelia. *Am J Physiol Lung Cell Mol Physiol* (2011) 300(1):L25–31. doi: 10.1152/ajplung. 00256.2010

Dvorak A, Tilley AE, Shaykhiev R, Wang R, Crystal RG. Do Airway Epithelium Air-Liquid Cultures Represent the *In Vivo* Airway Epithelium Transcriptome? *Am J Respir Cell Mol Biol* (2011) 44(4):465–73. doi: 10.1165/ rcmb.2009-0453OC

Travanty E, Zhou B, Zhang H, Peter Di Y, Alcorn JF, Wentworth DE, et al. Differential Susceptibilities of Human Lung Primary Cells to H1N1 Influenza Viruses. *J Virol* (2015) 89(23):11935–44. doi: 10.1128/JVI.01792-15

Aguiar JA, Tremblay BJ, Mansfield MJ, Woody O, Lobb B, Banerjee A, et al. Gene Expression and *in Situ* Protein Profiling of Candidate SARS-CoV-2 Receptors in Human Airway Epithelial Cells and Lung Tissue. *Eur Respir J* (2020) 56(3):2001123. doi: 10.1183/13993003.01123-2020

Smith JC, Sausville EL, Girish V, Yuan ML, Vasudevan A, John KM, et al. Cigarette Smoke Exposure and Inflammatory Signaling Increase the Expression of the SARS-CoV-2 Receptor ACE2 in the Respiratory Tract. *Dev Cell* (2020) 53(5):514–29.e3. doi: 10.1016/j.devcel.2020.05.012

Peretz J, Pekosz A, Lane AP, Klein SL. Estrogenic Compounds Reduce Influenza a Virus Replication in Primary Human Nasal Epithelial Cells Derived From Female, But Not Male, Donors. *Am J Physiol Lung Cell Mol Physiol* (2016) 310(5):L415–25. doi: 10.1152/ajplung.00398.2015

Salka K, Arroyo M, Chorvinsky E, Abutaleb K, Perez GF, Wolf S, et al. Innate IFN-Lambda Responses to dsRNA in the Human Infant Airway Epithelium and Clinical Regulatory Factors During Viral Respiratory Infections in Early Life. *Clin Exp Allergy* (2020) 50(9):1044–54. doi: 10.1111/cea.13701

Dominguez SR, Shrivastava S, Berglund A, Qian Z, Góes LGB, Halpin RA, et al. Isolation, Propagation, Genome Analysis and Epidemiology of HKU1 Betacoronaviruses. *J Gen Virol* (2014) 95(PART 4):836–48. doi: 10.1099/vir.0.059832-0

Sims AC, Burkett SE, Yount B, Pickles RJ. SARS-CoV Replication and Pathogenesis in an *In Vitro* Model of the Human Conducting Airway Epithelium. *Virus Res* (2008) 133(1):33–44. doi: 10.1016/j.virusres.2007.03.013

Hou YJ, Okuda K, Edwards CE, Martinez DR, Asakura T, Dinnon 3KH, et al. SARS-CoV-2 Reverse Genetics Reveals a Variable Infection Gradient in the Respiratory Tract. *Cell* (2020) 182(2):429–46.e14. doi: 10.1016/j.cell.2020.05.042

Pickles RJ. Human Airway Epithelial Cell Cultures for Modeling Respiratory Syncytial Virus Infection. *Curr Top Microbiol Immunol* (2013) 372:371–87. doi: 10.1007/978-3-642-38919-1_19

Schaap-Nutt A, Liesman R, Bartlett EJ, Scull MA, Collins PL, Pickles RJ, et al. Human Parainfluenza Virus Serotypes Differ in Their Kinetics of Replication and Cytokine Secretion in Human Tracheobronchial Airway Epithelium. *Virology* (2012) 433(2):320–8. doi: 10.1016/j.virol.2012.08.027

Gillen AE, Yang R, Cotton CU, Perez A, Randell SH, Leir SH, et al. Molecular Characterization of Gene Regulatory Networks in Primary Human Tracheal and Bronchial Epithelial Cells. *J Cyst Fibros* (2018) 17 (4):444–53. doi: 10.1016/j.jcf.2018.01.009

Mihaylova VT, Kong Y, Fedorova O, Sharma L, Dela Cruz CS, Pyle AM, et al. Regional Differences in Airway Epithelial Cells Reveal Tradeoff Between Defense Against Oxidative Stress and Defense Against Rhinovirus. *Cell Rep* (2018) 24(11):3000 –7. e3. doi: 10.1016/ j.celrep.2018.08.033

Zhao Y, Jamaluddin M, Zhang Y, Sun H, Ivanciuc T, Garofalo RP, et al. Systematic Analysis of Cell-Type Differences in the Epithelial Secretome Reveals Insights Into the Pathogenesis of Respiratory Syncytial Virus- Induced Lower Respiratory Tract Infections. *J Immunol* (2017) 198 (8):3345–64. doi: 10.4049/jimmunol.1601291

Broadbent L, Manzoor S, Zarcone MC, Barabas J, Shields MD, Saglani S, et al. Comparative Primary Paediatric Nasal Epithelial Cell Culture Differentiation and RSV-Induced Cytopathogenesis Following Culture in Two Commercial Media. Tripp RA, Editor. *PloS One* (2020) 15(3):e0228229. doi: 10.1371/journal.pone.0228229

Jia HP, Look DC, Shi L, Hickey M, Pewe L, Netland J, et al. ACE2 Receptor Expression and Severe Acute Respiratory Syndrome Coronavirus Infection Depend on Differentiation of Human Airway Epithelia. *J Virol* (2005) 79 (23):14614–21. doi: 10.1128/JVI.79.23.14614-14621.2005

Chan MC, Chan RW, Tsao GS, Peiris JS. Replication and Pathogenesis of Avian Influenza A (H5N1) Virus Infection in Polarised Human Bronchial and Alveolar Epithelium. *Hong Kong Med J* (2013) 19 Suppl 4:24–8.

Lopez-Souza N, Dolganov G, Dubin R, Sachs LA, Sassina L, Sporer H, et al. Resistance of Differentiated Human Airway Epithelium to Infection by Rhinovirus. *Am J Physiol Lung Cell Mol Physiol* (2004) 286(2 30-2):L373–81. doi: 10.1152/ajplung.00300.2003

Chan RWY, Yuen KM, Yu WCL, Ho CCC, Nicholls JM, Malik Peiris JS, et al. Influenza H5N1 and H1N1 Virus Replication and Innate Immune Responses in Bronchial Epithelial Cells are Influenced by the State of Differentiation. *PloS One* (2010) 5(1):e8713. doi: 10.1371/journal.pone.0008713

Reeves SR, Barrow KA, White MP, Rich LM, Naushab M, Debley JS. Stability of Gene Expression by Primary Bronchial Epithelial Cells Over Increasing Passage Number. *BMC Pulm Med* (2018) 18(1):91. doi: 10.1186/s12890-018- 0652-2

Gray TE, Guzman K, Davis CW, Abdullah LH, Nettesheim P. Mucociliary Differentiation of Serially Passaged Normal Human Tracheobronchial Epithelial Cells. *Am J Respir Cell Mol Biol* (1996) 14(1):104–12. doi: 10.1165/

ajrcmb.14.1.8534481

Gardner DE. *Toxicology of the Lung. 4th edition*. Boca Raton, Florida, United States: CRC Press (2005). p. 124.

Jonsdottir HR, Marti S, Geerts D, Rodriguez R, Thiel V, Dijkman R. Establishment of Primary Transgenic Human Airway Epithelial Cell Cultures to Study Respiratory Virus-Host Interactions. *Viruses* (2019) 11 (8):747. doi: 10.3390/v11080747

Kurose M, Kojima T, Koizumi J, Kamekura R, Ninomiya T, Murata M, et al. Induction of Claudins in Passaged hTERT-Transfected Human Nasal Epithelial Cells With an Extended Life Span. *Cell Tissue Res* (2007) 330 (1):63–74. doi: 10.1007/s00441-007-0453-z

Toouli CD, Huschtscha LI, Neumann AA, Noble JR, Colgin LM, Hukku B, et al. Comparison of Human Mammary Epithelial Cells Immortalized by Simian Virus 40 T-Antigen or by the Telomerase Catalytic Subunit. *Oncogene* (2002) 21(1):128–39. doi: 10.1038/sj.onc.1205014

Wu X, Wang S, Li M, Li J, Shen J, Zhao Y, et al. Conditional Reprogramming: Next Generation Cell Culture. *Acta Pharm Sin B* (2020) 10(8):1360–81. doi: 10.1016/j.apsb.2020.01.011

Lehmann R, Lee CM, Shugart EC, Benedetti M, Charo RA, Gartner Z, et al. Human Organoids: A New Dimension in Cell Biology. *Mol Biol Cell* (2019) 30(10):1129–37. doi: 10.1091/mbc.E19-03-0135

Sato T, Vries RG, Snippert HJ, van de Wetering M, Barker N, Stange DE, et al. Single Lgr5 Stem Cells Build Crypt-Villus Structures *In Vitro* Without a Mesenchymal Niche. *Nature* (2009) 459(7244):262–5. doi: 10.1038/ nature07935

Wong AP, Bear CE, Chin S, Pasceri P, Thompson TO, Huan LJ, et al. Directed Differentiation of Human Pluripotent Stem Cells Into Mature Airway Epithelia Expressing Functional CFTR Protein. *Nat Biotechnol* (2012) 30(9):876–82. doi: 10.1038/nbt.2328

Chen YW, Huang SX, De Carvalho ALRT, Ho SH, Islam MN, Volpi S, et al.A Three-Dimensional Model of Human Lung Development and Disease From Pluripotent Stem Cells. *Nat Cell Biol* (2017) 19(5):542–9. doi: 10.1038/ncb3510

Porotto M, Ferren M, Chen YW, Siu Y, Makhsous N, Rima B, et al. Authentic Modeling of Human Respiratory Virus Infection in Human Pluripotent Stem Cell-Derived Lung Organoids. *MBio* (2019) 10(3):1360– 81. doi: 10.1128/mBio.00723-19

Evans KV, Lee JH. Alveolar Wars: The Rise of *In Vitro* Models to Understand Human Lung Alveolar Maintenance, Regeneration, and Disease. *Stem Cells Transl Med* (2020) 9(8):867–81. doi: 10.1002/sctm.19-0433

Vazin T, Freed WJ. Human Embryonic Stem Cells: Derivation, Culture, and Differentiation: A Review. *Restor Neurol Neurosci* (2010) 28(4):589–603. doi: 10.3233/RNN-2010-0543

Medvedev SP, Shevchenko AI, Zakian SM. Induced Pluripotent Stem Cells: Problems and Advantages When Applying Them in Regenerative Medicine. *Acta Naturae* (2010) 2(2):18–28. doi: 10.32607/20758251-2010-2-2-18-27

Huang SX, Islam MN, O'Neill J, Hu Z, Yang YG, Chen YW, et al. Efficient Generation of Lung and Airway Epithelial Cells From Human Pluripotent Stem Cells. *Nat Biotechnol* (2014) 32(1):84–91. doi: 10.1038/nbt.2754

Hombach-Klonisch S, Panigrahi S, Rashedi I, Seifert A, Alberti E, Pocar P, et al. Adult Stem Cells and Their Trans-Differentiation Potential- Perspectives and Therapeutic Applications. *J Mol Med* (2008) 86 (12):1301–14. doi: 10.1007/s00109-008-0383-6

Sachs N, Papaspyropoulos A, Zomer-van Ommen DD, Heo I, Böttinger L, Klay D, et al. Long-Term Expanding Human Airway Organoids for Disease Modeling. *EMBO J* (2019) 38(4):e100300. doi: 10.15252/embj.2018100300

Lamers MM, van der Vaart J, Knoops K, Riesebosch S, Breugem TI, Mykytyn AZ, et al. An Organoid-Derived Bronchioalveolar Model for SARS-CoV-2 Infection of Human Alveolar Type II-Like Cells. *EMBO J* (2021) 40(5): e105912. doi: 10.15252/embj.2020105912

Salahudeen AA, Choi SS, Rustagi A, Zhu J, van Unen V, de la O SM, et al. Progenitor Identification and SARS-CoV-2 Infection in Human Distal Lung Organoids. *Nature* (2020) 588(7839):670–5. doi: 10.1038/s41586-020-3014-1

Youk J, Kim T, Evans KV, Jeong YI, Hur Y, Hong SP, et al. Three- Dimensional Human Alveolar Stem Cell Culture Models Reveal Infection Response to SARS-CoV-2. *Cell Stem Cell* (2020) 27(6):905–19.e10. doi: 10.1016/j.stem.2020.10.004

Katsura H, Sontake V, Tata A, Kobayashi Y, Edwards CE, Heaton BE, et al. Human Lung Stem Cell-Based Alveolospheres Provide Insights Into SARS- CoV-2-Mediated Interferon Responses and Pneumocyte Dysfunction. *Cell Stem Cell* (2020) 27(6):890–904.e8. doi: 10.1016/j.stem.2020.10.005

Zhou J, Li C, Sachs N, Chiu MC, Wong BHY, Chu H, et al. Differentiated Human Airway Organoids to Assess Infectivity of Emerging Influenza Virus. *Proc Natl Acad Sci USA* (2018) 115(26):6822–7. doi: 10.1073/pnas. 1806308115

Hui KPY, Ching RHH, Chan SKH, Nicholls JM, Sachs N, Clevers H, et al. Tropism, Replication Competence, and Innate Immune Responses of Influenza Virus: An Analysis of Human Airway Organoids and Ex-Vivo Bronchus Cultures. *Lancet Respir Med* (2018) 6(11):846–54. doi: 10.1016/ S2213-2600(18)30236-4

Villenave R, O'Donoghue D, Thavagnanam S, Touzelet O, Skibinski G, Heaney LG, et al. Differential Cytopathogenesis of Respiratory Syncytial Virus Prototypic and Clinical Isolates in Primary Pediatric Bronchial Epithelial Cells. *Virol J* (2011) 8:43. doi: 10.1186/1743-422X-8-43

Iketani S, Shean RC, Ferren M, Makhsous N, Aquino DB, des Georges A, et al. Viral Entry Properties Required for Fitness in Humans Are Lost Through Rapid Genomic Change During Viral Isolation. *MBio* (2018) 9(4): e00898–18. doi: 10.1128/mBio.00898-18

Terajima M, Yamaya M, Sekizawa K, Okinaga S, Suzuki T, Yamada N, et al. Rhinovirus Infection of Primary Cultures of Human Tracheal Epithelium: Role of ICAM-1 and IL-1*b*. *Am J Physiol Lung Cell Mol Physiol* (1997) 273(4 17-4):L749–59. doi: 10.1152/ajplung.1997.273.4.L749

Schroth MK, Grimm E, Frindt P, Galagan DM, Konno SI, Love R, et al. Rhinovirus Replication Causes RANTES Production in Primary Bronchial Epithelial Cells. *Am J Respir Cell Mol Biol* (1999) 20(6):1220–8. doi: 10.1165/ ajrcmb.20.6.3261

Papi A, Stanciu LA, Papadopoulos NG, Teran LM, Holgate ST, Johnston SL. Rhinovirus Infection Induces Major Histocompatibility Complex Class I and Costimulatory Molecule Upregulation on Respiratory Epithelial Cells. *J Infect Dis* (2000) 181(5):1780–4. doi: 10.1086/315463

Papadopoulos NG, Bates PJ, Bardin PG, Papi A, Leir SH, Fraenkel DJ, et al. Rhinoviruses Infect the Lower Airways. *J Infect Dis* (2000) 181(6):1875–84. doi: 10.1086/315513

Suzuki T, Yamaya M, Sekizawa K, Hosoda M, Yamada N, Ishizuka S, et al. Erythromycin Inhibits Rhinovirus Infection in Cultured Human Tracheal Epithelial Cells. *Am J Respir Crit Care Med* (2002) 165(8):1113–8. doi: 10.1164/ajrccm.165.8.2103094

Griggs TF, Bochkov YA, Basnet S, Pasic TR, Brockman-Schneider RA, Palmenberg AC, et al. Rhinovirus C Targets Ciliated Airway Epithelial Cells. *Respir Res* (2017) 18(1):84. doi: 10.1186/s12931-017-0567-0

Chen YX, Xie GC, Pan D, Du YR, Pang LL, Song JD, et al. Three- Dimensional Culture of Human Airway Epithelium in Matrigel for Evaluation of Human Rhinovirus C and Bocavirus Infections. *BioMed Env Sci* (2018) 31(2):136–45. doi: 10.3967/bes2018.016

Jamieson KC, Wiehler S, Michi AN, Proud D. Rhinovirus Induces Basolateral Release of IL-17C in Highly Differentiated Airway Epithelial Cells. *Front Cell Infect Microbiol* (2020) 10:103. doi: 10.3389/fcimb. 2020.00103

Veerati PC, Troy NM, Reid AT, Li NF, Nichol KS, Kaur P, et al. Airway Epithelial Cell Immunity Is Delayed During Rhinovirus Infection in Asthma and COPD. *Front Immunol* (2020) 11:974. doi: 10.3389/fimmu.2020.00974

Raj VS, Mou H, Smits SL, Dekkers DHW, Müller MA, Dijkman R, et al. Dipeptidyl Peptidase 4 is a Functional Receptor for the Emerging Human Coronavirus-EMC. *Nature* (2013) 495(7440):251–4. doi: 10.1038/nature12005

Wang G, Deering C, Macke M, Shao J, Burns R, Blau DM, et al. Human Coronavirus 229E Infects Polarized Airway Epithelia From the Apical Surface. *J Virol* (2000) 74(19):9234–9. doi: 10.1128/JVI.74.19.9234-9239.2000

Dijkman R, Jebbink MF, Koekkoek SM, Deijs M, Jonsdottir HR, Molenkamp R, et al. Isolation and Characterization of Current Human Coronavirus Strains in Primary Human Epithelial Cell Cultures Reveal Differences in Target Cell Tropism. *J Virol* (2013) 87(11):6081–90. doi: 10.1128/JVI.03368-12

Huang X, Dong W, Milewska A, Golda A, Qi Y, Zhu QK, et al. Human Coronavirus HKU1 Spike Protein Uses O-Acetylated Sialic Acid as an Attachment Receptor Determinant and Employs Hemagglutinin-Esterase Protein as a Receptor-Destroying Enzyme. *J Virol* (2015) 89(14):7202–13. doi: 10.1128/JVI.00854-15

Lamers MM, Beumer J, van der Vaart J, Knoops K, Puschhof J, Breugem TI, et al. SARS-CoV-2 Productively Infects Human Gut Enterocytes. *Science* (2020) 369(6499):50–4. doi: 10.1126/science.abc1669

Pei R, Feng J, Zhang Y, Sun H, Li L, Yang X, et al. Host Metabolism Dysregulation and Cell Tropism Identification in Human Airway and Alveolar Organoids Upon SARS-CoV-2 Infection. *Protein Cell* (2020) 12:1–17. doi: 10.1007/s13238-020-00811-w

Qian Z, Ou X, Góes LGB, Osborne C, Castano A, Holmes KV, et al. Identification of the Receptor-Binding Domain of the Spike Glycoprotein of Human Betacoronavirus HKU1. *J Virol* (2015) 89(17):8816–27. doi: 10.1128/JVI.03737-14

Jang Y, Seo SH. Gene Expression Pattern Differences in Primary Human Pulmonary Epithelial Cells Infected With MERS-CoV or SARS-CoV-2. *Arch Virol* (2020) 165(10):2205–11. doi: 10.1007/s00705-020-04730-3

Loo SL, Wark PAB, Esneau C, Nichol KS, Hsu ACY, Bartlett NW. Human Coronaviruses 229E and OC43 Replicate and Induce Distinct Antiviral Responses in Differentiated Primary Human Bronchial Epithelial Cells.

Am J Physiol Lung Cell Mol Physiol (2020) 319(6):L926–31. doi: 10.1152/ajplung.00374.2020

Vanderheiden A, Ralfs P, Chirkova T, Upadhyay AA, Zimmerman MG, Bedoya S, et al. Type I and Type III Interferons Restrict SARS-CoV-2 Infection of Human Airway Epithelial Cultures. *J Virol* (2020) 94(19): e00985–20. doi: 10.1101/2020.05.19.105437

Bui CHT, Chan RWY, Ng MMT, Cheung MC, Ng KC, Chan MPK, et al. Tropism of Influenza B Viruses in Human Respiratory Tract Explants and Airway Organoids. *Eur Respir J* (2019) 54(2):1900008. doi: 10.1183/ 13993003.00008-2019

Bhowmick R, Derakhshan T, Liang Y, Ritchey J, Liu L. Gappa-Fahlenkamp H. A Three-Dimensional Human Tissue-Engineered Lung Model to Study Influenza A Infection. *Tissue Eng Part A* (2018) 24(19–20):1468–80. doi: 10.1089/ten.tea.2017.0449

Ioannidis I, McNally B, Willette M, Peeples ME, Chaussabel D, Durbin JE, et al. Plasticity and Virus Specificity of the Airway Epithelial Cell Immune Response During Respiratory Virus Infection. *J Virol* (2012) 86(10):5422–36. doi: 10.1128/JVI.06757-11

Lin YT, Lin CF, Yeh TH. Influenza A Virus Infection Induces Indoleamine 2,3-Dioxygenase (IDO) Expression and Modulates Subsequent Inflammatory Mediators in Nasal Epithelial Cells. *Acta Otolaryngol* (2020) 140(2):149–56. doi: 10.1080/00016489.2019.1700304

Jeong KI, Piepenhagen PA, Kishko M, DiNapoli JM, Groppo RP, Zhang L, et al. CX3CR1 Is Expressed in Differentiated Human Ciliated Airway Cells and Co-Localizes With Respiratory Syncytial Virus on Cilia in a G Protein- Dependent Manner. *PloS One* (2015) 10(6):e0130517. doi: 10.1371/ journal.pone.0130517

Johnson SM, McNally BA, Ioannidis I, Flano E, Teng MN, Oomens AG, et al. Respiratory Syncytial Virus Uses CX3CR1 as a Receptor on Primary Human Airway Epithelial Cultures. *PLoS Pathog* (2015) 11(12):e1005318. doi: 10.1371/journal.ppat.1005318

Griffiths CD, Bilawchuk LM, McDonough JE, Jamieson KC, Elawar F, Cen Y, et al. IGF1R Is an Entry Receptor for Respiratory Syncytial Virus. *Nature* (2020) 583(7817):615–9. doi: 10.1038/s41586-020-2369-7

Zhang L, Peeples ME, Boucher RC, Collins PL, Pickles RJ. Respiratory Syncytial Virus Infection of Human Airway Epithelial Cells is Polarized, Specific to Ciliated Cells, and Without Obvious Cytopathology. *J Virol* (2002) 76(11):5654–66. doi: 10.1128/JVI.76.11.5654-5666.2002

Hong GP, Canning P, Douglas I, Villenave R, Heaney LG, Coyle PV, et al. Relative Respiratory Syncytial Virus Cytopathogenesis in Upper and Lower Respiratory Tract Epithelium. *Am J Respir Crit Care Med* (2013) 188(7):842– 51. doi: 10.1164/rccm.201304-0750OC

Persson BD, Jaffe AB, Fearns R, Danahay H. Respiratory Syncytial Virus can Infect Basal Cells and Alter Human Airway Epithelial Differentiation. *PloS One* (2014) 9(7):e102368. doi: 10.1371/journal.pone.0102368

Porotto M, Ferren M, Chen YW, Siu Y, Makhsous N, Rima B, et al. Authentic Modeling of Human Respiratory Virus Infection in Human Pluripotent Stem Cell-Derived Lung Organoids. *MBio* (2019) 10(3):e00723–19. doi: 10.1128/mBio.00723-19

Loevenich S, Malmo J, Liberg AM, Sherstova T, Li Y, Rian K, et al. Cell- Type-Specific Transcription of Innate Immune Regulators in Response to Hmpv Infection. *Mediat Inflammation* (2019) 4964239. doi: 10.1155/ 2019/4964239

Bao X, Liu T, Spetch L, Kolli D, Garofalo RP, Casola A. Airway Epithelial Cell Response to Human Metapneumovirus Infection. *Virology* (2007) 368 (1):91–101. doi: 10.1016/j.virol.2007.06.023

Yu X, Lakerveld AJ, Imholz S, Hendriks M, ten Brink SCA, Mulder HL, et al. Antibody and Local Cytokine Response to Respiratory Syncytial Virus Infection in Community-Dwelling Older Adults. *mSphere* (2020) 5(5): e00577–20. doi: 10.1128/mSphere.00577-20

Villenave R, Thavagnanam S, Sarlang S, Parker J, Douglas I, Skibinski G, et al. *In Vitro* Modeling of Respiratory Syncytial Virus Infection of Pediatric Bronchial Epithelium, the Primary Target of Infection In Vivo. *Proc Natl Acad Sci USA* (2012) 109(13):5040–5. doi: 10.1073/pnas.1110203109

Villenave R, Broadbent L, Douglas I, Lyons JD, Coyle PV, Teng MN, et al. Induction and Antagonism of Antiviral Responses in Respiratory Syncytial Virus-Infected Pediatric Airway Epithelium. *J Virol* (2015) 89(24):12309–18. doi: 10.1128/JVI.02119-15

Das S, Palmer OP, Leight WD, Surowitz JB, Pickles RJ, Randell SH, et al. Cytokine Amplification by Respiratory Syncytial Virus Infection in Human Nasal Epithelial Cells. *Laryngoscope* (2005) 115(5):764–8. doi: 10.1097/01.MLG.0000159527.76949.93

Okabayashi T, Kojima T, Masaki T, Yokota S-I, Imaizumi T, Tsutsumi H, et al. Type-III Interferon, Not Type-I, is the Predominant Interferon Induced by Respiratory Viruses in Nasal Epithelial Cells. *Virus Res* (2011) 160:360– doi: 10.1016/j.virusres.2011.07.011

Kogure T, Suzuki T, Takahashi T, Miyamoto D, Hidari KIPJ, Guo CT, et al. Human Trachea Primary Epithelial Cells Express Both Sialyl(*a*2-3)Gal Receptor for Human Parainfluenza Virus Type 1 and Avian Influenza Viruses, and Sialyl(*a*2-6)Gal Receptor for Human Influenza Viruses. *Glycoconjugate J* (2006) 23(1–2):101–6. doi: 10.1007/s10719-006-5442-z

Zhang L, Bukreyev A, Thompson CI, Watson B, Peeples ME, Collins PL, et al. Infection of Ciliated Cells by Human Parainfluenza Virus Type 3 in an *In Vitro* Model of Human Airway Epithelium. *J Virol* (2005) 79(2):1113–24. doi: 10.1128/JVI.79.2.1113-1124.2005

Zhang H, Newman DR, Sannes PL. HSULF-1 Inhibits ERK and AKT Signaling and Decreases Cell Viability *In Vitro* in Human Lung Epithelial Cells. *Respir Res* (2012) 13:69. doi: 10.1186/1465-9921-13-69

Zhang L, Collins PL, Lamb RA, Pickles RJ. Comparison of Differing Cytopathic Effects in Human Airway Epithelium of Parainfluenza Virus 5 (W3A), Parainfluenza Virus Type 3, and Respiratory Syncytial Virus. *Virology* (2011) 421(1):67–77. doi: 10.1016/j.virol.2011.08.020

Schaap-Nutt A, D'Angelo C, Scull MA, Amaro-Carambot E, Nishio M, Pickles RJ, et al. Human Parainfluenza Virus Type 2 V Protein Inhibits Interferon Production and Signaling and Is Required for Replication in non-Human Primates. *Virology* (2010) 397(2):285–98. doi: 10.1016/j.virol.2009.11.018

Lam E, Ramke M, Warnecke G, Schrepfer S, Kopfnagel V, Dobner T, et al. Effective Apical Infection of Differentiated Human Bronchial Epithelial Cells and Induction of Proinflammatory Chemokines by the Highly Pneumotropic Human Adenovirus Type 14p1. *PloS One* (2015) 10(7): e0131201. doi: 10.1371/journal.pone.0131201

Meyer-Berg H, Zhou Yang L, Pilar de Lucas M, Zambrano A, Hyde SC, Gill DR. Identification of AAV Serotypes for Lung Gene Therapy in Human Embryonic Stem Cell-Derived Lung Organoids. *Stem Cell Res Ther* (2020) 11 (1):488. doi: 10.1186/s13287-020-01950-x

Yang TI, Li WL, Chang TH, Lu CY, Chen JM, Lee PI, et al. Adenovirus Replication and Host Innate Response in Primary Human Airway Epithelial Cells. *J Microbiol Immunol Infect* (2019) 52(2):207–14. doi: 10.1016/ j.jmii.2018.08.010

Raj VS, Lamers MM, Smits SL, Demmers JA, Mou H, Bosch BJ, et al. Identification of Protein Receptors for Coronaviruses by Mass Spectrometry. *Methods Mol Biol* (2015) 1282:165–82. doi: 10.1007/978-1-4939-2438-7_15

Barrass SV, Butcher SJ. Advances in High-Throughput Methods for the Identification of Virus Receptors. Vol. 209, Medical Microbiology and Immunology. *Springer;* (2020) 209(3):309–23. doi: 10.1007/s00430-019-00653-2

Wang S, Qiu Z, Hou Y, Deng X, Xu W, Zheng T, et al. AXL is a Candidate Receptor for SARS-CoV-2 That Promotes Infection of Pulmonary and Bronchial Epithelial Cells. *Cell Res* (2021) 31(2):126–40. doi: 10.1038/ s41422-020-00460-y

Yeager CL, Ashmun RA, Williams RK, Cardellichio CB, Shapiro LH, Look AT, et al. Human Aminopeptidase N Is a Receptor for Human Coronavirus 229E. *Nature* (1992) 357(6377):420–2. doi: 10.1038/357420a0

Vlasak R, Luytjes W, Spaan W, Palese P. Human and Bovine Coronaviruses Recognize Sialic Acid-Containing Receptors Similar to Those of Influenza C Viruses. *Proc Natl Acad Sci USA* (1988) 85(12):4526–9. doi: 10.1073/pnas.85.12.4526

Li W, Moore MJ, Vasilieva N, Sui J, Wong SK, Berne MA, et al. Angiotensin-Converting Enzyme 2 is a Functional Receptor for the SARS Coronavirus. *Nature* (2003) 426(6965):450–4. doi: 10.1038/nature02145

Hofmann H, Pyrc K, van der Hoek L, Geier M, Berkhout B, Pöhlmann S. Human Coronavirus NL63 Employs the Severe Acute Respiratory Syndrome Coronavirus Receptor for Cellular Entry. *Proc Natl Acad Sci USA* (2005) 102 (22):7988–93. doi: 10.1073/pnas.0409465102

Hoffmann M, Kleine-Weber H, Schroeder S, Krüger N, Herrler T, Erichsen S, et al. SARS-CoV-2 Cell Entry Depends on ACE2 and TMPRSS2 and Is Blocked by a Clinically Proven Protease Inhibitor. *Cell* (2020) 181(2):271– 280.e8. doi: 10.1016/j.cell.2020.02.052

Pyrc K, Sims AC, Dijkman R, Jebbink M, Long C, Deming D, et al. Culturing the Unculturable: Human Coronavirus HKU1 Infects, Replicates, and Produces Progeny Virions in Human Ciliated Airway Epithelial Cell Cultures. *J Virol* (2010) 84(21):11255–63. doi: 10.1128/JVI.00947-10

Staunton DE, Merluzzi VJ, Rothlein R, Barton R, Marlin SD, Springer TA. A Cell Adhesion Molecule, ICAM-1, is the Major Surface Receptor for Rhinoviruses. *Cell* (1989) 56(5):849–53. doi: 10.1016/0092-8674(89)90689-2

Hofer F, Gruenberger M, Kowalski H, Machat H, Huettinger M, Kuechler E, et al. Members of the Low Density Lipoprotein Receptor Family Mediate Cell Entry of a Minor-Group Common Cold Virus. *Proc Natl Acad Sci USA* (1994) 91(5):1839–42. doi: 10.1073/pnas.91.5.1839

Marlovits TC, Abrahamsberg C, Blaas D. Very-Low-Density Lipoprotein Receptor Fragment Shed From HeLa Cells Inhibits Human Rhinovirus Infection. *J Virol* (1998) 72(12):10246–50. doi: 10.1128/JVI.72.12.10246- 10250.1998

Suzuki T, Yamaya M, Kamanaka M, Jia YX, Nakayama K, Hosoda M, et al. Type 2

Rhinovirus Infection of Cultured Human Tracheal Epithelial Cells: Role of LDL Receptor. *Am J Physiol Lung Cell Mol Physiol* (2001) 280(3 24- 3):L409–20. doi: 10.1152/ajplung.2001.280.3.L409

Bochkov YA, Palmenberg AC, Lee WM, Rathe JA, Amineva SP, Sun X, et al. Molecular Modeling, Organ Culture and Reverse Genetics for a Newly Identified Human Rhinovirus C. *Nat Med* (2011) 17(5):627–32. doi: 10.1038/nm.2358

Johnson JE, Gonzales RA, Olson SJ, Wright PF, Graham BS. The Histopathology of Fatal Untreated Human Respiratory Syncytial Virus Infection. *Mod Pathol* (2007) 20(1):108–19. doi: 10.1038/modpathol.3800725

Tayyari F, Marchant D, Moraes TJ, Duan W, Mastrangelo P, Hegele RG. Identification of Nucleolin as a Cellular Receptor for Human Respiratory Syncytial Virus. *Nat Med* (2011) 17(9):1132 5. doi: 10.1038/nm.2444

Chang A, Masante C, Buchholz UJ, Dutch RE. Human Metapneumovirus (HMPV) Binding and Infection Are Mediated by Interactions Between the HMPV Fusion Protein and Heparan Sulfate. *J Virol* (2012) 86(6):3230–43. doi: 10.1128/JVI.06706-11

Cox RG, Erickson JJ, Hastings AK, Becker JC, Johnson M, Craven RE, et al. Human Metapneumovirus Virus-Like Particles Induce Protective B and T Cell Responses in a Mouse Model. *J Virol* (2014) 88(11):6368–79. doi: 10.1128/JVI.00332-14

Bergelson JM, Cunningham JA, Droguett G, Kurt-Jones EA, Krithivas A, Hong JS, et al. Isolation of a Common Receptor for Coxsackie B Viruses and Adenoviruses 2 and 5. *Science* (1997) 275(5304):1320–3. doi: 10.1126/ science.275.5304.1320

Dominguez SR, Travanty EA, Qian Z, Mason RJ. Human Coronavirus HKU1 Infection of Primary Human Type II Alveolar Epithelial Cells: Cytopathic Effects and Innate Immune Response. *PloS One* (2013) 8(7): e70129. doi: 10.1371/journal.pone.0070129

Qian Z, Travanty EA, Oko L, Edeen K, Berglund A, Wang J, et al. Innate Immune Response of Human Alveolar Type II Cells Infected With Severe Acute Respiratory Syndrome-Coronavirus. *Am J Resp Cell Mol Biol* (2013) 48 (6):742–8. doi: 10.1165/rcmb.2012-0339OC

Jakiela B, Brockman-Schneider R, Amineva S, Lee WM, Gern JE. Basal Cells of Differentiated Bronchial Epithelium Are More Susceptible to Rhinovirus Infection. *Am J Respir Cell Mol Biol* (2008) 38(5):517–23. doi: 10.1165/rcmb.2007-0050OC

Mosser AG, Brockman-Schneider R, Amineva S, Burchell L, Sedgwick JB, Busse WW, et al. Similar Frequencyaa of Rhinovirus-Infectible Cellsasas in Upper and Lower Airway Epithelium. *J Infect Dis* (2002) 185(6):734–43xxzx. doi: 10.1086/339339

Nakagome K, Bochkov YA, Ashraf S, Brockman-Schneider RA, Evans MD, Pasic TR, et al. Effects of Rhinovirus Species on Viral Replication and Cytokine Production. *J Allergy Clin Immunol* (2014) 134(2):332–41.e10. doi: 10.1016/j.jaci.2014.01.029

Yeo NK, Jang YJ. Rhinovirus Infection-Induced Alteration of Tight Junction and Adherens Junction Components in Human Nasal Epithelial Cells. *Laryngoscope* (2010) 120(2):346–52. doi: 10.1002/lary.20764

Teng MN, Whitehead SS, Collins PL. Contribution of the Respiratory Syncytial Virus G Glycoprotein and its Secreted and Membrane-Bound Forms to Virus Replication *In Vitro* and *In Vivo*. *Virology* (2001) 289 (2):283–96. doi: 10.1006/viro.2001.1138

de Graaf M, Herfst S, Aarbiou J, Burgers PC, Zaaraoui-Boutahar F, Bijl M, et al. Small Hydrophobic Protein of Human Metapneumovirus Does Not Affect Virus Replication and Host Gene Expression In Vitro. *PloS One* (2013) 8(3):e58572. doi: 10.1371/journal.pone.0058572

Geiser J, Boivin G, Huang S, Constant S, Kaiser L, Tapparel C, et al. RSV and HMPV Infections in 3D Tissue Cultures: Mechanisms Involved in Virus-Host and Virus-Virus Interactions. *Viruses* (2021) 13(1):139. doi: 10.3390/v13010139

Rijsbergen LC, Rennick LJ, Laksono BM, van Run PRWA, Kuiken T, Duprex WP, et al. *In Vivo* Comparison of a Laboratory-Adapted and Clinical-Isolate-Based Recombinant Human Respiratory Syncytial Virus. *J Gen Virol* (2020) 101(10):1037–46. doi: 10.1099/jgv.0.001468

Liesman RM, Buchholz UJ, Luongo CL, Yang L, Proia AD, DeVincenzo JP, et al. RSV-Encoded NS2 Promotes Epithelial Cell Shedding and Distal Airway Obstruction. *J Clin Invest* (2014) 124(5):2219–33. doi: 10.1172/ JCI72948

Deng Y, Herbert JA, Robinson E, Ren L, Smyth RL, Smith CM. Neutrophil-Airway Epithelial Interactions Result in Increased Epithelial Damage and Viral Clearance During Respiratory Syncytial Virus Infection. *J Virol* (2020) 94(13):e2161–19. doi: 10.1128/JVI.02161-19

Piedimonte G, Perez MK. Respiratory Syncytial Virus Infection and Bronchiolitis. *Pediatr Rev* (2014) 35(12):519–30. doi: 10.1542/pir.35-12-519

Kindler E, Jonsdottir HR, Muth D, Hamming OJ, Hartmann R, Rodriguez R, et al. Efficient Replication of the Novel Human Betacoronavirus EMC on Primary Human Epithelium Highlights its Zoonotic Potential. *MBio* (2013) 4(1):e00611–12. doi: 10.1128/mBio.00611-12

Montgomery ST, Frey DL, Mall MA, Stick SM, Kicic A. Rhinovirus Infection Is Associated With Airway Epithelial Cell Necrosis and Inflammation *via* Interleukin-1 in Young Children With Cystic Fibrosis. *Front Immunol* (2020) 11:596. doi: 10.3389/fimmu.2020.00596

Montgomery ST, Stick SM, Kicic A. An Adapted Novel Flow Cytometry Methodology to Delineate Types of Cell Death in Airway Epithelial Cells. *J Biol Methods* (2020) 7(4):e139. doi: 10.14440/jbm.2020.336

Liu A, Zhang X, Li R, Zheng M, Yang S, Dai L, et al. Overexpression of the SARS-CoV-2 Receptor ACE2 is Induced by Cigarette Smoke in Bronchial and Alveolar Epithelia. *J Pathol* (2021) 253(1):17–30. doi: 10.1002/path.5555

Radzikowska U, Ding M, Tan G, Zhakparov D, Peng Y, Wawrzyniak P, et al. Distribution of ACE2, CD147, CD26, and Other SARS-CoV-2 Associated Molecules in Tissues and Immune Cells in Health and in Asthma, COPD, Obesity, Hypertension, and COVID-19 Risk Factors. *Allergy Eur J Allergy Clin Immunol* (2020) 75(11):2829–45. doi: 10.1111/all.14429

Zhang H, Rostami MR, Leopold PL, Mezey JG, O'Beirne SL, Strulovici-Barel Y, et al. Expression of the SARS-CoV-2 ACE2 Receptor in the Human Airway Epithelium. *Am J Respir Crit Care Med* (2020) 202(2):219–29. doi: 10.1164/rccm.202003-0541OC

Lukassen S, Chua RL, Trefzer T, Kahn NC, Schneider MA, Muley T, et al. SARS-CoV-2 Receptor ACE2 and TMPRSS2 Are Primarily Expressed in Bronchial Transient Secretory Cells. *EMBO J* (2020) 39(10):e105114. doi: 10.15252/embj.20105114

Kormuth KA, Lin K, Prussin AJ, Vejerano EP, Tiwari AJ, Cox SS, et al. Influenza Virus Infectivity Is Retained in Aerosols and Droplets Independent of Relative Humidity. *J Infect Dis* (2018) 218(5):739–47. doi: 10.1093/infdis/ jiy221

Ilyushina NA, Ikizler MR, Kawaoka Y, Rudenko LG, Treanor JJ, Subbarao K, et al. Comparative Study of Influenza Virus Replication in MDCK Cells and in Primary Cells Derived From Adenoids and Airway Epithelium. *J Virol* (2012) 86(21):11725–34. doi: 10.1128/JVI.01477-12

Hawksworth A, Lockhart R, Crowe J, Maeso R, Ritter L, Dibben O, et al. Replication of Live Attenuated Influenza Vaccine Viruses in Human Nasal Epithelial Cells Is Associated With H1N1 Vaccine Effectiveness. *Vaccine* (2020) 38(26):4209–18. doi: 10.1016/j.vaccine.2020.04.004

Hou YJ, Chiba S, Halfmann P, Ehre C, Kuroda M, Dinnon KH, et al. SARS- CoV-2 D614G Variant Exhibits Efficient Replication Ex Vivo and Transmission *In Vivo*. *Science* (2020) 370(6523):1464–8. doi: 10.1101/ 2020.09.28.317685

Komabayashi K, Matoba Y, Seto J, Ikeda Y, Tanaka W, Aoki Y, et al. Isolation of Human Coronaviruses OC43, HKU1, NL63, and 229E in Yamagata, Japan, Using Primary Human Airway Epithelium Cells Cultured by Employing an Air-Liquid Interface Culture. *Jpn J Infect Dis* (2020) 74 (4):285–92. doi: 10.7883/yoken.JJID.2020.776

Benam KH, Villenave R, Lucchesi C, Varone A, Hubeau C, Lee H-H, et al. Small Airway-on-a-Chip Enables Analysis of Human Lung Inflammation and Drug Responses In Vitro. *Nat Methods* (2016) 13(2):151–7. doi: 10.1038/ nmeth.3697

Bhatia SN, Ingber DE. Microfluidic Organs-on-Chips. *Nat Biotechnol* (2014) 32(8):760–72. doi: 10.1038/nbt.2989

Kaarj K, Yoon JY. Methods of Delivering Mechanical Stimuli to Organ-On- a-Chip. *Micromachines (Basel)* (2019) 10(10):700. doi: 10.3390/mi10100700

Nickol ME, Lyle SM, Dennehy B, Kindrachuk J. Dysregulated Host Responses Underlie 2009 Pandemic Influenza-Methicillin Resistant Staphylococcus Aureus Coinfection Pathogenesis at the Alveolar-Capillary Barrier. *Cells* (2020) 9(11):1–19. doi: 10.3390/cells9112472

Wu A, Mihaylova VT, Landry ML, Foxman EF. Interference Between Rhinovirus and Influenza A Virus: A Clinical Data Analysis and Experimental Infection Study. *Lancet Microbe* (2020) 1(6):e254–62. doi: 10.1016/S2666-5247(20)30114-2

Cebrián G, Condón S, Mañas P. Physiology of the Inactivation of Vegetative Bacteria by Thermal Treatments: Mode of Action, Influence of Environmental Factors and Inactivation Kinetics. *Foods* (2017) 6(12):107. doi: 10.3390/foods6120107

Gulraiz F, Bellinghausen C, Dentener MA, Reynaert NL, Gaajetaan GR, Beuken EV, et al. Efficacy of IFN-*l*1 to Protect Human Airway Epithelial Cells Against Human Rhinovirus 1B Infection. *PloS One* (2014) 9(4):e95134. doi: 10.1371/journal.pone.0095134

Bellinghausen C, Gulraiz F, Heinzmann AC, Dentener MA, Savelkoul PH, Wouters EF, et al. Exposure to Common Respiratory Bacteria Alters the Airway Epithelial Response to Subsequent Viral Infection. *Respir Res* (2016) 17(1):68. doi: 10.1186/s12931-016-0382-z

Sajjan U, Wang Q, Zhao Y, Gruenert DC, Hershenson MB. Rhinovirus Disrupts the Barrier Function of Polarized Airway Epithelial Cells. *Am J Respir Crit Care Med* (2008) 178(12):1271–81. doi: 10.1164/rccm.200801-136OC

Wang JH, Kwon HJ, Jang YJ. Rhinovirus Enhances Various Bacterial Adhesions to Nasal Epithelial Cells Simultaneously. *Laryngoscope* (2009) 119(7):1406–11. doi: 10.1002/lary.20498

Golda A, Malek N, Dudek B, Zeglen S, Wojarski J, Ochman M, et al. Infection With

Human Coronavirus NL63 Enhances Streptococcal Adherence to Epithelial Cells. *J Gen Virol* (2011) 92(6):1358–68. doi: 10.1099/vir.0.028381-0

Avadhanula V, Rodriguez CA, De Vincenzo JP, Wang Y, Webby RJ, Ulett GC, et al. Respiratory Viruses Augment the Adhesion of Bacterial Pathogens to Respiratory Epithelium in a Viral Species- and Cell Type- Dependent Manner. *J Virol* (2006) 80(4):1629–36. doi: 10.1128/ JVI.80.4.1629-1636.2006

Min S, Kim S, Cho SW. Gastrointestinal Tract Modeling Using Organoids Engineered With Cellular and Microbiota Niches. *Exp Mol Med* (2020) 52 (2):227–37. doi: 10.1038/s12276-020-0386-0

Choi KG, Wu BC, Lee AH, Baquir B, Hancock REW. Utilizing Organoid and Air-Liquid Interface Models as a Screening Method in the Development of New Host Defense Peptides. *Front Cell Infect Microbiol* (2020) 10:228. doi: 10.3389/ fcimb.2020.00228

Habibi MS, Thwaites RS, Chang M, Jozwik A, Paras A, Kirsebom F, et al. Neutrophilic Inflammation in the Respiratory Mucosa Predisposes to RSV Infection. *Science* (2020) 370(6513):eaba:9301. doi: 10.1126/ science.aba9301

Stark JM, Van Egmond AWA, Zimmerman JJ, Carabell SK, Tosi MF. Detection of Enhanced Neutrophil Adhesion to Parainfluenza-Infected Airway Epithelial Cells Using a Modified Myeloperoxidase Assay in a Microtiter Format. *J Virol Methods* (1992) 40(2):225–42. doi: 10.1016/ 0166-0934(92)90071-K

Tosi MF, Stark JM, Hamedani A, Smith CW, Gruenert DC, Huang YT. Intercellular Adhesion Molecule-1 (ICAM-1)-Dependent and ICAM-1- Independent Adhesive Interactions Between Polymorphonuclear Leukocytes and Human Airway Epithelial Cells Infected With Parainfluenza Virus Type 2. *J Immunol* (1992) 149(10):3345–9.

Jornot L, Cordey S, Caruso A, Gerber C, Vukicevic M, Tapparel C, et al. T Lymphocytes Promote the Antiviral and Inflammatory Responses of Airway Epithelial Cells. *PloS One* (2011) 6(10):e29293. doi: 10.1371/ journal. pone.0026293

Rahmatpanah F, Agrawal S, Jaiswal N, Ngyuen HM, McClelland M, Agrawal Airway Epithelial Cells Prime Plasmacytoid Dendritic Cells to Respond to Pathogens *via* Secretion of Growth Factors. *Mucosal Immunol* (2019) 12 (1):77–84. doi: 10.1038/s41385-018-0097-1

Ugonna K, Bingle CD, Plant K, Wilson K, Everard ML. Macrophages are Required for Dendritic Cell Uptake of Respiratory Syncytial Virus From an Infected Epithelium. *PloS One* (2014) 9(3):e91855. doi: 10.1371/journal. pone.0091855

Papazian D, Würtzen PA, Hansen SW. Polarized Airway Epithelial Models for Immunological Co-Culture Studies. *Int Arch Allergy Immunol* (2016) 170 (1):1–21. doi: 10.1159/000445833

van der V J, L MM, H BL, C H. Advancing Lung Organoids for COVID-19 Research. *Dis Model Mech* (2021) 14(6):dmm049060. doi: 10.1242/ dmm.049060

Suksatu A, Sangsawad W, Thitithanyanont A, Smittipat N, Fukuda MM, Ubol S. Characteristics of Stork Feces-Derived H5N1 Viruses That are Preferentially Transmitted to Primary Human Airway Epithelial Cells. *Microbiol Immunol* (2009) 53(12):675–84. doi: 10.1111/j.1348-0421. 2009.00177.x

Kim J-S, Heo P, Yang T-J, Lee K-S, Cho D-H, Kim BT, et al. Selective Killing of Bacterial Persisters by a Single Chemical Compound Without Affecting Normal Antibiotic-Sensitive Cells. *Antimicrob Agents Chemother* (2011) 55 (11):5380–3. doi: 10.1128/AAC.00708-11

Huang DTN, Lu CY, Chi YH, Li WL, Chang LY, Lai MJ, et al. Adaptation of Influenza A (H7N9) Virus in Primary Human Airway Epithelial Cells. *Sci Rep* (2017) 7(1):11300. doi: 10.1038/s41598-017-10749-5

Anthony SJ, Gilardi K, Menachery VD, Goldstein T, Ssebide B, Mbabazi R, et al. Further Evidence for Bats as the Evolutionary Source of Middle East Respiratory Syndrome Coronavirus. *MBio* (2017) 8(2):e00373–17. doi: 10.1128/ mBio.00373-17

Forbes B, Ehrhardt C. Human Respiratory Epithelial Cell Culture for Drug Delivery Applications. *Eur J Pharm Biopharm* (2005) 60(2):193–205. doi: 10.1016/j. ejpb.2005.02.010

Fang Y, Eglen RM. Three-Dimensional Cell Cultures in Drug Discovery and Development. *SLAS Discovery* (2017) 22(5):456–72. doi: 10.1177/ 1087057117696795

21

Prevalence of Bandemia in Respiratory Viral Infections: A Pediatric Emergency Room Experience

Estela Noyola[1], *Asif Noor*[1*], *Nicole Sweeney*[1], *Joshua Chan*[1], *Rahul Ramesh*[1], *Rose Calixte*[1,2] *and Leonard R. Krilov*[1]

[1] *Department of Pediatrics, NYU Long Island School of Medicine, Mineola, NY, United States,* [2] *Department of Community Health and Social Medicine, The City University of New York (CUNY) School of Medicine, New York, NY, United States*

***Correspondence:**
Asif Noor
asif.noor@nyulangone.org

Objective: The aim of this study was to examine the prevalence of bandemia in confirmed respiratory viral infections in febrile infants and children presenting to the emergency department.

Methods: An observational retrospective study from January 1, 2016, through December 31, 2016, was conducted in patients between the ages of $\geq$ 1 month and $\leq$ 5 years presenting to the emergency room with fever and who had a complete blood cell count performed. Patients were separated into seven groups based on the type of respiratory viral infection. Inclusion criteria strictly counted children with viral infections and absence of clinical and laboratory evidence of a bacterial coinfection.

Results: A total of 419 patients had a documented viral infection. A significant proportion of these children were found to have bandemia; children with adenovirus (17%), respiratory syncytial virus (RSV) (14.9%), human metapneumovirus (hMPV) (13%), and parainfluenza virus (7.9%) had the highest prevalence when the cutoff for bandemia was set at 10%. The prevalence increased to 35.3, 30.9, 40.3, and 15.8% for adenovirus, RSV, hMPV, and parainfluenza virus, respectively, when this cutoff was lowered further to 5%.

Conclusion: Band neutrophils are detected frequently in confirmed respiratory viral infections particularly during early stages.

Keywords: bandemia, respiratory viral infections, fever, complete blood cell (CBC) count, absolute neutrophil count (ANC), absolute band count, film array

INTRODUCTION

Respiratory viral infections, either confirmed or presumed, account for the majority of febrile illnesses in healthy infants and young children (1, 2). Common viral presentations include fever with upper respiratory signs and symptoms, clinical bronchiolitis, or fever without localizing signs (3). The diagnosis of a viral infection is mainly based on clinical grounds. The multiplex molecular respiratory panel (respiratory PCR assay) has enabled better identification of these respiratory viral infections and provides objective data. Many of these children would get non-specific laboratory markers performed, i.e., complete blood count (CBC), C-reactive protein (CRP), and erythrocyte sedimentation rate (ESR) to investigate a concomitant bacterial infection (4). Since the 1990's, there have been multiple studies and guidelines on the management of febrile infants, which indicated a low, but non-negligible, risk of serious bacterial infections (5–7). Infants > 1 month of age who present to the emergency room (ER) often get a CBC as part of the workup. This study sought to investigate the prevalence of bandemia in a cohort of children with confirmed viral infection.

METHODS

We conducted a retrospective study from January 1, 2016, through December 31, 2016, in children between the ages of ≥ 1 month and ≤ 5 years. These children presented to our Children's Medical Center, which is a suburban, tertiary-care academic hospital in the Northeast United States with 95 pediatric inpatient beds and 19,000 pediatric ED visits per year. They presented with documented fevers defined as a temperature of 100.4° Fahrenheit (38° C) or greater and had a complete blood cell count performed using Beckman Coulter ® LH 780 electric cell counter. A manual differential count of the peripheral blood smear was performed on every patient, which is standard protocol in patients 5 years or younger in our institution (**Figure 3**). Febrile children with confirmed viral infections (BioFire FilmArray® multiplex PCR) were included in the study. We excluded patients with chronic conditions (sickle cell disease, malignancy, and inflammatory bowel disease), immunodeficiencies, patients with diagnosed bacterial infections, and toxic appearing children as documented by attending physicians. We also excluded children with documented signs of acute otitis media because it is difficult to distinguish between viral or bacterial etiology. Cases where the chest x-ray was read as focal infiltrates due to atelectasis by the attending radiologists were included in the viral infection group and cases with chest x-ray findings of consolidation, effusion, or empyema were excluded to ensure that patients did not have a bacterial coinfection.

Cases with confirmed viral infections had nasopharyngeal specimens obtained and tested positive for Respiratory syncytial virus (RSV), adenovirus, influenza, parainfluenza, and human metapneumovirus (hMPV) on the Filmarray® multiplex PCR system. We excluded enterovirus and rhinovirus because of difficulty in distinguishing symptomatic infections from asymptomatic prolonged shedding. Also, results are reported together as enterovirus/rhinovirus (both are picornavirus) and it is difficult to determine which virus is the culprit. We also excluded coronavirus (non-SARS or MERS) as a majority of the cases were either asymptomatic or had mild upper respiratory symptoms.

In addition we collected data on a small sample of patients who presented to the ER with fever and were diagnosed with a bacterial infection, such as bacteremia, meningitis, bacterial gastroenteritis, and urinary tract infection (UTI). Bacteremia was defined as a positive blood culture (excluding contaminants: bacillus species [non-anthrax and non-cereus] coagulase negative staphylococcus or corynebacterium sp.). Meningitis was confirmed with positive CSF culture and enteritis with stool culture growth of a bacterial pathogen. Cases of urinary tract infection were diagnosed based on pyuria (>5 WBC on automated urinalysis) and >50,000 CFU of a single uropathogen.

The study was approved by the Institutional Review Board.

Abbreviations: CBC, complete blood count; WBC, white blood cell count; ANC, absolute neutrophil count; RSV, Respiratory syncytial virus; hMPV, human metapneumovirus; ER, emergency room; SBI, serious bacterial infection; PCR, polymerase chain reaction.

STATISTICAL ANALYSIS

Continuous variables, assumed to be normal, were analyzed using two-sample t-test and summarized using mean ± standard deviation. Continuous variables with skewed distribution were analyzed using the Wilcoxon rank-sum test and summarized using median and interquartile range. Categorical variables were summarized using frequency and percent, and analyzed using the Pearson's chi-square test of independence. When the asymptotic assumption of the chi-square distribution was violated, an exact chi-square p-value was computed. All analyses were done using SAS 9.4®, and p-value < 0.05 were considered significant for all analyses except for the planned comparisons within the viral group where significance was set at 0.025 after Bonferroni correction.

RESULTS

A total of 419 pediatric patients were included in the study (**Figure 1**). They all had documented viral infections with no evidence of bacterial coinfection: adenovirus (54), parainfluenza (114), influenza (77), hMPV (68), and RSV (175). Forty five of the cases were combination of the above.

Viral Group With Band ≥ 10% (Table 1)

In the viral group, patients with band proportions ≥10% had a significantly higher mean absolute neutrophil count (ANC), mean temperature, exposure to antibiotics, and rate of admission than their viral counterpart with band proportions <10%. Furthermore, these patients had significantly lower mean lymphocyte counts and lower mean lymphocyte proportions.

RSV Patients With Band ≥ 10% (Table 2)

Patients who were positive for RSV were significantly younger, had lower body temperature, were less likely to receive antibiotics, and were more likely to be admitted to the hospital than those negative for RSV.

Adenovirus Patients With Band ≥ 10%

Patients who were positive for adenovirus had higher ANC, body temperature, WBC, absolute neutrophil counts, and absolute monocyte counts. In addition, they were less likely to be admitted to the hospital than patients negative for adenovirus.

Parainfluenza Patients With Band ≥ 10%

Patients who were positive for parainfluenza virus had lower rates of admission to the hospital, and lower rate of patients with bandemia ≥ 10% when compared to patients

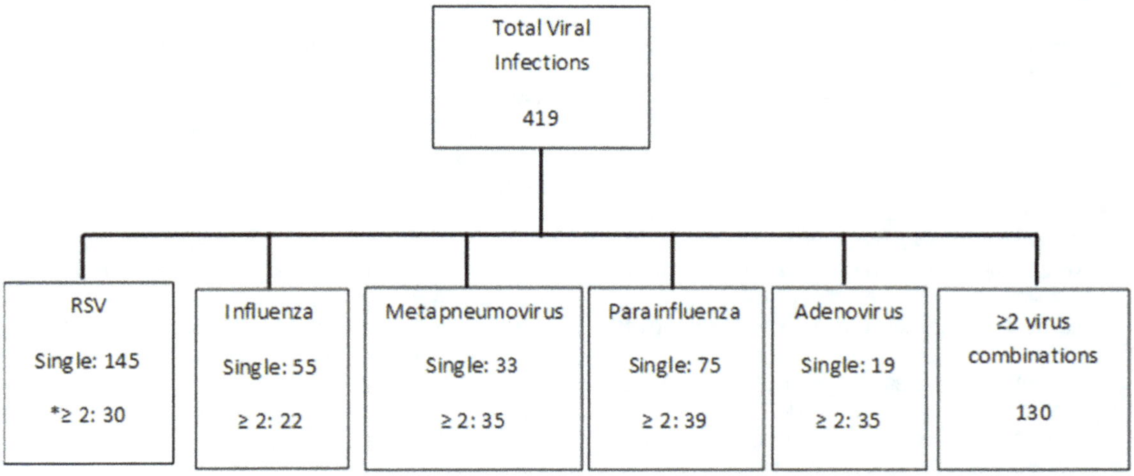

FIGURE 1 | Breakdown of viruses. *≥2 includes of combinations of viruses (most common combination was with enterovirus, rhinovirus, and coronavirus addition to be a combination of the above five viruses).

negative for parainfluenza. Of note, these patients had higher lymphocyte proportions.

Influenza Patients With Band ≥ 10%

Patients who were positive for influenza were older and had lower WBC, absolute lymphocyte counts, and absolute monocyte counts than patients negative for influenza.

Metapneumovirus Patients With Band ≥ 10%

Patients who were positive for hMPV had higher band proportions and exposure to antibiotics when compared to patients negative for hMPV.

Combination Group With Band ≥ 10%

Patients who were positive for 2 or more viruses had higher ANC, temperature, and WBC but had shorter length of stay in the hospital when compared to those positive with only one virus.

Bacterial vs. Viral Group

In our sample of 42 patients diagnosed with bacterial infections, there were urinary tract infections (36), Streptococcus pneumonia meningitis (2), bacteremia Escherichia coli (2), and Shigella enteritis (2).

We compared characteristics between the bacterial group and the viral group. Patients with a bacterial infection were significantly younger than patients with a viral infection. Patients with a bacterial infection had significantly higher mean ANC, mean WBC, mean neutrophil count, and higher exposure to antibiotics than their viral counterparts (**Table 3**). When comparing the absolute band count and band proportion between the viral group and the bacterial group, there was no statistically significant difference. When comparing the WBC and ANC between the viral group and the bacterial group, the bacterial group had a higher WBC and ANC which was significant ($p < 0.001$).

DISCUSSION

Bandemia or elevated immature neutrophil count (left shift) was detected in a cohort of febrile children presenting to the emergency department with confirmed respiratory viral infection without a concomitant bacterial infection. In our study, a significant proportion of these children were found to have bandemia. Adenovirus (17%), RSV (14.9%), human metapneumovirus (13%), and parainfluenza (7.9%) had the highest prevalence when the cutoff for bandemia was set at 10%. The prevalence increased to 35.3, 30.9, 40.3, and 15.8% for adenovirus, RSV, hMPV, and PIV, respectively when this cutoff was lowered further to 5%, which is the cutoff used by our institution (**Figure 2**).

Over the past decade, use of multiplex molecular respiratory panel has enabled better identification of respiratory viral infections. As a result, this information has allowed us to investigate the differential white blood cell count in common childhood viral infections (8). We reviewed the different cell lines, including immature neutrophils (bands), lymphocytes, and monocytes. We found that adenovirus had significantly ($p < 0.001$) higher ANC when compared to the other viruses with a mean value of 7,190.

Although identification of bandemia may represent a serious underlying bacterial infection (SBI) (9, 10) immature neutrophils are also associated with certain viral infections (11). Of note, in our study, we found viral cases with band proportions >10% which had significantly higher exposure to antibiotics and hospital admission rates ($p < 0.001$). The study results suggest

TABLE 1 | Bandemia (bands ≥ 10%) in viral infection.

	Bands < 10%	Bands ≥ 10%	Total	*P*-value
Number of participants	362	53	415	
Demographics				
Age (months)	16.5 (6.2–29.8)	15.5 (8.3–30.6)	16.0 (6.5–30.5)	0.756
Length of stay (days)	3.0 (2.0–4.0)	2.0 (2.0–5.0)	3.0 (2.0–4.0)	0.683
Duration of fever (days)	2.0 (1.0–4.0)	2.0 (1.0–3.0)	2.0 (1.0–4.0)	0.54
ANC	4219 (2745–7372)	6030 (4046–8909)	4556 (2835–7828)	0.008
Absolute band count	177.0 (0.0–396.0)	1340 (910.0–1780)	225.0 (0.0–591.0)	< 0.001
Initial temperature (°C)	100.6 ± 2.1	100.8 ± 2.2	100.6 ± 2.1	0.395
WBC absolute (1,000 K/μL)	11.7 ± 5.6	11.6 ± 5.9	11.7 ± 5.6	0.963
Neutrophil absolute	5.6 ± 4.4	5.4 ± 3.3	5.5 ± 4.3	0.797
Neutrophil proportion	45.2 ± 20.5	45.5 ± 15.1	45.2 ± 19.9	0.92
Lymphocyte absolute	4.8 ± 4.7	3.5 ± 2.1	4.7 ± 4.5	0.04
Lymphocyte proportion	41.7 ± 19.1	31.5 ± 13.8	40.4 ± 18.8	<0.001
Monocyte absolute	1.0 ± 0.7	1.2 ± 1.5	1.0 ± 0.8	0.353
Monocyte proportion	9.1 ± 4.8	8.9 ± 3.6	9.1 ± 4.7	0.807
Female (*N*, %)	185 (51.1%)	24 (45.3%)	209 (50.4%)	0.464
Antibiotics given (*N*, %)	87 (24.0%)	32 (60.4%)	119 (28.7%)	<0.001
Discharge from ED	204 (56.4%)	20 (37.7%)	224 (54.0%)	0.012
Admission to hospital (*N*, %)	158 (43.6%)	34 (64.2%)	192 (46.3%)	0.008
Toxic appearance (*N*, %)	4 (1.1%)	0 (0.0%)	4 (1.0%)	>0.999
Readmission (*N*, %)	7 (1.9%)	1 (1.9%)	8 (1.9%)	>0.999

that the traditional belief of bandemia and its association with SBI may persist in clinical practice.

What is bandemia? WBC is a component of the CBC. The WBC's differential measures the absolute number and proportion of granulocytes, lymphocytes, monocytes, basophils, and eosinophils (12). A neutrophil is a mature granulocyte and part of the innate immune system. Band is the most "mature" of the immature stages in the development of a neutrophil (**Figure 3**). In older children and adults, the normal blood circulation has 3–5% of bands which will mature into

TABLE 2 | Parameters in individual viruses.

	Positive	Negative	Total	*P*-value
RSV				
Number of participants	175	282	457	
Age (months)	11.6 (4.0–27.0)	17.2 (8.8–31.5)	15.9 (6.2–29.8)	0.001
ANC	4556 (2904–7372)	4612 (2745–8085)	4590 (2835–7828)	0.739
Absolute band count	256.0 (65.0–576.0)	185.5 (0.0–561.0)	218.0 (0.0–561.0)	0.029
Bandemia ≥ 10% (*N*, %)	26 (14.9%)	29 (10.4%)	55 (12.1%)	0.184
Bandemia ≥ 5% (*N*, %)	54 (30.9%)	76 (27.3%)	130 (28.7%)	0.456
Antibiotics given (*N*, %)	42 (24.0%)	89 (31.6%)	131 (28.7%)	0.089
Admission to hospital (*N*, %)	105 (60.0%)	106 (37.6%)	211 (46.2%)	<0.001
Adenovirus				
Number of participants	54	403	457	
Age (months)	14.9 (8.6–24.7)	15.9 (5.5–31.0)	15.9 (6.2–29.8)	0.902
ANC	7190 (4864–10465)	4154 (2662–7372)	4590 (2835–7828)	<0.001
Absolute band count	373.0 (77.0–813.0)	208.0 (0.0–489.0)	218.0 (0.0–561.0)	0.046
Antibiotics given (*N*, %)	13 (24.1%)	118 (29.3%)	131 (28.7%)	0.522
Admission to hospital (*N*, %)	15 (27.8%)	196 (48.6%)	211 (46.2%)	0.005
Bandemia ≥ 5% (*N*, %)	18 (35.3%)	112 (27.9%)	130 (28.7%)	0.324
Bandemia ≥ 10% (*N*, %)	9 (17.6%)	46 (11.4%)	55 (12.1%)	0.251
Influenza				
Number of participants	77	380	457	
Age (months)	26.3 (13.9–44.1)	14.3 (5.4–26.2)	15.9 (6.2–29.8)	<0.001
ANC	3500 (2312–6156)	4740 (3063–7901)	4590 (2835–7828)	0.004
Absolute band count	159.0 (0.0–395.0)	225.0 (0.0–590.5)	218.0 (0.0–561.0)	0.099
Band proportion	3.2 ± 4.1	3.7 ± 4.4	3.6 ± 4.4	0.373
A/T ratio	0.1 ± 0.1	0.1 ± 0.1	0.1 ± 0.1	0.339
Antibiotics given (*N*, %)	24 (31.2%)	107 (28.2%)	131 (28.7%)	0.583
Admission to hospital (*N*, %)	27 (35.1%)	184 (48.4%)	211 (46.2%)	0.034
Bandemia ≥ 5% (*N*, %)	23 (29.9%)	107 (28.5%)	130 (28.7%)	0.794
Bandemia ≥ 10% (*N*, %)	6 (7.8%)	49 (13.0%)	55 (12.1%)	0.252
Metapneumovirus				
Number of participants	68	389	457	

(Continued)

TABLE 2 | Continued

	Positive	Negative	Total	*P*-value
Age (months)	18.4 (9.0–31.1)	15.6 (5.5–29.2)	15.9 (6.2–29.8)	0.28
ANC	4011 (2552–7880)	4608 (2838–7821)	4590 (2835–7828)	0.667
Absolute band count	295.0 (93.5–691.5)	196.0 (0.0–530.0)	218.0 (0.0–561.0)	0.054
Band proportion	4.4 ± 5.0	3.5 ± 4.3	3.6 ± 4.4	0.092
Antibiotics given (*N*, %)	29 (42.6%)	102 (26.2%)	131 (28.7%)	0.009
Admission to hospital (*N*, %)	34 (50.0%)	177 (45.5%)	211 (46.2%)	0.512
Bandemia ≥ 5% (*N*, %)	27 (40.3%)	103 (26.7%)	130 (28.7%)	0.028
Bandemia ≥ 10% (*N*, %)	9 (13.4%)	46 (11.9%)	55 (12.1%)	0.688
Parainfluenza				
Number of participants	114	343	457	
Age (months)	15.9 (7.0–24.2)	15.9 (5.8–31.1)	15.9 (6.2–29.8)	0.361
ANC	4224 (2520–6966)	4615 (2916–7917)	4590 (2835–7828)	0.182
Absolute band count	132.5 (0.0–345.0)	252.0 (0.0–681.0)	218.0 (0.0–561.0)	<0.001
Band proportion	2.4 ± 3.5	4.0 ± 4.6	3.6 ± 4.4	0.001
A/T ratio	0.1 ± 0.1	0.1 ± 0.1	0.1 ± 0.1	0.008
Antibiotics given (*N*, %)	32 (28.1%)	99 (28.9%)	131 (28.7%)	0.905
Admission to hospital (*N*, %)	45 (39.5%)	166 (48.4%)	211 (46.2%)	0.105
Bandemia ≥ 5% (*N*, %)	18 (15.8%)	112 (33.0%)	130 (28.7%)	<0.001
Bandemia ≥ 10% (*N*, %)	9 (7.9%)	46 (13.6%)	55 (12.1%)	0.135

TABLE 3 | Demographic and clinical characteristic.

	Viral	Bacterial	Total	*P*-value
Number of participants	419	42	461	
Demographics Age (months)	15.9 (6.5–30.5)	7.1 (4.0–26.7)	15.6 (6.0–29.2)	0.008
Length of stay (days)	3.0 (2.0–4.0)	3.0 (3.0–4.0)	3.0 (2.0–4.0)	0.128
Duration of fever (days)	2.0 (1.0–4.0)	1.0 (1.0–3.0)	2.0 (1.0–3.0)	0.102
ANC	4558 (2835–7828)	8638 (4950–11700)	4717 (2904–8076)	<0.001
Absolute band count	222.0 (0.0–590.0)	248.5 (0.0–868.0)	225.0 (0.0–648.0)	0.275
Initial temperature (°C)	100.6 ± 2.1	100.6 ± 2.4	100.6 ± 2.1	0.974
WBC absolute (weeks)	11.7 ± 5.6	16.8 ± 7.5	12.1 ± 6.0	<0.001
Band proportion	3.7 ± 4.5	3.8 ± 4.8	3.7 ± 4.5	0.885
Neutrophil absolute	5.5 ± 4.3	7.4 ± 4.1	5.7 ± 4.3	0.009
Neutrophil proportion	45.3 ± 19.8	48.5 ± 18.4	45.6 ± 19.7	0.319
Lymphocyte absolute	4.7 ± 4.5	5.7 ± 4.1	4.8 ± 4.5	0.145
Lymphocyte proportion	40.3 ± 18.8	36.9 ± 16.2	40.0 ± 18.5	0.251
Monocyte absolute	1.0 ± 0.8	1.2 ± 1.0	1.1 ± 0.8	0.491
Monocyte proportion	9.1 ± 4.7	6.8 ± 5.3	8.9 ± 4.8	0.004
A/T ratio	0.1 ± 0.1	0.1 ± 0.1	0.1 ± 0.1	0.861
Female (*N*, %)	211 (50.4%)	25 (59.5%)	236 (51.2%)	0.331
Antibiotics given (*N*, %)	119 (28.4%)	39 (92.9%)	158 (34.3%)	<0.001
Admission to hospital (*N*, %)	192 (45.8%)	26 (61.9%)	218 (47.3%)	0.052
Toxic appearance (*N*, %)	4 (1.0%)	0 (0.0%)	4 (0.9%)	>0.999
Readmission (*N*, %)	9 (2.1%)	0 (0.0%)	9 (2.0%)	>0.999

neutrophils in the circulation. However, the majority of blasts undergo maturation in the marrow storage compartment. Any stress, whether an infection, inflammation, or a hypermetabolic state will lead to an increase in band count or bandemia (>10%) (13–15).

In our study, all differentials were performed manually. Manual band count requires the additional time-consuming, labor-intensive process of slide preparation and manual leukocyte tabulation. The interpretation is technician dependent, and its enumeration is associated with inaccuracy and imprecision. In addition, there exists a wide variation in reference ranges of bandemia (16). It has been reported in the literature that the percentage and absolute band count in healthy children between the ages of 15 days and 2 years of age is similar, but the response to infection may be different in young children of different ages (16).

What does presence of bandemia in viral infections mean? Bandemia has been reported in children with viral infections notably with lower respiratory tract infections, enteroviral infections, and rotavirus infections (6, 11, 17). Bandemia has also been reported in association with influenza and RSV infections (18).

We found bandemia (>10%) in about a quarter of cases of respiratory viral infections in the absence of concomitant bacterial infection (confirmed or presumed): RSV (14.9% 26/175), adenovirus (17.6% 9/54), hMPV (13.4% 9/68), influenza (7.8% 6/77), and parainfluenza virus (7.9% 9/114). The cutoff for bandemia in our laboratory is 5% which further increases the percentage of children classified with bandemia. This implies that a relatively higher band count is seen in viral infections that primarily cause lower respiratory tract disease and are associated with more parenchymal

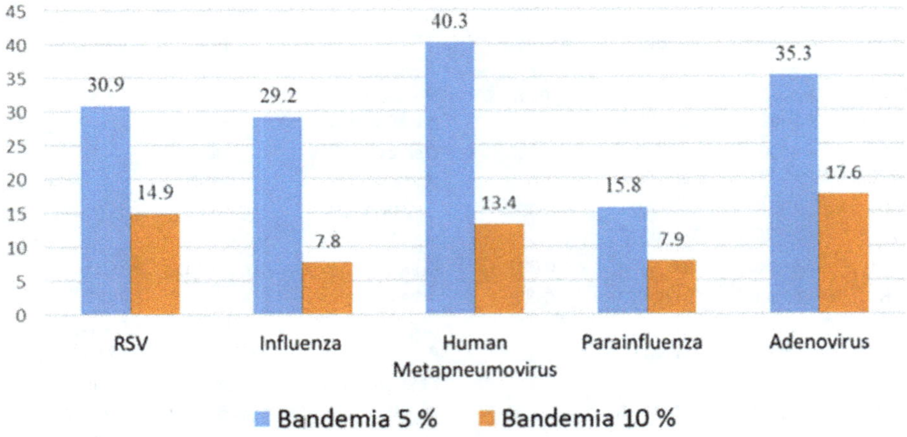

FIGURE 2 | % Bandemia in Respiratory viral Infections.

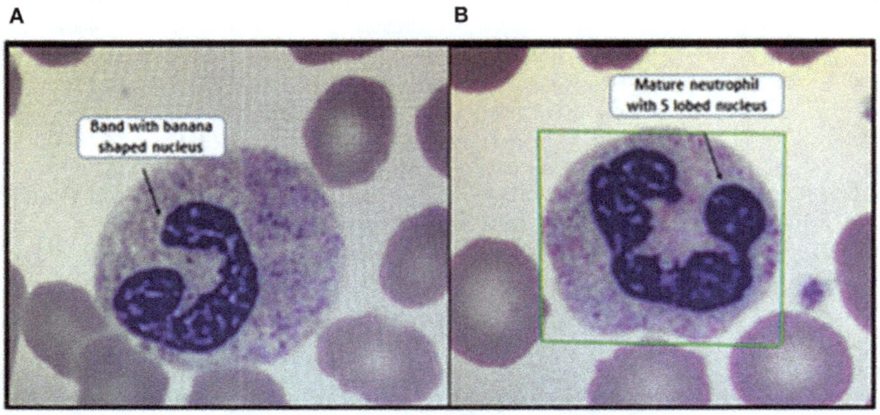

FIGURE 3 | (A) Immature neutrophil vs. **(B)** mature neutrophil.

inflammation at the time of ER presentation. In addition, our study is the first to report the prevalence of bandemia in hMPV infections.

In reviewing our data we noticed that patients admitted with a known viral infection, but high band count, were likely to receive antibiotics. Antibiotic exposure was seen in one quarter of the patients infected with hMPV (40.3%), followed by influenza (31%), parainfluenza (28%), RSV (24%), and adenovirus (17.6%). This lower antibiotic use in adenovirus can be attributed to the known association of bandemia in adenovirus by clinicians (**Table 4**).

We compared the bacterial group with the viral group and did not find a statistically significant difference in bandemia when comparing viral with bacterial infections in infants and young children. However, the bacterial group was a considerably smaller sample size so when comparing the groups, the results should be taken cautiously. Nevertheless, when comparing the absolute band count, band proportion, and A/T ratio between the viral group and the bacterial group, there was no statistical significant difference.

TABLE 4 | Bandemia in specific viruses with antibiotic prescription and hospitalization percent.

Viral group	Band > 5%	Band > 10%	Mean absolute band count	Antibiotic % (*n*)	Hospitalization % (*n*)
RSV	31%	15%	256	24% (42)	60 % (105)
Adenovirus	35%	17.6%	373	24% (13)	28 % (15)
Influenza	30%	7.8%	159	31 % (24)	35 % (27)
Parainfluenza	16%	7.9%	132	28 % (32)	39 % (45)
Metapneumo virus	40.3%	13%	295	42.6 % (29)	50 % (34)

This study has several limitations. First, it is a retrospective review conducted in a single center. Second, there were fewer patients in the bacterial group in comparison to the viral group; therefore, the incidence of true bandemia in the bacterial group might be under represented. In addition, we included only well-appearing children with confirmed viral infections, thus we cannot generalize our results to ill appearing patients.

CONCLUSIONS

Elevated band counts are seen in lower respiratory viral infections and clinicians should be aware of this association. While absolute neutrophil count and white blood cell count are reliable markers of bacterial infection, bandemia may also be present in viral infections. This is the first study comparing bandemia among different viral infections. We observed an elevated band count in many viral infections, specifically RSV, adenovirus, hMPV, influenza, and parainfluenza. Bandemia in well-appearing children with confirmed viral infections can be an area of opportunity to limit the use of antibiotics.

AUTHOR CONTRIBUTIONS

EN, AN, and RR was involved in manuscript writing and data collection of viral infections. JC was involved in data collection of bacterial infections. RC performed statistical analysis. NS was involved in manuscript writing, and LK supervised the project and was involved in revision of the manuscript. All authors contributed to the article and approved the submitted version.

REFERENCES

Byington CL, Enriquez FR, Hoff C, Tuohy R, Taggart EW, Hillyard DR, et al. Serious bacterial infections in febrile infants 1 to 90 days old with and without viral infections. *Pediatrics.* (2004) 113:1662. doi: 10.1542/peds.11 3.6.1662

Hall CB, Weinberg GA, Iwane MK, Blumkin AK, Edwards KM, Staat MA, et al. The burden of RSV infection in young children. *N Engl J Med.* (2009) 360:588–98. doi: 10.1056/NEJMoa0804877

Colvin JM, Muenzer JT, Jaffe DM, et al. Detection of viruses in young children with fever without an apparent source. *Pediatrics.* (2012) 130:e1455– 62. doi: 10.1542/peds.2012-1391

Librizzi J, McCulloh R, Koehn K, Alverson B. Appropriateness of testing for serious bacterial infection in children hospitalized with bronchiolitis. *Hosp Pediatr.* (2014) 4:33–8. doi: 10.1542/hpeds.2013-0073

Baker MD, Bell LM, Avner JR. Outpatient management without antibiotics of fever in selected infants. *N Engl J Med.* (1993) 329:1437–41. doi: 10.1056/NEJM199311113292001

Blaschke AJ, Korgenski EK, Wilkes J, Presson AP, Thorell EA, Pavia AT, et al. Rhinovirus in febrile infants and risk of bacterial infection. *Pediatrics.* (2018) 141:e20172384. doi: 10.1542/peds.2017-2384

Baraff LJ, Oslund SA, Schriger DL, Stephen ML. Probability of bacterial infections in febrile infants less than three months of age: a meta-analysis. *Pediatr Infect Dis J.* (1992) 11:257– 64. doi: 10.1097/00006454-199204000-00001

Echavarría M, Marcone DN, Querci M, Seoane A, Ypas M, Videla C, et al. Clinical impact of rapid molecular detection of respiratory pathogens in patients with acute respiratory infection. *J Clin Virol.* (2018) 108:90– 5. doi: 10.1016/j.jcv.2018.09.009

Hornik CP, Benjamin DK, Becker KC, Benjamin DK Jr, Li J, Clark RH, et al.Use of the complete blood cell count in early-onset neonatal sepsis. *Pediatr Infect Dis J.* (2012) 31:799–802. doi: 10.1097/INF.0b013e318256905c

Bone RC, Balk RA, Cerra FB, Dellinger RP, Fein AM, Knaus WA, et al. Definitions for sepsis and organ failure and guidelines for the use of innovative therapies in sepsis. The ACCP/SCCM consensus conference committee. American college of chest physicians/society of critical care medicine. *Chest.* (1992) 101:1644–55. doi: 10.1378/chest.101.6.1644

Kuppermann N, Walton EA. Immature neutrophils in the blood smears of young febrile children. *Arch Pediatr Adolesc Med.* (1999) 153:261– 6. doi: 10.1001/archpedi.153.3.261

Sacher RA, McPherson RA, Campos JM, Widmann FK. *Widmann's Clinical Interpretation of Laboratory Tests.* 11th ed. Philadelphia, PA: Davis (2000).

Morens DM. WBC count and differential. *AJDC.* (1979) 133:25– 27. doi: 10.1001/archpedi.1979.02130010031003

Baines KJ, Simpson JL, Gibson PG. Biology of neutrophils. *Middletons Allergy Princ. Pract.* 17:280–291. doi: 10.1016/B978-0-323-08593-9.00018-8

Mare TA, Treacher DF, Shankar-Hari M, Beale R, Lewis SM, Chambers DJ, et al. The diagnostic and prognostic significance of monitoring blood levels of immature neutrophils in patients with systemic inflammation. *Crit Care.* (2015) 19:57. doi: 10.1186/s13054-015-0778-z

Joanne Cornbleet P. Clinical utility of the band count. *Clin Lab Med.* (2002) 22:1. doi: 10.1016/S0272-2712(03)00069-6

Portnoy B, Hanes B, Salvatore MA, Eckert HL. The peripheral white blood count in respirovirus infection. *J Peditrics.* (1966) 68:181–8. doi: 10.1016/S0022-3476(66)80148-8

Wack RP, Demers DM, Bass JW. Immature neutrophils in the peripheral blood of children with viral infections. *Pediatric Infect Dis J.* (1994) 13:3. doi: 10.1097/00006454-199403000-00012

Low Frequency of Viral Respiratory Tract Infections during Family-Centered Neonatal Intensive Care: Results of a Prospective Surveillance Study

André Kidszun [1], Anna Neurohr [1], Britta Gröndahl [2], Susanne Tippmann [1], Daniel Schreiner [1], Julia Winter [1], Seyed Hamidreza Mahmoudpour [3,4], Stephan Gehring [2] and Eva Mildenberger [1]*

[1] Department of Neonatology, University Medical Center, Mainz, Germany, [2] Department of Pediatric Infectious Diseases, University Medical Center, Mainz, Germany, [3] Institute of Medical Biostatistics, Epidemiology, and Informatics, University Medical Center of the Johannes Gutenberg University Mainz, Mainz, Germany, [4] Center for Thrombosis and Hemostasis, University Medical Center of the Johannes Gutenberg University Mainz, Mainz, Germany

***Correspondence:**
André Kidszun
andre.kidszun@gmail.com

Background: Viral respiratory tract infections (VRTI) may cause severe respiratory and sepsis-like symptoms in infants hospitalized in the neonatal intensive care unit (NICU). Little is known about the frequencies of VRTI in relation to visiting policies in the NICU.

Objective: Aim of this study was to evaluate the frequency of symptomatic and asymptomatic VRTI in our family-centered NICU.

Methods: This was a 12-month, prospective, observational study from February 2018 to January 2019. Infants hospitalized ≥72 h were eligible for the study. To determine the frequency of VRTI, multiplexed point-of-care testing (mPOCT) of symptomatic infants was combined with a weekly screening of all infants. Our 10-bed NICU is 24/7 open to families and visitors. The number of simultaneous visitors is restricted to two per patient. Parents and visitors are instructed in hand hygiene and advised to avoid visits in cases of respiratory illness. Siblings irrespective of age may visit the NICU following a physical check-up.

Results Multiplexed point-of-care testing (71 symptomatic episodes) combined with the weekly screening (272 episodes) yielded in 21 positive samples from 2 of the 67 infants enrolled in the study. Both infants were first detected during symptomatic episodes. Rhino-/enterovirus were detected in all cases.

Conclusion: Respiratory viruses were detected during symptomatic and asymptomatic episodes but affected <3% of infants enrolled in the study. In our unit, a low frequency of VRTI was attained despite adherence to family integrated care including liberal visiting policies for younger siblings.

Keywords: family-centered, neonatology, infection, virus, surveillance

INTRODUCTION

Viral respiratory tract infections (VRTI) have been described to cause severe respiratory and sepsis-like symptoms in infants hospitalized in the neonatal intensive care unit (NICU) (1–3). During birth hospitalization, VRTI have also been associated with prolonged hospital stay, increase in home oxygen use and elevated rates of bronchopulmonary dysplasia (4, 5). However, and despite a growing body of literature, the magnitude of the problem is not sufficiently known (6). Evidence concerning frequency and impact of VRTI in the NICU is sparse and conflicting. While in one study, the incidence of VRTI was more than 50% in neonates <33 weeks of gestation (5), others only found four virus-positive cases in a cohort of 93 preterm infants (7). Study methodology varied markedly between available publications and so far only one study used a comprehensive, albeit blinded surveillance design (5). In particular, the significance of clinically asymptomatic VRTI remains unclear. Overall, evidence appears insufficient to inform clinicians and policy makers concerning indications for virus testing and visiting policies (6, 8). Aim of this study was to evaluate the frequency of symptomatic and asymptomatic VRTI in our family-centered NICU.

METHODS

This was a 12-month, prospective, observational study from February 2018 to January 2019. Infants hospitalized postnatally ≥72 h in the NICU were eligible for the study.

Surveillance of VRTI consisted of multiplexed point-of-care testing (mPOCT) of symptomatic infants, which was combined with a weekly screening of all infants. Infants were considered symptomatic if they were started on intravenous antibiotics due to suspicion of a bacterial infection or if they exhibited new and not otherwise explicable respiratory symptoms (i.e., nasal congestion, FiO_2 increase of ≥0.1, increased pressure support or intubation).

Virus samples were collected via flocked nasopharyngeal swabs with a sterile viral transport medium and analyzed with the BioFire® FilmArray® Respiratory RP2 Panel (mPOCT) and an in-house multiplexed PCR (weekly screening). The RP2 Panel detects adenovirus, coronaviruses (HKU1, NL63, 229E and OC43), human metapneumovirus, human rhinovirus/enterovirus, influenza (A, A/H1, A/H3, A/H1-2009, and B), parainfluenza virus 1–4 and respiratory syncytial virus. Clinicians performed mPOCT as soon as possible after sample collection and were not blinded to the test results. Analysis was performed in the NICU. Results were usually available within 2–6 h. At each individual episode, clinicians were asked to indicate whether they felt that the test results were useful or not regarding hygiene measures, antibiotic therapy, or establishing a diagnosis. Clinicians were blinded to the results of the weekly screening tests. The 19-valent in-house multiplexed PCR method detects a similar range of viruses and was performed as previously described (9). Infants' clinical characteristics were recorded as was the frequency of parents' and siblings' visits.

Our 10-bed NICU is a tertiary care facility that is located near to the delivery suite and the maternity ward. The unit primarily cares for preterm infants with a birthweight <1,500 g and more mature infants with respiratory or circulatory support. The majority of neonates admitted to the NICU are transferred to a 20-bed special care unit following initial stabilization. Most infants are inborn and are admitted immediately after birth. However, the unit also accepts infants transferred from other hospitals, readmissions from the special care unit and in some cases, infants after discharge home. The NICU consists of three patient rooms, a 5-bed, a 4-bed, and a single room. The shared rooms are rather small with an average distance between the incubators of 2–3 m. For this reason, no permanent rooming-in for parents or families is possible. Nevertheless, we encourage mothers and fathers to do kangaroo care whenever, and as long as possible, also during night time. Parents have a lounge area in close proximity to the NICU. A separate family home is provided for overnight stays. The unit makes comprehensive efforts to integrate parents and to support their role as primary caregivers for their infants. Areas of family-centered care include, but are not limited to, communication, involvement in care, peer-to-peer support, and parent education.

The NICU is 24/7 open to families and visitors (e.g., other family members, close friends). The number of simultaneous visitors is restricted to two per patient. Parents and visitors are instructed in hand hygiene and advised to avoid visits in cases of respiratory illness. Siblings irrespective of age may visit the NICU following a physical check-up by the NICU physicians at least once a week. The duration of sibling visits is not restricted. Siblings are allowed to stay with their parents during kangaroo care, but we usually allow only parents to do kangaroo care.

Prompt isolation measures are implemented in virus-positive cases, which include single room accommodation if possible, cohorting of positive infants, care with gloves and gowns, and a detailed parent's instruction in hygiene measures.

The local ethics committee of the Rhineland-Palatinate Medical Association approved this study. Legal guardians of the infants provided written informed consent before inclusion in the study.

RESULTS

During the study period, 366 infants were admitted to the NICU. Of those, 70 were eligible for the study. Three parents declined participation, so 67/70 infants (96%) were finally enrolled and analyzed. **Table 1** summarizes the infants' characteristics.

In total, 75 symptomatic episodes and 272 weekly screening episodes were recorded. Complete data were available for 71 of the 75 (94.7%) symptomatic and all 272 (100%) screening episodes. Via mPOCT, two infants were diagnosed with VRTI. Infant A was born at 26+1 weeks of gestation with a birth weight of 1100g. He was tested positive in May 2018 on day of life (DOL) 63. Major clinical symptoms were increased work of breathing and re-introduction of nasal continuous airway pressure. Infant B was born at 25+6 weeks of gestation with a birth weight of 410 g. He was first tested positive in October 2018 on DOL 25. His

TABLE 1 | Demographic characteristics.

Characteristic	
No. of enrolled infants	67
Gestational age, week, median (IQR)	29.4 (26.4–32.9)
Gestational age, ≤ 32 weeks, *n* (%)	47 (70.1)
Gestational age, ≤ 28 weeks, *n* (%)	24 (35.8)
Female, *n* (%)	33 (49.3)
Birth weight, mean (SD), g	1,524.8 ± 980.6
nCPAP, *n* (%)	58 (86.6)
Intubation, *n* (%)	47 (70.1)
Bronchopulmonary dysplasia, *n* (%)	17 (25.4)
Discharge on home oxygen, *n* (%)	2 (3)
Death before discharge, *n* (%)	1 (1.5)

nCPAP, nasal continuous airway pressure; IQR, interquartile range; SD, standard deviation.

TABLE 2 | Clinician's evaluation of mPOCT results.

Condition	mPOCT results judged as useful [all results*]	Negative mPOCT results judged as useful	Positive mPOCT results judged as useful
Hygiene measures	21/68 (30.9%)	13/60 (21.7%)	8/8 (100%)
Antibiotic treatment	10/68 (14.7%)	7/60 (11.7%)	3/8 (37.5%)
Diagnostic certainty	19/68 (27.9%)	14/60 (23.3%)	5/8 (62.5%)

**Data available for 68 of 71 episodes; multiple answers possible.*
mPOCT, multiplexed point-of-care test.

clinical symptoms were rising FiO_2 on nasal continuous airway pressure and frequent apneas. Subsequently, that infant was repeatedly tested positive during several symptomatic episodes (9 positive samples) and also during the weekly screening (11 positive samples). Human rhinovirus/enteroviruses were detected in all cases.

No new VRTI were diagnosed during asymptomatic episodes.

Frequency of parents' visits was recorded in 233 of the 272 weekly screening episodes. Daily parents' visits were seen during 208 of those 233 (89.3%) episodes. Visits of siblings younger than 12 years of age were recorded in 25 of 233 (10.7%) episodes, respectively. During 21 weeks of the 52-week study period, at least one sibling younger than 12 years of age was present in the NICU.

Clinicians' perceptions of usefulness of mPOCT results are presented in **Table 2**. All positive virus tests were considered useful concerning isolation measures, whereas overall usefulness of mPOCT, especially when negative, was judged low.

DISCUSSION

In this study, VRTI were rare in the NICU. This is in contrast to the findings of Bennett et al. (5) who detected VRTI in many of their NICU patients, but similar to those of Caserta et al. (7) and Shui et al. (10).

Our findings suggest that routine surveillance is not warranted in asymptomatic infants whereas symptomatic infants should be tested for possible VRTI. That may include infants with new respiratory symptoms, respiratory deterioration, and infants with suspected bacterial sepsis (2, 11, 12).

Our study also suggests that surveillance of VRTI might play a role in the prevention of viral spread. In the study of Bennett et al., clinicians were blinded to the results of the virus tests and so unable to isolate or cohort positive infants. However, because viruses may persist for weeks, these measures may be crucial for the prevention of virus transmissions or outbreaks in the NICU.

Other factors that might explain differing frequencies of virus-positive infants may be the size of the NICU and local visiting policies. Previous evidence from retrospective analysis suggested that restriction of young sibling visitation is associated with less respiratory syncytial virus positive infants in the NICU (13). In Bennet's study, children younger than <17 years were even excluded from visiting the NICU (5). In contrast, in our family-centered setting, the frequency of VRTI was low and virus transmission did not occur despite one infant being virus-positive for several weeks. In order to maintain family-centered care and foster family–child interaction, we suggest that virus testing, isolation of positive cases and enhancing hygiene measures should be preferred over restricting visiting policies. Our results are in line with those of Horikoshi et al. (14) whose retrospective analysis detected no correlation between sibling visits and the rate of nosocomial viral infections in a Japanese NICU. In our study, clinicians' judgements supported this assumption. Although clinicians judged mPOCT as unhelpful with respect to antibiotic treatment and establishing a diagnosis, all positive test results were considered helpful regarding hygiene measures.

The study's main limitations are its single-center design and limited sample size. Larger units will have more visitor traffic and more health care personnel involved. In addition, the study period was outside an epidemic viral season, with an average viral community burden. Previous observational data indicated that restricting visitors to NICUs may reduce the incidence of VRTI during pandemic times (15). Hence, more large-scale studies are needed across periods of high community burden to establish if our findings are generalizable.

In summary, VRTI affected <3% of NICU infants enrolled in this study. In our unit, a low frequency of VRTI was attained despite adherence to family-centered care including liberal visiting policies for younger siblings. Testing for VRTI may help preventing viral spread from positive infants as it allows early detection and prompt implementation of isolation and enhanced hygiene measures.

ETHICS STATEMENT

This study involving human participants was reviewed and approved by Ethics committee of the Rhineland-Palatinate Medical Association. Written informed consent to participate in this study was provided by the participants' legal guardian/next of kin.

AUTHOR CONTRIBUTIONS

AK: methodology (lead), conceptualization (equal), writing—original draft (lead), writing—review, and editing (equal). AN: resources (supporting), formal analysis (supporting), writing—original draft (supporting), writing—review, and editing (equal). BG: resources (lead), software (lead), writing—review, and editing (equal). ST: resources (supporting), formal analysis (supporting), writing—review, and editing (equal). DS: conceptualization (supporting), writing—review, and editing (equal). JW: validation (supporting), writing—review, and editing (equal). SM: formal analysis (lead), writing—review, and editing (equal). SG: resources (supporting), conceptualization (supporting), methodology (supporting), writing—review, and editing (equal). EM: supervision (lead), validation (lead), methodology (equal), conceptualization (equal), writing—original draft (supporting), writing—review, and editing (equal). All authors contributed to the article and approved the submitted version.

ACKNOWLEDGMENTS

Parts of the study results have been presented as an abstract at the 3rd jENS Congress of joint European Neonatal Societies in September 2019 in Maastricht, Netherlands. Study results are part of the doctoral thesis of one co-author (AN).

REFERENCES

Kidszun A, Klein L, Winter J, Schmeh I, Gröndahl B, Gehring S, et al. Viral infections in neonates with suspected late-onset bacterial sepsis-a prospective cohort study. *Am J Perinatol.* (2017) 34:1–7. doi: 10.1055/s-0036-1584150

Ronchi A, Michelow IC, Chapin KC, Bliss JM, Pugni L, Mosca F, et al. Viral respiratory tract infections in the neonatal intensive care unit: the VIRIoN-I study. *J Pediatr.* (2014) 165:690–6. doi: 10.1016/j.jpeds.2014.05.054

Steiner M, Strassl R, Straub J, Böhm J, Popow-Kraupp T, Berger A. Nosocomial rhinovirus infection in preterm infants. *Pediatr Infect Dis J.* (2012) 31:1302– 4. doi: 10.1097/INF.0b013e31826ff939

Zinna S, Lakshmanan A, Tan S, McClaughry R, Clarkson M, Soo S, et al. Outcomes of nosocomial viral respiratory infections in high-risk neonates. *Pediatrics.* (2016) 138:e20161675. doi: 10.1542/peds.2016-1675

Bennett NJ, Tabarani CM, Bartholoma NM, Wang D, Huang D, Riddell SW, et al. Unrecognized viral respiratory tract infections in premature infants during their birth hospitalization: a prospective surveillance study in two neonatal intensive care units. *J Pediatr.* (2012) 161:814– 8. doi: 10.1016/j.jpeds.2012.05.001

Taylor C, Tan S, McClaughry R, Sharkey D. Hospital-acquired viral respiratory tract infections in the neonatal unit: a comparison with other inpatient groups. *Neonatology.* (2020). doi: 10.1159/000506427. [Epub ahead of print].

Caserta MT, Yang H, Gill SR, Holden-Wiltse J, Pryhuber G. Viral respiratory infections in preterm infants during and after hospitalization. *J Pediatr.* (2017) 182:53–8.e3. doi: 10.1016/j.jpeds.2016.11.077

Tan S, Clarkson M, Sharkey D. Variation in visiting and isolation policies in neonatal units: a U.K. Nationwide Survey. *Pediatr Infect Dis J.* (2018) 37:e20–e2. doi: 10.1097/INF.0000000000001820

Puppe W, Weigl J, Gröndahl B, Knuf M, Rockahr S, von Bismarck P, et al. Validation of a multiplex reverse transcriptase PCR ELISA for the detection of 19 respiratory tract pathogens. *Infection.* (2013) 41:77– 91. doi: 10.1007/s15010-012-0298-6

Shui JE, Messina M, Hill-Ricciuti AC, Maykowski P, Leone T, Sahni R, et al. Impact of respiratory viruses in the neonatal intensive care unit. *J Perinatol Off J Calif Perinat Assoc.* (2018) 38:1556–65. doi: 10.1038/s41372-018-0197-5

Cerone JB, Santos RP, Tristram D, Lamson DM, Stellrecht KA, St George K, et al. Incidence of respiratory viral infection in infants with respiratory symptoms evaluated for late-onset sepsis. *J Perinatol Off J Calif Perinat Assoc.* (2017) 37:922–6. doi: 10.1038/jp.2017.69

Kidszun A, Hansmann A, Winter J, Gröndahl B, Knuf M, Weise K, et al. Detection of respiratory viral infections in neonates treated for suspicion of nosocomial bacterial sepsis: a feasibility study. *Pediatr Infect Dis J.* (2014) 33:102–4. doi: 10.1097/INF.0000000000000008

Peluso AM, Harnish BA, Miller NS, Cooper ER, Fujii AM. Effect of young sibling visitation on respiratory syncytial virus activity in a NICU. *J Perinatol Off J Calif Perinat Assoc.* (2015) 35:627–30. doi: 10.1038/jp.2015.27

Horikoshi Y, Okazaki K, Miyokawa S, Kinoshita K, Higuchi H, Suwa J, et al. Sibling visits and viral infection in the neonatal intensive care unit. *Pediatr Int Off J Jpn Pediatr Soc.* (2018) 60:153–6. doi: 10.1111/ped.13470

Szatkowski L, McClaughry R, Clarkson M, Sharkey D. Restricted visiting reduces nosocomial viral respiratory tract infections in high-risk neonates. *Eur Respir J.* (2019) 53:1801874. doi: 10.1183/13993003.01874-2018

Permissions

All chapters in this book were first published by Frontiers; hereby published with permission under the Creative Commons Attribution License or equivalent. Every chapter published in this book has been scrutinized by our experts. Their significance has been extensively debated. The topics covered herein carry significant findings which will fuel the growth of the discipline. They may even be implemented as practical applications or may be referred to as a beginning point for another development.

The contributors of this book come from diverse backgrounds, making this book a truly international effort. This book will bring forth new frontiers with its revolutionizing research information and detailed analysis of the nascent developments around the world.

We would like to thank all the contributing authors for lending their expertise to make the book truly unique. They have played a crucial role in the development of this book. Without their invaluable contributions this book wouldn't have been possible. They have made vital efforts to compile up to date information on the varied aspects of this subject to make this book a valuable addition to the collection of many professionals and students.

This book was conceptualized with the vision of imparting up-to-date information and advanced data in this field. To ensure the same, a matchless editorial board was set up. Every individual on the board went through rigorous rounds of assessment to prove their worth. After which they invested a large part of their time researching and compiling the most relevant data for our readers.

The editorial board has been involved in producing this book since its inception. They have spent rigorous hours researching and exploring the diverse topics which have resulted in the successful publishing of this book. They have passed on their knowledge of decades through this book. To expedite this challenging task, the publisher supported the team at every step. A small team of assistant editors was also appointed to further simplify the editing procedure and attain best results for the readers.

Apart from the editorial board, the designing team has also invested a significant amount of their time in understanding the subject and creating the most relevant covers. They scrutinized every image to scout for the most suitable representation of the subject and create an appropriate cover for the book.

The publishing team has been an ardent support to the editorial, designing and production team. Their endless efforts to recruit the best for this project, has resulted in the accomplishment of this book. They are a veteran in the field of academics and their pool of knowledge is as vast as their experience in printing. Their expertise and guidance has proved useful at every step. Their uncompromising quality standards have made this book an exceptional effort. Their encouragement from time to time has been an inspiration for everyone.

The publisher and the editorial board hope that this book will prove to be a valuable piece of knowledge for researchers, students, practitioners and scholars across the globe.

List of Contributors

Shuwen Feng, Dongxin Zeng, Junwen Zheng and Dongchi Zhao
Department of Pediatrics, Children's Digital Health and Data Center, Zhongnan Hospital of Wuhan University, Wuhan, China

Merle Höpken
Klinik für Hals-, Nasen- und Ohrenheilkunde, Kliniken der Stadt Köln, Klinikum der Privaten Universität Witten/Herdecke mit Sitz in Köln, Cologne, Germany
Institut für Pathologie, Kliniken der Stadt Köln, Klinikum der Privaten Universität Witten/Herdecke mit Sitz in Köln, Cologne, Germany

Isabel Förster, Michael Brockmann, Oliver Schildgen and Verena Schildgen
Institut für Pathologie, Kliniken der Stadt Köln, Klinikum der Privaten Universität Witten/Herdecke mit Sitz in Köln, Cologne, Germany

Steffen Maune
Klinik für Hals-, Nasen- und Ohrenheilkunde, Kliniken der Stadt Köln, Klinikum der Privaten Universität Witten/Herdecke mit Sitz in Köln, Cologne, Germany

Anne Birgitta Versluys
Blood and Marrow Transplantation Program, Princess Maxima Center for Pediatric Oncology, Utrecht, Netherlands

Jaap Jan Boelens
Stem Cell Transplant and Cellular Therapies Program, Pediatrics, Memorial Sloan Kettering Cancer Center, New York, NY, United States

Zetao Cheng, Yuqian Yan, Shuping Jing, Jing Zhang, Min Li, Shan Zhao, Na Cao, Junxian Ou, Suhui Zhao and Xianbo Wu
Guangzhou Key Laboratory of Drug Research for Emerging Virus Prevention and Treatment, Guangdong Provincial Key Laboratory of Tropical Disease Research, School of Public Health, Southern Medical University, Guangzhou, China

Wen-Gang Li and Wei-Wei Chen
Treatment and Research Center for Infectious Diseases, 302 Military Hospital of China, Beijing, China

Bin Cao
Department of Pulmonary and Critical Care Medicine, China-Japan Friendship Hospital, Beijing, China

Qiwei Zhang
Guangzhou Key Laboratory of Drug Research for Emerging Virus Prevention and Treatment, Guangdong Provincial Key Laboratory of Tropical Disease Research, School of Public Health, Southern Medical University, Guangzhou, China
Dermatology Hospital, Southern Medical University, Guangzhou, China

Dongyin Wang and Dong Wang
Department of Hepatology, The First Hospital of Jilin University, Jilin University, Changchun, China
Institute of Virology and AIDS Research, The First Hospital of Jilin University, Changchun, China

Haoran Guo and Wei Wei
Institute of Virology and AIDS Research, The First Hospital of Jilin University, Changchun, China

Junliang Chang
Institute of Virology and AIDS Research, The First Hospital of Jilin University, Changchun, China
Changchun Institute of Biological Products, Changchun, China

Bin Liu
Department of Hand Surgery, The First Hospital of Jilin University, Changchun, China

Pujun Gao
Department of Hepatology, The First Hospital of Jilin University, Jilin University, Changchun, China

Peiyu Li
Key Laboratory of Medical Molecular Virology of MOE/MOH, School of Basic Medical Sciences & Shanghai Public Health Clinical Center, Fudan University, Shanghai, China
Wellman Center for Photomedicine, Massachusetts General Hospital, Department of Dermatology, Harvard Medical School, Boston, MA, United States
Department of Infectious Diseases and the Key Lab of Endogenous Infection, Shenzhen Nanshan People's Hospital, Guangdong Medical University, Shenzhen, China

Ji Wang
Wellman Center for Photomedicine, Massachusetts General Hospital, Department of Dermatology, Harvard Medical School, Boston, MA, United States
The First Affiliated Hospital of Sun Yat-sen University, Sun Yat-sen University, Guangzhou, China

Miao Cao and and Lu Lu
Key Laboratory of Medical Molecular Virology of MOE/MOH, School of Basic Medical Sciences & Shanghai Public Health Clinical Center, Fudan University, Shanghai, China

Qiwen Deng
Department of Infectious Diseases and the Key Lab of Endogenous Infection, Shenzhen Nanshan People's Hospital, Guangdong Medical University, Shenzhen, China

Shibo Jiang
Key Laboratory of Medical Molecular Virology of MOE/MOH, School of Basic Medical Sciences & Shanghai Public Health Clinical Center, Fudan University, Shanghai, China
Lindsley F. Kimball Research Institute, New York Blood Center, New York, NY, United States

Mei X. Wu
Wellman Center for Photomedicine, Massachusetts General Hospital, Department of Dermatology, Harvard Medical School, Boston, MA, United States
Harvard-MIT Division of Health Sciences and Technology, Cambridge, MA, United States

Heidi L. Tessmer and Kimihito Ito
Division of Bioinformatics, Research Center for Zoonosis Control, Hokkaido University, Sapporo, Japan

Ryosuke Omori
Division of Bioinformatics, Research Center for Zoonosis Control, Hokkaido University, Sapporo, Japan
Precursory Research for Embryonic Science and Technology (PRESTO), Japan Science and Technology Agency, Saitama, Japan

Xianmiao Ye, Jinlin Wang, Tao Shu and Qian Wang
State Key Laboratories of Respiratory Diseases, Guangzhou Institutes of Biomedicine and Health, Chinese Academy of Sciences, Guangzhou, China
University of Chinese Academy of Sciences, Beijing, China
Shanghai Public Health Clinical Center and School of Basic Medical Sciences, Key Laboratory of Medical Molecular Virology of MOE/MOH, Fudan University, Shanghai, China

Lijun Xiao
Center for Disease Control and Prevention of Chenzhou, Chenzhou, China

Xuehua Zheng, Xinglong Liu and Liqiang Feng
State Key Laboratories of Respiratory Diseases, Guangzhou Institutes of Biomedicine and Health, Chinese Academy of Sciences, Guangzhou, China

Ying Feng and Chufang Li
The First Affiliated Hospital of Guangzhou Medical University, Guangzhou, China

Wan Su
State Key Laboratories of Respiratory Diseases, Guangzhou Institutes of Biomedicine and Health, Chinese Academy of Sciences, Guangzhou, China
School of Biomedical Sciences, Huaqiao University, Quanzhou, China

Ling Chen
State Key Laboratories of Respiratory Diseases, Guangzhou Institutes of Biomedicine and Health, Chinese Academy of Sciences, Guangzhou, China
The First Affiliated Hospital of Guangzhou Medical University, Guangzhou, China

Wen Zhang, Si-Tai Chen, Qiu-Yan He, Xiao-Hong Liu and Geng Li
Laboratory Animal Center, Guangzhou University of Chinese Medicine, Guangzhou, China

Li-Quan Huang
The First Affiliated Hospital of Zhejiang Chinese Medical University, Hangzhou, China

Xiong Li
Guangdong Provincial Academy of Chinese Medical Sciences, Guangzhou, China

Xiao-Ping Lai
Laboratory Animal Center, Guangzhou University of Chinese Medicine, Guangzhou, China
Dongguan Mathematical Engineering Academy of Chinese Medicine, Guangzhou University of Traditional Chinese Medicine, Dongguan, China

Shao-Feng Zhan and Hui-Ting Huang
The First Affiliated Hospital of Guangzhou University of Chinese Medicine, Guangzhou, China

Jianguo Wu
Key Laboratory of Virology, Institute of Medical Microbiology, Jinan University, Guangzhou, China
Guangdong Longfan Biological Science and Technology Company, Ltd., Foshan, China

Shubhagata Das and Sherry Dunbar
Global Scientific Affairs, Luminex Corporation, Austin, TX, United States

Yi-Wei Tang
Department of Laboratory Medicine, Memorial Sloan Kettering Cancer Center, Weill Medical College of Cornell University, New York, NY, United States
Department of Pathology and Laboratory Medicine, Memorial Sloan Kettering Cancer Center, Weill Medical College of Cornell University, New York, NY, United States

Wei Xu, Shuai Xia, Jing Pu, Peiyu Li and Lu Lu
Shanghai Public Health Clinical Center and School of Basic Medical Sciences, Key Laboratory of Medical Molecular Virology of MOE/MOH, Fudan University, Shanghai, China

Yanjie Zhao, Roujian Lu and Wenjie Tan
Key Laboratory of Laboratory Medicine, Ministry of Education, Institute of Medical Virology, Wenzhou Medical University, Wenzhou, China
National Institute for Viral Disease Control and Prevention, Chinese Center for Disease Control and Prevention, Beijing, China

Jun Shen
Infectious Disease Department, Children's Hospital of Fudan University, Shanghai, China

Bingjie Wu and Gaoshan Liu
Key Laboratory of Laboratory Medicine, Ministry of Education, Institute of Medical Virology, Wenzhou Medical University, Wenzhou, China

Hayley Cassidy, Randy Poelman, Marjolein Knoester, Coretta C. Van Leer-Buter and Hubert G. M. Niesters
Department of Medical Microbiology and Infection Prevention, Division of Clinical Virology, University of Groningen, University Medical Center Groningen, Groningen, Netherlands

Karin Kosulin and René Geyeregger
Molecular Microbiology, Children's Cancer Research Institute, Vienna, Austria

Herbert Pichler and Anita Lawitschka
Stem Cell Transplant Unit, St. Anna Children's Hospital, Vienna, Austria

Thomas Lion
Molecular Microbiology, Children's Cancer Research Institute, Vienna, Austria
Department of Pediatrics, Medical University of Vienna, Vienna, Austria

Karin Pichler and Angelika Berger
Division of Neonatology, Intensive Care and Neuropediatrics, Department of Pediatrics and Adolescent Medicine, Medical University of Vienna, Vienna, Austria

Ojan Assadian
Department for Hospital Epidemiology and Infection Control, Medical University of Vienna, Vienna, Austria

Yingchen Wang, Tuo Dong, Lixin Qu, Wei Liang, Binbin Qi, Zhe Zhang, Lei Shang, Hong Gao, Xiqiao Du, Bing Lu, Zhenwei Liu, Huisong Yu, Qi Cui, Xiaocen Wang and Ye Li
Department of Microbiology, Public Health College, Harbin Medical University, Harbin, China

Guiyun Qi and Weiyuan Guo
Department of Clinical Laboratory, The Second Affiliated Hospital of Harbin Medical University, Harbin, China

Yan Guo
Department of Ear Nose Throat, The Second Affiliated Hospital of Harbin Medical University, Harbin, China

Zhangyi Qu
Department of Microbiology, Public Health College, Harbin Medical University, Harbin, China
Department of Natural Focus Disease Control, Institute of Environment-Associated Disease, Sino-Russia Joint Medical Research Center, Harbin Medical University, Harbin, China

Ashrafali M. Ismail, Ji Sun Lee, James Chodosh and Jaya Rajaiya
Howe Laboratory, Massachusetts Eye and Ear, Harvard Medical School, Boston, MA, United States

Jeong Yoon Lee
Howe Laboratory, Massachusetts Eye and Ear, Harvard Medical School, Boston, MA, United States
Molecular Virology Laboratory, Korea Zoonosis Research Institute, Jeonbuk National University, Jeonju, South Korea

Gurdeep Singh
Howe Laboratory, Massachusetts Eye and Ear, Harvard Medical School, Boston, MA, United States
Department of Cell and Systems Biology, University of Toronto, Toronto, ON, Canada

David W. Dyer
Department of Microbiology and Immunology, University of Oklahoma Health Sciences Center, Oklahoma City, OK, United States

Donald Seto
Bioinformatics and Computational Biology Program, School of Systems Biology, George Mason University, Manassas, VI, United States

Diego R. Hijano and Gabriela Maron
Department of Infectious Diseases, St Jude Children's Research Hospital, Memphis, TN, United States

Randall T. Hayden
Department of Pathology, St Jude Children's Research Hospital, Memphis, TN, United States

Prasanth Manohar
Zhejiang University-University of Edinburgh Institute, Zhejiang University, Haining, China
The Second Affiliated Hospital, School of Medicine, Zhejiang University, Hangzhou, China

Belinda Loh
Zhejiang University-University of Edinburgh Institute, Zhejiang University, Haining, China

Sudarsanan Athira and Ramesh Nachimuthu
Antibiotic Resistance and Phage Therapy Laboratory, School of Biosciences and Technology, Vellore Institute of Technology, Vellore, India

Xiaoting Hua
Department of Infectious Diseases, Sir Run Run Shaw Hospital, School of Medicine, Zhejiang University, Hangzhou, China
Key Laboratory of Microbial Technology and Bioinformatics of Zhejiang Province, Hangzhou, China

Susan C. Welburn
Zhejiang University-University of Edinburgh Institute, Zhejiang University, Haining, China
Infection Medicine, Biomedical Sciences, Edinburgh Medical School, College of Medicine and Veterinary Medicine, The University of Edinburgh, Edinburgh, United Kingdom

Sebastian Leptihn
Zhejiang University-University of Edinburgh Institute, Zhejiang University, Haining, China
Department of Infectious Diseases, Sir Run Run Shaw Hospital, School of Medicine, Zhejiang University, Hangzhou, China
Infection Medicine, Biomedical Sciences, Edinburgh Medical School, College of Medicine and Veterinary Medicine, The University of Edinburgh, Edinburgh, United Kingdom

Laurine C. Rijsbergen, Laura L. A. van Dijk, Rory D. de Vries and Rik L. de Swart
Department of Viroscience, Postgraduate School of Molecular Medicine, Erasmus MC, University Medical Centre Rotterdam, Rotterdam, Netherlands

Maarten F. M. Engel
Medical Library, Erasmus MC, University Medical Centre Rotterdam, Rotterdam, Netherlands

Estela Noyola, Asif Noor, Nicole Sweeney, Joshua Chan, Rahul Ramesh and Leonard R. Krilov
Department of Pediatrics, NYU Long Island School of Medicine, Mineola, NY, United States

Rose Calixte
Department of Pediatrics, NYU Long Island School of Medicine, Mineola, NY, United States
Department of Community Health and Social Medicine, The City University of New York (CUNY) School of Medicine, New York, NY, United States

André Kidszun, Anna Neurohr, Susanne Tippmann, Daniel Schreiner, Julia Winter and Eva Mildenberger
Department of Neonatology, University Medical Center, Mainz, Germany

Britta Gröndahl and Stephan Gehring
Department of Pediatric Infectious Diseases, University Medical Center, Mainz, Germany

Seyed Hamidreza Mahmoudpour
Institute of Medical Biostatistics, Epidemiology, and Informatics, University Medical Center of the Johannes Gutenberg University Mainz, Mainz, Germany
Center for Thrombosis and Hemostasis, University Medical Center of the Johannes Gutenberg University Mainz, Mainz, Germany

Index